SpringerWienNewYork

Lars-Peter Kamolz, Marc G. Jeschke,
Raymund E. Horch, Markus Küntscher,
Pavel Brychta *(editors)*

Handbook of Burns

Reconstruction and Rehabilitation

Volume 2

SpringerWienNewYork

Lars-Peter Kamolz, M.D., M.Sc.
Plastische, Aesthetische und Rekonstruktive Chirurgie, Landesklinikum Wiener Neustadt,
Wiener Neustadt, Austria

Marc G. Jeschke, M.D., Ph.D.
Sunnybrook Health Sciences Centre, Department of Surgery, Division of Plastic Surgery University of
Toronto, Sunnybrook Research Institute, Toronto, ON, Canada

Raymund E. Horch, M.D., Ph.D.
Universitätsklinikum Erlangen, Plastisch- und Handchirurgische Klinik, Erlangen, Germany

Markus Küntscher, M.D., Ph.D.
Evangelische Elisabeth Klinik Krankenhausbetriebs gGmbH, Berlin, Germany

Pavel Brychta, M.D., Ph.D., C.Sc.
Prednosta Kliniky popálenin, a rekonstrukcní chirurgie, FN Brno, Czech Republic

© 2012 Springer-Verlag/Wien
Printed in Austria

SpringerWienNewYork is part of
Springer Science+Business Media
springer.at

Typesetting: Jung Crossmedia Publishing GmbH, 35633 Lahnau, Germany
Printing: Holzhausen Druck GmbH, 1140 Wien, Austria

Printed on acid-free and chlorine-free bleached paper
SPIN: 12679652

With 175 (partly coloured) figures

Library of Congress Control Number: 2011943501

ISBN 978-3-7091-0314-2 SpringerWienNewYork

Preface

Dear Colleagues,

Over the past decades, extraordinary advances have been made in the understanding of cellular and molecular processes involved in acute wound healing. This knowledge has led to wound care innovations and new developments concerning burn care; burn care has improved to the extent that persons with burns can frequently survive.

The trend in current treatment extends beyond the preservation of life; the ultimate goal is the return of burn victims, as full participants, back into their families and communities.

The possibility of surviving burn injuries has changed dramatically over the past decades. One of the milestones was a more aggressive approach concerning surgery; early wound debridement and early wound coverage has led to a higher survival rate, but also to a higher number of patients, who will require reconstructive surgery and specialized after care.

I would like to express my deep appreciation to my co-editors, colleagues and friends for their distribution to this new book on burn reconstruction and rehabilitation. The authors have tried to achieve the highest degree in actuality and practical relevance within the field of burn reconstruction and rehabilitation.

Moreover, this book demonstrates that successful burn treatment with good long time result is only possible as a result of teamwork between different specialists and disciplines. This book offers a quick orientation, but also profound overview about burn reconstruction and rehabilitation.

Sincere appreciation goes to Günther Meissl, who was my teacher and mentor for many years; he has aroused my interest concerning burn care and burn research. Moreover, I like to thank David Herndon and his staff for the interesting and meaningful time in Galveston.

I am grateful to the Springer publishing staff for their support and cooperation in the development and preparation of this new handbook. I wish to recognize Katrin Stakemeier, who guided this book throughout the development process.

Finally, I would like to thank my wife, Birgit, and my kids, Emilia and Moritz, for their invaluable support. I love you.

Lars-Peter Kamolz

Contents

List of contributers

Oskar C. Aszmann, M.D., Ph.D.
Division of Plastic and Reconstructive Surgery
Department of Surgery
Medical University of Vienna
Vienna, Austria

Monica C. T. Bloemen, M.D.
Association of Dutch Burn Centers
Beverwijk, The Netherlands

Burn Center, Red Cross Hospital
Beverwijk, The Netherlands

Antonio Brancati, M.D.
Burns Unit, Wound Healing Unit
Lapeyronie Hospital
Montpellier University Hospital
Montpellier Cedex, France

Andrew Burd, M.D., Ph.D.
Division of Plastic, Reconstructive and
Aesthetic Surgery, Department of Surgery
The Chinese University of Hong Kong
Prince of Wales Hospital
Hong Kong, China

Erhan Demir, M.D.
Department of Plastic Surgery and Hand Surgery
Burn Center University Hospital RWTH Aachen
Aachen University of Technology
Aachen, Germany

Hans Dietl, Ph.D.
Division of Research & Development
Otto Bock HealthCare Products
Vienna, Austria

Johannes Dirnberger, M.Sc.
Johannes Kepler University Linz
RISC Software GmbH
Division of Medical Informatics
Hagenberg, Austria

Adelheid Elbe-Bürger, Ph.D.
Department of Dermatology
Division of Immunology
Allergy and Infectious Diseases (DIAID)
Medical University of Vienna
Vienna, Austria

Manfred Frey, M.D., Ph.D.
Division of Plastic and Reconstructive Surgery
Department of Surgery
Medical University of Vienna
Vienna, Austria

Guenter Germann, M.D., Ph.D.
ETHIANUM
Clinic for Plastic, Aesthetic & Preventive Medicine
at Heidelberg
University Hospital
Heidelberg, Germany

Michael Giretzlehner, Ph.D., M.Sc.
Johannes Kepler University Linz
RISC Software GmbH
Division of Medical Informatics
Hagenberg im Mühlkreis, Austria

Riccardo E. Giunta M.D., Ph.D.
Department Hand Surgery
Plastic and Aesthetic Surgery
Ludwig-Maximilians Universität München
Munich, Germany

Bernd Hartmann M.D.
Zentrum für Schwerbrandverletzte mit
Plastischer Chirurgie
Unfallkrankenhaus Berlin
Berlin, Germany

Andreas Heckmann M.D.
Department of Plastic, Hand, and Reconstructive
Surgery
Medizinische Hochschule Hannover
Hannover, Germany

Raymund E. Horch, M.D., Ph.D.
Department of Plastic and Hand Surgery
University of Erlangen-Nürnberg Medical Center
Erlangen, Germany

Marc G. Jeschke, M.D., Ph.D., FACS, FRCSC
Sunnybrook Health Sciences Centre
Ross Tilley Burn Centre
Toronto, Canada

Lars-Peter Kamolz, M.D., Ph.D., M.Sc.
Section of Plastic, Aesthetic and Reconstructive
Surgery
Department of Surgery
Landesklinikum Wiener Neustadt
Wiener Neustadt, Austria

Division of Plastic and Reconstructive Surgery
Department of Surgery
Medical University of Vienna
Vienna, Austria

Birgit Karle, M.D.
Division of Plastic and Reconstructive Surgery
Department of Surgery
Medical University of Vienna
Vienna, Austria

Maike Keck, M.D.
Division of Plastic and Reconstructive Surgery
Department of Surgery
Medical University of Vienna
Vienna, Austria

Hugo Benito Kitzinger M.D.
Division of Plastic and Reconstructive Surgery
Department of Surgery
Medical University of Vienna
Vienna, Austria

Eva Koellensperger, M.D.
Department for Hand-, Plastic- and
Reconstructive Surgery
Intensive Burn Care Unit
BG-Trauma Centre Ludwigshafen

Department for Plastic- and Hand Surgery
The University of Heidelberg
Ludwigshafen, Germany

Karen J. Kowalske, M.D.
Department of Physical Medicine
and Rehabilitation
University of Texas Southwestern Medical Center
Dallas, TX USA

David B. Lumenta, M.D.
Division of Plastic and Reconstructive Surgery
Department of Surgery
Medical University of Vienna
Vienna, Austria

Serina J. McEntire, M.D.
Shriners Hospitals for Children, and Department
of Surgery
University of Texas Medical Branch
Galveston, TX, USA

Walter J. Meyer III, M.D.
Department of Psychological and
Psychiatric Services
Shriners Hospitals for Children
Galveston, TX, USA

Maria Michaelidou, M.D.
Division of Plastic and Reconstructive Surgery
Department of Surgery
Medical University of Vienna
Vienna, Austria

Esther Middelkoop, Ph.D.
Department of Plastic, Reconstructive, and
Hand Surgery
VU Medical Centre Amsterdam
Amsterdam, The Netherlands

Rainer Mittermayr, M.D.
Burns Unit, Wound Healing Unit
Lapeyronie Hospital
Montpellier University Hospital
Montpellier Cedex, France

Sami Otman, M.D.
Burns Unit, Wound Healing Unit
Lapeyronie Hospital
Montpellier University Hospital
Montpellier Cedex, France

Christian Ottomann M.D.
Plastische Chirurgie und Handchirurgie
Intensiveinheit für Schwerbrandverletzte
Universitätsklinikum Schleswig-Holstein
Campus Lübeck, Lübeck, Germany

Robert Owen, M.Sc.
Johannes Kepler University Linz
RISC Software GmbH
Division of Medical Informatics
Hagenberg im Mühlkreis, Austria

Tatjana Paternostro, M.D., Ph.D.
Department of Physiotherapy and Rehabilitation
Medical University of Vienna
Vienna, Austria

Norbert Pallua, M.D., Ph.D.
Department of Plastic Surgery and Hand Surgery
Burn Center University Hospital RWTH Aachen
Aachen University of Technology
Aachen, Germany

Thilo Schenck, M.D.
Klinik und Poliklinik für Plastische Chirurgie
und Handchirurgie
Klinikum rechts der Isar
Technische Universität München
München, Germany

Volker J. Schmidt, M.D.
Department of Plastic and Hand Surgery
University of Erlangen-Nürnberg Medical Center
Erlangen, Germany

Harald Selig, M.D.
Section of Plastic, Aesthetic and Reconstructive
Surgery
Department of Surgery
Landesklinikum Wiener Neustadt
Wiener Neustadt, Austria

Oscar E. Suman, M.D.
Shriners Hospitals for Children, and Department
of Surgery
University of Texas Medical Branch
Galveston, TX, USA

Sherri Sharp, M.D.
Child Psychiatry
Department of Psychiatry and Behavioral Sciences
Departments of Pediatrics and Human Biological
Chemistry and Genetics
The University of Texas Medical Branch
Galveston, TX, USA

Maria Siemionow, M.D., Ph.D., DSc
Department of Plastic Surgery
Cleveland Clinic
Cleveland, OH, USA

Timo A. Spanholtz M.D.
Department Hand Surgery
Plastic and Aesthetic Surgery
Ludwig-Maximilians Universität München
Munich Germany

Luc Teot, M.D., Ph.D.
Burns Unit, Wound Healing Unit
Lapeyronie Hospital
Montpellier University Hospital
Montpellier Cedex, France

Peter M. Vogt, M.D., Ph.D.
Department of Plastic, Hand, and
Reconstructive Surgery
Medizinische Hochschule Hannover
Hannover, Germany

Martijn B. A. van der Wal, M.D.
Association of Dutch Burn Centres Beverwijk
Beverwijk, The Netherlands

Burn Centre, Red Cross Hospital Beverwijk
Beverwijk, The Netherlands

Paul P. M. van Zuijlen, M.D.
Department of Plastic
Reconstructive, and Hand Surgery
Red Cross Hospital Beverwijk
Beverwijk, The Netherlands

Pauline D. H. M. Verhaegen, M.D.
Association of Dutch Burn Centres Beverwijk
Beverwijk, The Netherlands

Department of Plastic, Reconstructive, and
Hand Surgery, Red Cross Hospital Beverwijk
Beverwijk, The Netherlands

Burn Centre, Red Cross Hospital Beverwijk
Beverwijk, The Netherlands

Department of Plastic, Reconstructive, and
Hand Surgery
Academical Medical Centre Amsterdam
Amsterdam, The Netherlands

Shelley Wiechman, Ph.D.
University of Washington School of Medicine
Department of Rehabilitation Medicine
Harborview Burn Center
Seattle, WA, USA

Fatih Zor, M.D.
Gulhane Military Medical Academy
Department of Plastic Surgery
Etlik, Ankara, Turkey

Burn injuries and their psychosocial and long time consequences

Acute stress disorder and post traumatic stress disorder in individuals suffering from burn injury

Sherri Sharp[1,2], Walter J. Meyer[1,2]

[1] Child Psychiatry, Department of Psychiatry and Behavioral Sciences; Departments of Pediatrics and Human Biological Chemistry and Genetics, The University of Texas Medical Branch, Galveston, TX, USA
[2] Department of Psychological and Psychiatric Services, Shriners Hospitals for Children, Galveston, TX, USA

Introduction

An individual's recovery from a burn includes many aspects. One of which is their psychological healing. Emotional well-being plays an important role in one's physical recovery [108]. Some burn victims do not experience any negative psychological reactions while others experience numerous issues. These negative reactions can vary from short-term to long and from mild to debilitating. Psychological reaction to trauma can interfere with one's medical recovery [55]. This can be a problem during the recovery of an injury as critical as a burn. Such intrusive symptoms could interfere with a patient's ability to participate in necessary medical cares (e. g. lying still so as not to tear a graft, bathing with water). Management of these symptoms would allow the individual to focus more exclusively on his/her medical needs. There are numerous psychiatric disorders which need to be distinguished to determine the most appropriate treatment. Typical maladaptive behaviors can include the signs and symptoms of anxiety and/or depression. While these can be normal instinctive coping mechanisms, part of the body's natural response to trauma, the symptoms can escalate into an experience more intrusive and debilitating.

Definition and symptoms

Acute Stress Disorder (ASD) and Posttraumatic Stress Disorder (PTSD) are types of negative psychological reactions post trauma. La Greca et al. [41] suggested that symptoms of PTSD were a common reaction to trauma such as physical burn. In order to warrant such a diagnosis, the initial experience must include exposure to a terrifying event or ordeal in which there was the potential for serious physical harm or death. ASD is an acute emotional reaction, within two to thirty days after a trauma. The reaction must involve fear, helplessness, or horror. In children it may appear more like disorganized or agitated behavior. This response would include anxiety, concentration difficulty, emotional numbness, irritability, flashbacks, restlessness, and sleep disturbance. It is primarily associated with dissociative symptoms, which may include: depersonalization, derealization, difficulty experiencing pleasure, numbing, and/or temporary amnesia. Individuals may say things like: "It was as though I wasn't even there", "Time was standing still", "I felt like I was watching things happening from above" or "I can't remember most of what happened". These symptoms must last at least 2 days and cause significant distress or impairment in social, occupational, or other important areas of functioning [1]. The presentation of symptoms may vary depending upon the characteristics of the event and the individual (e. g. age, previous exposure to trauma).

If these symptoms appear or persist after 30 days post-trauma, then a diagnosis of Posttraumatic Stress Disorder (PTSD) would be given instead of ASD. The principle difference between these two diagnoses, aside from duration, is that PTSD does not include a set of dissociative symptoms [1]. So, the two main differences are the timing and nature of the symptoms. PTSD has been divided into two subcategories: the initial phase called "acute" and the "chronic" phase after symptoms have persisted for three or more months.

PTSD was recognized as a disorder in the DSM-III in 1980. There was a "surge of research" after its inclusion [47]. ASD was not recognized as an official trauma-related diagnosis until 1994 in the DSM-IV. According to Bryant and Harvey [10] dispute continues to exist as to whether or not the criteria for an ASD diagnosis reflects a pathological reaction to trauma or instead a normal reaction. It has also been suggested that the DSM-IV requirement of having three of five dissociative symptoms in order to receive the ASD diagnosis might be too stringent, causing false negatives. The thought was that this may exclude a number of individuals experiencing an "identifiable trauma-related syndrome" and may later achieve a diagnosis of PTSD [47]. This has led many clinicians to begin treatment before the full criteria are met.

Assessment

Distress after a trauma can be assessed in several ways. The method is dependant on the current status and functional ability of the individual. The first step in an assessment is to determine the individual's mental status (e. g. orientation to person, place, and time). If the patient presents with a poor mental status (e. g. confused, not oriented), then delirium should be suspected. Since the evaluation and treatment of delirium is very different from that of ASD or PTSD, distinguishing delirium is very important.

Delirium

Delirium is a state that tends to fluctuate across time in which there is (1) a diminished awareness of the environment, accompanied by difficulty fo-

cusing and maintaining attention, and (2) a reduction in cognitive performance (e. g. deficits of memory, language, or orientation) [1]. If symptoms of delirium are present, it is key to first rule-out potential medical causes (e. g. fever, metabolic disruption, blood pressure abnormalities, drug effects). Delirium is usually an early reaction that can occur during the immediate postburn phase when patients may be intubated, heavily medicated with narcotic analgesics, overstimulated, or sleep and sensory deprived. These factors make reliable diagnoses of delirium difficult. To date, studies suggest that true delirium may occur in roughly one fifth of burn patients. Levenson [43] stated, "it is very difficult to determine how much of a burn patient's agitation is due to delirium versus pain versus acute anxiety, especially since most patients will have all three to varying degrees during hospitalization in the burn unit". For that reason, adequate pain management must be vigorously addressed first. Patients who developed PTSD were more likely than those without the diagnosis to have experienced an episode of delirium [61]. Therefore, ascertaining the presence of delirium is important because, if left untreated, the experience can impact psychological recovery.

Obstacles to assessment

Symptoms of distress can be assessed via clinical interview or a number of symptom checklists. Information is ideally obtained from the individual experiencing the symptoms. However, this is not always possible due to the current medical status, severity of the distress symptoms, and/or the age of the person. Perhaps the greatest challenge of assessment in children, is gaining an objective assessment of their functioning. Infants and young children have difficulty verbalizing their feelings. Older children may also still be unable to conceptualize and communicate their experiences. In such cases, observations can be provided by caregivers and/or medical professionals tending to the patient.

As with any critically ill population, assessment on an intensive care burn unit can have its obstacles. Pain is often a large part of the post-burn experience and, if not controlled adequately, can be an overwhelming symptom. The physical and psychological manifestations of pain symptoms can appear very similar to that of anxiety and/or depression [44]. Control of pain decreases the stress response, lowering cortisol and catecholamines. Success in managing pain may decrease the risk of posttraumatic stress, anxiety, and depression [65].

Even just finding adequate patient time to conduct an evaluation can be difficult. Patients' awake time can be very busy with surgeries, tubbing, rehabilitation, etc. To further compound this, medications given before and/or during the activities can also leave the patient fairly sedated or drowsy afterward. However, it is important to prioritize frequent assessment of patients, especially those with large burns. Two early descriptive studies suggested that poor adjustment or psychiatric complications occurred in 50 % to 65 % of hospitalized burn patients [1, 89]. In both studies, poor hospital adjustment was associated with premorbid psychopathology and a high total body surface area (TBSA) burned.

Available assessment instruments

Different measures exist for the evaluation of ASD versus PTSD due to the slightly different diagnostic criteria; however, there is a large overlap between instruments. Gibson [31] suggested two measures with the "strongest psychometric properties" for the assessment of ASD. These included the Acute Stress Disorder Interview (ASDI) and the Acute Stress Disorder Scale (ASDS). The ASDI structured clinical interview that has been validated against DSM-IV criteria for ASD [11] While the ASDS is a self-report measure that correlates highly with symptom clusters found on the first instrument [12].

There are also several instruments utilized frequently in children with burn injury. The Acute Stress Disorder Symptom Checklist [71] is 12-item DSM-IV based instrument that was developed in a pediatric burn intensive care unit to expedite the assessment of posttraumatic distress. This scale is for in-hospital use and does not assess avoidance. The Child Stress Reaction Checklist has a Burn Version (CSRS). It is a 36-item observer-report instrument that measures acute stress and posttraumatic symptoms in children [77].

PTSD can be measured in a similar manner. The Structured Clinical Interview for DSM-IV Axis I Disorders (SCID-I), PTSD module is a semi-structured interview [27]. There is a self-report PTSD Checklist (PCL-C; [105]). The Diagnostic Interview for Children and Adolescents (DICA; [106]) or the MAGIC [68] are frequently utilized in younger populations. As indicated previously, the Child Stress Reaction Checklist, Burn Version (CSRS) is an observer-report instrument that measures posttraumatic symptoms in children [77].

Prevalence

ASD and PTSD are common diagnoses received after traumatic events. The prevalence of ASD varies between 6–33 % depending on the type of trauma [102]. ASD is a relatively new diagnosis and, as such, there is only a limited amount of research on the disorder to date. This may account for some of the variability in the reported incidence. Research on PTSD is fairly abundant however. A review of the literature by Caffo and Belaise [14] found PTSD to be the most frequently experienced psychiatric disorder after traumatic injuries. Approximately 8 % of men and 20 % of women develop PTSD post- trauma, and approximately 30 % of those individuals develop chronic PTSD [102].

Prevalence in burn populations

The incidence of ASD in adults who have been burned varies from 10–23 % [20, 35]. While the prevalence of ASD is from 8–31 % in children who have sustained burns [67, 78, 94]. This frequency is in spite of regimented medication management for pain and anxiety [67, 71].

Burn injuries can share similar characteristics to non-burn medical conditions as both can result in chronic psychological morbidity [51, 61, 97]. The prevalence of PTSD in adult burn survivors has shown some variability across years following the trauma. The incidence of PTSD has been reported to be 24–40 % at four to six months [24, 50, 62, 74], 15–45 % at 12 months [50, 62, 104], and 25 % at two years [50]. Additionally, 36 % of adults described themselves to be experiencing current PTSD eight years after their burn injury [20]. With regards to pediatric burn survivors, 2–19 % of those who were still children at the time of follow-up met DSM-IV criteria for current PTSD and 30 % for lifetime PTSD [42, 75, 92, 100]. For pediatric burn survivors who were young adults at follow up, the current and lifetime rates of PTSD were nearly 9 % and 21 %, respectively [53] with both rates higher than those found in epidemiological samples.

There are different possible explanations as to why there was variability in the incidence rates. One theory is related to the diversity in the approach to the studies in which the information was obtained (e. g. assessment tool used, sample characteristics and size, study design, presence or absence of treatment interventions). Another hypothesis is regarding the amount of time elapsed between burn trauma and the evaluation of symptoms. Blakeney et al. [6] study recognized the importance of time in psychological adaptation. Similarly, La Greca et al. [41] found that in school-aged children distressed by a natural disaster, posttraumatic stress symptoms decreased and changed over time. A comparison of current versus lifetime rates of PTSD by Meyer et al. [53] also supports the notion that PTSD decreases with time.

Risk factors

There has not been a definitive set of risk factors established to predict the development of ASD and/or PTSD. Studies to date tended to focus more on the prevalence rates rather than variables that influence psychological adjustment [58]. Identifying impact variables could be helpful in identifying those burn patients who are most at risk for developing psychological sequalae post-trauma. What we do know is that the presentation of symptoms may vary depending upon the characteristics of the event and the individual (e. g. age, previous exposure to trauma).

Relationship between ASD and PTSD

Multiple investigators have found that individuals with high levels of posttraumatic symptoms early on are at risk of subsequent PTSD [36, 47, 88] While a number of patients with ASD never develop PTSD, a diagnosis of ASD in adults has proven to be a strong predictor of having a PTSD diagnosis later [19, 20, 22, 50]. The diagnostic criterion that have been found to be most strongly correlated are dissociative [104] and avoidant [19] symptoms. Saxe et al. [79] found acute phase dissociative symptoms to be predictive of PTSD in school-age children. Rosenberg in an extensive study involving 140 children has found that ASD per say does not predict PTSD in children who are burn survivors [75].

Specific burn characteristics

While the literature suggests that the greater the exposure to a traumatic event the more likely one is to develop acute stress symptoms, there is no consensus on which factors specific to the individual or the event are predictive of developing posttraumatic distress [12]. The occurrence of PTSD has not been found to be statistically higher in the presence of a more severe injury [26, 38]. In other words, apart from one study [104], total burned surface area has not been found to be a significant predictor of PTSD in adults [22, 50, 58]. On the other hand, burn size has been found to be a predictor of acute and later onset of posttraumatic distress in pre-school [94] and school-age children [79].

The burn survivor is somewhat unique in that he/she recovers from his/her acute illness but he/she is usually left with visible scars. The location of the burn was found to be strongly associated with post-burn adjustment [58]. Almost all burns over 30 % TBSA involve either the hands or the face and cause significant scarring. A burn injury to the head or neck was found to be predictors of ASD in adults, but no data was found regarding children and adolescents [50]. A large burn injury is thought to be a chronic stressor rather than a one-time traumatic event because of this scarring and because the initial treatment is painful and occurs over weeks to months. Pain was determined to be associated with the experience of acute stress symptoms in pre-school age children [94] and of PTSD in school-age children [79]. In addition to pain, functionality was also affected by the location of the burn injury. Both pain and limited range of motion have been found to increase the likelihood of psychological distress [60 a, 90].

As burned children and adolescents evolve through various stages of life, past issue may resurface. Pediatric burn survivors may have difficulty transitioning to adult roles [70]. For example, intimacy anxiety could be caused by concern about revealing hidden scars. This could contribute to higher prevalence rates of PTSD than ASD in burn survivors. However, another possible explanation for the lower rate of ASD than PTSD is the intensive pain and anxiety management that patients are now receiving during the acute phase of recovery [18, 61].

Individual characteristics that contribute to post-burn adjustment

An individual's history, life circumstances, personal traits, and genetics play some role in determining the risk of posttraumatic maladjustment, as does the nature of the trauma itself [102]. Risk factors include:
▶ pre-burn emotional disorder(s)
  • DSM-IV-TR Axis I psychiatric disorder [64]
  • personality trait of neuroticism [25]
  • pre-burn affective disorder [108]
  • undergoing treatment [50]
▶ poor relationship with others
  • poor support system, perceived or real [43, 108]
  • for children, parent's level of stress [21, 78, 94]
  • for school-age children, acute phase separation anxiety [78]
▶ internal issues
  • preexisting maladaptive coping skills [43]
  • for school-age children, poor body image [78]
▶ other
  • socioeconomically disadvantaged [43]

Comorbidity

PTSD has been found to have a strong comorbidity with other psychological disorders, approximately 80 % (lifetime rates [29]). Frequent comorbid conditions can include anxiety, mood, sleep, and conduct problems [14]. Anxiety is frequent psychological reaction to burn injury across the age spectrum [61, 90], especially in children [90, 91, 100].

Depression is also common psychological reaction in children to burn injury [61, 90, 96]. In a study by El Hamaoui et al. [23] twenty-three percent of the participants met the diagnostic criteria for PTSD and 55 % for major depressive disorder. The more concerning reactions include suicidal ideation, self-rejection, aggressiveness, irritability, and withdrawal [15, 23, 93]. Additionally, pediatric burn patients reported experiencing anger, grief, and guilt [90].

Other post-burn comorbid issues include sleep disturbances [101] and, in children, attention problems, memory difficulties, learning disabilities, and/or unhealthy coping behaviors [102].

Treatment

If left untreated, posttraumatic symptoms can follow a long, difficult course [32, 99]. Bradley et al. [7] conducted a meta-analysis that revealed that psychotherapy for PTSD leads to a large initial improvement from baseline. More than half of patients who complete treatment improve. "The goals of treatment for individuals with a diagnosis of ASD or PTSD include reducing the severity of ASD or PTSD symptoms, preventing or treating trauma-related comorbid conditions that may be present or emerge, improving adaptive functioning and restoring a psychological sense of safety and trust, limiting the generalization of the danger experienced as a result of the traumatic situation(s), and protecting against relapse" (p. 12, APA 2004).

Initial intervention

The acute phase post-injury, the focus tends to be on crisis intervention. This can include supportive services, case management, and psycho-education about the possible symptoms and course of posttraumatic distress. During this time, individuals are encouraged to rely on their innate strengths and support system. This alone may reduce the need for further psychological intervention (APA 2004).

Early pain and anxiety management

Another aspect of early intervention may include frequent pain assessment and more aggressive management of the patient's pain and anxiety. Ratcliff et al. [67] found a 25 % reduction in the incidence of ASD with pediatric burn patients since the implementation of a structured pain protocol. They documented that an increase in the use of morphine and benzodiazepine across an eight year span also found a simultaneous decrease (from 12.1 % to 8.7 %) in PTSD symptoms. This benefit of managing pain with higher doses morphine was also confirmed in a later study conducted with very young children [95].

Therapeutic intervention

Cognitive Behavior Therapy (CBT)

The prevailing method of treatment for posttraumatic distress has been psychotherapy. Cognitive-behavior therapy (CBT), exposure therapy in particular, has shown the best evidence as an effective treatment for PTSD [80]. During CBT, patients are exposed in a gradual manner to the feared stimulus. Exposure may be done in vivo or in imagination. Exposure in imagination involves the person describing traumatic memories (e.g. storytelling, writing, etc) until they become less distressing. This component of the therapy is based on the idea of habituation. During the exposure, the person is to utilize anxiety management techniques. These are skills that help individuals cope with their reaction to the exposure both physically and mentally. The skills are learned prior to the exposure component of therapy, practiced repetitiously until they become automatic, and reinforced throughout. Anxiety management techniques include: breathing training, relaxation, assertiveness training, positive thinking and self-talk, and thought stopping. CBT may also address distorted thoughts through cognitive restructuring.

CBT has been shown to reduce posttraumatic symptoms in adults [7, 28, 59, 84], as well as children and adolescents [14] There is no evidence to date that indicates that early intervention with CBT is more effective than later intervention [12].

Bisson and Andrew (2007) conducted a meta-analysis of the randomized control trials available to date assessing the efficacy of various psychological treatment approaches post trauma. Thirty-three studies conducted with adults were reviewed [5]. They found PTSD symptoms to be more significantly reduced with trauma-focused CBT than with support-

ive therapy, non-directive counseling, psychodynamic therapy, and/or hypnotherapy. However, there was no significant difference found between trauma-focused CBT and stress management or eye-movement desensitization and reprocessing (EMDR). Additionally, some evidence was present to suggest that individuals who received trauma-focused CBT and EMDR faired better at between 2 and 5 months post-treatment. Similar results were revealed in a meta-analysis of twenty-five studies examining the effectiveness of interventions to treat posttraumatic symptoms that arise within 3 months of a traumatic event [73]. Trauma-focused CBT was found to be efficacious for individuals with traumatic stress symptoms, especially those who meet the criteria for Post Traumatic Stress Disorder.

Kornør et al. [39] reviewed 7 studies examining 5 random controlled trials comparing trauma-focused CBT to supportive therapy in adults with an initial ASD diagnosis. Results of these studies supported trauma-focused CBT as being more efficient than supportive therapy in reducing the occurrence of chronic PTSD, as well as symptoms of anxiety and depression. In a study with individuals who were diagnosed with PTSD and either a mood disorder, schizophrenia, or schizoaffective disorder, those who received CBT as opposed to "treatment as usual" improved significantly more at blinded post treatment, 3-month, and 6-month follow-up assessments [56]. Similar results were found by Roberts et al. [73].

Younger children may not have the verbal skills and self-awareness to participate in CBT. Therefore play therapy may be more developmentally appropriate [33]. This approach allows indirect or symbolic expressions of emotion and events through the use of dolls, toys, art, and/or music. Play therapy can be considered an age-appropriate form of exposure therapy.

Other forms of therapy

In addition to CBT, there are other alternative approaches to treatment that have yet to gain adequate validation through research (e.g. hypnosis, yoga, acupuncture). Eye movement desensitization and reprocessing (EMDR) is another intervention for posttraumatic symptoms. EMDR combines talk therapy with therapist-guided eye movements. Studies have found mixed results with EMDR. The benefit of the eye movement component of the treatment has not been consistently found [16].

Psychological debriefing is a brief intervention lasting about 3–4 hours administered within days of a crisis [66]. The aim is to encourage the individual(s) to talk about his/her feelings and reactions to the event [54]. The approach has not been shown to benefit and has, in fact, been found to be detrimental to one's recovery [5, 48, 73].

Having a strong support system is crucial in the recovery of burn patients both acutely and long-term [108]. While it can be difficult for friends and family to see their loved one suffering, they can provide important emotional support. They can also help the patient to utilize their learned CBT skills (e. g. reminding them to implement their breathing training and positive self-talk).

Medication intervention

Acutely burned patients may initially not be able to fully engage in psychotherapy. Robert et al. [71] stated that the "acutely burned patient is often too physically impaired to engage in counseling, unable to focus cognitively, developmentally unable to process emotions verbally, or too distraught or agitated to verbalize emotions. Thus, psychopharmacologic treatment may be the only option" (p. 255). Medications, while not originally developed for treatment of ASD/PTSD, can be helpful in controlling these symptoms [3, 69].

After the Vietnam War, PTSD was recognized as a major sequelae of the war and a need for treating thousands of troops was appreciated. At the same time, a number of new antidepressants became available. These medications proved to be extremely effective in treating the symptoms of PTSD. Tricyclic antidepressants, such as imipramine, and monoamine oxidase inhibitors were effective in some studies at 67–100 % [30, 87]. In the 1990's, the selective serotonin reuptake inhibitor (SSRI) fluoxetine was introduced as therapy and found to be very effective [57, 83, 103]. That was followed by other SSRIs, citalopram and sertraline, which were also found to be effective [8a, 81, 85].

In addition, imipramine and fluoxetine have been found to significantly reduce ASD symptoms in more than 80 % of the subjects [98]. In that study of 130 children, children with very large burns (> 60 % TBSA) did not respond as consistently as those with smaller burns. Robert et al. [71] demonstrated that imipramine was superior to chlorohydrate. However, the benefit of antidepressants could not be replicated in a subsequent study utilizing a randomized double blind match controlled study which compared medication with placebo [72]. This study suggests that ASD will often disappear on its own without intervention. Perhaps the 2 days of symptoms required for the diagnosis is not long enough to substantiate the diagnosis of ASD.

For symptoms of ASD and PTSD, SSRIs are often the first medication utilized [107]. There is also evidence to suggest that benzodiazepines and/or morphine will also reduce such symptoms [79]. However, the use of benzodiazepines has demonstrated mixed results [46]. Patients are often taking this medication when their symptoms of ASD and/or PTSD exhibit themselves [71]. Anticonvulsants have been used as second line medications [4]. A medication that has recently reported some success with children in particular is risperidone [34, 37, 52]. It has also been an effective augmentation of SSRI treatment in adults [76]. Pregabalin has been used to augment antidep-ressants for PTSD [60 b] Seroquel has also been shown to be effective in PTSD [40]. Depakote has not been found to be helpful [17].

The immediate post-trauma administration of adrenergic antagonists, such as propranolol, has demonstrated mixed results in the short and long-term. The theory behind utilizing a medication such as propranolol is based on the idea that post-traumatic stress is illustrated by atypical neuronal activation [86]. Interrupting the brain and nervous systems' natural reaction to "overlearn" the physiological response to a memory may be beneficial in the treatment of ASD/PTSD [18, 63]. This pairing of non-threatening stimuli with unpleasant stimuli is thought to be increased by prolonged production of beta-adrenergic chemicals [45]. Studies to date are limited and have found mixed results on the benefit of propranolol on ASD and PTSD in adults and children (e. g. [8b, 37, 49, 82]).

Summary and conclusions

A burn can be a complex and traumatic injury. Special care in needed to assist individuals with their recovery both short and long term. A multidisciplinary approach to treatment seems warranted. While some patients recover without emotional distress, many experience ASD and/or PTSD. Certainly, adequate pain and anxiety management during the acute phase of treatment seems to aid in the prevention of ASD and PTSD development. If ASD or PTSD develops, those symptoms often respond to with therapeutic interventions (CBT) and medication (antidepressants, SSRIs). However, no convergent treatment has been established to date. More research is needed to determine the most effective intervention protocol to address these potentially debilitating symptoms.

References

[1]   American Psychiatric Association (2000) Diagnostic and statistical manual of mental disorders, 4th edn, text revision. Author, Washington, DC

[2]   Andreasen NJ, Noyes R Jr, Hartford CE (1972) Factors influencing adjustment of burn patients during hospitalization. Psychosom Med 34: 517–525

[3]   Baker GB, Nievergelt CM, Risbrough VB (2009) Post-traumatic stress disorder: emerging concepts of pharmacotherapy. Expert Opin Emerg Drugs 14: 251–272

[4]   Berger W, Mendlowicz MV, Marques-Portella C, Kinrys G, Fontenelle LF, Marmar CR, Figueira I (2009) Pharmacologic alternatives to antidepressants in post-traumatic stress disorder: a systematic review. Prog Neuropsychopharmacol Biol Psychiatry 33: 169–180

[5]   Bisson J, Andrew M (2007) Psychological treatment of post-traumatic stress disorder (PTSD). Cochrane Database Syst Rev 18(3): CD003388

[6]   Blakeney P, Meyer W, Robert R, Desai M, Wolf S, Herndon D (1998) Long-term psychosocial adaptation of children who survive burns involving 80 % or greater total body surface area. J Trauma 44: 625–633

[7]   Bradley R, Greene J, Russ E, Dutra L, Westen D (2005) A multidimensional meta-analysis of psychotherapy for PTSD. Am J Psychiatry 162(2): 214–227

[8a]   Brady K, Pearlstein T, Asnis GM, Baker D, Rothbaum B, Sikes C, Farfel G (2000) Efficacy and safety of sertraline treatment of posttraumatic stress disorder a randomized controlled trial. JAMA 283(14): 1837–1844

[8b]   Brunet A, Orr SP, Tremblay J, Robertson K, Nader K, Pitman RK (2008) Effect of post-retrieval propranolol on psychophysiologic responding during subsequent script-driven traumatic imagery in post-traumatic stress disorder. J Psychiatr Res 42(6): 503–506

[9]   Bryant RA (2006) Cognitive-behavioral therapy for acute stress disorder. In: Follette AM, Ruzeck JI (eds) Cognitive-behavioral therapies for trauma, 2nd edn. Guilford Press, New York, pp 201–227

[10]   Bryant RA, Harvey AG (2000) Acute stress disorder: A handbook of theory, assessment, and treatment. American Psychological Association, Washington, DC

[11]   Bryant RA, Harvey AG, Dang ST, Sackville (1998) Assessing acute stress disorder: Psychometric properties of a structured clinical interview. Psychol Assessment 10: 215–220

[12]   Bryant RA, Harvey AG, Guthrie RM, Moulds ML (2000) A prospective study of psychophysiological arousal, acute stress disorder, and posttraumatic stress disorder. J Abnorm Psychol 109: 341–344

[13]   Bryant RA, Moulds ML, Guthrie RM (2000) Acute stress disorder scale: A self-report measure of acute stress disorder. Psychol Assessment 12: 61–68

[14]   Caffo E, Belaise C (2003) Psychological aspects of traumatic injury in children and adolescents. Child Adolesc Psychiatr Clin N Am 12(3): 493–535

[15]   Carvajal HF (1990) Burns in children and adolescents: initial management as the first step in successful rehabilitation. Pediatrician 17(4): 237–243

[16]   Davidson PR, Parker KC (2001) Eye movement desensitization and reprocessing (EMDR): a meta-analysis. J Consult Clin Psychol 69(2): 305–316

[17]   Davis LL, Davidson JR, Ward LC, Bartolucci A, Bowden CL, Petty F (2008) Divalproex in the treatment of post-traumatic stress disorder: a randomized, double-blind, placebo-controlled trial in a veteran population. J Clin Psychopharmacol 28(1): 84–88

[18]   Debiec J, LeDoux JE (2006) Noradrenergic signaling in the amygdala contributes to the reconsolidation of fear memory: treatment implications for PTSD. Ann N Y Acad Sci 1071: 521–524

[19]   Difede J, Barocas D (1999) Acute intrusive and avoidant PTSD symptoms as predictors of chronic PTSD following burn injury. J Trauma Stress 12(2): 363–369

[20]   Difede J, Ptacek JT, Roberts J, Barocas D, Rives W, Apfeldorf W, Yurt R (2002) Acute stress disorder after burn injury: a predictor of posttraumatic stress disorder? Psychosom Med 64(5): 826–834

[21]   Drake JE, Stoddard FJ Jr, Murphy JM, Ronfeldt H, Snidman N, Kagan J, Saxe G, Sheridan R (2006) Trauma severity influences acute stress in young burned children. J Burn Care Res 27(2): 174–182

[22]   Ehde DM, Patterson DR, Wiechman SA, Wilson LG (2000) Post-traumatic stress symptoms and distress 1 year after burn injury. J Burn Care Rehabil 21(2): 105–111

[23] El hamaoui Y, Yaalaoui S, Chihabeddine K, Boukind E, Moussaoui D (2002) Post-traumatic stress disorder in burned patients. Burns 28(7): 647–650

[24] Fauerbach JA, Lawrence J, Haythornthwaite J, Richter D, McGuire M, Schmidt C, Munster A (1997) Preburn psychiatric history affects posttrauma morbidity. Psychosomatics 38(4): 374–385

[25] Fauerbach JA, Lawrence JW, Schmidt CW Jr, Munster AM, Costa PT Jr (2000) Personality predictors of injury-related posttraumatic stress disorder. J Nerv Ment Dis 188(8): 510–517

[26] Fein JA, Kassam-Adams N, Gavin M, Huang R, Blanchard D, Datner EM (2002) Persistence of post-traumatic stress in violently injured youth seen in the emergency department. Arch Pediatr Adolesc Med 156(8): 836–840

[27] First MB, Spitzer RL, Gibbon M, Williams JB (1996) Structured clinical interview for the DSM-IV axis I disorders. American Psychiatric Publishing, Inc

[28] Foa EB (2006) Psychosocial therapy for posttraumatic stress disorder. J Clin Psychiatry 67 [Suppl 2]: 40–45

[29] Foa EB (2009) Treatment of PTSD and comorbid disorders. In: Effective treatments for PTSD. Guilford Press, New York, pp 606–613

[30] Frank J, Kosen T, Giller E, Dan E (1988) A randomized clinical trial of phenelzine and imipramine for PTSD. Am J Psychiatry 145: 759–769

[31] Gibson LE (2009) Acute stress disorder. Washington, DC: U. S. Department of Veterans Affairs. http://www.ptsd.va.gov/professional/pages/acute-stress-disorder.asp

[32] Gillies M, Barton J, Di Gallo A (2003) Follow-up of young road accident victims. J Trauma Stress 16(5): 523–526

[33] Goodyear-Brown P (2009) Play therapy with traumatized children: A prescriptive approach. John Wiley & Sons, Hoboken, NJ

[34] Hamner MB, Faldowski RA, Ulmer HG, Frueh BC, Huber MG, Arana GW (2003) Adjunctive risperidone treatment in PTSD: A preliminary controlled trial of effects on comorbid psychotic symptoms. Int Clin Psychopharmacol 18(1): 1–8

[35] Harvey AG, Bryant RA (1999) Acute stress disorder across trauma populations. J Nerv Ment Dis 187(7): 443–446

[36] Harvey AG, Bryant RA (1999) The relationship between acute stress disorder and posttraumatic stress disorder: a 2-year prospective evaluation. J Consult Clin Psychol 67: 985–988

[37] Jiménez JIP, Romero CC, Diéguez NG, Aliño JJ (2007) Pharmacological treatment of acute stress disorder with propranolol and hypnotics. Actas Esp Psiquiatr 35(6): 351–358

[38] Kassam-Adams N, Winston FK (2004) Predicting child PTSD: the relationship between acute stress disorder and PTSD in injured children. J Am Acad Child Adolesc Psychiatry 43(4): 403–411

[39] Kornør H, Winje D, Ekeberg Ø, Weisaeth L, Kirkehei I, Johansen K, Steiro A (2008) Early trauma-focused cognitive-behavioural therapy to prevent chronic post-traumatic stress disorder and related symptoms: a systematic review and meta-analysis. BMC Psychiatry 8: 81

[40] Kozaric-Kovacic D, Pivac N (2007) Quetiapine treatment in an open trial in combat-related post-traumatic stress disorder with psychotic features. Int J Neuropsychop 10: 253–261

[41] La Greca A, Silverman WK, Vernberg EM, Prinstein MJ (1996) Symptoms of posttramatic stress in children after hurricane Andrew. J Consult Clin Psychol 64: 712–723

[42] Landolt MA, Buehlmann C, Maag T, Schiestl C (2009) Brief report: quality of life is impaired in pediatric burn survivors with posttraumatic stress disorder. J Pediatr Psychol 34(1): 14–21

[43] Levenson J (2007) Psychiatric issues in surgery – Part 2: Specific topics. Prim Psychiatry 14(7): 40–43

[44] Main C, Spanswick C (2000) Pain management: An interdisciplinary approach. Harcourt Publishers Limited, Endinburgh, UK

[45] Marmar CR, Neylan TC, Schoenfeld FB (2002) New directions in the pharmacotherapy of posttraumatic stress disorder. Psychiatr Quart 73: 259–270

[46] Marshall RD, Pierce D (2000) Implications of recent findings in posttraumatic stress disorder and the role of pharmacotherapy. Harv Rev Psychiatry 7(5): 247–256

[47] Marshall RD, Spitzer R, Liebowitz MR (1999) Review and critique of the new DSM-IV diagnosis of acute stress disorder. Am J Psychiatry 156(11): 1677–1685

[48] Mayou RA, Ehlers A, Hobbs M (2000) Psychological debriefing for road traffic accident victims. Three year follow-up of a randomised controlled trial. Br J Psychiatry 176: 589–593

[49] McGhee LL, Maani CV, Garza TH, Desocio PA, Gaylord KM, Black IH (2009) The effect of propranolol on post-traumatic stress disorder in burned service members. J Burn Care Res 30(1): 92–97

[50] McKibben JB, Bresnick MG, Wiechman Askay SA, Fauerbach JA (2008) Acute stress disorder and posttraumatic stress disorder: a prospective study of prevalence, course, and predictors in a sample with major burn injuries. J Burn Care Res 29(1): 22–35

[51] McLoughlin E, McGuire A (1990) The causes, cost, and prevention of childhood burn injuries. Am J Dis Child 144: 677–683

[52] Meighen KG, Hines LA, Lagges AM (2007) Risperidone treatment of preschool children with thermal burns and acute stress disorder. J Child Adol Psychop 17(2): 223–232

[53] Meyer WJ, Blakeney P, Thomas CR, Russell W, Robert RS, Holzer CE (2007) Prevalence of major psychiatric illness in young adults who were burned as children. Psychosom Med 69(4): 377–382

[54] Mitchell JT (1983) When disaster strikes: The critical incident stress debriefing process. J Emerg Med Serv 8(1): 36–39

[55] Morgan J, Roufeil L, Kaushik S, Bassett M (1998) Influence of coping style and precolonoscopy information on pain and anxiety of colonoscopy. Gastrointest Endosc 48(2): 119–127

[56] Mueser KT, Rosenberg SD, Xie H, Jankowski MK, Bolton EE, Lu W, Hamblen JL, Rosenberg HJ, McHugo GJ, Wolfe R (2008) A randomized controlled trial of cognitive-behavioral treatment for posttraumatic stress disorder in severe mental illness. J Consult Clin Psychol 76(2): 259–271

[57] Nagy L, Morgan C, Southwick, S, Charney D (1993) Open prospective trial of fluoxetine for posttraumatic stress disorder. J Clin Psychopharmacol 13: 107–113

[58] Noronha DO, Faust J (2007) Identifying the variables impacting post-burn psychological adjustment: a meta-analysis. J Pediatr Psychol 32(3): 380–391

[59] Norton PJ, Price EC (2007) A meta-analytic review of adult cognitive-behavioral treatment outcome across the anxiety disorders. J Nerv Ment Dis 195(6): 521–531

[60 a] Nover RA (1973) Pain and the burned children. Am Acad Child Psychiatry 12: 499–505

[60 b] Pae C, Marks DM, Han C, Masand PS, Patkar AA (2009) Pregabalin augmentation of antidepressants in patients with accident-related posttraumatic stress disorder: an open label pilot study. Int Clin Psychopharmacol 24: 29–33

[61] Patterson DR, Everett JJ, Bombardier CH, Questad KA, Lee VK, Marvin JA (1993) Psychological effects of severe burn injuries. Psychol Bull 113: 362–378

[62] Perry S, Difede J, Musngi G, Frances AJ, Jacobsberg L (1992) Predictors of posttraumatic stress disorder after burn injury. Am J Psychiatry 149(7): 931–935

[63] Pitman RK, Delahanty DL (2005) Conceptually driven pharmacologic approaches to acute trauma. CNS Spectr 10(2): 99–106

[64] Powers PS, Cruse CW, Boyd F (2000) Psychiatric status, prevention, and outcome in patients with burns: a prospective study. J Burn Care Rehabil 21(1,Pt 1): 85–88

[65] Ptacek JT, Patterson DR, Montgomery BK, Heimbach DM (1995) Pain, coping, and adjustment in patients with burns: preliminary findings from a prospective study. J Pain Symptom Manage 10(6): 446–455

[66] Raphael B, Wilson JP (2000) Psychological debriefing: Theory, practice, evidence. Cambridge University Press, Cambridge, UK

[67] Ratcliff SL, Brown A, Rosenberg L, Rosenberg M, Robert R, Cuervo LJ, Villarreal C, Thomas C, Meyer III WJ (2006) The effectiveness of a pain and anxiety protocol to treat the acute pediatric burn patient. Burns 32: 554–562

[68] Reich W, Licht P, Lehman H, Sathyan S, Unger K (1997) Missouri Assessment of Genetics Interview for Children (MAGIC). Washington University Press, St. Louis

[69] Reinblatt SP, Riddle MA (2007) The pharmacological management of childhood anxiety disorders: A review. Psychopharmacology 191(1): 67–86

[70] Robert R, Meyer III WJ, Bishop S, Rosenberg L, Murphy L, Blakeney PE (1999) Disfiguring burn scars and adolescent self-esteem. Burns 25: 581–558

[71] Robert R, Meyer W, Villareal C, Blakeney P, Desai M, Herndon D (1999) An approach to the timely treatment of Acute Stress Disorder. J Burn Care Rehabil 20(3): 250–258

[72] Robert R, Tcheung WJ, Rosenberg L, Rosenberg M, Mitchell C, Villarreal C, Thomas C, Holzer C, Meyer WJ 3rd (2008) Treating thermally injured children suffering symptoms of acute stress with imipramine and fluoxetine: a randomized, double-blind study. Burns 34(7): 919–928

[73] Roberts NP, Kitchiner NJ, Kenardy J, Bisson JI (2009) Systematic review and meta-analysis of multiple-session early interventions following traumatic events. Am J Psychiatry 166(3): 293–301

[74] Roca RP, Spence RJ, Munster AM (1992) Posttraumatic adaptation and distress among adult burn survivors. Am J Psychiatry 149(9): 1234–1238

[75] Rosenberg L, Rosenberg M, Perry J, Sharp S, Richardson L, Holzer III C, Meyer III W (2009) Long-term psychosocial adjustment of pediatric burn survivors previously diagnosed and treated for acute stress disorder. In: Proceedings of the ABA Annual Conference, San Antonio, TX

[76] Rothbaum BO, Killeen TK, Davidson JR, Brady KT, Connor KM, Heekin MH (2008) Placebo-controlled trial of risperidone augmentation for selective serotonin reuptake inhibitor-resistant civilian posttraumatic stress disorder. J Clin Psychiatry 69(4): 520–525

[77] Saxe G, Chawla N, Stoddard F, Kassam-Adams N, Courtney D, Cunningham K, Lopez C, Hall E, Sheridan R, King D, King L (2003) Child stress disorders checklist: A measure of ASD and PTSD in children. J Am Acad Child Adolesc Psychiatry 42(8): 972–978

[78] Saxe G, Miller A, Bartholomew D, Hall E, Lopez C, Kaplow J, Koenen K, Bosquet M, Allee L, Erikson I, Moulton S (2005) Incidence of and risk factors for acute stress disorder in children with injuries. J Traum 59(4): 946–953

[79] Saxe GN, Stoddard F, Hall E, Chawla N, Lopez C, Sheridan R, King D, King L, Yehuda R (2005) Pathways to PTSD, part I: Children with burns. Am J Psychiatry 162(7): 1299–1304

[80] Schnyder U (2003) Post-traumatic stress disorders: diagnostic and therapeutic principles. Praxis 92(8): 337–343

[81] Seed S, Stein D, Ziervogel C, Middleton T, Kaminer D, Emsley R, Rosouw W (2002) Comparison of response to a selective serotonin reuptake inhibitor in children, adolescents and adults with posttraumatic stress disorder. J Child Adolesc Psychopharmacol 12: 37–46

[82] Sharp S, Thomas C, Meyer III W (2010) The effectiveness of propranolol in controlling symptoms of acute stress disorder. J Trauma 68(1): 193–197

[83] Shay J (1992) Fluoxetine reduces explosiveness and elevates mood on Vietnam combat vets with PTSD. J Traumatic Stress 5: 97–110

[84] Sherman JJ (1998) Effects of psychotherapeutic treatments for PTSD: a meta-analysis of controlled clinical trials. J Trauma Stress 11(3): 413–435

[85] Simon NM, Connor KM, Lang AJ, Rauch S, Krulewicz S, LeBeau RT, Davidson JRT, Stein MB, Otto MW, Foa EB, Pollack MH (2008) Paroxetine CR augmentation for posttraumatic stress disorder refractory to prolonged exposure therapy. J Clin Psychiatry 69: 400–405

[86] Southwick SM, Paige S, Morgan CA 3rd, Bremner JD, Krystal JH, Charney DS (1999) Neurotransmitter alterations in PTSD: catecholamines and serotonin. Semin Clin Neuropsychiatry 4(4): 242–248

[87] Southwick SM, Yehuda R, Giller E, Charney, DS (1994) Use of tricyclics and monoamine oxidase inhibitors in the treatment of PTSD: A quantitative review. In: Marburg MM (ed) Catecholamine function in post traumatic stress disorder: Emerging concepts. Washington D.C. American Psychiatric Press, pp 293–305

[88] Staab JP, Grieger TA, Fullerton CS, Ursano RJ (1996) Acute stress disorder, subsequent posttraumatic stress disorder and depression after a series of typhoons. Anxiety 2: 219–225

[89] Steiner H, Clark WR (1977) Psychiatric complications of burned adults: A classification. J Trauma 17: 134–143

[90] Stoddard FJ (1982) Body image development in the burned child. J Am Acad Child Psychiatry 21(5): 502–507

[91] Stoddard FJ, Chedekel DS, Remensnyder JP (1984) Psychological reactions of a boy to severe electrical burns including the loss of his penis. J Am Acad Child Psychiatry 23(2): 219–221

[92] Stoddard FJ, Norman DK, Murphy JM, Beardslee WR (1989) Psychiatric outcome of burned children and adolescents. J Am Acad Child Adolesc Psychiatry 28(4): 589–595

[93] Stoddard FJ, O'Connell KG (1983) Dysphoria in children with severe burns. Journal of Children in Contemporary Society 15: 41–50

[94] Stoddard FJ, Saxe G, Ronfeldt H, Drake JE, Burns J, Edgren C, Sheridan R (2006) Acute stress symptoms in young children with burns. J Am Acad Child Adolesc Psychiatry 45(1): 87–93

[95] Stoddard FJ Jr, Sorrentino EA, Ceranoglu TA, Saxe G, Murphy JM, Drake JE, Ronfeldt H, White GW, Kagan J, Snidman N, Sheridan RL, Tompkins RG (2009) Preliminary evidence for the effects of morphine on posttraumatic stress disorder symptoms in one- to four-year-olds with burns. J Burn Care Res 30(5): 836–843

[96] Stoddard FJ, Stroud L, Murphy JM (1992) Depression in children after recovery from severe burns. J Burn Care Rehabil 13(3): 340–347

[97] Tarnowski KJ, Rasnake LK, Gavaghan-Jones MP, Smith L (1991) Psychosocial sequelea of pediatric burn injuries. A Review. Clin Psychol Rev 11: 399–418

[98] Tcheung WJ, Robert R, Rosenberg L, Rosenberg M, Villarreal C, Thomas C, Holzer CE 3rd, Meyer WJ 3rd (2005) Early treatment of acute stress disorder in children with major burn injury. Pediatr Crit Care Med 6(6): 676–681

[99] Terr LC (1983) Chowchilla revisited: the effects of psychic trauma four years after a school-bus kidnapping. Am J Psychiatry 140(12): 1543–1550

[100] Thomas CR, Blakeney P, Holzer III CE, Meyer III WJ (2009) Psychiatric disorders in long term adjustment of at risk adolescent burn survivors. J Burn Care Res 30: 458–463

[101] Thomas CR, Meyer III WJ, Blakeney PE (2007) Psychiatric disorders associated with burn injury In: Herndon D (ed) Total burn care. Saunders, Philadelphia, pp 819–828

[102] US Department of Veteran Affairs, National Center for Post Traumatic Stress Disorder (2009) Acute Stress Disorder: A brief description. Washington, DC: U.S. Department of Veterans Affairs. http://www.ptsd.va.gov/public/pages/acute-stress-disorder.asp

[103] Van der Kolk B, Dryfuss D, Michaels M, Shera D. Berkowitz R, Fisler R, Sax G (1994) Fluoxetine in posttraumatic stress disorder. J Clin Psychiatry 55: 517–522

[104] Van Loey NE, Maas CJ, Faber AW, Taal LA (2003) Predictors of chronic posttraumatic stress symptoms following burn injury: results of a longitudinal study. J Trauma Stress 16(4): 361–369

[105] Weathers FW, Huska JA, Keane TM (1991) The PTSD Checklist-Civilian Version (PCL-C). Available from F.W. Weathers, National Center for PTSD, Boston Veterans Affairs Medical Center, 150 S. Huntington Avenue, Boston, MA 02130

[106] Welner Z, Reich W, Herjanic B, Jung KG, Amado H (1987) Reliability, validity, and parent-child agreement studies of the Diagnostic Interview for Children and Adolescents (DICA). J Am Acad Child Adolesc Psychiatry 26(5): 649–653

[107] Yehuda R, McFarlane AC (2000) PTSD is a valid diagnosis: Who benefits from challenging its existence? Aust N Z J Psychiatry 34(6): 940–953

[108] Yu B, Dimsdale J (1999) Postraumatic stress disorder in patients with burn injuries. J Burn Care Rehabil 20(5): 426–433

Correspondence: Walter J. Meyer, III, M.D., Head, Department of Psychological and Psychiatric Services, Shriners Hospitals for Children, 815 Market St, Galveston, Texas 77550–2725, USA, E-mail: wmeyer@utmb.edu

Long term consequences of burn injuries

Shelley Wiechman

University of Washington School of Medicine, Seattle, WA, USA

Acknowledgements

This manuscript was supported by a grant from the National Institute of Health (1RO3HD052 584 – 01A2), and the from the National Institute on Disability and Rehabilitation Research in the Office of Special Education and Rehabilitative Services in the U. S. Department of Education (H133A070 047).

Introduction

Data from the National Burn Repository of the American Burn Association [2], has revealed that between the years of 1998 – 2009, more patients are surviving large burns despite multiple complications. The mortality rate for all burn injuries is 4 %. The average length of stay declined during this time period from 11 days, in the decade prior, to 9 days. This is just over one day of hospitalization per 1 % burn. As a result, these patients are being discharged with multiple, long term physical and psychological challenges, such as scarring, contractures, amputations, pain and poor psychological adjustment. In the past, most of the literature on burn injuries was devoted to the acute phase of hospitalization, particularly resuscitation efforts and surgical interventions. In recent years, issues associated with long term adjustment have been recognized as a priority for research and clinical practice. Because of the relative infancy of the field of burn rehabilitation, there is little research on the efficacy of interventions that can help with the long-term challenges, such as pain, depression and PTSD that these survivors face once they are discharged from the hospital.

The post-acute phase of recovery typically begins when patients leave the hospital and are challenged to reintegrate into society. For patients with severe burn injuries, this phase likely involves continued physical rehabilitation, along with possible continuation of procedures such as dressing changes and cosmetic surgery, all performed in outpatient clinics. Patients may encounter daily pain during rehabilitation, and they may also be forced to confront cosmetic or other existential changes that have occurred as a result of their injury. There is also increasing evidence that patients may develop chronic neuropathic pain [13, 48]. This is a period when patients slowly regain a sense of competence while simultaneously adjusting to the practical limitations of a burn injury. Studies have shown that the first year after hospitalization is a psychologically unique period of high distress [56]. In this chapter, we will begin by examining the role that the initial physical stress caused by the burn injury has in maintaining ongoing distress. We will then introduce a biopsychosocial model that can be used to guide our understanding of the complex factors that determine a person's long term adjustment to injury. Finally, we will look at the various long term outcomes, both positive and negative, that people face following a burn injury. We will conclude with recommendations for treatment.

Allostatic load

The stress that the body endures as a result of a traumatic injury such as a burn can be explained in terms of allostasis. The concept of allostatic load can be useful in explaining the mechanisms of how a traumatic injury can have an impact on a person months to years later. Sterling and Eyer [71] first defined allostasis as the adaptation that the body makes in response to potentially stressful events. The process involves activation of several physiological systems, including the immune system, and is essentially the body's ability to maintain "stability through change". The body is able to cope effectively with these stressors when adaptations are activated infrequently. But there is the potential for this system to become overloaded. McEwen and Stellar [50] describe what happens to the body when these allostatic systems are overstimulated and first used the term "allostatic load". There are three types of allostatic load, including frequent activation of allostasis (e. g. daily wound debridements and painful physical therapy), the body's inability to turn off allostasis when the stressor is removed (e. g. anticipatory anxiety, PTSD symptoms), and an inadequate response to the stressor (e. g. inadequate coping resources). Please see [49] for more detailed discussion of allostatic load. Simply, it is the measure of cumulative wear and tear on the body. It is important to view allostatic load as an interaction between genetic, environmental and social factors. One could argue that the intense acute phase of burn recovery places such extensive load on the body that it taxes resources and continues to have an impact for several months to years after physical recovery is complete.

The identification of the body's physiological response to stressors sparked a large body of research examining the potential harmful effects of allostatic load on the body over time. Most relevant to the study of burn injuries is the body of literature that has shown slowed wound healing under psychological stress [11, 39]. More importantly, this research was extended to examining the effects of un-

controlled pain on wound healing in surgical patients and again, it was shown that higher post surgical pain levels delayed healing of wounds from a punch biopsy. This relationship between high pain levels and delayed wound healing was maintained even after controlling for presurgery depressive symptoms and other post surgical medical complications. Although there have been no specific studies looking at the relationship between stress and the healing of burn wounds, the underlying mechanisms are the same. Burn injury recovery requires the restoration of tissue perfusion for wound healing to occur and to defend against infection. One of the strongest arguments in support of the theory that stress can impair healing and recovery in burn injuries is the body of research showing the impact that high acute pain levels can predict long term outcomes. The physiologic stress of inadequate pain control during wound care will likely impact the healing of burn wounds. For example, one study [60] showed that pain during hospitalization predicted psychological adjustment up to two years following the burn injury. They found that pain during hospitalization was a stronger predictor of adjustment than either the size of the burn injury or the length of hospitalization. Further, Edwards et al. [16] found that pain severity at discharge was the sole consistent predictor of suicidal ideation at both six months and one year post discharge. Finally, several researchers have emphasized the complex, bidirectional interactions between pain, depression and physical function [16, 79]. This body of research emphasizes the importance of early pain control during the acute phase of hospitalization. Poor pain control during this period can set the stage for negative outcomes, such as slower healing time, hypertrophic scarring, PTSD and depression.

Biopsychosocial models of injury

A person's response to allostasis is a function of their personality style and coping mechanisms and how these interact over time with the environmental factors that are present. Univariate models are insufficient to explain a person's response to a burn injury and their long term outcome. In order to advance the field, more sophisticated, theory-driven biopsycho-

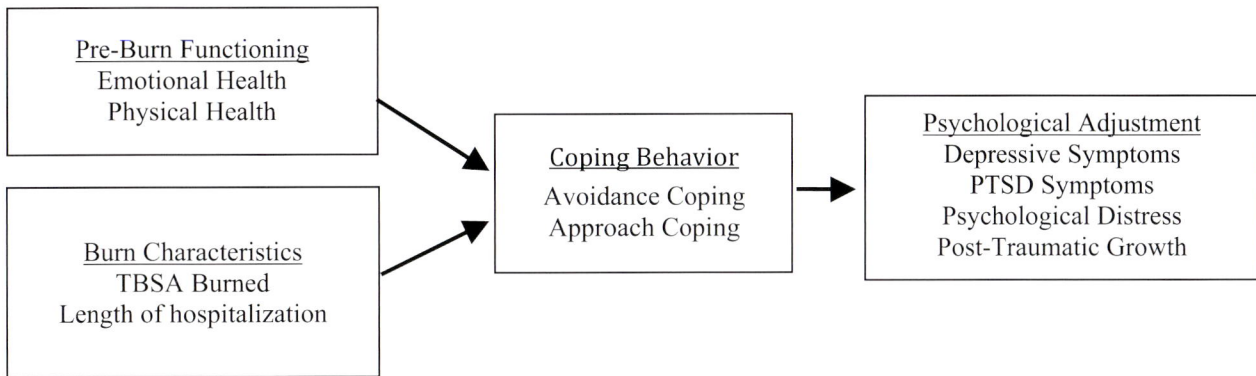

Fig. 1. Hypothesized model of psychological adjustment to burn injury

social models are needed to explain outcomes of burn injury. Researchers have identified pre-burn affective disorders, injury characteristics (e. g. burn size and location, inpatient pain), dispositional variables and coping styles as risk factors for the development of post-injury mood disorders and adjustment. Based on current literature, we have proposed the following conceptual model (see Fig. 1) to better understand the complex interplay of factors that can potentially affect burn recovery.

Lazarus and Folkman [45] first conceptualized the transactional model of stress. This model is based on the assumption that a body's response to stress is based on the interaction between our appraisal of the situation and its demands, our resources to cope with the demands of the situation, and the value that we place on the consequences of the situation. In other words, it is not the situation itself that is either stressful or non-stressful, but the complex interplay between the person and the situation. What is stressful to one person may not be as stressful to another person in the same situation. This is precisely why we cannot make blanket statements on how patients who suffer burn injuries will cope with the situation and what their long term outcome will be. The complexity of this interaction again forces us to consider a biopsychosocial model when predicting burn outcomes.

Preburn emotional and physical health

It is well known amongst clinicians that a person's preburn level of physical and emo tional functioning can greatly impact their course of recovery from

their ICU stay to years beyond discharge. For example, those patients with diabetes, COPD and other medical comorbidities have lower survival rates, longer lengths of stay and fair poorer overall. The available research largely supports the impression that individuals with burns severe enough to warrant hospital care often have preexisting chaos and dysfunction in their lives. In several reviews of the literature it was found that the incidence of mental illness and personality disorders was higher in burn unit patients than the general population [40, 56, 58]. For example, Patterson et al. [56] estimated that the presence of premorbid psychiatric disorders ranged between 28 % and 75 %, higher than expected in the general population. These disorders include depression, personality disorders, and substance abuse. Another study by Patterson et al. [58] found patients with burn injuries scored higher on premorbid levels of psychological distress, anxiety, depression, and loss of behavioral and emotional control when compared to a national normative sample. These studies also found that individuals with pre-existing psychopathology often cope with hospitalization through previously established, dysfunctional and often disruptive patterns. Such dysfunctional coping styles, in turn, had an adverse impact on hospital course that increased length of stay and led to more serious psychopathology upon discharge. As an example, a burn injury and its subsequent treatment can often exacerbate depression in previously depressed patients. Patients with personality disorders can also struggle to cope with their burn injury and have relationship patterns with staff that are dysfunctional and cause great difficulty for the staff. Mental health professionals need to be an integral part of the team and help to educate burn team members about preexisting conditions and understand that a person with a burn injury will not be "cured" of their personality disorder, mental illness, depression, etc. while on the burn unit.

Burn characteristics

Researchers have begun to focus on potential variables from acute hospitalization that may have a long-term impact on adjustment. As mentioned earlier, the amount of pain that a person reports in the hospital supersedes both the size of their burn and the length of hospitalization as predictors of long-term outcome at six months, one year and two years post discharge [60, 63]. Total Burn Surface Area (TBSA), length of hospitalization, and days spent in the ICU or on a ventilator have been used as indicators of the severity of a burn injury. Research on the relation between these variables and outcomes has been equivocal. Patterson et al. [56] cautioned against using TBSA as the sole predictor of emotional outcome, citing studies that have shown significant emotional distress in persons with relatively small burns, and little to no distress in persons with large burns. Location of the burn has been found to predict adjustment, with those persons with burns on their face or hands showing more emotional distress than those with more hidden burns [82].

Coping

Early work on coping by Lazarus and Folkman [45] proposed a comprehensive model of stress and coping that is based on the notion that a person's appraisal of the demands and consequences of a situation and the amount of control they perceive to have over the situation, will lead to selection of a particular coping strategy. A number of organizing frames and taxonomies have been used to categorize and delineate coping processes [73]. The extent to which a coping strategy involves approaching a particular stressor, versus avoidance, is a widely used classification [72]. For instance, active strategies such as problem-solving, information seeking, and social support seeking can be construed as approach-oriented coping, and strategies that involve disengagement, denial, or distraction can be viewed as avoidance-oriented efforts. Neither approach-oriented nor avoidance-oriented coping behaviors are inherently adaptive or maladaptive; coping effectiveness is better determined by the characteristics of the individual and the situation [45]. However, reviews of the literature on coping with chronic illness have suggested a salutary effect of approach-oriented coping on physical and emotional health outcomes in medical populations [70].

According to theory, selection of a specific coping strategy will depend on the individual's appraisal of the amount of control they have over the situation. For example, some research has suggested that if a person appraises the situation as being more controllable, then they will use a strategy in which they will attempt to actively problem-solve or mobilize resources; if they appraise low levels of control, then they will likely employ strategies in which they distract their attention away from the stressor [28]. Little research has attempted to characterize the adaptiveness of specific coping strategies in burn patients over time. It is also unknown if a person can be taught a specific coping style, especially when under such considerable stress as recovering from a burn injury.

Long term outcomes

Patients have long reported that the first year following a burn injury is a time of substantial distress. An accumulating body of research on the psychosocial effects of a burn injury has supported these reports [16, 20, 25, 56, 79]. Clearly, mood disorders [20, 29, 47, 62, 76, 82] and anxiety disorders [5, 17, 20, 29, 47, 76] are the most common symptoms of distress, however, patients may also experience a myriad of other problems, including sleep disturbance [8, 37, 43], body image concerns [23] and sexual problems [7]. All of these symptoms potentially contribute to decreased quality of life [24, 59] Depression and post-traumatic stress disorder (PTSD) are two of the more commonly reported psychological problems in burn survivors and we will focus our discussion on these two disorders.

Depression

Research that has attempted to identify rates of depressive disorders following a burn injury has been fraught with challenges. In their comprehensive review, Thombs et al. [77] found that most of the studies have been at single centers with small sample sizes with poor rates of recruitment and retention. In addition, the multiple approaches and measures used have lead to a wide variation in reported rates of depressive symptoms and diagnosable disorders. For example, the range of reported symptoms in the first year after a burn injury is 2–22 % and the prevalence rate after one year is 3–54 % [78]. There seem to be much lower prevalence rates of depression when a structured interview is used as compared to a standardized measure. But even when standardized measures are used the rates vary widely. The most common standardized measures are the Hospital Anxiety and Depression Scale (depression subscale) [87] and the Beck Depression Inventory [6]. The HADS does not include questions with somatic symptoms, but the BDI does. Oftentimes it is difficult to differentiate between what symptoms can be attributed to the medical disorder and what are somatic symptoms of depression, which could account for the higher reported rates of depression when using the BDI versus the HADS. The field is still debating whether or not a measure of depression that is specific to those with burn injuries needs to be designed and validated. The 9-item Patient Health Questionnaire [69] is a widely used screening tool in primary care and other medical specialty clinics and may prove to be useful in the burn setting.

Several studies have also found that scores tend to be stable from discharge to at least the first year following a burn injury [62]. Although it is commonly assumed that these rates will decrease after the first year, no longitudinal studies have looked at depression rates longer than one year post-injury. Thombs et al. [78] found seven studies that reported on risk factors for depression following a burn injury. As mentioned earlier, many of the identified risk factors encompass premorbid functioning, such as employment status, medical illness and prior depression. Those who suffered from depressive symptoms in the year prior to the burn injury were 5 times more likely to be diagnosed with a mood disorder at discharge

[20]. Other risk factors include female gender, and a visible burn [85]. Although research in this area has been fraught with methodological problems making it difficult to pin down actual rates of depressive disorders, we can confidently recommend a brief screen for depressive symptoms both during the inpatient hospitalization and at discharge and at follow up clinic visits. Referrals to mental health professionals can be made for more in-depth assessments if warranted by the responses on the screening tool.

PTSD

The reported frequency of acute stress disorder (ASD) following a burn injury ranges from 11–32 % of patients [9, 15, 26, 42, 18, 47, 80]. While the frequency of post-traumatic stress disorder (PTSD) is approximately 23–33 % of patients 3 to 6 months after a burn injury [15, 19]. That percentage ranges from 15–45 % at one year following the injury [14, 20, 47, 80]. In contrast, community-based studies show that the lifetime prevalence of persons with PTSD is 1–14 % [3]. The large variability in reported rates of diagnosed ASD/PTSD is likely due to differences in measurement strategies and measurement timepoints. However, most researchers and clinicians agree that even if patients do not meet a formal diagnosis of ASD or PTSD, the majority of burn survivors are having at least some of the symptoms of this disorder (e. g. nightmares, intrusive thoughts, hypervigilance, avoidance) that negatively impacts their quality of life. When identifying possible risk factors for the development of PTSD, pre-existing anxiety or depressive disorders have been associated with an increased risk of developing post-traumatic stress disorder. Further, the baseline symptoms of Acute Stress Disorder (ASD) at discharge and at one month predict presence of post-traumatic stress disorder at one year [51], suggesting that symptoms do not decrease over time if left untreated. In addition, burn patients who have a comorbid diagnosis of PTSD are higher utilizers of medical services. Injury-related characteristics such as total body surface area burned and the location of the injury have repeatedly failed to predict who will suffer from such trauma. In contrast, issues such as the patient's mental health history, social support and coping style hold significant promise as predictive factors.

Clearly, burn injuries cause various forms of psychological distress. One study sought to determine the root causes of this distress. Wiechman et al. [82] used a form of qualitative methodology that asked burn survivors to rate their top reasons for distress. Four distinct groups emerged. The primary source of distress from the first group appeared to be from chronic, physical discomfort related to scars, decreased motion, pain, open donor sites and itching. Their distress appeared to be oriented more toward the present and their current physical discomfort. Those in the second group indicated that physical stress, such as pain, temperature changes, decreased range of motion and sleep disturbance, are troublesome. However, they were also concerned about non-physical stressors caused by burn injuries, such as financial and insurance concerns, decrease in pleasurable activities and the health/well-being of other family members. In other words, the direct physical distress is mixed in with the toll it has taken on the family. The third group seemed to be more focused on the appearance of the burn and their future, such as the financial, legal and insurance concerns and the rude behavior of others. They were more concerned with the long-term realities of the disability.

Finally, the fourth group seemed to be equally focused on both psychological (fear of re-injury and hypervigilance, financial concerns, health and well-being of family members, impatience/irritability) and physical matters (itching and uncomfortable scars, decreased strength, changes in sensations). This mix of concerns implied that they were experiencing helplessness and anxiety, as many of the concerns were out of their control. This data indicated that reasons for post-burn distress are complicated and vary widely across groups and over time. Interventions need to specifically target the various concerns.

Body image dissatisfaction

Burn survivors frequently list the change in appearance as a major concern and source of distress. Burn injuries can cause significant changes in appearance through scarring, contractures, changes in skin pigmentation, or amputations. The impact that these physical changes have on self-esteem and body image has only recently been studied [22]. Several studies of risk factors for the development of poor body image found that burn characteristics, such as the visibility of the scar, depression, female gender and coping style best predicted body image dissatisfaction [1, 22, 44]. An additional predictor of body image dissatisfaction is the importance that a patient placed on their appearance before the burn injury. If an individual did not place much importance on their appearance before the burn, they tend to be much less distressed by the consequences of disfigurement [22].

A variety of approaches have been used to address cosmetic concerns in those who present in the treatment setting [21, 61]. Surprisingly, there have been no published studies to date on the efficacy of these various treatments. Most treatments focus on cognitive-behavioral strategies to address a person's appraisal of their appearance, to teach adaptive coping strategies, and to introduce social skills that enhance self esteem and improve social competence. Two programs designed to enhance self-esteem are the Changing Faces program in Great Britain [55], and the BEST program in the US [38]. Both of these programs include a hospital-based social skills program, along with a series of publications for patients dealing with aspects of disfigurement. These programs allow people to explore their internal reactions to the response of others towards their disfigurement and also to access a number of adaptive behaviors in response to the inevitable negative societal responses to disfigurement.

Sleep

One of the most commonly identified complications of burn injuries is sleep disturbance, yet it is often overlooked and untreated. One of the biggest predictors of post-burn sleep disturbance is a person's preburn sleep quality. Abnormal sleep patterns are common in the general population, with up to 50 % of non-burn adults in the US reporting sleep problems [4]. Poor sleep can affect issues such as therapy performance, pain control, mood, and even wound healing. A burn injury and its treatment present a multitude of factors that can interfere with sleep. A series of studies by Gottschlich et al. has shown that a burn injury changes sleep architecture [30, 33, 34]. They monitored polysomnogram (PSG) in burn survivors and reported increased total sleep time, decreases in stage 3 and 4 sleep, decreased rapid eye movement (REM) sleep and increased arousals when compared to age-matched controls [31, 32, 64]. Environmental factors can also impact sleep quality. Early in care, the hospital setting and nature of care can be highly disruptive factors. Frequent painful and intrusive treatments, noisy settings, metabolic imbalance and awakening to take vital signs can all lead to poor sleep. As wounds heal pruritus (itch) can become extremely unpleasant and can disrupt sleep. Anxiety and depression also contribute to poor sleep and the medications used to treat these disorders impact sleep. It is not surprising then that patients with burn injuries will experience impaired sleep long after discharge from the hospital. Rose and colleagues [65] followed 82 children with severe burn injuries and reported serious sleep disturbance one year after injury. Sleep disturbances included nightmares, bedwetting and sleep walking. 63 % of the sample complained of needing daytime names with is far greater than the norm [41].

With respect to treatment for sleep disorders after burn injuries, there are various nonpharmacological and pharmacological options available. It is recommended that clinicians work with the patients on nonpharmacological interventions before turning to medication. Nonpharmacologic options include sleep hygiene, stimulus control, sleep restriction, relaxation therapy, cognitive-behavioral therapy and light therapy. Sleep hygiene interventions include changing the environment (e. g. quiet rooms), reducing day time naps, establishing regular sleep/wake schedules, reducing stimulants from late afternoon to prior to bedtime when appropriate (e. g. caffeine, candy, nicotine, alcohol), decreasing stimuli at night (e. g. internet, TV) and proper timing of food and exercise. Stimulus control involves creating the bed as a stimulus for sleep by having the patient go to bed only when sleepy and removing competing stimuli from the room (e. g. television). Sleep restriction focuses on limiting the amount of hours a person can sleep. Cognitive-behavioral therapy can help patients work with the dysfunctional thoughts that disrupt sleep and include relaxation training. Although

these techniques have primarily been applied to patients in the outpatient setting, many of these options are appropriate in the hospital setting as well.

If sleep problems persist after attempting the non-pharmacologic approaches then time-limited trials of medication may be warranted. Benzodiazepines such as diazepam and lorazepam were introduced as a treatment for insomnia in the 1960s. A newer class of drugs, the nonbenzodiazepine benzodiazepine receptor agonists, were introduced in the 1990s. This class of drugs has been regarded as preferable. They are effective at promoting sleep [53, 68, 81] but have shorter half-lives relative to more traditional benzodiazepines. They are also thought to be less addictive, have a lower impact on cognition and create less "hangover" effects [35, 36, 81]. Examples of this class of drug are zolpidem, zaleplon, and eszopicione. There is little question that this class of drugs have a high habit-forming potential.

If patients cannot remain asleep with nonbenzodiazepine, benzodiazepine receptor agonists, or if they are remaining on these agents for a prolonged period of time then it may be appropriate to consider an antidepressant for sleep, particularly if they have current depressive symptoms. Several of these agents are used for sleep management because they have sedating and sleep-promoting properties. A full review of the issues discussed above regarding sleep after burn injuries is reported by Jaffee and Patterson [37].

Post-traumatic growth

Although it is important to study distress and negative affect following a trauma, it is equally important to study positive emotions and growth. Standardized measures need to include questions of positive, as well as negative emotions; and interventions for PTSD and depression should take into account the potential for posttraumatic growth.

Post traumatic growth (PTG) was defined by Tedeschi and Calhoun [10, 74] as a positive psychological change experienced as a result of the struggle with highly challenging life circumstances. Other terms have been used to refer to this positive psychology model, including adversarial growth, benefit finding, optimism, hardiness and resiliency. Tedeschi and Calhoun [75] have indentified five components of

PTG. These include a greater appreciation of life and changed priorities; warmer, more intimate relations with others; a greater sense of personal strength, recognition of new possibilities, and spiritual development.

Although PTG has been studied in several medical populations, such as those diagnosed with cancer [12], HIV [52], multiple sclerosis [54] and heart disease [67], we found only one study that looked at PTG following burn injuries. Rosenbach and Renneberg [66] looked at PTG in burn patients at time of discharge and attempted to identify correlates facilitating or preventing PTG. Their sample included 149 adults who had been discharged from the burn center at least three months prior to the study. They were sent self report questionnaires that included the Post-Traumatic Growth Inventory, and other inventories assessing coping, social support, health related quality of life and psychological distress. Fifty-seven percent of their sample was men and the mean total burn surface area (TBSA) was 32 %. Percentage of TBSA was used as an indicator of injury severity where those with a TBSA greater than 30 % was classified as higher severity of injury than those with a TBSA less than 30 %. An active coping style, social support, and female gender were the strongest predictors of who would experience PTG. The severity of injury, the absence of distress and quality of life were not found to be associated with PTG. In fact, this study confirmed the findings of other studies that PTG and distress can co-occur. Their sample experienced a high degree of PTG as a whole, yet reported high levels of distress and lower quality of life. In general, participants in this study showed the most growth in more appreciation of life, enhancement of personal relationships and a greater sense of personal strength dimensions of PTG. PTG is not something that can be forced upon a patient. A skillful clinician needs to listen carefully for opening and clues that a person is ready to acknowledge potential growth.

Summary and recommendations

The last 20 years of research have helped us understand the frequency of psychological disorders and distress symptoms in the burn survivor population. Research that has been guided by biopsychosocial models has shown us that burn survivors face a combination of physical, emotional and social factors that impact quality of life. Adjustment to a burn injury involves a complex interplay between the preinjury characteristics of the survivor, the moderating environmental factors, and the nature of the injury and ensuing medical care. Actual rates of Axis I disorders such as major depressive disorder and PTSD are hard to pinpoint due to discrepancies in the literature. These discrepancies are likely from the use of different assessment tools and measurement at different time points, as well as various methodological problems. For most people with burns large enough to require hospitalization, symptoms of depression and PTSD are common and considered to be in the realm of normal adjustment [15, 18, 20]. However, this does not mean that symptoms should not be treated. Patients may be so distressed by their symptoms that it affects their quality of life.

In addition to Axis 1 disorders, burn survivors report difficulties with body image, ongoing physical challenges such as scarring and contractures, financial stressors and difficulty in returning to school or employment. Also, the impact of the burn injury on family members and the family structure should not be overlooked.

Treatment interventions must be sophisticated and flexible enough to account for the large variability in causes of distress. We recommend screening for distress symptoms both during inpatient hospitalization and again during outpatient clinic visits and treating as indicated. A thorough psychological intake should include a brief history and an assessment of pain level, quality of sleep, and symptoms of depression and PTSD. We have also found success in using brief screening tools such as the PHQ-9 [69] to supplement the intake.

Since there have been very few randomized controlled clinical trials specific to patients with burn injuries, treatments should be used that have been effective for non-burn patients with these psychological problems. For example, depressed burn survivors may benefit from a combination of medication, cognitive-behavior therapy and exercise to treat depression. Exposure-based therapies may be effective for burn survivors with PTSD [27], particularly after discharge from the hospital setting. A multidisciplinary team approach should also be used as patients can benefit from support from a vocational or rehabilitation counselor to address issues related to return to work. Social workers will also be needed to assist with a variety of matters, including financial resources. Support groups and peer counseling visitation may also be useful if carefully monitored by trained professionals [82]. Finally, we should not overlook the opportunity for post-traumatic growth. A burn injury is a life-changing event and some patients find that their life has changed for the better. This message of hope can be particularly powerful to new burn survivors, especially when the message is relayed directly from a survivor.

References

[1]   Abdullah A, Blakeney P, Hunt R, Broemeling L, Phillips L, Herndon D N et al (1994) Visible scars and self-esteem in pediatric patients with burns. J Burn Care Rehabil 15(2): 164–168

[2]   American Burn Association (2010) National burn repository: Report of data from 2000–2009, from http://www. ameriburn. org/2009NBRAnnualReport. pdf?PHPSESSID=c2099c30cd05c31bd5b13 650c95b4677

[3]   American Psychiatric Association (1994) Diagnostic and statistical manual of mental disorders, 4th edn. American Psychiatric Association, Washington, DC

[4]   Ancoli-Israel S, Roth T (1999) Characteristics of insomnia in the United States: Results of the 1991 National Sleep Foundation Survey I. Sleep 22(2): S347-S353

[5]   Bauer K, Hardy P, Van Sorsten V (1998) Posttraumatic stress disorder in burn populations: A critical review of the literature. J Burn Care Rehabil 19: 230–240

[6]   Beck A, Steer RA, Brown G (1996) BDI-II manual,2nd edn. The Psychological Corporation, San Antonio, TX

[7]   Bianchi TL (1997) Aspects of sexuality after burn injury: outcomes in men. J Burn Care Rehabil 18(2): 183–186; discussion 182

[8]   Boeve SA, Aaron LA, Martin-Herz SP, Peterson A, Cain V, Heimbach DM et al (2002) Sleep disturbance after burn injury. J Burn Care Rehabil 23(1): 32–38

[9]   Bryant R (1996) Predictors of post-traumatic stress disorder following burn injury. Burns 22: 89–92

[10] Calhoun LG, Tedeschi RG (1999) Facilitating posttraumatic growth: a clinician's guide. Lawrence Erlbaum Associates, New Jersey

[11] Christian LM, Graham JE, Padgett DA, Glaser R, Kiecolt-Glaser JK (2006) Stress and wound healing. Neuroimmunomodulation 13(5–6): 337–346

[12] Cordova MJ, Cunningham LL, Carlson CR, Andrykowski MA (2001) Posttraumatic growth following breast cancer: a controlled comparison study. Health Psychol 20(3): 176–185

[13] Dauber A, Osgood PF, Breslau AJ, Vernon HL, Carr DB (2002) Chronic persistent pain after severe burns: a survey of 358 burn survivors. Pain Med 3(1): 6–17

[14] Difede J, Barocas D (1999) Acute intrusive and avoidant PTSD symptoms as predictors of chronic PTSD following burn injury. J Trauma Stress 12(2): 363–369

[15] Difede J, Ptacek JT, Roberts J, Barocas D, Rives W, Apfeldorf W et al (2002) Acute stress disorder after burn injury: a predictor of posttraumatic stress disorder? Psychosom Med 64(5): 826–834

[16] Edwards RR, Magyar-Russell G, Thombs B, Smith MT, Holavanahalli RK, Patterson D R et al (2007) Acute pain at discharge from hospitalization is a prospective predictor of long-term suicidal ideation after burn injury. Arch Phys Med Rehabil 88[12 Suppl 2]: S36–42

[17] Ehde D, Patterson D, Wiechman S, Wilson L (2000) Post-traumatic stress symptoms and distress one year after burn injury. J Burn Care Rehabil 21(2): 105–111

[18] Ehde DM, Patterson DR, Wiechman SA, Wilson LG (1999) Post-traumatic stress symptoms and distress following acute burn injury. Burns 25: 587–592

[19] El hamaoui Y, Yaalaoui S, Chihabeddine K, Boukind E, Moussaoui D (2002) Post-traumatic stress disorder in burned patients. Burns 28(7): 647–650

[20] Fauerbach J, Lawrence J, Haythornthwaite J, Richter D, McGuire M, Schmidt C (1997) Pschiatric history affects post trauma morbidity in a burn injured adult sample. Psychosomatics 38: 374–385

[21] Fauerbach J, Spence R, Patterson D (eds) (2006) Adult burn injury. Lippincott Williams and Wilkins, Philadelphia, PA

[22] Fauerbach JA, Heinberg LJ, Lawrence JW, Bryant AG, Richter L, Spence RJ (2002) Coping with body image changes following a disfiguring burn injury. Health Psychol 21(2): 115–121

[23] Fauerbach JA, Heinberg LJ, Lawrence JW, Munster AM, Palombo DA, Richter D et al (2000) Effect of early body image dissatisfaction on subsequent psychological and physical adjustment after disfiguring injury. Psychosom Med 62(4): 576–582

[24] Fauerbach JA, Lawrence JW, Munster AM, Palombo DA, Richter D (1999) Prolonged adjustment difficulties among those with acute posttrauma distress following burn injury. J Behav Med 22(4): 359–378

[25] Fauerbach JA, McKibben J, Bienvenu OJ, Magyar-Russell G, Smith MT, Holavanahalli R et al (2007) Psychological distress after major burn injury. Psychosom Med 69(5): 473–482

[26] Fleming MP, Difede J (1999) Effects of varying scoring rules of the Clinician Administered PTSD Scale (CAPS) for the diagnosis of PTSD after acute burn injury. J Trauma Stress 12(3): 535–542

[27] Foa EB (ed) (1995) PDS (Posttraumatic Stress Diagnostic Scale) Manual. Natl. Comput. Syst., Minneapolis

[28] Folkman S, Lazarus RS (1980) An analysis of coping in a middle-aged community sample. J Health Soc Behav 21: 219–239

[29] Fukunishi I (1999) Relationship of cosmetic disfigurement to the severity of posttraumatic stress disorder in burn injury or digital amputation. Psychother Psychosom 68(2): 82–86

[30] Gottschlich MM, Jenkins M, Mayes T, Khoury J, Kagan R, Warden GD (1997a) Lack of effect of sleep on energy expenditure and physiologic measures in critically ill burn patients. J Am Diet Assoc 97(2): 131–139

[31] Gottschlich MM, Jenkins M, Mayes T, Khoury J, Kagan R, Warden GD (1997b) Lack of effect of sleep on energy expenditure and physiologic measures in critically ill burn patients. J Am Diet Assoc 97(2): 131–139

[32] Gottschlich MM, Jenkins ME, Mayes T, Khoury J, Kramer M, Warden GD et al (1994a) The 1994 Clinical Research Award. A prospective clinical study of the polysomnographic stages of sleep after burn injury. J Burn Care Rehabil 15(6): 486–492

[33] Gottschlich MM, Jenkins ME, Mayes T, Khoury J, Kramer M, Warden GD et al (1994b) The 1994 Clinical Research Award. A prospective clinical study of the polysomnographic stages of sleep after burn injury. J Burn Care Rehabil 15(6): 486–492

[34] Gottschlich MM, Khoury J, Warden GD, Kagan RJ (2009) An evaluation of the neuroendocrine response to sleep in pediatric burn patients. JPEN J Parenter Enteral Nutr 33(3): 317–326

[35] Holbrook A, Crowther R, Lotter A, Endeshaw Y (2001) The role of benzodiazepines in the treatment of insomnia: meta-analysis of benzodiazepine use in the treatment of insomnia. J Am Geriatr Soc 49(6): 824–826

[36] Holbrook AM, Crowther R, Lotter A, Cheng C, King D (2000) Meta-analysis of benzodiazepine use in the treatment of insomnia. Cmaj 162(2): 225–233

[37] Jaffe S, Patterson DR (2004) Treating sleep problems in patients with burn injuries: Practical considerations. J Burn Care Rehabil 25(3): 294–305

[38] Kammerer B (2010) BEST program provides key to successful community reintegration. Burn Support News, Winter 1–4

[39] Kiecolt-Glaser JK, Marucha PT, Malarkey WB, Mercado AM, Glaser R (1995) Slowing of wound healing by psychological stress. Lancet 346(8984): 1194–1196

[40] Kolman PBR (1983) The incidence of psychopathology in burned adult patients: A critical review. J Burn Care Rehabil 4: 430–436

[41] Kravitz M, McCoy BJ, Tompkins DM, Daly W, Mulligan J, McCauley RL et al (1993) Sleep disorders in children after burn injury. J Burn Care Rehabil 14(1): 83–90

[42] Lambert JF, Difede J, Contrada RJ (2004) The relationship of attribution of responsibility to acute stress disorder among hospitalized burn patients. J Nerv Ment Dis 192(4): 304–312

[43] Lawrence J, Fauerbach J, Eudell E, Ware L, Munster A (1998) Sleep disturbance following burn injury: A frequent yet understudied complication. J Burn Care Rehabil 19: 480–486

[44] Lawrence JW, Fauerbach JA, Heinberg L, Doctor M (2004) Visible vs hidden scars and their relation to body esteem. J Burn Care Rehabil 25(1): 25–32

[45] Lazarus RS, Folkman S (1984) Stress, appraisal and coping. Springer, New York

[46] Luszczynska A, Mohamed NE, Schwarzer R (2005) Self-efficacy and social support predict benefit finding 12 months after cancer surgery: the mediating role of coping strategies. Psychol Health Med 10: 365–375

[47] Madianos MG, Papaghelis M, Ioannovich J, Dafni R (2001) Psychiatric disorders in burn patients: a follow-up study. Psychother Psychosom 70(1): 30–37

[48] Malenfant A, Forget R, Papillon J, Amsel R, Frigon JY, Choiniere M (1996) Prevalence and characteristics of chronic sensory problems in burn patients. Pain 67(2–3): 493–500

[49] McEwen BS (1998) Protective and damaging effects of stress mediators. N Engl J Med 338(3): 171–179

[50] McEwen BS, Stellar E (1993) Stress and the individual. Mechanisms leading to disease. Arch Intern Med 153(18): 2093–2101

[51] McKibben JB, Bresnick MG, Wiechman Askay SA, Fauerbach JA (2008) Acute stress disorder and posttraumatic stress disorder: a prospective study of prevalence, course, and predictors in a sample with major burn injuries. J Burn Care Res 29(1): 22–35

[52] Milam JE (2004) Posttraumatic growth among HIV/AIDS patients. J Appl Soc Psychol 34: 2353–2376

[53] Nowell PD, Mazumdar S, Buysse DJ, Dew MA, Reynolds CF 3rd, Kupfer DJ (1997) Benzodiazepines and zolpidem for chronic insomnia: a meta-analysis of treatment efficacy. Jama 278(24): 2170–2177

[54] Pakenham KI (2005) Benefit finding in multiple sclerosis and associations with positive and negative outcomes. Health Psychol 24(2): 123–132

[55] Partridge J (1997) When burns affect the way you look. Changing Faces, London

[56] Patterson DR, Everett JJ, Bombardier CH, Questad KA, Lee VK, Marvin JA (1993) Psychological effects of severe burn injuries. Psychol Bull 113(2): 362–378

[57] Patterson DR, Finch CP, Wiechman SA, Bonsack R, Gibran N, Heimbach D (2003) Premorbid mental health status of adult burn patients: comparison with a normative sample. J Burn Care Rehabil 24(5): 347–350

[58] Patterson DR, Jensen M (2003) Hypnosis and clinical pain. Psychol Bull 129(4): 495–521

[59] Patterson DR, Ptacek JT, Cromes F, Fauerbach JA, Engrav L (2000) The 2000 Clinical Research Award. Describing and predicting distress and satisfaction with life for burn survivors. J Burn Care Rehabil 21(6): 490–498

[60] Patterson DR, Tininenko J, Ptacek JT (2006) Pain during burn hospitalization predicts long-term outcome. J Burn Care Res 27(5): 719–726

[61] Pruzinsky T, Cash T F (1990) Integrative themes in body-image development, deviance, and change. In: Cash TF, Pruzinsky T (eds) Body images: Development, deviance, and change. Guilford Press, New York, pp 337–349

[62] Ptacek J, Patterson D, Heimbach D (2002) Inpatient depression in persons with burns. J Burn Care Rehabilitation 23(1): 1–9

[63] Ptacek JT, Patterson DR, Montgomery BK, Ordonez NA, Heimbach DM (1995) Pain, coping, and adjustment in patients with severe burns: Preliminary findings from a prospective study. J Pain Symptom Manage 10: 446–455

[64] Robertson CF, Zuker R, Dabrowski B, Levison H (1985) Obstructive sleep apnea: a complication of burns to the head and neck in children. J Burn Care Rehabil 6(4): 353–357

[65] Rose M, Sanford A, Thomas C, Opp MR (2001) Factors altering the sleep of burned children. Sleep 24(1): 45–51

[66] Rosenbach C, Renneberg B (2008) Positive change after severe burn injuries. J Burn Care Res 29(4): 638–643

[67] Sheikh AI (2004) Posttraumatic growth in the context of heart disease. J Clin Psychol Med Settings 11: 265–273

[68] Smith MT, Perlis ML, Park A, Smith MS, Pennington J, Giles DE et al (2002) Comparative meta-analysis of pharmacotherapy and behavior therapy for persistent insomnia. Am J Psychiatry 159(1): 5–11

[69] Spitzer RL, Williams JB, Kroenke K, Hornyak R, McMurray J (2000) Validity and utility of the PRIME-MD patient health questionnaire in assessment of 3000 obstetric-gynecologic patients: the PRIME-MD Patient Health Questionnaire Obstetrics-Gynecology Study. Am J Obstet Gynecol 183(3): 759–769

[70] Stanton AL, Revenson TA, Tennen H (2007) Health psychology: psychological adjustment to chronic disease. Annu Rev Psychol 58: 565–592

[71] Sterling P, Eyer J (1988) Allostasis: a new paradigm to explain arousal pathology. In: Fisher S, Reason J (eds) Handbook of life stress, cognition and health. John Wiley & Son, New York, pp 629–649

[72] Suls J, Fletcher B (1985) The relative efficacy of avoidant and nonavoidant coping strategies: a meta-analysis. Health Psychol 4(3): 249–288

[73] Taylor SE, Stanton AL (2007) Coping resources, coping processes, and mental health. Annu Rev Clin Psychol 3: 377–401

[74] Tedeschi RG, Calhoun LG (1995) Trauma and transformation: growing in the aftermath of suffering. Sage Publications, Thousand Oaks, CA

[75] Tedeschi RG, Calhoun LG (1996) The posttraumatic growth inventory: measuring the positive legacy of trauma. J Trauma Stress 9(3): 455–471

[76] Tedstone JE, Tarrier N (1997) An investigation of the prevalence of psychological morbidity in burn-injured patients. Burns 23(7–8): 550–554

[77] Thombs BD, Bass EB, Ford DE, Stewart KJ, Tsilidis KK, Patel U et al (2006) Prevalence of depression in survivors of acute myocardial infarction. J Gen Intern Med 21(1): 30–38

[78] Thombs BD, Bresnick MG, Magyar-Russell G (2006) Depression in survivors of burn injury: a systematic review. Gen Hosp Psychiatry 28(6): 494–502

[79] Ullrich PM, Askay SW, Patterson DR (2009) Pain, depression, and physical functioning following burn injury. Rehabil Psychol 54(2): 211–216

[80] Van Loey NE, Maas CJ, Faber AW, Taal LA (2003) Predictors of chronic posttraumatic stress symptoms following burn injury: results of a longitudinal study. J Trauma Stress 16(4): 361–369

[81] Walsh J, Erman M, Erwin C et al (1998) Subjective hpynotic efficacy of trazodone and zolpidem in DSMI-II-R primary insomnia. Hum Psychopharmacol 13: 191–198

[82] Wiechman Askay SA, Patterson DR (2009) Psychological rehabilitation in burn injuries. In: Frank RG, Rosenthal M, Caplan B (eds) Handbook of rehabiliation psychology, 2nd edn. American Psychological Association, Washington, D. C.

[83] Wiechman Askay SA, Stricklin M, Carrougher G, Patterson DR, Klein MB, Esselman P et al (2009) Using QMethodology to identify reasons for distress in burn survivors postdischarge. J Burn Care Rehabil 30(1): 83–91

[84] Wiechman SA, Ptacek JT, Patterson DR, Gibran NS, Engrav LE, Heimbach DM (2001) Rates, trends, and depression following burn injuries. J Burn Care Rehabil 22: 417–424

[85] Williams EE, Griffiths TA (1991) Psychological consequences of burn injury. Burns 17(6): 478–480

[86] Williams RM, Patterson DR, Schwenn C, Day J, Bartman M, Engrav LH (2002) Evaluation of a peer consultation program for burn inpatients. 2000 ABA paper. J Burn Care Rehabil 23(6): 449–453

[87] Zigmond AS, Snaith RP (1983) The hospital anxiety and depression scale. Acta Psychiatr Scand 67(6): 361–370

Correspondence: Shelley Wiechman, Ph. D., University of Washington School of Medicine, Department of Rehabilitation Medicine, Harborview Burn Center, 325 Ninth Ave, Box 359 740, Seattle, WA 98 104, USA, E-mail: wiechman@u.washington.edu

.

Burn wound healing, documentation, scar management and rehabilitation

Skin architecture and function

Adelheid Elbe-Bürger

Department of Dermatology, Division of Immunology, Allergy and Infectious Diseases (DIAID), Medical University of Vienna, Vienna, Austria

Summary

From early life until death, a challenge for the well-being of all higher organisms is the detection and destruction of invading microorganisms, and the elimination of cells that undergo malignant transformation. This challenge has been met by defence mechanisms of the immune system, the most basic principle of which is the recognition of antigens. The mammalian immune system comprises innate (including factors such as complement, antimicrobial peptides, cytokines, chemokines, and cells like dendritic cells, macrophages, natural killer cells, polymorphonuclear leukocytes) and adaptive (T and B lymphocytes) functional components. Both possess different types of recognition receptors and differ in the speed in which they reply to a potential danger. Even though distinct, the innate and adaptive immune system interact and can influence the extent and type of their counterpart and act in synergy to defend the host against infection, cancer and autoimmunity. For higher organisms, the skin is the first barrier that protects the body from disorders caused by infectious or chemical agents, thermal and electromagnetic radiation, and mechanical trauma and is critically involved in immune reactivity. Immune responses in the skin involve an armamentarium of immune cells and soluble mediators. Professional antigen-presenting cells such as epidermal Langerhans cells and dermal dendritic cells in combination with T cells and other resident cells orchestrate the decision between immunity and tolerance. Such responses in the skin are part of the systemic immune system. Although the components of the epidermis and dermis work in concert to accomplish immune responses in the skin, the focus of this chapter will mainly be on the cells, receptors and mediators of the epidermal (immunologic) unit, the frontline of immune protection against harmful threats.

Skin structure

The skin – covering the whole surface of the body – accounts for about 15 % of the total adult body weight and is the largest organ. It exerts multiple crucial functions. It forms a protective barrier, shields our muscles, internal organs, and body fluids from bacteria, viruses, ultraviolet light and other environmental aggressors, protects the body from dehydration or massive absorption of water, functions as a thermo regulator and sense organ, and plays a crucial role in the body's defence mechanism, which is controlled by several types of immune cells. It associates tissues of various origins (epithelial, connective, vascular, muscular and nervous) which are organized in three layers including epidermis (outermost layer), dermis and the hypodermis (consisting of fatty tissue that

Fig. 1. Structure of the skin – the different layers and cell types. Collagen, elastin, and other components of the extracellular matrix of the dermis and the hypodermis are not represented. The stratum lucidum usually present in thick epidermis such as palms and soles is not included; it is normally located between the stratum granulosum and stratum corneum and consists of flattened cells with no nuclei. Merkel cells are not represented either (designed by Marion Prior)

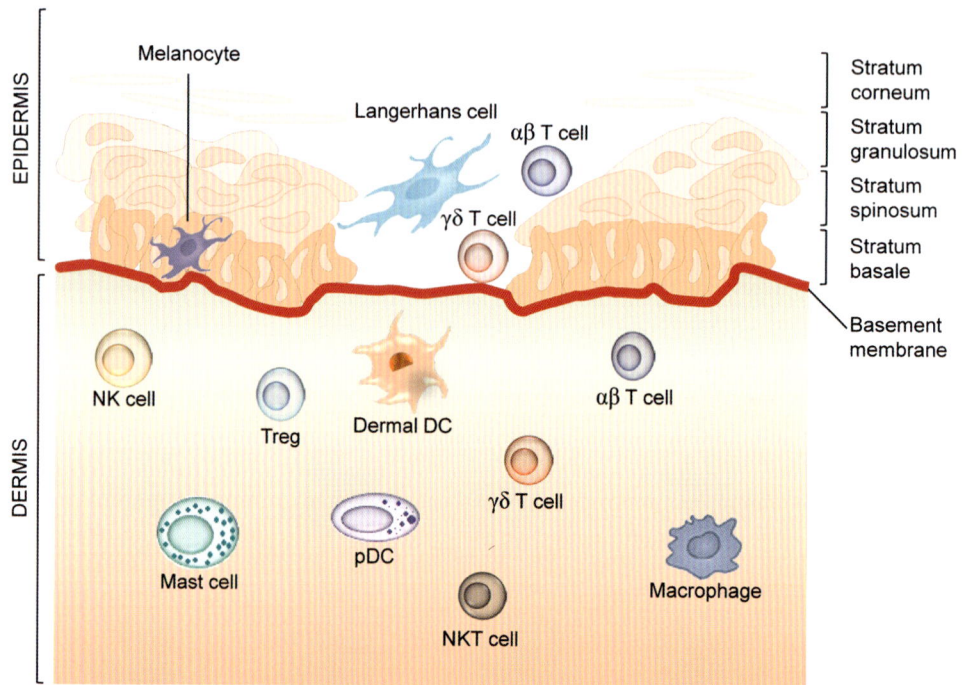

connects the dermis to underlying skeletal components) (Fig. 1). The epidermis and its appendages are of ectodermal origin whereas the dermis and the hypodermis are of mesenchymal origin. The epidermis and dermis are connected by the dermal-epidermal junction, which is synthesised by basal keratinocytes and dermal fibroblasts. The skin is not developed homogeneously and shows regional variations not only in thickness and distribution of epidermal appendages [41, 94].

Epidermis

The epidermis is a stratified, non-vascularized epithelium that undergoes a continuous process of renewal and loss through cell replication in the basal compartment and desquamation at the surface. The primary source of cell renewal is through proliferation of stem cells [20, 21, 153]. However, there seems to be some plasticity between stem cells and their early progeny, as most basal keratinocytes maintain their regenerative potential and are capable of regenerating epidermis [114]. Most recently, evidence has been provided that commitment to differentiation does not prohibit keratinocytes from re-entering the cell cycle, de-differentiation, and acquiring "stemness", suggesting that epidermis can use different strategies for homeostasis and tissue regeneration [119].

Many cell types can be found in the epidermis, the majority (~90%) of which are keratinocytes. They undergo morphological and biochemical differentiation (keratinisation), resulting in the production of corneocytes that shed from the skin surface with time (~30 days). There are a few other distinct cell populations which have specific functions such as Langerhans cells (LCs) – resident immune cells, melanocytes – which produce the pigment melanin, Merkel cells – mediators of mechanotransduction of the skin, and infrequent T cells.

The epidermis consists of a multilayered sheet of keratinocytes (from the bottom up) interspersed by hair follicles [41]. The stratum basale (also known as stratum germinativum) is a single layer of cells attached to a noncellular basement membrane that separates the epidermis from the dermis. It consists mostly of basal keratinocytes, Merkel cells and melanocytes. The stratum spinosum (5–15 layers) contains irregular polyhedral keratinocytes with limited capacity for cell division and LCs. This cell layer provides the mechanical strength necessary to resist physical trauma. The stratum granulosum (1–3 layers) contains flattened, polyhedral keratinocytes producing keratohyalin granules. Tight junctions in this layer play an essential role in retaining the water content of the body [164]. The stratum corneum contains many sheets of flattened, nonviable scale like corneocytes responsible for the actual protection of the skin [51] (Fig. 1). In some body areas (palmoplantar region) there is an additional layer between the stratum granulosum and the stratum corneum – the stratum lucidum [61]. The thickness of the epidermis varies among body areas [thinnest sites: face, trunk (20–60 μm), thicker areas: arms, legs, back of hand, upper foot (40–80 μm), thickest sites: soles of the feet, fingertips (160–560 μm)] [186]. Furthermore, the epidermis contains the superficial part of the eccrine sweat glands.

Dermis

Below the epidermis is the dermis which is much thicker (2–4 mm) than the epidermis and can be divided into a papillary (superficial) dermis and a reticular (deep) dermis. It is a supportive, compressible and elastic connective tissue protecting the epidermis, its appendages and the nervous and vascular plexuses. The dermis contains an extracellular matrix composed of fibrous and non-fibrous proteins, a wide network of blood vessels – providing nutrient supply for the stratum basale of the epidermis, lymphatic vessels, nerve endings, sweat glands, excretory glands (sebaceous, eccrine and apocrine), muscles, hair follicles, nails, resident and trafficking cells [41]. The main cell type of the dermis is the fibroblast. The dermis also hosts cells of the immune system such as interstitial dendritic cells (DCs), plasmacytoid DCs, macrophages, mast cells, natural killer (NK) cells and T cells [TCR $\alpha\beta^+$ T cells (T helper 1 (T_H1) cells, T_H2 cells, CD8$^+$ T cells, T_H17 cells), regulatory T cells (Tregs), natural killer T (NKT) cells, and TCR $\gamma\delta^+$ T cells] (Fig. 1) [38, 103, 145]. The thickness of the dermis varies depending on the anatomic region (back, palms and soles have a much thicker dermis than the eyelids). Collagen (mainly of types I and III, but types IV and VII can also be found) provides the skin with tensile strength and tissue integrity whereas elastin provides elastic-

ity and resiliency. The dermal extracellular ground substance consists of a complex mixture of glycoproteins (laminin, fibronectin etc.), proteoglycans (versican, perlecan), glycosaminoglycans (keratin sulphate, heparin, chondroitin etc.), water, and hyaluronic acid [41, 94].

Hypodermis (subcutanous fat, panniculus adiposus)

The hypodermis is a subcutaneous tissue and in fact not part of the skin. It connects the dermis to the underlying bones or muscles, stores lipids, regulates the body temperature, insulates and cushions the body. The main cell type is the adipocyte showing pericellular expression of S100 protein and vimentin [94]. Fibroblasts, mast cells, sweat gland endings, vessels and nerves contribute to the formation of the corresponding dermal plexuses.

Skin (stem) cells – A promising source for tissue engineering and regenerative medicine?

Within the next decade, therapeutic applications of stem cells in regenerative medicine can be anticipated to be part of clinical medicine. With regard to skin, the focus of stem cell research is and will be on the epidermis and the hair follicle. Under normal conditions, the interfollicular epidermis and sebaceous glands are constantly self-renewing, while the hair follicles undergo cyclic changes of growth, involution and resting phases [5, 62]. For hair follicle stem cells it has been described that they not only reside in the stem cell niche called "bulge" and express CD34, cyotokeratin 15, CD200 [22, 82, 117, 139, 150, 191] and retain DNA or histone labels [29, 42, 193], but that they are also present in other areas [83, 88, 89 147]. Most recently, Hans Clevers and his group found that a stem cell cluster in a hair follicle, characterized by the expression of leucine-rich-repeat-containing G protein-coupled receptor 6 (Lgr6), a close homolog of the Lgr5 marker for stem cells in the small intestine and colon, resides directly above the hair bulge and gives rise to all cell lineages of the mouse skin [169]. In experiments with wounded mice, they found that Lrg6 stem cells around the wound initiated wound repair [169]. The isolation of the human variant could dramatically improve clinical trials in patients. Today we are already able to grow new skin in vitro using skin cells from patients with severe burns, but the new hairless skin is often dry and fragile. With the discovery of the "mother" stem cell it could be possible to re-establish the normal anatomy and function of the skin and its appendages in burn and wound patients.

Mesenchymal stem cells (MSCs) residing within the dermis were first isolated in 2001 and named "skin-derived precursors" (SKPs). They have the capacity to differentiate into adipocytes, osteocytes, chondrocytes, smooth muscle cells, neurons, glia cells such as Schwann cells as well as hematopoietic cells of myeloid and erythroid lineage [53, 54, 65, 79, 81, 91, 102, 112, 125, 188, 189, 204, 209]. They also seem to be able to differentiate into insulin-producing pancreatic cells, keratinocytes, hepatocytes and other cells [118, 127, 166]. However, this needs a more careful investigation. The dermal papilla of hair follicles represent the likely anatomical niche for these multipotent dermal cells [18, 54, 78, 80, 85, 109]. Because of their easy isolation and culture, multipotency and highly expansive properties, dermal MSCs have the potential to function as an easily accessible, autologous source for several therapeutic applications. These comprise the treatment of graft-versus-host disease, idiopathic pulmonary fibrosis, systemic lupus erythematosus, arthritis, neurodegenerative disorders, traumatic spinal injury and others [165, 178]. The most immediate impact can be expected in the field of wound healing. Many studies have suggested a contribution of MSCs to reconstitute skin in cutaneous wounds, but problems still need resolution before MSCs can be widely used clinically [59, 175].

During the last years a new technology has been developed to de-differentiate and reprogram adult somatic cells (in the skin from keratinocytes, dermal fibroblasts, dermal papilla cells, etc.) into a stem cell-like state which have been named induced pluripotent stem (iPS) cells. Originally performed in mice and later established also in humans, researchers took a few genes and incorporated them into the nucleus of cells to induce pluripotency [1, 180, 181, 192, 205]. Such lines could be expanded indefinitely and could differentiate to form numerous kinds of different tissues. Even though several limitations currently preclude their use in a clinical setting, this discovery opens up the possibility of generating patient-specific pluripotent cells for autologous regenerative medicine.

Keratinocytes – Immune competent epithelial cells

The predominant cell type of the epidermis is the keratinocyte with morphological variations within epidermal layers. Keratinocytes of the stratum basale are anchored by hemidesmosomes to the basement membrane that separates the epidermis from the dermis (Fig. 1). Adjacent keratinocytes of all layers are generally interconnected by desmosomes, tight junctions, and adherens junctions. Basal keratinocytes contain melanosomes, to store the skin colour pigment melanin, which is synthesised by melanocytes. The basal layer contains stem cells and cycling keratinocytes, expressing proliferation antigens such as Ki67 and PCNA. The stratum corneum consists of corneocytes which are devoid of a nucleus and of cytoplasmic organelles and are shed from the skin surface, thus contributing to the barrier function of the skin. Keratins (K) are fibrous proteins belonging to the family of intermediate filaments and are parts of the cytoskeleton. Their primary function is to protect epithelial cells from mechanical and nonmechanical stresses that result in cell death. Other emerging functions include roles in cell signalling, the stress response and apoptosis, as well as unique roles that are keratin specific and tissue specific. Two types of keratins can be distinguished, based on their pH-value. Type 1 keratins are acidic, whereas type 2 keratins are neutral/basic [43, 60]. Keratinocytes express keratin polypeptides in pairs, composed of a type 1 and a type 2 keratin. Within normal epidermis, K5 and K14/K15 are expressed in basal keratinocytes wheras K1 and K10 are expressed in suprabasal keratinocytes. Stratum granulosum cells express K2 and K11, and those in the plantar region express K9 [93].

Keratinocytes are not inert but are able to function as immune sentinels. They can recognize foreign and dangerous agents such as conserved pathogen-associated molecular patterns (PAMPs) which are shared by numerous microorganisms, danger-associated molecular patterns such as toxins and irritants and ultraviolet light through a variety of pattern recognition receptors (PRRs). These include Toll-like receptors (TLRs), nucleotide-binding domain, leucine-rich repeat (NLRs) proteins, scavenger receptors, and C-type lectin receptors and are instrumental in both launching innate immune responses and influencing adaptive immunity of the skin as well as being vital players in infectious and inflammatory skin diseases [45, 84, 122, 123, 124, 185]. Their activation triggers signaling pathways that result in the production of antimicrobial peptides, cytokines, chemokines, and costimulatory molecules which induce inflammatory responses and protective immunity against pathogens [2, 124, 145]. Originally recognized for their expression on immune cells, TLRs have also been identified on keratinocytes. Basal keratinocytes express TLR2/TLR4 mRNA and proteins and suprabasal keratinocytes express TLR1–5, TLR7, and TLR10 mRNA [14, 55, 170], suggesting that keratinocytes in different layers of the epidermis also express different TLRs. A most recent study suggests, that rather than stimulating inflammation in response to injury, some commensal organisms actually help to limit the inflammatory response by acting as negative regulators of TLR3 signalling [107]. Another reason for the natural resistance to commensals, is a "barrier" consisting of antimicrobial peptides and proteins, which are produced either constitutively or upon induction through various stimuli (β-defensins, RNase 7, psoriasin, cathelicidin LL-37) [108, 161, 162].

In unperturbed skin, keratinocytes produce only a few cytokines such as Interleukin (IL)-1, IL-7 and transforming growth factor (TGF)-β constitutively. They alert the host to delivery of certain noxious or potentially hazardous stimuli (trauma, non-ionizing radiation, chemicals) by the production of a plethora of proinflammatory and immunomodulatory cytokines [IL-1, -6, -7, -10, -12, -15, -17, -18, -20, tumor necrosis factor (TNF)-α], chemokines [CC-chemokine ligand (CCL)2, CCL5, CCL27, CXC-chemokine ligand (CXCL)8] and colony-stimulating factors [granulocyte-colony stimulating factor (G-CSF) and granulocyte-macrophage colony-stimulating factor (GM-CSF)] [70]. This activation has multiple consequences. It causes the migration of cells into and out of the skin, has systemic effects, influences keratinocyte proliferation and differentiation and affects the production of other cytokines [131]. More specifically, activated keratinocytes attract several cell types into the skin such as LC precursors via the expression of CCL20 [32, 46]. They can also recruit effector T cells to the skin by expressing CCL20, CXCL9–11, whereas neutrophils are attracted through CXCL1 and CXCL8 [4]. The fact that keratinocytes express many cytokine receptors and respond to cytokines clearly demonstrates that their functional properties can be regulated by cells of the immune system.

Keratinocytes also secrete neuropeptides, eicosanoids, reactive oxygen species, complement and related receptors. These mediators have potent inflammatory and immunomodulatory properties [131]. Dysregulation and abnormal expression of inflammatory mediators or their receptors in keratinocytes are relevant to the pathogenesis of chronic inflammatory skin diseases such as psoriasis, atopic dermatitis and allergic contact dermatitis.

Melanocytes – Pigment cells with immune properties

Human skin exists in a wide range of different colours and gradations. This is due to the presence of a chemically inert and stable pigment known as melanin, the biosynthesis of which appears in melanocytes within membrane-bound organelles known as melanosomes. The latter can be divided into four maturation stages, determined by their structure and the quantity, quality and arrangement of the melanin produced. Melanocytes transfer melanosomes through their dendrites to adjacent keratinocytes, where they form caps that protect the keratinocyte from harmful ultraviolet light and other environmental stimuli [101]. The anatomical relationship between keratinocytes and melanocytes is known as the "epidermal melanin unit" [41]. Melanocytes represent 2–5% of all epidermal cells, descend from neural crest and migrate into the basal cell layer of the epidermis where they are regularly distributed [94, 158] (Fig. 1). Each melanocyte is in contact with ~ 40 keratinocytes in the basal and suprabasal layers

[41]. They have a dendritic morphology and express S100, bcl-2, vimentin, c-kit/CD117 and other markers [93, 94, 148]. The density of melanocytes is constant in human skin. Various skin colors result from different quantities of produced and stored melanin [90]. Human melanocytes are not simply pigment-producing cells but also have phagocytic capacity and constitutively secrete a number of cytokines such as IL-1, IL-3, IL-6, GM-CSF, TNF-α and TGF-β [158, 121]. Recently, it has been shown that melanocytes express a panel of TLRs (1–4, 6, 7 and 9) most of which are also functional [206]. These properties can turn melanocytes into active players of the skin innate immunity.

Merkel cells – Essential for light-touch responses

The skin is also a sensory organ. Four main classes of sensory receptors in mammalian skin mediate different aspects of the sense of touch [92]. One of these specialized structures, the Merkel cell–neurite complex, is thought to be important for two-point discrimination and the detection of texture, shape and curvature [116]. These receptors consist of Merkel cells, a distinct cell population located in the basal layer of the epidermis and in the epithelial sheath of hair follicles [93], and the afferent somatosensory fibers that innervate them. Merkel cell–neurite complexes are found in touch-sensitive areas of the skin including whisker follicles, glabrous (hair-less) skin surfaces such as the hands and feet, and specialized epithelial structures in the hairy skin called touch domes [72]. Since their discovery in 1875, the functions of Merkel cells are still unclear. Using Merkel cell-deficient mice, it has been shown recently that they are required for the characteristic neurophysiological response of Merkel cell–neurite complexes to tactile stimuli [120]. Merkel cells are characterized by dense-core granules that contain a variety of neuropeptides, plasma membrane spines and cytoskeletal filaments consisting of cytokeratins like K20 and desmosomes [26, 132]. Furthermore, Merkel cells express many components of the presynaptic machinery and transcription factors involved in neuronal cell fate determination [71]. Their density shows regional variations [106]. In hair follicles, Merkel cells are rarely associated with nerve endings, whereas those in the epidermis are in close contact with terminal nerves. Merkel cells not in close association with nerve terminals have an endocrine function [26, 115, 136].

Two hypotheses heat up an intense controversy about the developmental origin of Merkel cells since their discovery in 1875 [26, 115, 136]. The neural crest hypothesis proposes, that Merkel cells are derived from neural crest stem cells based on the findings that they synthesize neuropeptides, express presynaptic molecules and proneural transcription factors, and from observations in lineage-tracing experiments in animals [68, 179, 202]. The epidermal origin hypothesis is based on their location in the basal layer and the presence of cytokeratin 20, the observation of their temporal appearance, and their presence in the epidermis before the appearance of other neural crest derivatives such as nerve endings of the skin [33, 133–135, 144, 197]. Genetic lineage tracing and conditional knockout techniques provided conclusive evidence for an epidermal origin of Merkel cells [140, 196]. With this definitive assignment of the origin of this cell population, insights into the pathogenesis of human diseases such as Merkel cell carcinoma could be possible [167].

Dendritic cells – Key regulators of the immune response

DCs – the most potent antigen-presenting cells (APCs) – translate innate to adaptive immunity [174]. They are present in an immature state in minute numbers (1–3%) in most peripheral tissues. Encounter with antigens or other stimuli by phagocytosis, macropinocytosis and receptor-mediated endocytosis causes their migration towards T cell rich areas of the secondary lymphoid organs via afferent lymphatics. During this migration process, DCs mature, lose their ability to capture antigens and acquire the capacity to present antigens to naive T cells, which then start to proliferate [16, 172]. To avoid an excessive immune response, activated T cells can induce apoptosis in DCs by expressing Fas Ligand, TNF-α 4 and TNF-related apoptosis-inducing ligand (TRAIL) [113]. DCs can direct a T cell-mediated adaptive immune response towards a type-1 and/or type-2 reaction [187] and have the unique ability to cross-present antigens to naive T cells [141]. Beyond these skills, DCs are involved in the induction of tolerance in the thymus and in lymphoid organs [172–174]. A small number of DCs move from the periphery to the lymph nodes, even in the absence of invading pathogens in the steady state [141]. These tolerogenic DCs neither activate T cells nor lead to a clonal expansion, because of the release of IL-10 and catabolizing enzyme ideolamine 2,3-dioxygenase (IDO) which enable T cell anergy, T cell death and Treg cell proliferation [138]. Even though a remarkable phenotypic heterogeneity of DCs has been long recognized, it has been only possible to clearly relate DC phenotype to DC function in a few instances. In the skin, DCs can be divided according to their anatomical localisation. In the epidermis one can detect LCs, and in the dermis interstitial DCs.

Langerhans cells – Required for induction of immunity and/or tolerance?

Paul Langerhans, a medical student in Berlin, who was especially interested in the anatomy of cutaneous nerves, inoculated gold into human skin and discovered in 1868 a population of dendritically-shaped cells in the epidermis which he supposed to be nerve cells [110]. More then one century later it was appreciated, that he discovered leukocytes which are now recognized as a member of the DC system. Landmark papers and several excellent reviews on skin DCs have been published over decades and are discussed and cited by Nikolaus Romani et al. in a most recent review [156].

LCs represent the most striking example of an extensively studied tissue DC subpopulation. They reside in basal and suprabasal epidermal layers and mucosa epithelium and extend their protrusions, known as dendrites, through the tight seals between keratinocytes to comprise a dense network that covers the entire body surface (Fig. 2A). LCs account for 3–5% of epidermal cells and originate from haematopoietic stem cells in the bone marrow [58, 97, 152, 199]. The defining marker for LCs is an intracytoplasmic organelle, known as Birbeck granule, with a tennis-racket or, more often, rod-shaped morphology

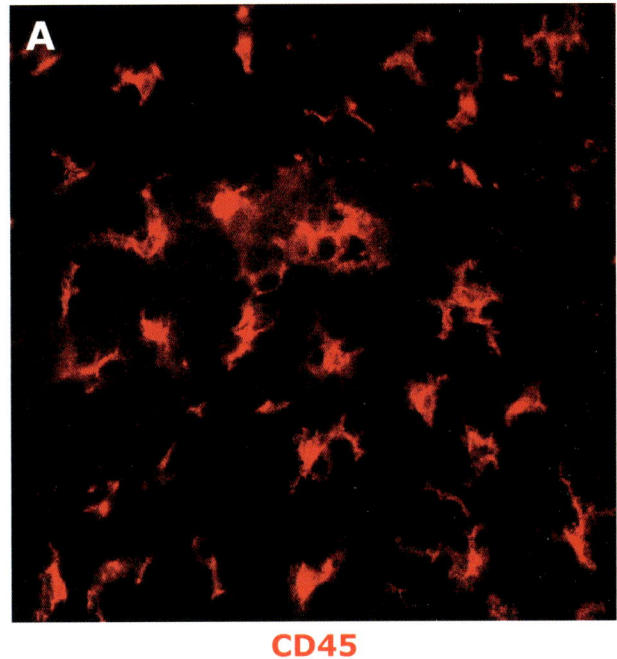

CD45

Fig. 2A. LCs form a dense network in the epidermis as visualized here with an anti-CD45 staining on an epidermal human sheet (Courtesy of Christopher Schuster, MD)

[19]. In humans, LCs also express a characteristic set of cell surface molecules such as membrane ATPase (CD39), CD1a (plays a role in presentation of microbial lipid antigens), E-cadherin/CD324 (mediates LC attachment to keratinocytes), Langerin/CD207 (responsible for the generation of Birbeck granules), CC chemokine receptor (CCR)6 (responsible for their migration to the epithelium), and the skin homing antigen named cutaneous lymphocyte-associated antigen (CLA) (Fig. 2B) [131]. Furthermore, they are equipped with a large array of conserved PRRs including TLRs, C-type lectin receptors, and NLRs that recognize microbial products as well as other intracellular danger signals [55, 104, 151, 155, 182, 195]. The poor reactivity of LCs to various PAMPs may potentially explain why commensal bacteria do not continuously trigger inflammation in skin. It is conceivable that keratinocytes may initially respond instead of LCs and then secrete cytokines to modulate LC functions indirectly [12]. LCs are also characterized by the absence of the macrophage mannose receptor (MMR/CD206), DC-SIGN/CD209 and the coagulation factor XIIIa, molecules that can be found on dermal APCs (Fig. 2C) [131].

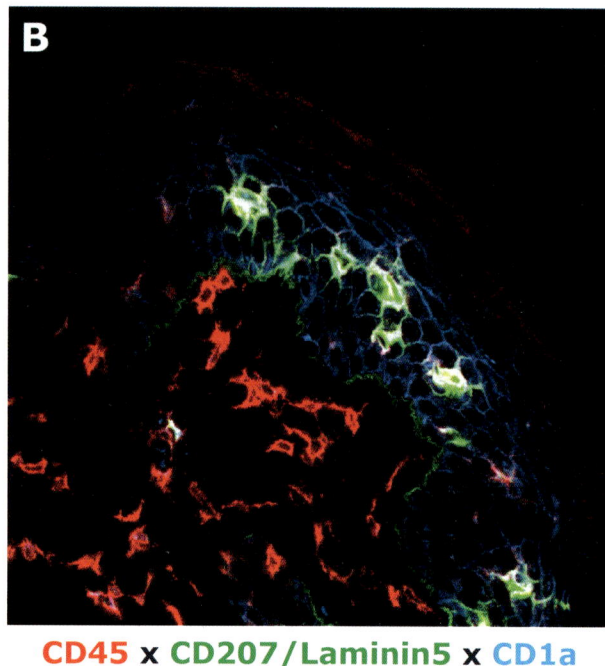

CD45 x CD207/Laminin5 x CD1a

Fig. 2B. CD45+ (red) cells with a dendritic morphology are present in the epidermis and dermis. CD1a+ (blue) and CD207+ (green) cells, presumably LCs, are located in the epidermis as demonstrated in a human skin tissue section (Courtesy of Christopher Schuster, MD)

For a long time it was believed that LCs are continually replenished by circulating haematopoietic bone marrow-derived precursors cells during adult life. Elegant studies from Miriam Merad and her colleagues have shown that LCs are maintained locally independently of circulating precursors in the steady state [129]. Over the years, several researchers have confirmed this finding and evidence has been provided that this happens via self-renewal and/or specialized local LC precursors as reviewed by Romani et al. [156]. For example, CD14+ LC-precursors reside in the human dermis [111] and it has been shown that their migration step into the epidermis is controlled by the release of keratinocyte-derived macrophage-inflammatory protein-3α/CCL20 and CXCL14 [32, 46, 160].

In contrast, in inflamed situations (infection [50], contact sensitizers [201], physical damage from heat [64], gentle tape stripping [76], ultraviolet and ionising radiation [44, 87], chemokine stimuli [198], or exposure to TLR agonists [15, 151]) LCs leave the epidermis. In a mouse model it has been shown that

LCs are replaced by circulating Gr-1+ monocytes in a M-CSFR-dependent manner [67].

As TGF-β is critical for LC development [11, 23, 86, 96, 177] and the production of TGF-β in developing prenatal human epidermis correlates with the appearance of markers such as CD207 and CD1a [163], it is possible that TGF-β also plays an important role for the acquisition of the LC phenotype in human epidermis. In addition, the increasing staining intensity of these markers in prenatal human skin may reflect the consistently increasing total amount of TGF-β in the developing epidermis [163].

Despite years of intensive research, the function of LCs remains enigmatic. Recent data from three LC-deficient mouse models established from three independent groups have begun to challenge the dogma that there is a requirement for LCs for the induction of certain types of cell-mediated immune responses such as contact hypersensitivity [95, 99, 128]. Rather than establishing an exact role for LCs, the groups found unchanged, diminished or enhanced contact hypersensitivity using their mouse models, implying that LCs may have regulatory/downregulating properties that serve to contain and constrain adaptive immune responses in the skin. Other observations provide evidence for a strong immunogenic function of LCs under certain conditions. Thus, their role in the skin immune system seems to be manifold, depending on the state of the skin condition (steady state versus inflammation), the doses of antigens, the type of pathogen, and other variables as proposed by Romani et al. [156]. Several questions remain unsolved, and new questions have arisen as a result of this recent progress.

Dermal dendritic cell subsets – Possess diverse functions

The human dermis contains three distinct subsets of APCs. HLA-DRbrightCD1a+CD14-CD1b+CD1c+CD207- DCs, HLA-DRbrightCD1a-CD14+ DCs and HLA-DRdim-CD1a-CD14+CD1c-FXIIIa+CD163+ dermal macrophages [7, 8, 74, 126, 146, 149, 194, 208]. CD1a+CD14- DCs are located close to lymphatic vessels in the upper layers of the dermis and are clearly distinct from migrating LCs [8, 74]. They can induce the proliferation of allogeneic T cells though less efficient than LCs

[100, 208]. CD14[+] cells include both migratory DCs and nonmigratory macrophages and evidence has been provided that they are from distinct lineages [74]. CD14[+] dermal DCs are able to prime CD4[+] T cells into cells that can induce naive B cells to perform an isotype-switch and to become cells secreting large amounts of immunoglobulins thereby controlling humoral immunity [100]. Some rare migrating LCs, expressing markers such as CD1a, CD1b, CD207, and CD208 can be identified in healthy human dermis [7–10].

Plasmacytoid DCs are present but rare in healthy human skin [17], while lesional skin samples from patients with psoriasis vulgaris and contact dermatitis contain high numbers of these cells [203]. They express IL-3Rα/CD123, blood dendritic cell antigen (BDCA)-4/CD304 and, the only exclusive marker for plasmacytoid DCs, BDCA-2/CD303. A special feature of plasmacytoid DCs is that they express a wide range of TLRs which makes them very competent to recognize microbial pathogens. Furthermore, they are very potent producers of type I interferons in case of a viral infection [39].

In mice, but not yet in humans, a novel CD207[+] DC subset has recently been described in the dermis. Some of the major immune functions historically assigned to LCs are now recognized as being performed with greater efficiency by these cells and other dermal DC cell subsets [30, 66, 143, 154].

In conclusion, the diverse range and function of skin APCs, even though not entirely clear, has significant implications most particularly for the development of novel human vaccines [100].

Resident skin T cells – Major players in skin homeostasis and pathology

T cells have a variety of functions that mediate the body's immune responses to infections. Depending on the type of infection, T cells react by secreting specific cytokine patterns, which provide important signals to other subsets of immune cells. It has been suspected for a long time that T cells are also present in healthy human skin [6]. Approximately 1 million T cells are present per 1 cm[2] of normal human adult skin, resulting in 20 billion T cells per individual, which is more than twice the total number of T cells in the

blood [36]. Initially, it was thought that T cells circulate between the skin and skin-draining lymph nodes and thus can quickly respond to antigen challenges [105, 176]. Recently, it has been shown that skin is steadily colonized by long-lived populations of memory T cells [28, 40, 63, 200] and it has been proposed that these cells but not recruited T cells have a major role in skin immune homeostasis and pathology [27].

The vast majority of skin-associated T cells in normal adult human skin are located in the dermis, whereas only small numbers reside in the epidermis. Nearly all skin-resident T cells express TCR αβ heterodimers. TCR γδ[+] T cells make up a small proportion of the total T cells in the skin [48, 56, 183]. Less than 5% of the T cells resident in normal adult human skin are CD45RA[+] naive T cells, whereas over 95% are CD45RO memory T cells. Most express the skin homing addressin CLA which is the ligand for E- and P-selectin. Skin-specific memory T cells acquire skin-homing properties after a process known

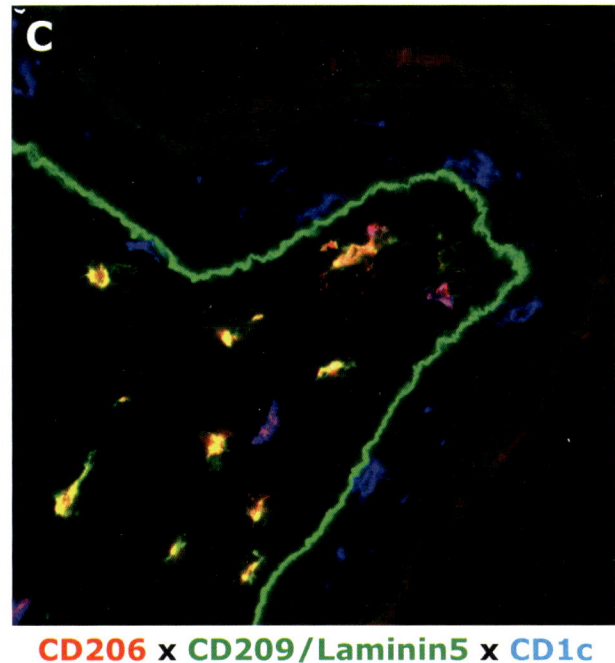

CD206 x CD209/Laminin5 x CD1c

Fig. 2C. Dendritic-appearing cells expressing monocyte/macrophage markers such as CD206 (red) and CD209 (green) are only located in the dermis and not in the epidermis. CD1c[+] (blue) cells exist in the epidermis and dermis. An Alexa Fluor 488-labeled Laminin 5/332 (green) mAb visualizes the dermo-epidermal junction (Courtesy of Christopher Schuster, MD)

as imprinting, which involves contact with tissue-derived DCs and lymph node stromal cells [49, 137]. Thus, effector T cells are programmed during differentiation to migrate to the tissue from which their cognate antigen was originally derived. While the distribution of naive and memory T cells in adult peripheral blood is quite similar to the skin, only 10% of the CD3+ blood cells are positive for CLA [35, 190]. To regulate the trafficking of T cells to cutaneous sites, chemokine receptors play an important role. Approximately 50% of CLA+ T cells express CCR8 and only a subset expresses CCR7 and CCR10 [31, 35, 77, 160]. Vitamin D has been proposed to have a crucial role in the direction of memory T cells to the skin via upregulation of CCR10 expression [168].

In the dermis, T cells are preferentially located around postcapillary venules and are often situated just beneath the dermo-epidermal junction of adjacent cutaneous appendages. TCR αβ+ cells are primarily single positive for CD4 or CD8 co-receptors, showing either an equal distribution or preference for the CD4+ subset [25].

Epidermal T cells account for about 2% of the CD3+ population in normal skin [24, 25, 57]. They primarily reside within the basal and suprabasal keratinocyte layer often in close apposition to LCs [57]. The epidermal TCR αβ+ T cell population is primarily represented by single CD4+ or CD8+ cells [24, 171]. Spetz et al. not only have shown that CD8+ TCR αβ-bearing epidermal T cells express the CD8αα homodimer at higher frequencies compared with peripheral blood, but have also found CD4-CD8-TCR αβ+ cells in the epidermis [171]. A minor population of epidermal T cells display TCR γδ heterodimers. Most of them are negative for CD4 and CD8 markers [3, 57, 69].

Not too much is known about the function of TCR γδ+ T cells in human skin. Increased numbers have been shown in a wide range of human skin pathologies. TCR γδ+ skin T cells primarily express the Vδ1 chain, whereas TCR γδ+ T cells in peripheral blood express the Vδ2 chain [190]. It has been proposed that Vδ1+ skin T cells act as immune sentinels by responding to stressed epithelial cells, thus controlling epithelial cell integrity [75]. Human TCR γδ+ epidermal T cells produce growth factors such as insulin-like growth factor 1 upon activation and contribute to the effective healing of acute wounds [190].

Our immune system not only has to mount immune responses to pathogens but also has to maintain tolerance to self and non-self antigens. Tregs which are characterized by the expression of the transcription factor FOXP3, maintain self-tolerance and function by suppressing the activation, cytokine production and proliferation of other T cells [157]. Clark et al. have described that between 5 and 10% of the T cells resident in normal human skin are FOXP3+ Tregs [37, 38]. These cells not only protect against autoimmune reactions to self antigens and assist in the resolution of cutaneous inflammation, but unfortunately, can also protect tumors from immune detection, allow latent infections to persist and can dysfunction under conditions present in inflammatory diseases [34].

Also NK cells are present in the dermis which express receptors for homing to noninflamed skin and for recognition of allogeneic tumor cells [48].

Dermal-epidermal junction – Engaged with multiple functions

The dermal-epidermal junction is a complex basement membrane (Fig. 1) which is continuous along the epidermis and skin appendages, including sweat glands, hair follicles, and sebaceous glands. From the surface to the depth, the dermal-epidermal junction can be divided into three zones including the keratin filament-hemidesmosome complex of the basal cells, the lamina lucida, and the lamina densa [47, 98]. The major components of all basement membranes are collagenous and non-collagenous glycoproteins and proteoglycans such as collagen IV, laminins, nidogens, perlecan, fibulins, and fibronectin [52, 184, 207]. Collagen IV is a heterotrimer of three α chains each of which contains three distinct domains [142, 184]. Laminins are very large heterotrimeric glycoproteins (600–950 kd) composed of an α, β, and γ chain [207]. To date, five distinct α, four β, and three γ laminin chains have been identified that can combine to form 15 different isoforms. As the old nomenclature from laminin 1 to laminin 15 (according to their discovery) appeared impractical, a new simplified nomenclature, based on the chain composition and the number of each chain is used today. For example, the major laminin of the epidermal basement membrane, the previous laminin 5, with an α-chain composition α3β3γ2, is now called laminin 332 [13, 73] and can be detected on frozen tissue specimens by a specific antibody (Fig. 2C). The function of laminins are not yet fully understood, but through interactions with other surface components they control cellular activities such as adhesion, migration, proliferation etc. [13, 130]. Some molecules demonstrate a restricted distribution. For example, collagens VII and XVII are associated with skin but are not found in glomerular and alveolar membranes. Based on ultrastructural and biochemical studies several functions have been proposed for the basement membrane. It may be a structural source for the secure attachment and polarity of the epidermal basal cells and may have a barrier function, separating the dermis and epidermis. Furthermore, the basement membrane is most likely responsible for a firm attachment of the dermis to the epidermis through a continuous system of structural elements, and modifies several cellular functions [47, 98].

Acknowledgements

I thank Marion Prior and Karin Pfisterer (Department of Dermatology, Vienna) for editorial comments and Nikolaus Romani and Patrizia Stoitzner (Department of Dermatology, Innsbruck) for their continued help with "skin-related" questions. Supported by the Jubiläumsfonds der Österreichischen Nationalbank (Nr. 12 958) and a research grant of the Austrian Science Fund (FWF, P19 474-B13).

References

[1] Aasen T, Raya A, Barrero MJ, Garreta E, Consiglio A, Gonzalez F, Vassena R, Bilic J, Pekarik V, Tiscornia G, Edel M, Boue S, Izpisua Belmonte JC (2008) Efficient and rapid generation of induced pluripotent stem cells from human keratinocytes. Nat Biotechnol 26: 1276–1284

[2] Akira S, Uematsu S, Takeuchi O (2006) Pathogen recognition and innate immunity. Cell 124: 783–801

[3] Alaibac M, Morris J, Yu R, Chu AC (1992) T lymphocytes bearing the γδ T-cell receptor: a study in normal human skin and pathological skin conditions. Br J Dermatol 127: 458–462

[4] Albanesi C, Scarponi C, Giustizieri ML, Girolomoni G (2005) Keratinocytes in inflammatory skin diseases. Curr Drug Targets Inflamm Allergy 4: 329–334

[5] Alonso L, Fuchs E (2006) The hair cycle. J Cell Sci 119: 391–393

[6] Andrew CE, Andrew NV (1949) Lymphocytes in the normal epidermis of the rat and man. Anat Rec 104: 217–241

[7] Angel CE, Chen CJ, Horlacher OC, Winkler S, John T, Browning J, MacGregor D, Cebon J, Dunbar PR (2009) Distinctive localization of antigen-presenting cells in human lymph nodes. Blood 113: 1257–1267

[8] Angel CE, George E, Brooks AES, Ostrovsky LL, Brown TLA, Dunbar PR (2006) CD1a+ antigen-presenting cells in human dermis respond rapidly to CCR7 ligands. J Immunol 176: 5730–5734

[9] Angel CE, George E, Ostrovsky LL, Dunbar PR (2007a) Comprehensive analysis of MHC-II expression in healthy human skin. Immunol Cell Biol 85: 363–369

[10] Angel CE, Lala A, Chen CJ, Edgar SG, Ostrovsky LL, Dunbar PR (2007b) CD14+ antigen-presenting cells in human dermis are less mature than their CD1a+ counterparts. Int Immunol 19: 1271–1279

[11] Annes JP, Munger JS, Rifkin DB (2003) Making sense of latent TGFbeta activation. J Cell Sci 116: 217–224

[12] Asahina A, Tamaki K (2006) Role of Langerhans cells in cutaneous protective immunity: is the reappraisal necessary? J Dermatol Sci 44: 1–9

[13] Aumailley M, Bruckner-Tuderman L, Carter WG, Deutzmann R, Edgar D, Ekblom P, Engel J, Engvall E, Hohenester E, Jones JC, Kleinman HK, Marinkovich MP, Martin GR, Mayer U, Meneguzzi G, Miner JH, Miyazaki K, Patarroyo M, Paulsson M, Quaranta V, Sanes JR, Sasaki T, Sekiguchi K, Sorokin LM, Talts JF, Tryggvason K, Uitto J, Virtanen I, von de Mark K, Wewer UM, Yamada Y, Yurchenco PD (2005) A simplified laminin nomenclature. Matrix Biol 24: 326–332

[14] Baker BS, Ovigne JM, Powles AV, Corcoran S, Fry L (2003) Normal keratinocytes express Toll-like receptors (TLRs) 1, 2 and 5: modulation of TLR expression in chronic plaque psoriasis. Br J Dermatol 148: 670–679

[15] Ban E, Dupre L, Hermann E, Rohn W, Vendeville C, Quatannens B, Ricciardi-Castagnoli P, Capron A, Riveau G (2000) CpG motifs induce Langerhans cell migration in vivo. Int Immunol 12: 737–745

[16] Banchereau J, Briere F, Caux C, Davoust J, Lebecque S, Liu Y-J, Pulendran B, Palucka K (2000) Immunobiology of dendritic cells. Annu Rev Immunol 18: 767–811

[17] Bangert C, Friedl J, Stary G, Stingl G, Kopp T (2003) Immunopathologic features of allergic contact dermatitis in humans: participation of plasmacytoid dendritic cells in the pathogenesis of the disease? J Invest Dermatol 121: 1409–1418

[18] Biernaskie J, Paris M, Morozova O, Fagan BM, Marra M, Pevny L, Miller FD (2009) SKPs derive from hair follicle precursors and exhibit properties of adult dermal stem cells. Cell Stem Cell 5: 610–623

[19] Birbeck MS, Breathnach AS, Everall JD (1961) An electron microscopic study of basal melanocytes and high level clear cells (Langerhans cell) in vitiligo. J Invest Dermatol 37: 51–64

[20] Blanpain C, Fuchs E (2009) Epidermal homeostasis: a balancing act of stem cells in the skin. Nat Rev Mol Cell Biol 10: 207–217

[21] Blanpain C, Horsley V, Fuchs E (2007) Epithelial stem cells: turning over new leaves. Cell 128: 445–458

[22] Blanpain C, Lowry WE, Geoghegan A, Polak L, Fuchs E (2004) Self-renewal, multipotency, and the existence of two cell populations within an epithelial stem cell niche. Cell 118: 635–648

[23] Borkowski TA, Letterio JJ, Farr AG, Udey MC (1996) A role for endogenous transforming growth factor β1 in Langerhans cell biology: the skin of transforming growth factor β1 null mice is devoid of epidermal Langerhans cells. J Exp Med 184: 2417–2422

[24] Bos JD, de Boer OJ, Tibosch E, Das PK, Pals ST (1993) Skin-homing T lymphocytes: detection of cutaneous lymphocyte-associated antigen (CLA) by HECA-452 in normal human skin. Arch Dermatol Res 285: 179–183

[25] Bos JD, Zonneveld I, Das PK, Krieg SR, van der Loos CM, Kapsenberg ML (1987) The skin immune system (SIS): distribution and immunophenotype of lymphocyte subpopulations in normal human skin. J Invest Dermatol 88: 569–573

[26] Boulais N, Misery L (2007) Merkel cells. J Am Acad Dermatol 57: 147–165

[27] Boyman O, Conrad C, Tonel G, Gilliet M, Nestle FO (2007) The pathogenic role of tissue-resident immune cells in psoriasis. Trends Immunol 28: 51–57

[28] Boyman O, Hefti HP, Conrad C, Nickoloff BJ, Suter M, Nestle FO (2004) Spontaneous development of psoriasis in a new animal model shows an essential role for resident T cells and tumor necrosis factor-α. J Exp Med 199: 731–736

[29] Braun KM, Niemann C, Jensen UB, Sundberg JP, Silva-Vargas V, Watt FM (2003) Manipulation of stem cell proliferation and lineage commitment: visualisation of label-retaining cells in wholemounts of mouse epidermis. Development 130: 5241–5255

[30] Bursch LS, Wang L, Igyarto B, Kissenpfennig A, Malissen B, Kaplan DH, Hogquist KA (2007) Identification of a novel population of Langerin+ dendritic cells. J Exp Med 204: 3147–3156

[31] Campbell JJ, Murphy KE, Kunkel EJ, Brightling CE, Soler D, Shen Z, Boisvert J, Greenberg HB, Vierra MA, Goodman SB, Genovese MC, Wardlaw AJ, Butcher EC, Wu L (2001) CCR7 expression and memory T cell diversity in humans. J Immunol 166: 877–884

[32] Charbonnier AS, Kohrgruber N, Kriehuber E, Stingl G, Rot A, Maurer D (1999) Macrophage inflammatory protein 3alpha is involved in the constitutive trafficking of epidermal Langerhans cells. J Exp Med 190: 1755–1768

[33] Cheng Chew SB, Leung PY (1994) Ultrastructural study of the Merkel cell and its expression of met-enkephalin immunoreactivity during fetal and postnatal development in mice. J Anat 185: 511–520

[34] Clark RA (2010) Skin-resident T cells: the ups and downs of on site immunity. J Invest Dermatol 130: 362–370

[35] Clark RA, Chong B, Mirchandani N, Brinster NK, Yamanaka K, Dowgiert RK, Kupper TS (2006a) The vast majority of CLA+ T cells are resident in normal skin. J Immunol 176: 4431–4439

[36] Clark RA, Chong BF, Mirchandani N, Yamanaka K, Murphy GF, Dowgiert RK, Kupper TS (2006b) A novel method for the isolation of skin resident T cells from normal and diseased human skin. J Invest Dermatol 126: 1059–1070

[37] Clark RA, Huang SJ, Murphy GF, Mollet IG, Hijnen D, Muthukuru M, Schanbacher CF, Edwards V, Miller DM, Kim JE, Lambert J, Kupper TS (2008) Human squamous cell carcinomas evade the immune response by down-regulation of vascular E-selectin and recruitment of regulatory T cells. J Exp Med 205: 2221–2234

[38] Clark RA, Kupper TS (2007) IL-15 and dermal fibroblasts induce proliferation of natural regulatory T cells isolated from human skin. Blood 109: 194–202

[39] Colonna M, Krug A, Cella M (2002) Interferon-producing cells: on the front line in immune responses against pathogens. Curr Opin Immunol 14: 373–379

[40] Conrad C, Boyman O, Tonel G, Tun-Kyi A, Laggner U, de Fougerolles A, Kotelianski V, Gardner H, Nestle FO (2007) Alpha1beta1 integrin is crucial for accumulation of epidermal T cells and the development of psoriasis. Nat Med 13: 836–842

[41] Costin GE, Hearing VJ (2007) Human skin pigmentation: melanocytes modulate skin color in response to stress. FASEB J 21: 976–994

[42] Cotsarelis G, Sun TT, Lavker RM (1990) Label-retaining cells reside in the bulge area of pilosebaceous unit: implications for follicular stem cells, hair cycle, and skin carcinogenesis. Cell 61: 1329–1337

[43] Coulombe PA, Omary MB (2002) 'Hard' and 'soft' principles defining the structure, function and regulation of keratin intermediate filaments. Curr Opin Cell Biol 14: 110–122

[44] Cummings RJ, Mitra S, Foster TH, Lord EM (2009) Migration of skin dendritic cells in response to ionizing radiation exposure. Radiat Res 171: 687–697

[45] Curry JL, Qin JZ, Bonish B, Carrick R, Bacon P, Panella J, Robinson J, Nickoloff BJ (2003) Innate immune-related receptors in normal and psoriatic skin. Arch Pathol Lab Med 127: 178–186

[46] Dieu-Nosjean MC, Massacrier C, Homey B, Vanbervliet B, Pin JJ, Vicari A, Lebecque S, Dezutter-Dambuyant C, Schmitt D, Zlotnik A, Caux C (2000) Macrophage inflammatory protein 3alpha is expressed at inflamed epithelial surfaces and is the most potent chemokine known in attracting Langerhans cell precursors. J Exp Med 192: 705–718

[47] Eady RA, McGrath JA, McMillan JR (1994) Ultrastructural clues to genetic disorders of skin: the dermal-epidermal junction. J Invest Dermatol 103: 13S-18S

[48] Ebert LM, Meuter S, Moser B (2006) Homing and function of human skin gammadelta T cells and NK cells: relevance for tumor surveillance. J Immunol 176: 4331-4336

[49] Edele F, Molenaar R, Gutle D, Dudda JC, Jakob T, Homey B, Mebius R, Hornef M, Martin SF (2008) Cutting edge: instructive role of peripheral tissue cells in the imprinting of T cell homing receptor patterns. J Immunol 181: 3745-3749

[50] Eidsmo L, Allan R, Caminschi I, van Rooijen N, Heath WR, Carbone FR (2009) Differential migration of epidermal and dermal dendritic cells during skin infection. J Immunol 182: 3165-3172

[51] Elias PM (2005) Stratum corneum defensive functions: an integrated view. J Invest Dermatol 125: 183-200

[52] Erickson AC, Couchman JR (2000) Still more complexity in mammalian basement membranes. J Histochem Cytochem 48: 1291-1306

[53] Fernandes KJ, Kobayashi NR, Gallagher CJ, Barnabe-Heider F, Aumont A, Kaplan DR, Miller FD (2006) Analysis of the neurogenic potential of multipotent skin-derived precursors. Exp Neurol 201: 32-48

[54] Fernandes KJ, McKenzie IA, Mill P, Smith KM, Akhavan M, Barnabe-Heider F, Biernaskie J, Junek A, Kobayashi NR, Toma JG, Kaplan DR, Labosky PA, Rafuse V, Hui CC, Miller FD (2004) A dermal niche for multipotent adult skin-derived precursor cells. Nat Cell Biol 6: 1082-1093

[55] Flacher V, Bouschbacher M, Verronese E, Massacrier C, Sisirak V, Berthier-Vergnes O, Saint-Vis B, Caux C, Dezutter-Dambuyant C, Lebecque S, Valladeau J (2006) Human Langerhans cells express a specific TLR profile and differentially respond to viruses and Gram-positive bacteria. J Immunol 177: 7959-7967

[56] Foster CA, Elbe A (1997) Lymphocyte subpopulations of the skin. In: Bos JD (ed) Skin immune system (SIS), 2 edn. CRC Press, Boca Raton New York, pp 85-108

[57] Foster CA, Yokozeki H, Rappersberger K, Koning F, Volc-Platzer B, Rieger A, Coligan JE, Wolff K, Stingl G (1990) Human epidermal T cells predominately belong to the lineage expressing αβ T cell receptor. J Exp Med 171: 997-1013

[58] Frelinger JG, Hood L, Hill S, Frelinger JA (1979) Mouse epidermal Ia molecules have a bone marrow origin. Nature 282: 321-323

[59] Fu X, Li H (2009) Mesenchymal stem cells and skin wound repair and regeneration: possibilities and questions. Cell Tissue Res 335: 317-321

[60] Fuchs E (1995) Keratins and the skin. Annu Rev Cell Dev Biol 11: 123-153

[61] Fuchs E (2007) Scratching the surface of skin development. Nature 445: 834-842

[62] Fuchs E (2008) Skin stem cells: rising to the surface. J Cell Biol 180: 273-284

[63] Gebhardt T, Wakim LM, Eidsmo L, Reading PC, Heath WR, Carbone FR (2009) Memory T cells in nonlymphoid tissue that provide enhanced local immunity during infection with herpes simplex virus. Nat Immunol 10: 524-530

[64] Ghaznawie M, Papadimitriou JM, Heenan PJ (1999) The repopulation of murine Langerhans cells after depletion by mild heat injury. Br J Dermatol 141: 206-210

[65] Gingras M, Champigny MF, Berthod F (2007) Differentiation of human adult skin-derived neuronal precursors into mature neurons. J Cell Physiol 210: 498-506

[66] Ginhoux F, Collin MP, Bogunovic M, Abel M, Leboeuf M, Helft J, Ochando J, Kissenpfennig A, Malissen B, Grisotto M, Snoeck H, Randolph G, Merad M (2007) Blood-derived dermal langerin+ dendritic cells survey the skin in the steady state. J Exp Med 204: 3133-3146

[67] Ginhoux F, Tacke F, Angeli V, Bogunovic M, Loubeau M, Dai XM, Stanley ER, Randolph GJ, Merad M (2006) Langerhans cells arise from monocytes in vivo. Nat Immunol 7: 265-273

[68] Grim M, Halata Z (2000) Developmental origin of avian Merkel cells. Anat Embryol (Berl) 202: 401-410

[69] Groh V, Porcelli S, Fabbi M, Lanier LL, Picker LJ, Anderson T, Warnke RA, Bhan AK, Strominger JL, Brenner MB (1989) Human lymphocytes bearing T cell receptor γδ are phenotypically diverse and evenly distributed throughout the lymphoid system. J Exp Med 169: 1277-1294

[70] Grone A (2002) Keratinocytes and cytokines. Vet Immunol Immunopathol 88: 1-12

[71] Haeberle H, Fujiwara M, Chuang J, Medina MM, Panditrao MV, Bechstedt S, Howard J, Lumpkin EA (2004) Molecular profiling reveals synaptic release machinery in Merkel cells. Proc Natl Acad Sci USA 101: 14503-14508

[72] Halata Z, Grim M, Bauman KI (2003) Friedrich Sigmund Merkel and his "Merkel cell", morphology, development, and physiology: review and new results. Anat Rec A Discov Mol Cell Evol Biol 271: 225-239

[73] Hallmann R, Horn N, Selg M, Wendler O, Pausch F, Sorokin LM (2005) Expression and function of laminins in the embryonic and mature vasculature. Physiol Rev 85: 979-1000

[74] Haniffa M, Ginhoux F, Wang XN, Bigley V, Abel M, Dimmick I, Bullock S, Grisotto M, Booth T, Taub P, Hilkens C, Merad M, Collin M (2009) Differential rates of replacement of human dermal dendritic cells and macrophages during hematopoietic stem cell transplantation. J Exp Med 206: 371-385

[75] Holtmeier W, Kabelitz D (2005) Gammadelta T cells link innate and adaptive immune responses. Chem Immunol Allergy 86: 151-183

[76] Holzmann S, Tripp CH, Schmuth M, Janke K, Koch F, Saeland S, Stoitzner P, Romani N (2004) A model system using tape stripping for characterization of Langerhans cell-precursors in vivo. J Invest Dermatol 122: 1165-1174

[77] Homey B, Alenius H, Muller A, Soto H, Bowman EP, Yuan W, McEvoy L, Lauerma AI, Assmann T, Bunemann E, Lehto M, Wolff H, Yen D, Marxhausen H, To W, Sedgwick J, Ruzicka T, Lehmann P, Zlotnik A (2002) CCL27-CCR10 interactions regulate T cell-mediated skin inflammation. Nat Med 8: 157–165

[78] Hoogduijn MJ, Gorjup E, Genever PG (2006) Comparative characterization of hair follicle dermal stem cells and bone marrow mesenchymal stem cells. Stem Cells Dev 15: 49–60

[79] Hunt DP, Jahoda C, Chandran S (2009) Multipotent skin-derived precursors: from biology to clinical translation. Curr Opin Biotechnol 20: 522–530

[80] Hunt DP, Morris PN, Sterling J, Anderson JA, Joannides A, Jahoda C, Compston A, Chandran S (2008) A highly enriched niche of precursor cells with neuronal and glial potential within the hair follicle dermal papilla of adult skin. Stem Cells 26: 163–172

[81] Hunt DP, Sajic M, Phillips H, Henderson D, Compston A, Smith K, Chandran S (2010) Origins of gliogenic stem cell populations within adult skin and bone marrow. Stem Cells Dev 19: 1055–1065

[82] Inoue K, Aoi N, Sato T, Yamauchi Y, Suga H, Eto H, Kato H, Araki J, Yoshimura K (2009) Differential expression of stem-cell-associated markers in human hair follicle epithelial cells. Lab Invest 89: 844–856

[83] Ito M, Kizawa K, Hamada K, Cotsarelis G (2004) Hair follicle stem cells in the lower bulge form the secondary germ, a biochemically distinct but functionally equivalent progenitor cell population, at the termination of catagen. Differentiation 72: 548–557

[84] Iwasaki A, Medzhitov R (2010) Regulation of adaptive immunity by the innate immune system. Science 327: 291–295

[85] Jahoda CA, Whitehouse J, Reynolds AJ, Hole N (2003) Hair follicle dermal cells differentiate into adipogenic and osteogenic lineages. Exp Dermatol 12: 849–859

[86] Jaksits S, Kriehuber E, Charbonnier AS, Rappersberger K, Stingl G, Maurer D (1999) CD34+ cell-derived CD14+ precursor cells develop into Langerhans cells in a TGF-beta 1-dependent manner. J Immunol 163: 4869–4877

[87] Janssens AS, Pavel S, Out-Luiting JJ, Willemze R, de Gruijl FR (2005) Normalized ultraviolet (UV) induction of Langerhans cell depletion and neutrophil infiltrates after artificial UVB hardening of patients with polymorphic light eruption. Br J Dermatol 152: 1268–1274

[88] Jensen KB, Collins CA, Nascimento E, Tan DW, Frye M, Itami S, Watt FM (2009) Lrig1 expression defines a distinct multipotent stem cell population in mammalian epidermis. Cell Stem Cell 4: 427–439

[89] Jensen UB, Yan X, Triel C, Woo SH, Christensen R, Owens DM (2008) A distinct population of clonogenic and multipotent murine follicular keratinocytes residing in the upper isthmus. J Cell Sci 121: 609–617

[90] Jimbow K, Quevedo WC, Jr, Fitzpatrick TB, Szabo G (1976) Some aspects of melanin biology: 1950–1975. J Invest Dermatol 67: 72–89

[91] Joannides A, Gaughwin P, Schwiening C, Majed H, Sterling J, Compston A, Chandran S (2004) Efficient generation of neural precursors from adult human skin: astrocytes promote neurogenesis from skin-derived stem cells. Lancet 364: 172–178

[92] Johnson KO (2001) The roles and functions of cutaneous mechanoreceptors. Curr Opin Neurobiol 11: 455–461

[93] Kanitakis J (1998) Immunohistochemistry of normal human skin. Eur J Dermatol 8: 539–547

[94] Kanitakis J (2002) Anatomy, histology and immunohistochemistry of normal human skin. Eur J Dermatol 12: 390–399

[95] Kaplan DH, Kissenpfennig A, Clausen BE (2008) Insights into Langerhans cell function from Langerhans cell ablation models. Eur J Immunol 38: 2369–2376

[96] Kaplan DH, Li MO, Jenison MC, Shlomchik WD, Flavell RA, Shlomchik MJ (2007) Autocrine/paracrine TGFbeta1 is required for the development of epidermal Langerhans cells. J Exp Med 204: 2545–2552

[97] Katz SI, Tamaki K, Sachs DH (1979) Epidermal Langerhans cells are derived from cells originating in bone marrow. Nature 282: 324–326

[98] Keene DR, Marinkovich MP, Sakai LY (1997) Immunodissection of the connective tissue matrix in human skin. Microsc Res Tech 38: 394–406

[99] Kimber I, Cumberbatch M, Dearman RJ (2009) Langerhans cell migration: not necessarily always at the center of the skin sensitization universe. J Invest Dermatol 129: 1852–1853

[100] Klechevsky E, Morita R, Liu M, Cao Y, Coquery S, Thompson-Snipes L, Briere F, Chaussabel D, Zurawski G, Palucka AK, Reiter Y, Banchereau J, Ueno H (2008) Functional specializations of human epidermal Langerhans cells and CD14+ dermal dendritic cells. Immunity 29: 497–510

[101] Kobayashi N, Nakagawa A, Muramatsu T, Yamashina Y, Shirai T, Hashimoto MW, Ishigaki Y, Ohnishi T, Mori T (1998) Supranuclear melanin caps reduce ultraviolet induced DNA photoproducts in human epidermis. J Invest Dermatol 110: 806–810

[102] Kroeze KL, Jurgens WJ, Doulabi BZ, van Milligen FJ, Scheper RJ, Gibbs S (2009) Chemokine-mediated migration of skin-derived stem cells: predominant role for CCL5/RANTES. J Invest Dermatol 129: 1569–1581

[103] Kryczek I, Bruce AT, Gudjonsson JE, Johnston A, Aphale A, Vatan L, Szeliga W, Wang Y, Liu Y, Welling TH, Elder JT, Zou W (2008) Induction of IL-17+ T cell trafficking and development by IFN-gamma: mechanism and pathological relevance in psoriasis. J Immunol 181: 4733–4741

[104] Kummer JA, Broekhuizen R, Everett H, Agostini L, Kuijk L, Martinon F, van Bruggen R, Tschopp J (2007) Inflammasome components NALP 1 and 3 show distinct but separate expression profiles in human tissues suggesting a site-specific role in the inflammatory response. J Histochem Cytochem 55: 443–452

[105] Kupper TS, Fuhlbrigge RC (2004) Immune surveillance in the skin: mechanisms and clinical consequences. Nat Rev Immunol 4: 211–222

[106] Lacour JP, Dubois D, Pisani A, Ortonne JP (1991) Anatomical mapping of Merkel cells in normal human adult epidermis. Br J Dermatol 125: 535–542

[107] Lai Y, Di NA, Nakatsuji T, Leichtle A, Yang Y, Cogen AL, Wu ZR, Hooper LV, Schmidt RR, von AS, Radek KA, Huang CM, Ryan AF, Gallo RL (2009) Commensal bacteria regulate Toll-like receptor 3-dependent inflammation after skin injury. Nat Med 15: 1377–1382

[108] Lai Y, Gallo RL (2009) AMPed up immunity: how antimicrobial peptides have multiple roles in immune defense. Trends Immunol 30: 131–141

[109] Lako M, Armstrong L, Cairns PM, Harris S, Hole N, Jahoda CA (2002) Hair follicle dermal cells repopulate the mouse haematopoietic system. J Cell Sci 115: 3967–3974

[110] Langerhans P (1868) Über die Nerven der menschlichen Haut. Virchows Arch 44: 325–337

[111] Larregina AT, Watkins SC, Erdos G, Spencer LA, Storkus WJ, Beer SD, Falo LD, Jr (2001) Direct transfection and activation of human cutaneous dendritic cells. Gene Ther 8: 608–617

[112] Lavoie JF, Biernaskie JA, Chen Y, Bagli D, Alman B, Kaplan DR, Miller FD (2009) Skin-derived precursors differentiate into skeletogenic cell types and contribute to bone repair. Stem Cells Dev 18: 893–906

[113] Leibbrandt A, Penninger JM (2008) RANK/RANKL: regulators of immune responses and bone physiology. Ann N Y Acad Sci 1143: 123–150

[114] Li A, Pouliot N, Redvers R, Kaur P (2004) Extensive tissue-regenerative capacity of neonatal human keratinocyte stem cells and their progeny. J Clin Invest 113: 390–400

[115] Lucarz A, Brand G (2007) Current considerations about Merkel cells. Eur J Cell Biol 86: 243–251

[116] Lumpkin EA, Bautista DM (2005) Feeling the pressure in mammalian somatosensation. Curr Opin Neurobiol 15: 382–388

[117] Lyle S, Christofidou-Solomidou M, Liu Y, Elder DE, Albelda S, Cotsarelis G (1998) The C8/144B monoclonal antibody recognizes cytokeratin 15 and defines the location of human hair follicle stem cells. J Cell Sci 111: 3179–3188

[118] Lysy PA, Smets F, Sibille C, Najimi M, Sokal EM (2007) Human skin fibroblasts: from mesodermal to hepatocyte-like differentiation. Hepatology 46: 1574–1585

[119] Mannik J, Alzayady K, Ghazizadeh S (2010) Regeneration of multilineage skin epithelia by differentiated keratinocytes. J Invest Dermatol 130: 388–397

[120] Maricich SM, Wellnitz SA, Nelson AM, Lesniak DR, Gerling GJ, Lumpkin EA, Zoghbi HY (2009) Merkel cells are essential for light-touch responses. Science 324: 1580–1582

[121] Mattei S, Colombo MP, Melani C, Silvani A, Parmiani G, Herlyn M (1994) Expression of cytokine/growth factors and their receptors in human melanoma and melanocytes. Int J Cancer 56: 853–857

[122] Maytin EV (1992) Differential effects of heat shock and UVB light upon stress protein expression in epidermal keratinocytes. J Biol Chem 267: 23 189–23 196

[123] McGirt LY, Beck LA (2006) Innate immune defects in atopic dermatitis. J Allergy Clin Immunol 118: 202–208

[124] McInturff JE, Modlin RL, Kim J (2005) The role of toll-like receptors in the pathogenesis and treatment of dermatological disease. J Invest Dermatol 125: 1–8

[125] McKenzie IA, Biernaskie J, Toma JG, Midha R, Miller FD (2006) Skin-derived precursors generate myelinating Schwann cells for the injured and dysmyelinated nervous system. J Neurosci 26: 6651–6660

[126] McLellan AD, Heiser A, Sorg RV, Fearnley DB, Hart DN (1998) Dermal dendritic cells associated with T lymphocytes in normal human skin display an activated phenotype. J Invest Dermatol 111: 841–849

[127] Medina RJ, Kataoka K, Takaishi M, Miyazaki M, Huh NH (2006) Isolation of epithelial stem cells from dermis by a three-dimensional culture system. J Cell Biochem 98: 174–184

[128] Merad M, Ginhoux F, Collin M (2008) Origin, homeostasis and function of Langerhans cells and other langerin-expressing dendritic cells. Nat Rev Immunol 8: 935–947

[129] Merad M, Manz MG, Karsunky H, Wagers A, Peters W, Charo I, Weissman IL, Cyster JG, Engleman EG (2002) Langerhans cells renew in the skin throughout life under steady-state conditions. Nature Immunol 3: 1135–1141

[130] Miner JH, Yurchenco PD (2004) Laminin functions in tissue morphogenesis. Annu Rev Cell Dev Biol 20: 255–284

[131] Modlin RL, Kim J, Maurer D, Bangert C, Stingl G (2007) Innate and adaptive immunity in the skin. In: Wolff K, Goldsmith LA, Katz SI, Gilchrest BA, Paller AS, Leffell DJ (eds) Fitzpatrick's Dermatology in General Medicine, 7 edn, McGraw Hill, New York, pp 95–114

[132] Moll I, Kuhn C, Moll R (1995) Cytokeratin 20 is a general marker of cutaneous Merkel cells while certain neuronal proteins are absent. J Invest Dermatol 104: 910–915

[133] Moll I, Lane AT, Franke WW, Moll R (1990) Intraepidermal formation of Merkel cells in xenografts of human fetal skin. J Invest Dermatol 94: 359–364

[134] Moll I, Moll R (1992) Early development of human Merkel cells. Exp Dermatol 1: 180–184

[135] Moll I, Moll R, Franke WW (1986) Formation of epidermal and dermal Merkel cells during human fetal skin development. J Invest Dermatol 87: 779–787

[136] Moll I, Roessler M, Brandner JM, Eispert AC, Houdek P, Moll R (2005) Human Merkel cells–aspects of cell biology, distribution and functions. Eur J Cell Biol 84: 259–271

[137] Mora JR, Cheng GY, Picarella D, Briskin M, Buchanan N, Von Andrian U (2005) Reciprocal and dynamic control of CD8 T cell homing by dendritic cells from skin- and gut-associated lymphoid tissues. J Exp Med 201: 303–316

[138] Morelli AE, Thomson AW (2007) Tolerogenic dendritic cells and the quest for transplant tolerance. Nat Rev Immunol 7: 610–621

[139] Morris RJ, Liu Y, Marles L, Yang Z, Trempus C, Li S, Lin JS, Sawicki JA, Cotsarelis G (2004) Capturing and profiling adult hair follicle stem cells. Nat Biotechnol 22: 411–417

[140] Morrison KM, Miesegaes GR, Lumpkin EA, Maricich SM (2009) Mammalian Merkel cells are descended from the epidermal lineage. Dev Biol 336: 76–83

[141] Mutyambizi K, Berger CL, Edelson RL (2009) The balance between immunity and tolerance: the role of Langerhans cells. Cell Mol Life Sci 66: 831–840

[142] Myllyharju J, Kivirikko KI (2004) Collagens, modifying enzymes and their mutations in humans, flies and worms. Trends Genet 20: 33–43

[143] Nagao K, Ginhoux F, Leitner WW, Motegi S, Bennett CL, Clausen BE, Merad M, Udey MC (2009) Murine epidermal Langerhans cells and langerin-expressing dermal dendritic cells are unrelated and exhibit distinct functions. Proc Natl Acad Sci USA 106: 3312–3317

[144] Narisawa Y, Hashimoto K (1991) Immunohistochemical demonstration of nerve-Merkel cell complex in fetal human skin. J Dermatol Sci 2: 361–370

[145] Nestle FO, Di MP, Qin JZ, Nickoloff BJ (2009) Skin immune sentinels in health and disease. Nat Rev Immunol 9: 679–691

[146] Nestle FO, Zheng XG, Thompson CB, Turka LA, Nickoloff BJ (1993) Characterization of dermal dendritic cells obtained from normal human skin reveals phenotypic and functionally distinctive subsets. J Immunol 151: 6535–6545

[147] Nijhof JG, Braun KM, Giangreco A, van Pelt C, Kawamoto H, Boyd RL, Willemze R, Mullenders LH, Watt FM, De Gruijl FR, van Ewijk W (2006) The cell-surface marker MTS24 identifies a novel population of follicular keratinocytes with characteristics of progenitor cells. Development 133: 3027–3037

[148] Norris A, Todd C, Graham A, Quinn AG, Thody AJ (1996) The expression of the c-kit receptor by epidermal melanocytes may be reduced in vitiligo. Br J Dermatol 134: 299–306

[149] Ochoa MT, Loncaric A, Krutzik SR, Becker TC, Modlin RL (2008) "Dermal dendritic cells" comprise two distinct populations: CD1+ dendritic cells and CD209+ macrophages. J Invest Dermatol 128: 2225–2231

[150] Ohyama M, Terunuma A, Tock CL, Radonovich MF, Pise-Masison CA, Hopping SB, Brady JN, Udey MC, Vogel JC (2006) Characterization and isolation of stem cell-enriched human hair follicle bulge cells. J Clin Invest 116: 249–260

[151] Peiser M, Koeck J, Kirschning CJ, Wittig B, Wanner R (2008) Human Langerhans cells selectively activated via Toll-like receptor 2 agonists acquire migratory and CD4+ T cell stimulatory capacity. J Leukoc Biol 83: 1118–1127

[152] Perreault C, Pelletier M, Landry D, Gyger M (1984) Study of Langerhans cells after allogeneic bone marrow transplantation. Blood 63: 807–811

[153] Potten CS, Booth C (2002) Keratinocyte stem cells: a commentary. J Invest Dermatol 119: 888–899

[154] Poulin LF, Henri S, de BB, Devilard E, Kissenpfennig A, Malissen B (2007) The dermis contains langerin+ dendritic cells that develop and function independently of epidermal Langerhans cells. J Exp Med 204: 3119–3131

[155] Renn CN, Sanchez DJ, Ochoa MT, Legaspi AJ, Oh CK, Liu PT, Krutzik SR, Sieling PA, Cheng G, Modlin RL (2006) TLR activation of Langerhans cell-like dendritic cells triggers an antiviral immune response. J Immunol 177: 298–305

[156] Romani N, Clausen BE, Stoitzner P (2010) Langerhans cells and more: langerin-expressing dendritic cell subsets in the skin. Immunol Rev 234: 120–141

[157] Sakaguchi S (2005) Naturally arising Foxp3-expressing CD25+CD4+ regulatory T cells in immunological tolerance to self and non-self. Nat Immunol 6: 345–352

[158] Salmon JK, Armstrong CA, Ansel JC (1994) The skin as an immune organ. West J Med 160: 146–152

[159] Schaerli P, Ebert L, Willimann K, Blaser A, Roos RS, Loetscher P, Moser B (2004) A skin-selective homing mechanism for human immune surveillance T cells. J Exp Med 199: 1265–1275

[160] Schaerli P, Willimann K, Ebert LM, Walz A, Moser B (2005) Cutaneous CXCL14 targets blood precursors to epidermal niches for Langerhans cell differentiation. Immunity 23: 331–342

[161] Schauber J, Gallo RL (2007) Expanding the roles of antimicrobial peptides in skin: alarming and arming keratinocytes. J Invest Dermatol 127: 510–512

[162] Schröder JM (1999) Epithelial antimicrobial peptides: innate local host response elements. Cell Mol Life Sci 56: 32–46

[163] Schuster C, Vaculik C, Fiala C, Meindl S, Brandt O, Imhof M, Stingl G, Eppel W, Elbe-Bürger A (2009) HLA-DR+ leukocytes acquire CD1 antigens in embryonic and fetal human skin and contain functional antigen-presenting cells. J Exp Med 206: 169–181

[164] Segre JA (2006) Epidermal barrier formation and recovery in skin disorders. J Clin Invest 116: 1150–1158

[165] Sellheyer K, Krahl D (2010) Cutaneous mesenchymal stem cells: current status of research and potential clinical applications. Hautarzt 61: 429–434

[166] Shi CM, Cheng TM (2004) Differentiation of dermis-derived multipotent cells into insulin-producing pancreatic cells in vitro. World J Gastroenterol 10: 2550–2552

[167] Sidhu GS, Chandra P, Cassai ND (2005) Merkel cells, normal and neoplastic: an update. Ultrastruct Pathol 29: 287–294

[168] Sigmundsdottir H, Butcher EC (2008) Environmental cues, dendritic cells and the programming of tissue-selective lymphocyte trafficking. Nat Immunol 9: 981–987

[169] Snippert HJ, Haegebarth A, Kasper M, Jaks V, van Es JH, Barker N, van de Wetering M, van den Born M, Begthel H, Vries RG, Stange DE, Toftgard R, Clevers H (2010) Lgr6 marks stem cells in the hair follicle that generate all cell lineages of the skin. Science 327: 1385–1389

[170] Song PI, Park YM, Abraham T, Harten B, Zivony A, Neparidze N, Armstrong CA, Ansel JC (2002) Human keratinocytes express functional CD14 and toll-like receptor 4. J Invest Dermatol 119: 424–432

[171] Spetz AL, Strominger J, Groh-Spies V (1996) T cell subsets in normal human epidermis. Am J Pathol 149: 665–674

[172] Steinman RM (2007) Dendritic cells: versatile controllers of the immune system. Nat Med 13: 1155–1159

[173] Steinman RM, Banchereau J (2007) Taking dendritic cells into medicine. Nature 449: 419–426

[174] Steinman RM, Hemmi H (2006) Dendritic cells: translating innate to adaptive immunity. Curr Top Microbiol Immunol 311: 17–58

[175] Stoff A, Rivera AA, Sanjib BN, Moore ST, Michael NT, Espinosa-de-Los-Monteros A, Richter DF, Siegal GP, Chow LT, Feldman D, Vasconez LO, Michael MJ, Stoff-Khalili MA, Curiel DT (2009) Promotion of incisional wound repair by human mesenchymal stem cell transplantation. Exp Dermatol 18: 362–369

[176] Streilein JW (1983) Skin-associated lymphoid tissues (SALT): origins and functions. J Invest Dermatol 80: 12s–16s

[177] Strobl H, Riedl E, Scheinecker C, Bello-Fernandez C, Pickl WF, Rappersberger K, Majdic O, Knapp W (1996) TGF-β1 promotes in vitro development of dendritic cells from CD34+ hemopoietic progenitors. J Immunol 157: 1499–1507

[178] Sun L, Akiyama K, Zhang H, Yamaza T, Hou Y, Zhao S, Xu T, Le A, Shi S (2009) Mesenchymal stem cell transplantation reverses multiorgan dysfunction in systemic lupus erythematosus mice and humans. Stem Cells 27: 1421–1432

[179] Szeder V, Grim M, Halata Z, Sieber-Blum M (2003) Neural crest origin of mammalian Merkel cells. Dev Biol 253: 258–263

[180] Takahashi K, Tanabe K, Ohnuki M, Narita M, Ichisaka T, Tomoda K, Yamanaka S (2007) Induction of pluripotent stem cells from adult human fibroblasts by defined factors. Cell 131: 861–872

[181] Takahashi K, Yamanaka S (2006) Induction of pluripotent stem cells from mouse embryonic and adult fibroblast cultures by defined factors. Cell 126: 663–676

[182] Takeuchi J, Watari E, Shinya E, Norose Y, Matsumoto M, Seya T, Sugita M, Kawana S, Takahashi H (2003) Down-regulation of Toll-like receptor expression in monocyte-derived Langerhans cell-like cells: implications of low-responsiveness to bacterial components in the epidermal Langerhans cells. Biochem Biophys Res Commun 306: 674–679

[183] Tamaki K, Sugaya M, Tada Y, Yasaka N, Uehira M, Nishimoto H, Nakamura K (2001) Epidermal and dermal gamma-delta T cells. Chem Immunol 79: 43–51

[184] Timpl R (1996) Macromolecular organization of basement membranes. Curr Opin Cell Biol 8: 618–624

[185] Ting JP, Duncan JA, Lei Y (2010) How the noninflammasome NLRs function in the innate immune system. Science 327: 286–290

[186] Tobin DJ (2006) Biochemistry of human skin–our brain on the outside. Chem Soc Rev 35: 52–67

[187] Toebak MJ, Gibbs S, Bruynzeel DP, Scheper RJ, Rustemeyer T (2009) Dendritic cells: biology of the skin. Contact Dermatitis 60: 2–20

[188] Toma JG, Akhavan M, Fernandes KJ, Barnabe-Heider F, Sadikot A, Kaplan DR, Miller FD (2001) Isolation of multipotent adult stem cells from the dermis of mammalian skin. Nat Cell Biol 3: 778–784

[189] Toma JG, McKenzie IA, Bagli D, Miller FD (2005) Isolation and characterization of multipotent skin-derived precursors from human skin. Stem Cells 23: 727–737

[190] Toulon A, Breton L, Taylor KR, Tenenhaus M, Bhavsar D, Lanigan C, Rudolph R, Jameson J, Havran WL (2009) A role for human skin-resident T cells in wound healing. J Exp Med 206: 743–750

[191] Trempus CS, Morris RJ, Bortner CD, Cotsarelis G, Faircloth RS, Reece JM, Tennant RW (2003) Enrichment for living murine keratinocytes from the hair follicle bulge with the cell surface marker CD34. J Invest Dermatol 120: 501–511

[192] Tsai SY, Clavel C, Kim S, Ang YS, Grisanti L, Lee DF, Kelley K, Rendl M (2010) Oct4 and klf4 reprogram dermal papilla cells into induced pluripotent stem cells. Stem Cells 28: 221–228

[193] Tumbar T, Guasch G, Greco V, Blanpain C, Lowry WE, Rendl M, Fuchs E (2004) Defining the epithelial stem cell niche in skin. Science 303: 359–363

[194] Turville SG, Cameron PU, Handley A, Lin G, Pohlmann S, Doms RW, Cunningham AL (2002) Diversity of receptors binding HIV on dendritic cell subsets. Nature Immunol 3: 975–983

[195] Van der Aar AM, Sylva-Steenland RM, Bos JD, Kapsenberg ML, de Jong EC, Teunissen MB (2007) Loss of TLR2, TLR4, and TLR5 on Langerhans cells abolishes bacterial recognition. J Immunol 178: 1986–1990

[196] Van Keymeulen A, Mascre G, Youseff KK, Harel I, Michaux C, de Geest N, Szpalski C, Achouri Y, Bloch W, Hassan BA, Blanpain C (2009) Epidermal progenitors give rise to Merkel cells during embryonic development and adult homeostasis. J Cell Biol 187: 91–100

[197] Vielkind U, Sebzda MK, Gibson IR, Hardy MH (1995) Dynamics of Merkel cell patterns in developing hair follicles in the dorsal skin of mice, demonstrated by a monoclonal antibody to mouse keratin 8. Acta Anat (Basel) 152: 93–109

[198] Villablanca EJ, Mora JR (2008) A two-step model for Langerhans cell migration to skin-draining LN. Eur J Immunol 38: 2975–2980

[199] Volc-Platzer B, Stingl G, Wolff K, Hinterberger W, Schnedl W (1984) Cytogenetic identification of allogeneic epidermal Langerhans cells in a bone marrow-graft recipient. N Engl J Med 310: 1123–1124

[200] Wakim LM, Waithman J, van Rooijen N, Heath WR, Carbone FR (2008) Dendritic cell-induced memory T cell activation in nonlymphoid tissues. Science 319: 198–202

[201] Weinlich G, Heine M, Stössel H, Zanella M, Stoitzner P, Ortner U, Smolle J, Koch F, Sepp NT, Schuler G, Romani N (1998) Entry into afferent lymphatics and maturation in situ of migrating murine cutaneous dendritic cells. J Invest Dermatol 110: 441–448

[202] Winkelmann RK (1977) The Merkel cell system and a comparison between it and the neurosecretory or APUD cell system. J Invest Dermatol 69: 41–46

[203] Wollenberg A, Wagner M, Gunther S, Towarowski A, Tuma E, Moderer M, Rothenfusser S, Wetzel S, Endres S, Hartmann G (2002) Plasmacytoid dendritic cells: a new cutaneous dendritic cell subset with distinct role in inflammatory skin diseases. J Invest Dermatol 119: 1096–1102

[204] Yang LY, Zheng JK, Liu XM, Hui GZ, Guo LH (2004) Culture of skin-derived precursors and their differentiation into neurons. Chin J Traumatol 7: 91–95

[205] Yu J, Vodyanik MA, Smuga-Otto K, Antosiewicz-Bourget J, Frane JL, Tian S, Nie J, Jonsdottir GA, Ruotti V, Stewart R, Slukvin II, Thomson JA (2007) Induced pluripotent stem cell lines derived from human somatic cells. Science 318: 1917–1920

[206] Yu N, Zhang S, Zuo F, Kang K, Guan M, Xiang L (2009) Cultured human melanocytes express functional toll-like receptors 2–4, 7 and 9. J Dermatol Sci 56: 113–120

[207] Yurchenco PD, Amenta PS, Patton BL (2004) Basement membrane assembly, stability and activities observed through a developmental lens. Matrix Biol 22: 521–538

[208] Zaba LC, Fuentes-Duculan J, Steinman RM, Krueger JG, Lowes MA (2007) Normal human dermis contains distinct populations of CD11c$^+$BDCA-1$^+$ dendritic cells and CD163$^+$FXIIIA$^+$ macrophages. J Clin Invest 117: 2517–2525

[209] Zhao Z, Liao L, Cao Y, Jiang X, Zhao RC (2005) Establishment and properties of fetal dermis-derived mesenchymal stem cell lines: plasticity in vitro and hematopoietic protection in vivo. Bone Marrow Transplant 36: 355–365

Correspondence: Adelheid Elbe-Bürger, Department of Dermatology, DIAID, Medical University of Vienna, Währinger Gürtel 18–20, 1090 Vienna, Austria, Phone: +43 1 40160 63001, E-mail: adelheid.elbe-buerger@meduniwien.ac.at

Burn wound healing: Pathophysiology

Luc Teot, Sami Otman, Antonio Brancati, Rainer Mittermayr

Burns Unit, Wound Healing Unit, Lapeyronie Hospital, Montpellier University Hospital Montpellier Cedex, France

Introduction

Burn injuries represent a specific wound entity with unique clinical features which range from the difficulty of initial assessment to the long-term tendency to develop pathologic scars. For long time considered as acute wounds, burns are in fact wounds showing a long term evolution transforming them into chronic wounds, if inadequately managed. The pathophysiological changes in the burn wound are characterized by effects caused by heat *per se* and complex superimposed local as well as systemic alterations. Due to profound disturbances of the immunostatus in general burn wounds are highly susceptible to infections upon completed keratinization. A common consensus among burn specialists emerges considering that a burn wound has to be covered within a period of two to three weeks, justifying a dogma of rapid excision and grafting, a surgical approach popularized by surgeons since the 70's. In fact, burn wounds which remained unhealed for several weeks or months, either due to skin graft infection or by accumulation of the high level of proteases included the wound after 3 to 4 weeks of non-healing.

Local biological events occurring after burns

The skin is supposed to be the largest organ realizing multiple functions. It maintains not only a physical but also an immunological protective barrier conserving the organism against physical abrasion, bacterial invasion, dehydration, and ultraviolet radiation. Body temperature is kept constant by adaptation of the blood flow in the dermal plexus in conjunction with the tight regulation of fluid homeostasis via the sweet glands (thermoregulation). The skin contains abundant nerve endings and receptors that detect stimuli related to temperature, touch, pressure, and pain (sensation). Finally it defines also the personal features of the social appearance. Exogenous aggressors such as burns result in either the loss or disruption of some or all of these functions.

Jackson first described three zones of burn injury [1].

1. **Zone of coagulation:** The area of maximum impact is located at the center of the wound and is characterized by irreversible tissue loss. Coagulation and denaturation of the constituent proteins and loss of plasma membrane integrity is observed, with a necrosis visible at the center of injury.

2. **Zone of stasis:** In the surrounding zone of stasis a compromised tissue perfusion could be observed, ranging from critical capillary vasoconstriction to ischemia. This zone may be easily transformed into necrosis due to the accumulated effects of decreased perfusion, edema and infection. However, when correctly managed these changes may be preserved.

3. **Zone of hyperemia:** The outer periphery of the burn wound represents the zone of hyperemia

characterized by viable cells and vasodilatation mediated by local inflammatory mediators. Tissue within this zone usually recovers completely unless complicated by infection or severe hypoperfusion.

Secondary to the tissue loss in the zone of coagulation due to direct heat induced protein denaturation, especially the zone of stasis and hyperemia further contribute to the local pathology of the burn injury. An intense activation of toxic inflammatory mediators such as oxidants and proteases further damage skin and capillary endothelial cells, thus aggravating severity of trauma by inducing further ischemic tissue necrosis [2].

Immediately after burn, microvessels in the mentioned zones lose their capacity to keep fluids apart from the interstitial area. Loss of fluid and proteins is intense and contemporary to shift in the ionic content of the cells. This induced ischemia could lead to an increase in depth and the aggravation of tissue loss. This microvascular injury is of dual origin, on one side due to the intensity of thermal injury and on the other hand due to vasoconstrictive substances. The microcirculatory changes induced by the thermal impact may be also related to an excessive hydrostatic pressure. The hypovolemic shock as well as the coexistent tissue trauma by itself create the burn shock, a specific situation, which increases the entire body inflammatory response and turning it into an accelerated multi-organ failure. The hypermetabolic response of burns injury should be managed accurately [3].

Inflammation

The inflammatory response following thermal injury is characterized by specific differences in comparison to the "normal" wound healing process. It is controlled by a large number of mediators originating from the major plasma enzyme systems and released from different kinds of leucocytes. Fast-acting mediators, such as vasoactive amines and the products of the kinin system, modulate the immediate response. The early phase of post-burn edema seems to be partly mediated by the vasoactive histamine [4]. It was shown that in thermal injury an increased activation of the kinin system occurs [5]. This may be attributed to excessive activation of the Hageman factor (F XII) [6] which not only leads to increased activation of the kallikrenin-bradykinin system but also has consequences on the arachidonic acid cascade, complement cascade, and the coagulation-fibrinolytic cascades. However, bradykinin as a product from the kinin system considerably contributes to the local edema formation due increased venular dilation and permeability.

On the other hand the biosynthesis of the metabolites from the arachidonic acid cascade, specifically prostaglandins, prostacyclin, and thromboxan A2, are also increased [7]. In this context prostacyclin could lead to perpetuation of burn edema formation, and thromboxan A2 may be responsible for vasoconstriction and local ischemia in burned tissue.

The alternative pathway to activate the complement system in burns seems to be favored although an activation by hydroxyl radicals were been shown also [8]. Depletion of complement components takes place, early after thermal injury, concomitant with reduction in the serum opsonic activity for various bacteria [9]. Increased levels of the activated complement components C3 a and C5 a (anaphylatoxins) in the plasma of burn patients are considered to regulate polymorphonuclear leucocytes function in these patients [10].

A hypercoagulability in thermally damaged tissue has been observed two to three hours following scalding due to a pronounced activation of the coagulation cascade [11]. These findings correlate well with the increase of kinins in the lymph, indicating that the Hageman factor may serve as a common activator of the kinin and the coagulation-fibrinolytic system.

As soon as leucocytes have arrived at the site of injury or infection, they release mediators which control the later accumulation and activation of other cells. Cytokines are involved in both inflammation and immunity. These mediators regulate the amplitude and duration of the inflammatory response and have multiple overlapping regulatory actions. Among the number of cytokines released by activated platelets, IGF-1 was to be reduced and correlated with the burn surface area [12]. This lower IGF-I level may contribute to the impaired wound healing in these patients. IGF-1 also lowers protein oxidation in patients with thermal injury.

In this context, the function of various cell types as a main source of such cytokines is also modified by the thermal impact.

Polymorphonuclear cells show dysfunction in chemotaxis, phagocytosis, oxidative metabolism, granular enzyme contents and intracellular killing. A proposed mechanism is an overall systemic catabolism of the contractile actin protein in these cells. One consequence could include a predisposition for infectious complications [13].

Immunosuppression is often seen in severe thermal injury [14]. In this context the cell-mediated immunity (lymphocytes) is usually severely impaired. The lymphocyte subpopulations were shown to be altered following injury by means of flow cytometry, where all T-lymphocyte subpopulations decrease (CD4 lymphocytes within 48h and a larger proportion of CD8 cells for the following 3 weeks). B-lymphocytes and CD16 (natural killer cells), however, were found to be unchanged following thermal injury. In addition, a severe thermal injury is of such a magnitude that the extent of immunosuppression appears to be greater than following other forms of trauma.

Mastcells also secrete a broad range of substances including chemoattractants (TNF-α, IL-8, LTB4, PAF), vasoactivators (histamine, PAF, kininogenase) and spasmogens (histamine, PGD2, LTC4, LTD4) [15]. Thus, following thermal injury the chemoattractants released from mast cells directly contribute to the recruitment and interstitial migration of leucocytes. Furthermore, the mast cell-dependent arteriolar constriction that produces temporary reduction of blood flow immediately after tissue injury may provide favourable haemodynamic conditions for blood clotting and leucocyte migration.

Monocytes (upon activation termed as macrophages) release beside others IL-1 and TNF-a having a stimulatory effect on T-cells but also an influence of the control of remote functions (production of e. g. acute phase proteins, IL-6, and fever) [16]. On the other hand induce the thermal impact changes in skin proteins which have a specific effect on monocyte IL-1 secretion. It has been suggested that blood monocytes are superstimulated following severe burns in vivo and produce large amounts of IL-1 leading to exhaustion of monocyte function.

Edema

Edema, occurring during the first 24 hours is by itself a source of secondary induced lesions. During the first day after injury, extravasation occurs in both the burned skin and the non burned tissues. The amount of edema in burned skin depends on the type and extent of injury, but also on the type and degree of resuscitation administered. When burns involve large areas, edema is intense and creates important secondary lesions in the surrounding zones. Chemical mediators (cytokines) as discussed previously are intensively released into the burn lesion during the first 24 hours. Large amounts of histamine are released into the burn area from mast cells, increasing vessel permeability in the early stage. Prostaglandins are released from burned tissues, and act as potent vasoactive mediators. Serotonin, coming from platelets, is also released in the burn area. Its role is supposed to increase hydrostatic pressure by limiting the vein diameter. Bradykinin plays also a substantial role in the inflammatory process and has important effects in terms of edema formation. However, the role of these mediators remains poorly understood, and anti-mediators used in clinical situations do not substantially affect the edema formation. Free oxygen radicals are released in large amounts after trauma in general and burns in particular. Antioxidants have been shown to be partially efficient in reducing the extent of edema formation [17].

Kramer and Herndon [18] analyzed the factors interrelating the physiological determinants of trans-microvascular fluid flux, and could determine that edema is a resulting factor of several items (increased capillary filtration, capillary pressure, interstitial hydrostatic pressure, osmotic reflection coefficient, plasma colloid osmotic pressure, and interstitial colloid osmotic pressure).

Burn wound conversion

Burn wound conversion is also attributed to the secondary consequences of burn injury (Fig. 1). As a unique property of burn injury the wound extension shows dynamic characteristics in the sub-acute postburn phase. Burn wounds initially assessed as superficial could further progress into deep(er) lesions involving previously unburned adjacent tissue. A multitude of associated factors are related to an over-expression of vasoactive and inflammatory mediators. An imbalance between vasodilatory and vasoconstrictory prostanoids potentially could threat-

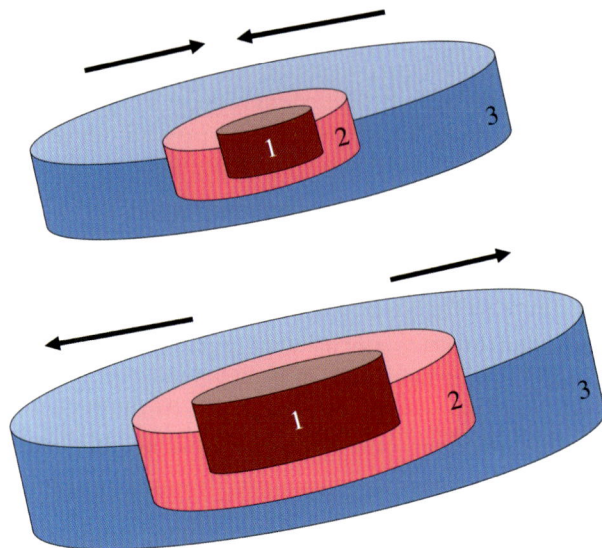

Fig. 1. Thermal burns covering limited areas (above) show recovery due to re-epithelialization after adequate management (arrows indicate recovery by re-epithelialization). If the burn wound exceeds a certain surface area (below) burn wound conversion is observed due to an overexpression of vasoactive and inflammatory mediators (arrows indicate progression of tissue downfall). (1) Zone of coagulation (2) Zone of stasis (3) Zone of hyperemia

en the viability of tissue in the zone of stasis [19]. However, also vasodilation is implicated in the progression of the burn wound. Up-regulation of inducible nitric oxide synthase causes peripheral vasodilation in the hyperemia and stasis zone thus perpetuating inflammation. Moreover, transcription factor nuclear factor KB (NF-κB), which is also up-regulated, induces increased downstream production of many inflammatory cytokines [20].

Toxic secondary products of activated xanthine oxidase as well as neutrophils, including hydrogen peroxide, superoxide and hydroxyl radicals, appear to directly damage dermal structures. A concomitant decrease in the physiological antioxidant mechanisms (e. g. superoxide dismutase, catalase, glutathione, α-tocopherol, and ascorbic acid levels) further impairs the local defense.

Hypoperfusion secondary to edema formation may also be linked to the conversion phenomenon. Increased vessel permeability whether as a reactive consequence of various factors (e. g. postaglandins, bradykinine, histamine) or celltoxic oxygen radicals

causes an interstitial fluid shift exacerbating hypoperfusion in vulnerable tissue, specifically in the zones of stasis and hyperemia [2].

Elevated levels of bradykinin are not only responsible for increased vascular permeability but also cause hypercoagulation thus resulting in microthrombosis. In combination with the procoagulant properties of thermal energy, bradykinin may stimulate microthrombosis in the zone of stasis and, as such, contribute to the burn wound progression.

Evolution of the burn wound and local consequences of burns

Burn wounds do not represent a static wound condition with determinate wound depth just after the thermal aggression.

If temperatures of a minimum of 45 °C for one minute are needed to create a deep burn, an exposure to a temperature of 100 °C for only one second leads to the same lesion. During the first 24 hours, several factors may lead to a local degradation. Jackson could distinguish three different zones: the burn lesion itself; an adjacent area of stasis; and the periwound area filled with edema. Depending on the general evolution of the patient and the local treatment, the zone of stasis may create an obstacle to revascularization and could emerge as an origin of secondary worsening of the burn wound.

On the contrary, a rigorous management of both the local wound and the general condition of the patient is of good prognosis factor. The burn impact induces a catecholamine surge, a hypermetabolic response, a shock. Adapted resuscitation measures may prevent a fatal outcome in severe burns. This period is at high risk of development of a local delay in healing leading to infection. Locally the most important factor impairing healing (as well as life threatening) remains infection. The general management of infection will be combined to a local use of a large variety of topical antimicrobials.

Common germs responsible for local infections are multiple and are sometimes difficult to treat. Rigorous isolation protocols and the use of new types of antibiotics (e. g. vancomycin and piperacillin/tazobactam) are capable to reduce both the local and the systemic infectivity of the multidrug resistant staphylococcus aureus. Pseudomonas aeruginosa and Acinetobacter are the main gram negative germs, on which colistin seems to act efficiently. Candida, Aspergillus and Fusarium are the most frequently encountered fungal pathogens, on which amphotericin B and voriconazole may sufficiently act. These germs interfere with the wound healing process and could further contribute to the extent of the necrotic tissue [21].

Hypergranulation may be observed when burns are not appropriately managed. Granulation tissue is present over large burns areas where epidermisation is lacking. Hypergranulation is an obstacle to epidermisation. An adapted local management, using corticosteroid will limit overgrowth and stabilize the granulation tissue at the same level than the surrounding epidermis.

Burns generate a high level of inflammation, impairing the whole healing process and in particular epidermisation. However, epidermisation should be obtained as fast as possible. Deep burns will need to be covered using surgical procedures of reconstructive skin surgery like skin grafts or flaps. More superficial wounds should be subjected to a quick surgical coverage using a combination of dermal and epidermal replacement. This constitutes the best local solution to obtain a stable non retractile scar. Total thickness skin grafts offer this type of solution, but the scarcity of sources especially in large burned individuals makes them unavailable to recover extended areas. Partial thickness skin grafts offer a good covering alternative in most clinical routine cases, subject to the condition that rehabilitation is started rapidly. When used on highly retractile areas like joints in fingers, the hand or wrist areas, the use of partial thickness skin graft may lead to retractile scars. The foot needs a dermal replacement thick enough to prevent hyperkeratosis and/or secondary dermabrasions. Nevertheless, one difference observed between burns and chronic wounds is that in chronic wounds the capacity for re-epidermisation is linked to the general condition of the patient, whose slow recovery issues to a very slow re-epidermisation process. In chronic burns, epidermisation is sometimes more difficult to achieve than in any other type of wound.

The last biological stage in burn healing is maturation of the wound, a period of time which describes the process of tissue remodeling resulting in a mature scar. This phase usually lasts for approximately 12 months, although sometimes prolonged (up to two years or longer in children, or in specific anatomical locations with high mechanostimulation, like the intermammary folds in women). On the other hand is an adequate mechanostimulation of scars a well accepted therapeutic approach to counteract the myofibroblast cell proliferation [22]. However, careful attention has to be drawn on adapted mechanical forces to manage scars resulting from burns sufficiently. Pathological scars are supposedly related to a disorder of wound healing [23]. The tendency to develop pathological scarring is more pronounced in burns of thermal origin. Joint retractions are often clinically observed when rehabilitation was not done correctly. Rehabilitation is mandatory to prevent pathological burns wound maturation.

If a burn wound is not adequately treated ending up in a chronic burn wound, healing will eventually also occur due to an intense skin contraction certainly as a consequence to the prolonged and intensive inflammatory process. These situations are still observed in emerging countries, issuing to extensive retractile scars, sources of important functional loss, particularly on the extremities. When burns occur early in life, these scars are source of intense deformities and irreversible loss of function (hand, wrist, elbow, shoulder being sometimes retracted together). These skin deformities generate in children an imbalance on the growing areas of bones at the extremities thus possibly resulting in irreversible changes in the skeletal shape.

General factors influencing the burn wound evolution

Skin lesions begin to appear after a heat exposure between 45 °C (1 hour) and 70 °C (a few seconds). A series of considerations in the wound management of thermal injuries should be taken into account.

Types of burns

Origin of burns can be thermal, electric or chemical.

▶ Thermal burns constitute the major group with an incidence of 80 % and present a specific profile. They are considered not only as wounds but also as a general disease with subsequent consequences on thermal regulation, glycemia control, immunological status, myocardial function and pulmonary hypertension. The resulting scars after thermal burns also present a higher tendency to develop hypertrophy and following congestion could last for a long period of time, longer than in any other type of burn injury.

▶ Electrical burns show a special feature, with two different types of lesion:
Flash burns, where the electrical current is spread on the surface of the skin. These lesions look like thermal burns.
Electrical passage burns show an entry point and an exit point, mostly found on the hand and the foot, the source of electricity being hung in the palm of the hand, the current running into the body, looking for a contact with earth, and exiting at the foot level. The heart may be also affected, with potential cardiac arrest due to a resonance effect between the amperage of the electrical current and the cardiac His bundle.

▶ Chemical burns often present a combination of chemical toxic effects on skin and thermal consequences. Basis and acids may attack the skin and the underlying tissues. The more concentrated the more invasive are the lesions, with a remnant effect sometimes which renders a simple lavage not sufficient for stopping progression of lesions towards the depth of the tissues. The development of amphotere solutions (Diphoterine gel, to be applied over mucosae as well as over skin lesions [24]), capable to react with both acid and basic aggressive products, has limited the interest of the "principle of neutralization" proned some decades ago. This attitude was more to rinse the fresh burns with a reverse base acid solution equivalent in concentration.

The systemic response to local burns

The release of cytokines and other inflammatory mediators at the site of injury has a systemic effect (Fig. 2) if burns involve more than 20 % of total body surface area (TBSA). Severe alterations of the cardiovascular function may determine the degree of the burn shock, an abnormal physiologic state in which tissue perfusion is insufficient to maintain adequate delivery of oxygen and nutrients and removal of cellular waste products [25].

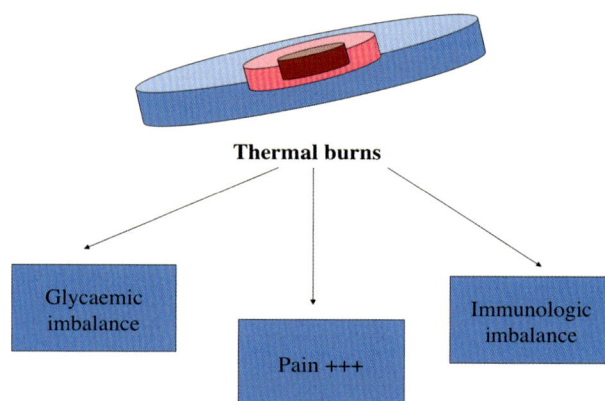

Fig. 2. Extended burn wounds (>20% TBSA) lead to a systemic response involving multiple organs and functional systems potentially leading to the burn shock

Influence of immediate care on burn wounds

The quality of immediate care has an important influence on the outcome of the burn wound. A superficial second degree burn observed during the initial evaluation can turn into a deep second degree burn the day after (burn wound conversion), either due to a poor general management or because the general condition worsens in the resuscitation unit. Problems inherent to immediate burn care will not be developed in this chapter; however, it is important to keep the importance of adapted resuscitation protocols during the initial stage in mind. Application of systemic antimicrobials is also of importance and has to be considered when dealing with general infections originating from the burn wound.

Pathophysiological consequences of choice of strategies concerning burn wound healing

In third degree burns, the strategy should remain univoqual. Early excision and skin grafting were adopted by most of the physicians since the last thirty years (Fig. 3). Nowadays the question is more which skin substitute is sufficiently able to minimize the scarring process. Dermal replacement is a real issue to prevent functional damages and cosmetic consequences. Options like choosing a two step procedure (delayed skin graft after a period of dermal re-vascularisation) or a single step procedure (immediate skin grafting after application of a dermal substitute) are linked to the angiogenetic capacities of the excised recipient wound bed to penetrate and to re-vascularize the inert material, sufficiently nourishing the freshly applied skin graft [26].

In second degree burns, difficulties concerning the adequate assessment and management of the infection risk still persist:

► Assessment of burns is considered to be insufficiently precise in more than 40 % of the cases evaluated by the specialists, especially during the first three days post burn. Hereby, primarily the assessment of the burn depth is at high risk to a false diagnosis. Some clinical key elements could be helpful to accurately evaluate the depth of the burn lesion initially. Superficial burns are characterized by severe pain at gauze passage, uniform redness of the surface, and vulnerability to bleeding. In contrast, deep second degree burns show a red-white aspect, a non hemorrhagic surface, and only a moderate pain at gauze passage.

► The adapted dressing should prevent in this period a pejorative evolution towards infection, and cover this risk. Topical antimicrobials are still first choice in the local treatment, and the most used agent is silversulfadiazine cream.

► A pending question is to change habits in using large quantities of antiseptics, still largely used in order to prevent infection in this situation, and abandon or change to milder concentrations as proposed in some new solutions like biguanides? It is still too early to answer these questions and large trials should be done in order to check the capacities of these new strategies to control infection and prevent skin damages.

The healing potential of burns: a chronic dilemna

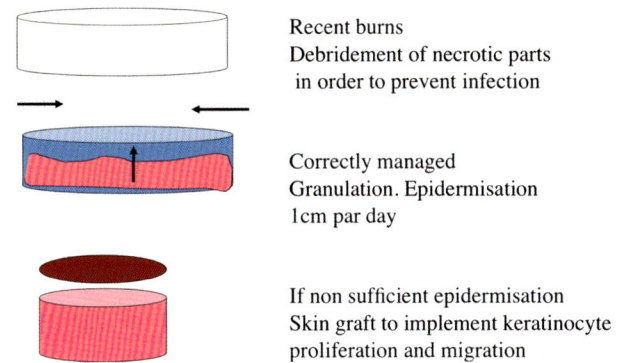

Recent burns
Debridement of necrotic parts
in order to prevent infection

Correctly managed
Granulation. Epidermisation
1cm par day

If non sufficient epidermisation
Skin graft to implement keratinocyte
proliferation and migration

Fig. 3. The healing potential of burns

Conclusion

The pathophysiology of burn wounds is univoqual for limited surfaces, and becomes dual when the TBSA is important, with a vicious circle between local and systemic effects. In this situation the local lesion will be aggravated by the intense inflammatory process and the impaired vascularization secondary to the large amount of edema. These changes, combined with local consequences of the general poor condition, create a rapid degradation of the patient's status, leading to the burn shock.

Early rescucitation, an adapted local management and the systematic prevention of infection (local and general) should be realized early, and combined with an aggressive debridement of deep burnt areas.

References

[1] Jackson DM(1953) [The diagnosis of the depth of burning]. Br J Surg 40: 588–596
[2] Kao CC, Garner WL (2000) Acute burns. Plast Reconstr Surg 105: 2482–2492
[3] Williams FN, Herndon DN, Jeschke MG (2009) The hypermetabolic response to burn injury and interventions to modify this response. Clin Plast Surg 36: 583–596
[4] Friedl HP, Till GO, Trentz O, Ward PA (1989) Roles of histamine, complement and xanthine oxidase in thermal injury of skin. Am J Pathol 135: 203–217
[5] Arturson G (1969) The plasma kinins in thermal injury. Scand J Clin Lab Invest [Suppl] 107: 153–161
[6] Arturson G (1996) Pathophysiology of the burn wound and pharmacological treatment. The Rudi Hermans Lecture, 1995. Burns 22: 255–274

[7]   Zweifach BW (1986) Dynamic sequelae of the acute in-flammatory process: a state-of-the-art review. In: Little RA, Frayn KN (eds) The scientific basis for the care of the critically ill. Manchester University Press, Manchester

[8]   Gelfand JA, Donelan M, Burke JF (1983) Preferential activation and depletion of the alternative complement pathway by burn injury. Ann Surg 198: 58–62

[9]   Bjornson AB, Altemeier WA, Bjornson HS (1980) Complement, opsonins, and the immune response to bacterial infection in burned patients. Ann Surg 191: 323–329

[10]   Davis CF, Moore FD, Jr, Rodrick ML, Fearon DT, Mannick JA (1987) Neutrophil activation after burn injury: contributions of the classic complement pathway and of endotoxin. Surgery 102: 477–484

[11]   Edery H, Lewis GP (1963) Kinin-forming activity and histamine in lymph after tissue injury. J Physiol 169: 568–583

[12]   Moller S, Jensen M, Svensson P, Skakkebaek NE(1991) Insulin-like growth factor 1 (IGF-1) in burn patients. Burns 17: 279–281

[13]   sko-Seljavaara S(1987) Granulocyte kinetics in burns. J Burn Care Rehabil 8: 492–495

[14]   O'Sullivan ST, O'Connor TP(1997) Immunosuppression following thermal injury: the pathogenesis of immunodysfunction. Br J Plast Surg 50: 615–623

[15]   Gordon JR, Burd PR, Galli SJ(1990) Mast cells as a source of multifunctional cytokines. Immunol. Today 11: 458–464

[16]   Schwacha MG (2003) Macrophages and post-burn immune dysfunction. Burns 29: 1–14

[17]   Demling RH (2005) The burn edema process: current concepts. J Burn Care Rehabil 26: 207–227

[18]   Kramer GC, Herndon DN, Linares HA, Traber DL (1989) Effects of inhalation injury on airway blood flow and edema formation. J Burn Care Rehabil 10: 45–51

[19]   Robson MC, Del Beccaro EJ, Heggers JP (1979) The effect of prostaglandins on the dermal microcirculation after burning, and the inhibition of the effect by specific pharmacological agents. Plast Reconstr Surg 63: 781–787

[20]   Rawlingson A (2003) Nitric oxide, inflammation and acute burn injury. Burns 29: 631–640

[21]   Branski LK et al (2009) Emerging infections in burns. Surg Infect (Larchmt) 10: 389–397

[22]   Desmouliere A, Chaponnier C, Gabbiani G (2005) Tissue repair, contraction, and the myofibroblast. Wound Repair Regen 13: 7–12

[23]   Shih B, Garside E, McGrouther DA, Bayat A(2010) Molecular dissection of abnormal wound healing processes resulting in keloid disease. Wound Repair Regen 18: 139–153

[24]   Hall AH, Cavallini M, Mathieu L, Maibach HI (2009) Safety of dermal diphoterine application: an active decontamination solution for chemical splash injuries. Cutan Ocul Toxicol 28: 149–156

[25]   Keck M, Herndon DH, Kamolz LP, Frey M, Jeschke MG (2009) Pathophysiology of burns. Wien Med Wochenschr 159: 327–336

[26]   Bloemen MC, van Leeuwen MC, van Vucht NE, van Zuijlen PP, Middelkoop E (2010) Dermal substitution in acute burns and reconstructive surgery: a 12-year follow-up. Plast Reconstr Surg 125: 1450–1459

Correspondence: Luc Teot, MD, PhD, Burns Unit, Wound Healing Unit, Lapeyronie Hospital, Montpellier University Hospital, 391 Avenue Doyen Giraud, 34 255 Montpellier Cedex, France, E-mail: lteot@aol.com

Burn scar treatment

Luc Teot, Sami Otman, Antonio Brancati, Rainer Mittermayr

Burns Unit, Wound Healing Unit, Lapeyronie Hospital, Montpellier University Hospital Montpellier Cedex, France

Physiological scarring

Scar formation is considered as an integrative part of the complex and dynamic process of normal physiological wound healing to restore skin integrity following injury and is referred as to the maturation phase. This phase is dominated by fibroblasts. The pivotal feature of this process is the synthesis, deposition, and remodeling of collagen, the major structural substance of connective tissue. The collagen deposition in normal wound healing peaks by the third week after injury. Collagen remodeling is characterized by a (balanced) continuous synthesis and degradation of collagen and is observed already early during the wound healing process. The degradation of wound collagen is controlled by a variety of enzymes such as collagenases (e. g. MMP-1) derived from granulocytes, macrophages, keratinocytes and fibroblasts. On the other hand the expression and activity of collagenases is tightly controlled by cytokines.

Wound contraction is a further inherent part of wound healing and is presented by an ongoing process resulting in part from the proliferation of a specialized fibroblast population termed as myofibroblasts containing myofilaments (α-SMA, desmin).

Overall, it has to be mentioned that scar tissue is never as strong as normal, uninjured skin. For the first 3 to 4 weeks after injury, the wound can easily be re-opened by minimal trauma. After 6 weeks, the scar has attained approximately half of its final strength. During the next 12 months, the scar gradually increases its ability to withstand injury, but it never attains normal strength (for review see [1]).

Pathological scarring

In some individuals, however, and particularly in burn victims, some of the wound healing processes may lead to production of overabundant extracellular matrix, resulting in abnormal scar formation, which is of altered composition (e. g. misbalanced collagen I/III ratio) and organization (e. g. non linear oriented collagen bundles). Causative factors which are implicated in pathological scar formation are a prolonged and subsequently dysregulated inflammatory phase, a misbalance between pro- and anti-fibrogenic factors, and the involvement of specific cell subpopulations.

Especially extended and deep wounds eliciting systemic responses, features of severe burn wounds, are prone to develop pathological scarring. While superficial burn wounds heal in a normal timely manner resulting in minimal scarring, deeper burns often result in pathological (hypertrophic) scarring necessitating further intervention. This is due to the fact that the majority of epidermal and dermal regenerative structures such as basal membrane, appendices, and hair follicles are destroyed and healing can only occur from the wound edges thus prolonging phases of wound healing. It was clinically shown that wounds which are not healed within a 3 weeks period have a high risk potential of hypertrophic scarring, independent of age, site and genetically predisposition [2]. Additionally, dermal fibroblasts were found to exhibit similar characteristics as fibroblasts cultured from hypertrophic scars, expressing higher TGF-β1, CTGF (connective tissue growth factor), and α-SMA levels [3–5].

Following the (thermal) impact the initial formed fibrin matrix serves as a scaffold for migrating cells. However, inadequate fibrin removal due to suppressed fibrinolysis controlled by the activity tissue plasminogen inhibitor-1 (is up-regulated by TGF-β1 and down regulated TGF-β3) impedes healing and might lead to fibrosis [6, 7]. Burns but also infected wounds (burn wounds are at high risk for infections) exaggerate especially the inflammatory phase thus leading to a misbalance in favor of a pro-fibrogenic status. Potential cytokines which are discussed in this context are PDGF, TGF-β, IGF-1, and IL-4.

PDGF is a degranulation product of platelets early during wound healing and is elevated in hypertrophic scar tissue. It has been shown as a potent promoter of fibroblast proliferation, extracellular matrix production, and the induction of the myofibroblast phenotype [1].

TGF-β is a cytokine well characterized as a fibrogenic factor and exists of three isoforms (TGF-β1 to 3). Following burn injury, TGF-β1 and 2 stimulate their own synthesis in an autocrine fashion and attract neutrophils monocytes as well as fibroblasts. In fibroblasts they stimulate the synthesis of collagen, fibronectin and certain glyosoaminoglycans partly via Smad transduction pathway [8].

TGF-β1 down regulates decorin, important for normal collagen fibrillogenesis, and up regulates versican and biglycan. Neovascularization is enhanced while different proteinases are modulated (MMP-1 down regulation).

In hypertrophic scars of post burn patients TGF-β is up-regulated locally and systemically [9].

A further factor which is also increased in hypertrophic scars is IGF-1, a cytokine with mitogenic activity on fibroblasts and endothelial cells with collagen synthesis stimulation of dermal fibroblasts [10].

Furthermore, it also decreases the expression of collagenase, thus aggravating the abnormal collagen deposition seen in hypertrophic scars [11].

Clinically, it has been well recognized that injuries associated with prolonged immune responses, such in burns, are predisposed to developing abnormal scarring. Therefore it is hypothesized that not the severity of inflammation predisposes to hypertrophic scarring but the type of immune response. The two subsets of CD41 cells present in wound healing, Th1 and Th2 cells, show antagonistic activity. While Th1 cytokine expression results in an antifibrotic phenotype (e. g. increased collagenase), Th2 cytokine profile results in pro-fibrotic milieu.

Studies evaluating the cytokine profile after burn injury show reduced Th1 cytokine synthesis (e. g. IL-2, IFN-γ) and increased Th2 cytokine profile [12, 13].

Th3, a further subtype of CD41 T-cells, is also pro-fibrotic, and was shown to be elevated in burn patients [14].

Therefore, it seems that early after burn injury a "Th2 immune response" leads to the pro-fibrotic Th3 cells which are capable to induce fibrosis, while inhibiting the antifibrotic Th1 activity [15].

Recently, a newly identified cell population, has been implicated in the pathopyhsiology of hypertrophic scars following thermal injury [16–18]. They exhibit both monocyte- and fibroblast like characteristics and originate from the bone marrow. They are thought to play a role in tissue repair by several mechanisms (e. g. ECM secretion, antigen presentation, cytokine production, angiogenesis). It is discussed that this cell population contribute to the myofibroblasts. In the peripheral blood of burn patients an increased percentage of fibrocytes were found compared to controls [17]. It was further shown that this fibrocytes from burned patients are able to modify dermal fibroblast function to increase the secretion for TGF-β and CTGF (Connective tissue growth factor), a factor stimulating the proliferation of fibroblasts and ECM protein synthesis and which may mediate many of the pro-fibrotic effects of TGF-β [19, 20].

There are many factors which lead in the outlined scar pathophysiology. In general, a higher prevalence of abnormal scarring is observed in burn patients (dependent upon burn extension), especially when caused by flame. The burn location is

Table 1. Scar classification from Mustoe et al. [21]

Scar type	Description
Mature scar	A light-colored, flat scar.
Immature scar	A red, sometimes itchy or painful, and slightly elevated scar in the process of remodeling. Many of these will mature normally over time and become flat, and assume a pigmentation that is similar to the surrounding skin, although they can be paler or slightly darker.
Linear hypertrophic (e.g., surgical/traumatic) scar	A red, raised, sometimes itchy scar confined to the border of the original surgical incision. This usually occurs within weeks after surgery. These scars may increase in size rapidly for 3–6 months and then, after a static phase, begin to regress. They generally mature to have an elevated, slightly rope-like appearance with increased width, which is variable. The full maturation process may take up to 2 years.
Widespread hypertrophic (e.g., burn) scar	A widespread red, raised, sometimes itchy scar that remains within the borders of the burn injury.
Minor keloid	A focally raised, itchy scar extending over normal tissue. This may develop up to 1 year after injury and does not regress on its own. Simple surgical excision is often followed by recurrence. There may be a genetic abnormality involved in keloid scarring. Typical sites include earlobes.
Major keloid	A large, raised (>0.5 cm) scar, possibly painful or pruritic and extending over normal tissue. This often results from minor trauma and can continue to spread over years.

also implied as a risk factor for pathological scar formation. However, both sexes show equal distribution, but hypertrophy is more common in children. Race as a risk factor is also discussed in the literature, with black patients bearing a higher risk compared to others.

To summarize, a lot of various factors of the normal physiological wound healing cascade are altered in a manner that finally result in abnormal scarring, which is primarily characterized by excessive disorientated collagen deposition.

Scar classification and grading

Classifying scars is essential for choosing the right treatment regime. Several approaches try to differentiate the pathological scars according to their appearance, histological patterns, and clinical symptoms. Recently, a schema was proposed by Mustoe et al. [21] with modified standard terminology to be clinically as relevant as possible (Table 1).

On the other hand, also a number of different grading systems were developed, in an effort to adjust treatment to the stage of the scar. The Vancouver Scar Scale is probably the most common and widely used, evaluating the burn scar in an objective manner subsequently providing assistance in prognosis and management.

However, to prevent the development of unsatisfactory outcomes such as hypertrophic scarring or keloids, clinicians should already initially develop a routine scar assessment program during the first 3 months after complete healing has occurred [22].

Scar treatment

Pathological scarring is seen in more than 50 % of healed deep burns thus making it an important entity in the long term run of burn victims. Several clinical as well as experimental attempts focus this specific problem ranging from conservative biophysical measures, surgical treatment, to pharmacological interventions.

According to the current knowledge of abnormal pathological scarring therapeutic approaches can target (1) the mechanical properties of wound repair, (2) misbalance between collagen synthesis and degradation, and (3) the altered inflammatory response.

Scar prevention

Prevention of a pathological event is usually more effective than treating them which is additionally often unsatisfying and associated with additional burden to health care expenses. As previously mentioned thermal injuries especially when extended in area and depth are prone to hypertrophic scarring and could potentially benefit from preventive burn scar management. However, focusing on burn treatment, prevention or treatment of pathological scarring can be conceptually and practically similar especially when considering the high percentage of pathological scarring in burns. Therefore, treatment regimes which are used as preventive means could also be used in treating manifest pathologies and vice versa.

Many preventive (and) treatment strategies have proven their efficacy due to extensive clinical use, applied whether as single or as a combination therapy. However, only few have reached a certain evidenced base medicine level.

Surgical treatment options

Surgery – Prevention

A well accepted classification system of burn injuries is oriented on the extent of the skin component involved. Second (dermal) degree burns are additionally subdivided in superficial or deep. In the first, necrosis occupies only the upper (superficial) dermis, with unaffected reticular dermis. These burns are usually managed conservatively (without excision and grafting) due to the good healing prognosis as well as low incidence of abnormal scarring.

In contrast, in deep dermal burns, necrosis involves the reticular dermis and the zone of stasis further extends deep into the dermis. These burns are generally best treated with excision and grafting, which can reduce the risk of long-term complications such as hypertrophic scarring and burn contractures [23].

Full-thickness (third-degree) burns involve the entire dermis and are generally managed with excision and grafting.

Degree of scarring is strongly dependent on the duration of healing and thus on the residues of dermal components (= burn depth). In particular, deep wounds (full thickness wounds or wounds with considerable dermal component involvement) are considered to heal unlikely within 21 days, and Deitch et al. showed a significantly enhanced risk of abnormal scarring if the wound is persistent for 10 days and that this risk rise to 80 % for wounds which show delayed healing beyond day 21 [2].

Therefore, each burn which is expected to take more than 3 weeks to heal (especially with knowledge of high risk scar formers) should be considered to be early skin grafted. Again, clinical correct assessment of the burn is mandatory to draw conclusions regarding the expected healing time.

Excision of burn wounds with an adequate technique and control of blood loss followed by early wound closure, primarily with autologous skin grafts, could effectively decrease severity of hypertrophic scarring, contraction, and allows faster rehabilitation [24, 25].

Skin grafts are widely accepted as a standard method in covering extended excised burn and scar areas. Over the past decades, great advances were made regarding the technique and tools for skin graft harvesting as well as graft meshing. Skin graft could generally be divided in subgroups dependent on the amount of dermis involved. Split thickness skin grafts, thin or thick, include only a portion of the dermis, whereas full thickness skin grafts consist of the epidermis and the entire dermal layer.

It is the thickness which determines also the postoperative degree of wound contraction. Normally, the thinner the skin graft applied the higher the degree of contraction which may occur at the recipient site. This is of clinical importance which skin graft should be used in which location. Split thickness skin grafts are more suitable to cover large burn areas or large defects originating from excised abnormal scars without involving mobile joint surfaces.

Split-thickness grafts also have significant disadvantages that must be considered. Split-thickness grafts are more fragile (dependent whether thin, intermediate, or thick is chosen), especially when applied over areas with few underlying nutritional support. The contraction is more pronounced, lacks elasticity and grows adequately with the individual. They tend to be abnormally pigmented, either pale or white, or alternatively hyper-pigmented, particularly in darker-skinned individuals.

On the other hand, full thickness skin grafts, which tend to less contraction, are particularly used over joints, in the face and in defects of the hand. Additionally, for smaller (profound) burns with sufficient donor sites or locations susceptible for contraction and scarring sheet grafts can be considered as a valuable tool.

However, the follow up management has to be carefully carried out due to the possibility of hematoma and seroma accumulation underneath this sheet grafts compromising graft survival with potentially graft loss.

Skin grafts can be further subdivided into sheet (unmeshed) and meshed grafts. Meshed grafts are fenestrated using mesh ratios ranging from 1:1 to 4:1 thus enabling to cover larger defect areas. The risk of hematoma or seroma formation is minimized due to the drainage via the fenestration. However, meshed grafts again show a certain degree of contraction and scarring (according to the mesh pattern) with prolonged healing times dependent on the ratio used, because of lacking dermal components in the mesh interstices. Further means such as allografts or other biological dressings can be applied over higher meshed grafts to prevent desiccation.

In areas where functional as well as cosmetic results are favorable such as face, neck, and hands sheet grafts are to prefer over meshed grafts.

Surgery – Treatment

Surgical excision of hypertrophic scars or keloids is a common management option whether to release associated scar contraction or to improve esthetical appearance. Small lesions can be excised in total and closed primarily but using essential principles to avoid re-scarring. This include minimizing trauma to the dermal edges, avoidance of excessive wound traction, adequate amount of suture material in the right location, and avoidance of wound tension. However, in larger areas of abnormal scarring, which are more common in burned patients, with considerable contractions, partial release of this contraction should be considered. Coverage of the resulting defect could be realized using skin graft of flaps. Flaps are more effective than grafting in term of prevention re-contraction.

However, excision alone for example of keloids without additional measures may result in a recurrence rate as high as 90 %. Therefore, adjunctive treatment modalities are recommended for hypertrophic scars as well as in the treatment of keloids, which are discussed later.

Additional surgical techniques to treat hypertrophic scars are Z- or W-plasty to release scar tension. A profound treatment should achieve both excision with narrowing the scars and change of the direction of the scars realized by Z- or W-plasty. The main principle of the Z-plasty is the extension of a reduced distance and the main scar axis is changed parallel to skin creases. The W-plasty causes a disruption of the scar thus making it less conspicuous. Every other scar shank can be positioned within the skin creases.

In keloids, however, simple excision is inadequate due to the stimulation of additional collagen synthesis thus resulting in fast and often more pronounced recurrences. Therefore, an intramarginal surgical excision is highly recommended to prevent this collagen synthesis. Moreover, especially in keloids surgical therapy should be combined with adjuvant therapies which were already shown to lower recurrence rates.

Stretching forces to wounds are considered to substantially contribute to abnormal scarring. Tension at the wound borders compromises microvascular perfusion, prolongs inflammation, and increases time of healing resulting in enhanced fibroplasias. Thus special attention has to be drawn on preventing these avoidable risk factors. However, wounds prone to tension forces can be effectively physically supported by intradermal sutures for at least 6 weeks. Recently, a new suture material (V-Loc®, Covidien) was introduced that allows distributing the tension throughout the wound by grasping the tissue at multiple points that spreads the tension across the wound. Moreover, due to the design with unidirectional, circumferential shallow barbs it allows avoiding knotting, and reduces foreign body material with associated complications. Some recent studies [26, 27] were published, with promising results in term of cost-efficacy.

Dermal substitutes

An intact basal membrane and the source of keratinocytes, like hair follicles and annexiae are essential in re-epithelialization and wound healing. Additionally, the dermis is recognized to play a pivotal role in contraction. Scars of limited depth normally preserve elasticity. Contrary, loss of dermal components in deep wounds results in the absence of elasticity, and fibroblastic cell proliferation issuing to hypertrophy and contraction.

The recent development of dermal substitutes could open a place for their use in pathologic scar prevention. Multiple devices, integrating different technologies, are now proposed for use in burns and reconstructive surgery. These artificial dermis formed either by a single layer of product (to be immediately covered by skin grafts), or a double layer (a collagen based product covered by a film, to be re-populated before a second procedure of skin grafting), some of them being of allogenic origin, or derived from synthetic compounds, sometimes having been previously repopulated by cells (fibroblasts, keratinocytes or both). Extensive researches are still to be done, both in fundamental research as in clinical trials establishing the real benefit of these technologies.

Bilayer non-cellularized dermal regeneration templates

Integra® was the first artificial dermis launched on the market in the 1990s. Composed of bovine collagen (prion-free, containing glyosoaminoglycans), bilayer Integra® is covered with a thin layer of silicone that prevents collagen desiccation. In a two step procedure, first full laminar adhesion is essential to initiate angiogenesis and remodeling which is characterized by a neodermis constituting an intermediate layer between the skin graft and the underlying wound bed. The second surgical procedure is performed when the collagen has been re-vascularized (within three weeks if no adjunct negative-pressure therapy is implemented, or 10 days if TPN is employed). Follow-ing removal of the silicone layer, a split thickness sheet graft is placed onto the scaffold. This technique has recently been proposed as an alternative method of covering burns with large surface areas [28].

Renoskin® is a bilayer artificial dermis. Like Integra®, it comprises a collagen layer covered with a thin layer of silicone. It is used in deep burns, and more recently in all reconstructive surgical applications. Renoskin® appears to improve the flexibility of scar tissue.

Hyalomatrix® promotes the formation of budding tissue formed by hyaluronic acid which enables skin grafting after one to two weeks. The dermis formed in this manner is impregnated with hyaluronic acid, the graft takes more effectively and the underlying area is improved (elasticity and flexibility are enhanced) [29, 30].

Single-layer cellularized dermal regeneration templates

Pelnac® is a porcine tendon collagen, neutralized and freeze-dried, available as sponge membranes. After debridement, the artificial dermis is applied to wounds, and ointment-impregnated gauze is applied to prevent wound desiccation. The adapted atelocollagen sponge promotes the early infiltration of mononuclear cells and fibroblasts and better growth of connective tissue strands and epithelium. Consequently, abundant granulation tissue develops on the wound surface, over which free skin grafting can be performed after about two weeks [31]

Matriderm® is an original matrix consisting of collagen and elastin. Available as a flexible sheet it adepts to the wound shape. Once applied, it exerts a mild haemostatic effect through suction of the underlying tissue. Matriderm® can be applied to viable sub-cutaneous cell tissue, tendons or bony tissue. In a one step procedure Matriderm® is first applied as a dermal sub-layer followed by the skin graft. The usage of a thin skin graft is preferred, and initial results show clear benefits of this artificial skin in terms of ease of use and elasticity [32, 33].

Single-layer Integra® is composed of collagen and glyosoaminoglycans. It exhibits the same properties as classic Integra®, but has no silicone layer, making it suitable for immediate application of a thin skin graft (one step procedure).

Alloderm™ and Strattice, Permaform is derived from porcine dermis. These products may be used as solid thick structures. Their capacity of being penetrated by vessels is lower than the previous ones. Used in dura matrix replacement, they can be proposed as fixation devices for abdominal wall reconstruction or internal brass in mammary ptosis or after breast reduction.

Gliader™ has recently been proposed by the Dutch skin bank. Clinical indications are burns coverage and trauma. The device is immediately covered using skin grafts during the same surgical procedure or some days after.

Non surgical treatment options

Among a long list of proposals, some of them are considered now as a classical approach, like silicone gel sheets, with some evidence behind, others are gaining evidence like 5-FU [34] injections and Avotermin (TGF-β3) [35].

Adhesive tapes

Multidirectional tension on wounds is meanwhile recognized as an important pathophysiological factor in developing abnormal scarring. Eliminating such stretching forces on wounds can be easily achieved by applying microporous hypoallergenic paper tapes [36].

This enables to control the wound tension forces and preventing hypertrophic scarring. Treatment should be initiated early after surgery and maintained for several weeks, as maximum strength of a scar is only achieved after at least 12 weeks post wounding [37].

Although the exact mechanism of efficacy is unknown a dual working hypothesis is suggested. The mechanical influence similar to that using pressure garments seems to be obvious and second may be an occlusive component analogous to the treatment with silicone gel sheets.

Nevertheless, paper tapes are non-invasive, inexpensive with minimal demands on patients and could be therefore used as a preventive mean at least in low risk patients.

Pressure garments

It was in the late 1960 when pressure treatment arose as a therapeutic standard means to prevent and treat abnormal scarring in burned patients [38]. Mechanism which are discussed to be involved in the effects of pressure therapy are decreased scar blood flow, decreased edema formation, decreased protein deposition including chondroitin sulfate, and increased lysis. Once edema formation is decreased it lower also the measured pressure and increases scar tissue temperature which is regarded to pertain positive effects. Increased temperature, even by 1 °C, will significantly increase collagenolysis and scar maturation [39–42].

The garments should be applied as soon as possible after the acute and subacute burn treatment.

Recommendations regarding the pressure which should be applied range between 24 to 30 mmHg for 6 to 12 months, although these recommendations are largely based on empiric clinical findings. Typically the garments which are used are custom-made from an elastic material with a high content of spandex. The use could be limited in difficult anatomic locations such as flexures or areas of high mobility (e. g. joints). Furthermore, patient discomfort could lead to a major problem with reports of non-compliant patients from 8.5 % to 59 % [40, 41].

A recently conducted meta-analysis on the effectiveness of pressure garment therapy for the prevention of abnormal scarring after burn injury was unable to demonstrate a difference to control scars [43].

Silicone gel sheeting

Since the early 1980s silicone gel sheeting became popular in the treatment of scar pathologies and has now good evidence in efficacy as demonstrated by several studies as a safe and effective management option [44–50].

More than 60 silicone elastomeric products have been marketed since 1990 [51].

Although the exact mechanism of silicone gel sheeting on improvement of abnormal scars is uncertain several hypothesis are proposed.

Possible mechanisms include increased temperature, hydration caused by occlusion of the underlying skin, increased oxygen tension, direct action of the silicone oil, and polarization of the scar tissue caused by the negative static electric charge generated by movement of the silicone [52–56].

The use of silicone gel sheeting is recommended to begin soon after the wound is entirely epithelialized and these sheets should be worn for at least 12 hours/day for a minimum of 2 months. Unfavorable events such as pruritus, rash, maceration, and odor can be managed by temporary interruption of treatment and regular washing of the sheet and the scar.

Many clinicians adopt a multimodal approach to the treatment and prevention of hypertrophic and keloid scars.

Corticosteroids

Intralesional corticosteroid injections are already used since the mid 1960s in scar management and are able to reduce scar volume while improving pliability, height and symptoms such as pruritus [57, 58].

Corticosteroid application has antimitotic effect on fibroblast thus decreasing fibroblast proliferation. This diminishes the collagen synthesis, and glyosoaminoglycans synthesis. Finally it suppresses pro-inflammatory mediators by inhibition of leukocytes and monocytes [59, 60].

The most common corticosteroid which is used for the treatment of scars is insoluble triamicinolone acetonide in a concentration of 10 to 40 mg/ml dependent on the scar pathology (10 mg/ml every 3 to 6 weeks in developing hypertrophic scars; 40 mg/ml 3 monthly in manifest keloids) [61].

Due to the painful sensations during intralesional injection the combination with a local anesthetic such as lidocain is recommended. Further common side effects include tissue atrophy, teleangiectasien, hypopigmentation, and rebound effects [57, 62].

However, due to broad variation in response rates from 50 to 100 % with recurrences of 9 to 50 % [42].

Combination with other therapies such as surgery, laser, and 5-fluorouracil may improve outcome [57, 63, 64].

Because of the poor absorption of topical administered corticosteroids usage is only of limited effect and thus preserved for superficial lesions only.

Radiotherapy

First reports using radiation for the treatment of keloids date back to 1906. But further evidence suggested that the monotherapy is inadequate [65] (response from 10 to 94 % with keloid recurrence rate of 50 to 100 %) [66].

Therefore radiotherapy was used in conjunction with other treatment modalities such as surgery and reported response rates varied between 65 and 99 % when compared

Proposed mode of efficacy is the direct apoptotic effect on cells in particular on fibroblast by using the suggested 15 to 20 Gy which should be fractionated over 5 to 6 treatment sessions in the early postoperative phase [67].

However, radiotherapy is still discussed controversially due to (anecdotal) reports of inducing malignancies especially when used as monotherapy. On the other hand large studies with long-term follow-up showed no evidence to substantiate the risk of carcinogenesis [68].

Nevertheless, radiotherapy remains a valuable and effective therapeutic option in severe keloids. It its suggested that a close team work up is carried out between surgeons and radiation oncologists before excluding radiotherapy in the treatment of keloids [69].

Laser therapy

Since the introduction of laser treatment in the indication of hypertrophic scars and keloids in the mid-1980s, more and more lasers with different wavelengths have been studied [70, 71].

Argon and CO2 lasers were examined in the treatment of hypertrophic scars with initially promising results but showed during follow-up high recurrence rate [72, 73].

More recent wavelength-specific lasers such as flashlamp-pulsed dye lasers (PDL) and the non-laser intense-pulsed light source were able to improve the scar texture, erythema, size and pliability of hypertrophic scar with the consequence that this lasers were used more frequently [74–77].

Currently, the PDL wavelengths 585 and 595 nm are most frequently used for therapeutic purposes.

For neodymium:yttrium-aluminum-garnet (Nd:YAG) lasers response rates between 36 and 47 percent are reported [73].

However, in a recent study determining Nd:YAG laser on keloids, nearly 60 % of the keloids were flattened after one treatment session. Additionally, these patients remained free of keloid scarring in the follow-up period of 5 years [78].

A study evaluating the pulsed erbium:yttrium-aluminum-garnet laser showed efficacy in the treatment of hypertrophic and depressed scars, without serious side effects [79].

Lasers have been shown also to be effective not only in the treatment of manifest abnormal scarring but also in the prevention of hypertrophic scars. In 1996, Gaston *et al* reported that a 585-nm PDL was effective in preventing the formation of hypertrophic scars in burn wounds [80].

This study is supported by other experimental studies, including incisional and burn wounds [81].

The mechanism of action by which laser irradiation improves proliferative scars is not known. Suggested theories are based on selective photothermolysis, in which the light energy emitted from a vascular laser (such as PDL) is absorbed by hemoglobin, generating heat and leading to coagulation necrosis thus inducing local hypoxia [82, 83].

It is also suggested that hypoxia induction by laser destruction of capillaries might also alter collagen synthesis by fibroblasts and degradation through metalloproteinase release [84].

Further factors which are discussed in conjunction with scar improvement are decreased fibroblast proliferation and collagen III deposition [85].

TGF-β1 is considered to induce and modulate collagen formation and PDL treatment is associated with the down regulation of TGF-β1 expression associated with an increase of MMP-13 (collagenase 3) activity [86].

Although lack of large controlled studies, laser therapy remains emerging technology, and further studies should be conducted to further evaluate efficacy in abnormal scar treatment.

Cryotherapy

Cryotherapy whether by contact or by spray using liquid nitrogen can effectively improve hypertrophic scars and keloids [87, 88].

When used as a single therapy it can result in flattening of keloids in 51 to 74 %, although several treatment sessions are necessary [88–90].

Application of cryotherapy induces local ischemia with subsequent necrosis of the hypertrophic scar tissue [63].

Due to the common side effect of permanent hypopigmentation as well as the long postoperative healing phase between the single applications this treatment modality is limited in general for small scars only. Other side effects include pain upon application, hyperpigmentation, and skin atrophy [87].

Recently, a new method has been developed to avoid drawbacks of the classical cryotherapy. An intralesional needle cryoprobe is inserted longitudinally in the scar axis to maximize the volume of tissue which can be frozen [88].

It was shown that a single application can achieve 50 % scar volume reduction, with only mild local edema and epidermiolysis, accompanied by mild pain or discomfort.

5-Fluorouracil

5-Fluorouracil (5-FU), a pyrimidine analog used in chemotherapy, has been shown to be converted intracellular into its active substrate and ultimately incorporated into DNA, thus inhibiting DNA synthesis [91].

Cells with a high turn-over, such as fibroblasts in dermal wounds responsible for excessive collagen production, are preferentially targeted by 5-FU, whose proliferation is inhibited. Scar softening was reported to be faster with intralesional 5-FU than with PDL alone [92].

However, 5-FU can be also used in combination with other treatment modalities such as corticosteroids.

Intralesional injection of 5-FU 50 mg/ml in combination with triamcinolone 10 mg/ml or with a very low concentration of betamethasone (5.7 mg/ml) may promote better regression without recurrence of keloid scars smaller than 2 cm in diameter [91, 93].

Limitations of the treatment are that the injection can be painful, purpura and ulcers may occur, and that the agent is expensive [94, 95].

There is to date no consensus concerning the dosage and exposure time and further studies are needed to improve efficacy of this potential treatment.

Interferon

It was outlined that Th2 polarized immune response contribute to abnormal scarring, thus newer therapeutics emerged to attempt the shift towards Th1 response. A Th1 cell product – interferons, which are divided into a, b, and g, inhibit types I and III collagen synthesis by dermal fibroblasts in a dose-dependent manner [96].

It could be shown in a study on keloids that intralesional application of IFN-g is able to reduce scar size, decreased collagen nodules, and more organized collagen bundles. The recurrence rate assessed after one year following injection was minimal [97]. This finding is supported by others which showed improved symptoms after intralesional IFN-g injection of 10 to 200 μg twice weekly for 4 weeks [98, 99].

However, injections are painful and may require local anesthesia. Furthermore, potential side effects include flu like syndromes characterized by headache, diffuse myalgia, low grade temperature, and fatigue [99].

Similarly, Tredget et al. report of significant improvement of hypertrophic scars when interferon-2b is injected three times weekly. Serum TGF-b levels were also reduced and continued to be low after treatment [9].

Reports further suggest that interferon treatment is significantly better than treamicinolone acetonide injection in preventing postsurgical recurrences of keloids [100]. However, other research groups could not reproduce such low recurrence rates associated with intralesional IFN-2a application [101, 102].

Thus, further studies are required to determine if these contradictory results may attributed to the dosage, delivery mode, differences of keloid location, or the combination of these factors.

Avotermin (TGF-β3)

The principle of preventing bad scarring was initiated by Renovo some years ago. Injections of TGF-β3 synthetic equivalent in the wound edges after closing the post operative wound were initiated and analyzed in RCTs. Fergusson et al. could recently demonstrate statistical differences on a meta-analysis of those different trials [103].

Conclusion

Pathological scarring is linked to different etiologies, among them the mechanical stimulation represents an important factor. The biological abnormal behavior of fibroblasts, with signaling imbalance, is also a pathway for new biological inhibitors.

These two issues are reflected in the catalogue of potentially valid solutions for scar management.

Mechanical stabilization of the scar, hydration and injection of products supposed to slow down inflammation and the permanence of the fibroblast proliferation are the basis of the recently proposed options in this domain. Surgical solutions like an extended use of dermal substitutes, skin grafts, flaps and the use of mechanically resistant sutures, taping the postoperative scar are also solutions having been proposed in the literature.

However, evidence is still weak and needs to be confirmed by prospective trials.

References

[1]   Werner S, Grose R (2003) Regulation of wound healing by growth factors and cytokines. Physiol Rev 83: 835–870

[2]   Deitch EA, Wheelahan TM, Rose MP, Clothier J, Cotter J (1983) Hypertrophic burn scars: analysis of variables. J Trauma 23: 895–898

[3]   Wang J, Dodd C, Shankowsky HA, Scott PG, Tredget EE (2008) Deep dermal fibroblasts contribute to hypertrophic scarring. Lab Invest 88: 1278–1290

[4]   Wang R et al (2000) Hypertrophic scar tissues and fibroblasts produce more transforming growth factor-beta1 mRNA and protein than normal skin and cells. Wound. Repair Regen 8: 128–137

[5]   Colwell AS, Phan TT, Kong W, Longaker MT, Lorenz PH (2005) Hypertrophic scar fibroblasts have increased connective tissue growth factor expression after trans-

forming growth factor-beta stimulation. Plast Reconstr Surg 116: 1387–1390

[6] Clark RA (2001) Fibrin and wound healing. Ann NY Acad Sci 936: 355–367

[7] Tuan TL et al (2003) Increased plasminogen activator inhibitor-1 in keloid fibroblasts may account for their elevated collagen accumulation in fibrin gel cultures. Am J Pathol 162: 1579–1589

[8] Ignotz RA, Massague J (1986) Transforming growth factor-beta stimulates the expression of fibronectin and collagen and their incorporation into the extracellular matrix. J Biol Chem 261. 4337–4345

[9] Tredget EE et al (1998)Transforming growth factor-beta in thermally injured patients with hypertrophic scars: effects of interferon alpha-2b. Plast Reconstr Surg 102. 1317–1328

[10] Ghahary A, Shen Q, Shen YJ, Scott PG, Tredget EE(1998) Induction of transforming growth factor beta 1 by insulin-like growth factor-1 in dermal fibroblasts. J Cell Physiol 174: 301–309

[11] Ghahary A et al (1996) Collagenase production is lower in post-burn hypertrophic scar fibroblasts than in normal fibroblasts and is reduced by insulin-like growth factor-1. J Invest Dermatol 106: 476–481

[12] O'Sullivan ST et al (1995)Major injury leads to predominance of the T helper-2 lymphocyte phenotype and diminished interleukin-12 production associated with decreased resistance to infection. Ann Surg 222: 482–490

[13] Horgan AF et al (1994) Altered gene transcription after burn injury results in depressed T-lymphocyte activation. Ann Surg 220: 342–351

[14] Wang J et al (2007) Increased TGF-beta-producing CD4+ T lymphocytes in postburn patients and their potential interaction with dermal fibroblasts in hypertrophic scarring. Wound Repair Regen 15. 530–539

[15] Ladak A, Tredget EE (2009) Pathophysiology and management of the burn scar. Clin Plast Surg 36: 661–674

[16] Yang L et al (2005) Identification of fibrocytes in post-burn hypertrophic scar. Wound Repair Regen 13: 398–404

[17] Yang L et al (2002) Peripheral blood fibrocytes from burn patients: identification and quantification of fibrocytes in adherent cells cultured from peripheral blood mononuclear cells. Lab Invest 82: 1183–1192

[18] Scott PG, Ghahary A, Tredget EE (2000) Molecular and cellular aspects of fibrosis following thermal injury. Hand Clin 16: 271–287

[19] Wang, J et al (2007) Accelerated wound healing in leukocyte-specific, protein 1-deficient mouse is associated with increased infiltration of leukocytes and fibrocytes. J Leukoc Biol 82: 1554–1563

[20] Grotendorst GR (1997)Connective tissue growth factor: a mediator of TGF-beta action on fibroblasts. Cytokine Growth Factor Rev 8. 171–179

[21] Mustoe TA et al (2002)International clinical recommendations on scar management. Plast Reconstr Surg 110: 560–571

[22] Teot L (2002) Clinical evaluation of scars. Wound Repair Regen 10: 93–97

[23] Silver GM et al (2007) Standard operating procedures for the clinical management of patients enrolled in a prospective study of Inflammation and the host response to thermal injury. J Burn Care Res 28:222–230

[24] Ramzy PI, Barret JP, Herndon DN (1999)Thermal injury. Crit Care Clin 15: 333–352, ix

[25] Atiyeh BS et al (2002)Benefit-cost analysis of moist exposed burn ointment. Burns 28: 659–663

[26] Tewari AK et al (2010) Use of a novel absorbable barbed plastic surgical suture enables a "Self-Cinching" technique of vesicourethral anastomosis during robot-assisted prostatectomy and improves anastomotic times. J Endourol 24: 1645–1650

[27] Demyttenaere SV et al (2009) Barbed suture for gastrointestinal closure: a randomized control trial. Surg Innov 16: 237–242

[28] Heimbach DM et al (2003)Multicenter postapproval clinical trial of Integra dermal regeneration template for burn treatment. J Burn Care Rehabil 24: 42–48

[29] Scuderi N et al (2008) The clinical application of autologous bioengineered skin based on a hyaluronic acid scaffold. Biomaterials 29: 1620–1629

[30] Gravante G et al (2007) The use of Hyalomatrix PA in the treatment of deep partial-thickness burns. J Burn Care Res 28: 269–274

[31] Fujioka M, Fujii T (1997) Maxillary growth following atelocollagen implantation on mucoperiosteal denudation of the palatal process in young rabbits: implications for clinical cleft palate repair. Cleft Palate Craniofac J 34: 297–308

[32] Ryssel H, Gazyakan E, Germann G, Ohlbauer M (2008) The use of MatriDerm in early excision and simultaneous autologous skin grafting in burns–a pilot study. Burns 34: 93–97

[33] Haslik W et al (2007) First experiences with the collagen-elastin matrix Matriderm as a dermal substitute in severe burn injuries of the hand. Burns 33: 364–368

[34] Wang XQ, Liu YK, Qing C, Lu SL (2009) A review of the effectiveness of antimitotic drug injections for hypertrophic scars and keloids. Ann Plast Surg 63: 688–692

[35] Ferguson MW et al (2009) Prophylactic administration of avotermin for improvement of skin scarring: three double-blind, placebo-controlled, phase I/II studies. Lancet 373: 1264–1274

[36] Reiffel RS (1995) Prevention of hypertrophic scars by long-term paper tape application. Plast Reconstr Surg 96: 1715–1718

[37] Atkinson JA, McKenna KT, Barnett AG, McGrath DJ, Rudd M (2005) A randomized, controlled trial to determine the efficacy of paper tape in preventing hypertrophic scar formation in surgical incisions that traverse Langer's skin tension lines. Plast Reconstr Surg 116: 1648–1656

[38] Linares HA, Larson DL, Willis-Galstaun BA (1993) Historical notes on the use of pressure in the treatment of hypertrophic scars or keloids. Burns 19: 17–21

[39] Rose MP, Deitch EA (1985) The clinical use of a tubular compression bandage, Tubigrip, for burn-scar therapy: a critical analysis. Burns Incl Therm Inj 12: 58–64

[40] Kealey GP, Jensen KL, Laubenthal KN, Lewis RW (1990) Prospective randomized comparison of two types of pressure therapy garments. J Burn Care Rehabil 11: 334–336

[41] Johnson J, Greenspan B, Gorga D, Nagler W, Goodwin C (1994) Compliance with pressure garment use in burn rehabilitation. J Burn Care Rehabil 15: 180–188

[42] Niessen FB, Spauwen PH, Schalkwijk J, Kon M (1999) On the nature of hypertrophic scars and keloids: a review. Plast Reconstr Surg 104: 1435–1458

[43] Anzarut A (2007) The evidence for and against the effectiveness of pressure garment therapy for scar management. Plast Reconstr Surg 120:1437–1438

[44] Ahn ST, Monafo WW, Mustoe TA (1989) Topical silicone gel: a new treatment for hypertrophic scars. Surgery 106:781–786

[45] Ahn ST, Monafo WW, Mustoe TA (1991) Topical silicone gel for the prevention and treatment of hypertrophic scar. Arch Surg 126:499–504

[46] Cruz-Korchin NI (1996) Effectiveness of silicone sheets in the prevention of hypertrophic breast scars. Ann Plast Surg 37:345–348

[47] Gold MH (1994) A controlled clinical trial of topical silicone gel sheeting in the treatment of hypertrophic scars and keloids. J Am Acad Dermatol 30:506–507

[48] Berman B, Flores F (1999) Comparison of a silicone gel-filled cushion and silicon gel sheeting for the treatment of hypertrophic or keloid scars. Dermatol Surg 25: 484–486

[49] Su CW, Alizadeh K, Boddie A, Lee RC (1998) The problem scar. Clin Plast Surg 25: 451–465

[50] Poston J (2000) The use of silicone gel sheeting in the management of hypertrophic and keloid scars. J Wound Care 9: 10–16

[51] Berman B et al (2007) A review of the biologic effects, clinical efficacy, and safety of silicone elastomer sheeting for hypertrophic and keloid scar treatment and management. Dermatol Surg 33: 1291–1302

[52] Hirshowitz B et al (1998) Static-electric field induction by a silicone cushion for the treatment of hypertrophic and keloid scars. Plast Reconstr Surg 101: 1173–1183

[53] Gilman TH (2003) Silicone sheet for treatment and prevention of hypertrophic scar: a new proposal for the mechanism of efficacy. Wound Repair Regen 11: 235–236

[54] Suetak T, Sasai S, Zhen YX, Tagami H (2000) Effects of silicone gel sheet on the stratum corneum hydration. Br J Plast Surg 53:503–507

[55] Branagan M, Chenery DH, Nicholson S (2000) Use of infrared attenuated total reflectance spectroscopy for the in vivo measurement of hydration level and silicone distribution in the stratum corneum following skin coverage by polymeric dressings. Skin Pharmacol Appl Skin Physiol 13: 157–164

[56] Musgrave MA, Umraw N, Fish JS, Gomez M, Cartotto RC (2002) The effect of silicone gel sheets on perfusion of hypertrophic burn scars. J Burn Care Rehabil 23: 208–214

[57] Manuskiatti W, Fitzpatrick RE (2002) Treatment response of keloidal and hypertrophic sternotomy scars: comparison among intralesional corticosteroid, 5-fluorouracil, and 585-nm flashlamp-pumped pulsed-dye laser treatments. Arch Dermatol 138: 1149–1155

[58] Kang N, Sivakumar B, Sanders R, Nduka C, Gault D (2006) Intra-lesional injections of collagenase are ineffective in the treatment of keloid and hypertrophic scars. J Plast Reconstr Aesthet Surg 59: 693–699

[59] Urioste SS, Arndt KA, Dover JS (1999) Keloids and hypertrophic scars: review and treatment strategies. Semin Cutan Med Surg 18: 159–171

[60] Sherris DA, Larrabee WF, Jr, Murakami CS (1995) Management of scar contractures, hypertrophic scars, and keloids. Otolaryngol Clin North Am 28: 1057–1068

[61] Brissett AE, Sherris DA (2001) Scar contractures, hypertrophic scars, and keloids. Facial Plast Surg 17:263–272

[62] Nemeth AJ (1993) Keloids and hypertrophic scars. J Dermatol Surg Oncol 19: 738–746

[63] Boutli-Kasapidou F, Tsakiri A, Anagnostou E, Mourellou O (2005) Hypertrophic and keloidal scars: an approach to polytherapy. Int J Dermatol 44: 324–327

[64] Asilian A, Darougheh A, Shariati F (2006) New combination of triamcinolone, 5-Fluorouracil, and pulsed-dye laser for treatment of keloid and hypertrophic scars. Dermatol Surg 32: 907–915

[65] Borok TL et al (1988) Role of ionizing irradiation for 393 keloids. Int J Radiat Oncol Biol Phys 15: 865–870

[66] Berman B, Bieley HC (1996) Adjunct therapies to surgical management of keloids. Dermatol Surg 22: 126–130

[67] Slemp AE, Kirschner RE (2006) Keloids and scars: a review of keloids and scars, their pathogenesis, risk factors, and management. Curr Opin Pediatr 18: 396–402

[68] Malaker K, Vijayraghavan K, Hodson I, Al YT (2004) Retrospective analysis of treatment of unresectable keloids with primary radiation over 25 years. Clin Oncol (R Coll Radiol) 16: 290–298

[69] Ogawa R, Yoshitatsu S, Yoshida K, Miyashita T (2009) Is radiation therapy for keloids acceptable? The risk of radiation-induced carcinogenesis. Plast Reconstr Surg 124: 1196–1201

[70] Castro DJ et al (1983) Effects of the Nd:YAG laser on DNA synthesis and collagen production in human skin fibroblast cultures. Ann Plast Surg 11: 214–222

[71] Apfelberg DB, Maser MR, Lash H, White D, Weston J (1984) Preliminary results of argon and carbon dioxide laser treatment of keloid scars. Lasers Surg Med 4: 283–290

[72] Henderson DL, Cromwell TA, Mes LG (1984) Argon and carbon dioxide laser treatment of hypertrophic and keloid scars. Lasers Surg Med 3: 271–277

[73] Abergel RP et al (1984) Control of connective tissue metabolism by lasers: recent developments and future prospects. J Am Acad Dermatol 11: 1142–1150

[74] Alster TS, Nanni CA (1998) Pulsed dye laser treatment of hypertrophic burn scars. Plast Reconstr Surg 102: 2190–2195

[75] Allison KP, Kiernan MN, Waters RA, Clement RM (2003) Pulsed dye laser treatment of burn scars. Alleviation or irritation? Burns 29: 207–213

[76] Kono T et al (2003) The flashlamp-pumped pulsed dye laser (585 nm) treatment of hypertrophic scars in Asians. Ann Plast Surg 51: 366–371

[77] Alster TS, Williams CM (1995) Treatment of keloid sternotomy scars with 585 nm flashlamp-pumped pulsed-dye laser. Lancet 345: 1198–1200

[78] Kumar K, Kapoor BS, Rai P, Shukla HS (2000) In-situ irradiation of keloid scars with Nd:YAG laser. J Wound Care 9: 213–215

[79] Kwon SD, Kye YC (2000) Treatment of scars with a pulsed Er:YAG laser. J Cutan Laser Ther 2: 27–31

[80] Gaston P, Humzah MD, Quaba AA (1996) The pulsed tuneable dye laser as an aid in the management of postburn scarring. Burns 22: 203–205

[81] Liew SH, Murison M, Dickson WA (2002) Prophylactic treatment of deep dermal burn scar to prevent hypertrophic scarring using the pulsed dye laser: a preliminary study. Ann Plast Surg 49: 472–475

[82] Anderson RR, Parrish JA (1983) Selective photothermolysis: precise microsurgery by selective absorption of pulsed radiation. Science 220: 524–527

[83] Reiken SR et al (1997) Control of hypertrophic scar growth using selective photothermolysis. Lasers Surg Med 21: 7–12

[84] Paquet P, Hermanns JF, Pierard GE (2001) Effect of the 585 nm flashlamp-pumped pulsed dye laser for the treatment of keloids. Dermatol Surg 27: 171–174

[85] Kuo YR et al (2005) Activation of ERK and p38 kinase mediated keloid fibroblast apoptosis after flashlamp pulsed-dye laser treatment. Lasers Surg Med 36: 31–37

[86] Kuo YR et al (2005) Suppressed TGF-beta1 expression is correl ated with up-regulation of matrix metalloproteinase-13 in keloid regression after flashlamp pulsed-dye laser treatment. Lasers Surg Med 36: 38–42

[87] Rusciani L, Rossi G, Bono R (1993) Use of cryotherapy in the treatment of keloids. J Dermatol Surg Oncol 19: 529–534

[88] Har-Shai Y, Amar M Sabo E (2003) Intralesional cryotherapy for enhancing the involution of hypertrophic scars and keloids. Plast Reconstr Surg 111: 1841–1852

[89] Ernst K, Hundeiker M (1995) [Results of cryosurgery in 394 patients with hypertrophic scars and keloids]. Hautarzt 46: 462–466

[90] Layton AM, Yip J, Cunliffe WJ (1994) A comparison of intralesional triamcinolone and cryosurgery in the treatment of acne keloids. Br J Dermatol 130: 498–501

[91] Apikian M, Goodman G (2004) Intralesional 5-fluorouracil in the treatment of keloid scars. Australas. J Dermatol 45: 140–143

[92] Nouri K, Vidulich K, Rivas MP (2006) Lasers for scars: a review. J Cosmet Dermatol 5: 14–22

[93] Lebwohl M (2000) From the literature: intralesional 5-FU in the treatment of hypertrophic scars and keloids: clinical experience. J Am Acad Dermatol 42: 677

[94] Gupta S, Kalra A (2002) Efficacy and safety of intralesional 5-fluorouracil in the treatment of keloids. Dermatology 204: 130–132

[95] Baisch A, Riedel F (2006) [Hyperplastic scars and keloids: part II: Surgical and non-surgical treatment modalities]. HNO 54: 981–992

[96] Jimenez SA, Freundlich B, Rosenbloom J (1984) Selective inhibition of human diploid fibroblast collagen synthesis by interferons. J Clin Invest 74: 1112–1116

[97] Granstein RD et al (1990) A controlled trial of intralesional recombinant interferon-gamma in the treatment of keloidal scarring. Clinical and histologic findings. Arch Dermatol 126: 1295–1302

[98] Pittet B et al (1994) Effect of gamma-interferon on the clinical and biologic evolution of hypertrophic scars and Dupuytren's disease: an open pilot study. Plast Reconstr Surg 93: 1224–1235

[99] Larrabee WF, Jr, East CA, Jaffe HS, Stephenson C, Peterson KE (1990) Intralesional interferon gamma treatment for keloids and hypertrophic scars. Arch Otolaryngol Head Neck Surg 116: 1159–1162

[100] Berman B, Flores F (1997) Recurrence rates of excised keloids treated with postoperative triamcinolone acetonide injections or interferon alfa-2b injections. J Am Acad Dermatol 37: 755–757

[101] Wong TW, Chiu HC, Yip KM (1994) Intralesional interferon alpha-2b has no effect in the treatment of keloids. Br J Dermatol 130: 683–685

[102] al-Khawajah MM (1996) Failure of interferon-alpha 2b in the treatment of mature keloids. Int J Dermatol 35: 515–517

[103] Occleston NL, Fairlamb D, Hutchison J, O'Kane S, Ferguson MW (2009) Avotermin for the improvement of scar appearance: a new pharmaceutical in a new therapeutic area. Expert Opin Investig Drugs 18: 1231–1239

Correspondence: Luc Teot, MD, PhD, Burns Unit, Wound Healing Unit, Lapeyronie Hospital, Montpellier University Hospital, 391 Avenue Doyen Giraud, 34 255 Montpellier Cedex, France, E-mail: lteot@aol.com

Scar assessment

Pauline D. H. M. Verhaegen[1-4,*], Martijn B. A. van der Wal[1,3,*], Esther Middelkoop[1,3,5],
Paul P. M. van Zuijlen[1-5]

[1] Association of Dutch Burn Centres Beverwijk, Beverwijk, The Netherlands
[2] Department of Plastic, Reconstructive, and Hand Surgery, Red Cross Hospital Beverwijk, Beverwijk, The Netherlands
[3] Burn Centre, Red Cross Hospital Beverwijk, Beverwijk, The Netherlands
[4] Department of Plastic, Reconstructive, and Hand Surgery, Academical Medical Centre Amsterdam, Amsterdam, The Netherlands
[5] Department of Plastic, Reconstructive, and Hand Surgery, VU Medical Centre Amsterdam, Amsterdam, The Netherlands

Scar assessment tools

Scars may lead to an array of functional, cosmetic, and psychological consequences. Scar tissue is usually distinguished from normal skin by an aberrant color, increased thickness, irregular surface area, and poor functional quality, caused by loss of pliability and contraction or expansion of the surface area. All separate scar features are relevant and attribute to the quality and general opinion on a scar.

An ideal assessment of a scar should include both subjective and objective aspects [99]. Scar assessment scales are frequently used to generate a systematic judgment by observers on the following aspects: color, thickness, relief, pliability, and the surface area. A judgment by the patient is obligatory to include pruritus and pain in the assessment. These items are particularly relevant when scars become hypertrophic [127]. Complaints and cosmetic disfigurement caused by scars may lead patients to suffer from psychosocial problems, which in turn may result in a decreased quality of life [12]. Both subjective and objective measurements of scar features are nowadays mandatory to practice evidence-based medicine. Therefore, in this chapter an overview will be given of the most important subjective and objective measurement tools for scar evaluation.

Scar features

Color: Generally, disturbance in the color of a scar is created by the components vascularization and pigmentation. Vascularization or erythema is caused by an increase of capillary blood flow. In the early maturation phase, an increase in redness is an indicator of scar activity (Fig. 1 A). Secondly, pigmentation is caused by a decrease or increase of melanin produced by melanocytes of the epidermis. Erythema usually diminishes after several months or sometimes years, whereas pigmentation mismatching often remains (Fig. 1 B).

Thickness: An increase in scar thickness e. g. hypertrophy can be a frequent and cosmetically disfiguring sequela of scarring (Fig. 1 A). Hypertrophic scars are often misdiagnosed as keloids. The difference between the two is that keloids proliferate beyond the boundaries of the original lesion, while hypertrophic scars become raised, but stay within their confines [93]. In addition, hypertrophic scars typically decrease in thickness over time as opposed to keloids, which may have phases of reactivation [15].

Relief: Previous research has shown that the overall opinion of a scar, given by a clinician, is significantly influenced by relief [31]. Surface irregu-

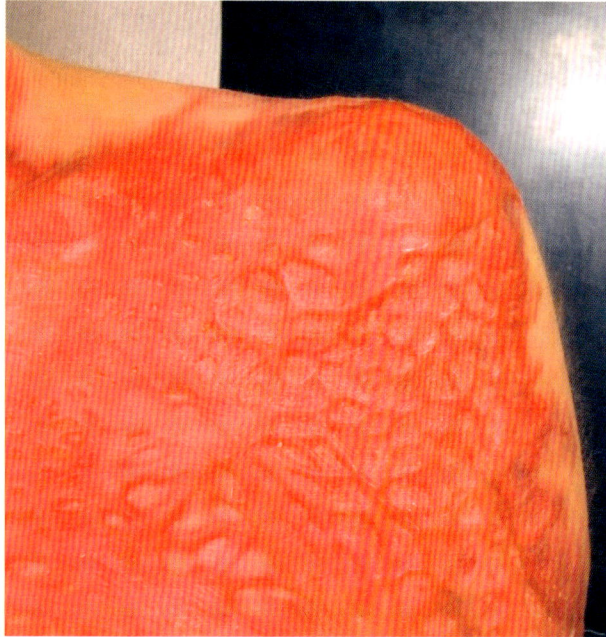

Fig. 1 A. A red and raised scar after a burn injury of the shoulder

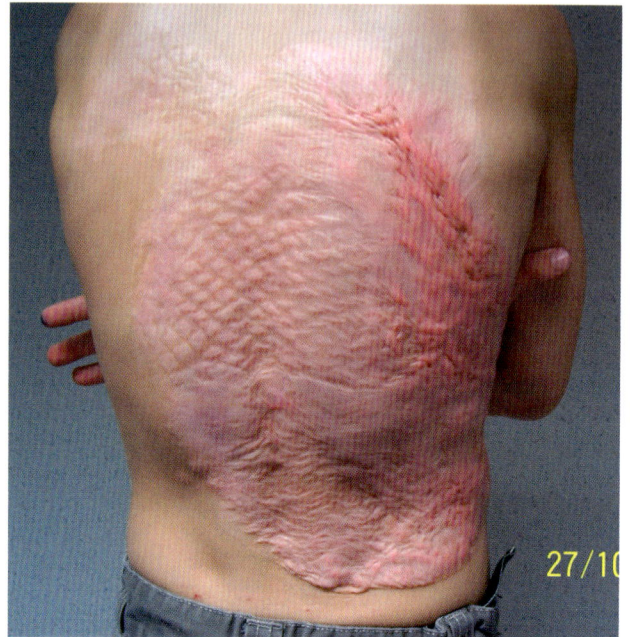

Fig. 1 C. Relief of a matured burn scar after skin transplantation of the back

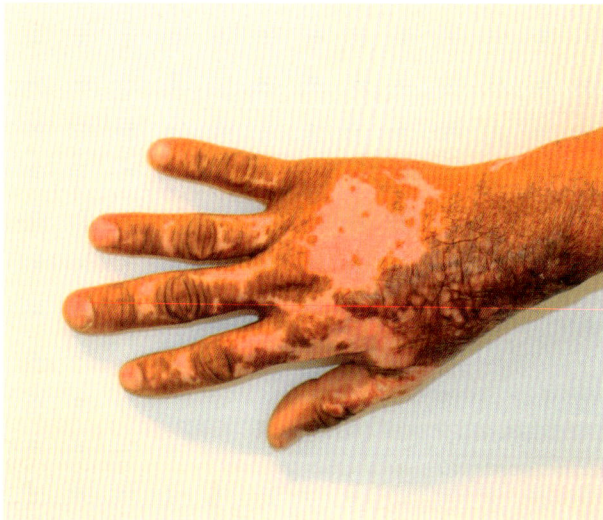

Fig. 1 B. Hypopigmentation after a burn injury of the hand

larities of a scar are especially seen after burn treatment, when a skin transplantation is needed and a meshed split skin graft is applied on the burned area. Often the areas in between the meshed split skin graft become raised [52]. As shown in Fig. 1 C such irregularities will remain.

Pliability: Loss of pliability is a major cause of functional impairment. Especially when a scar is situated adjacent to joints, scar stiffness may result in a limited range of motion. In addition, loss of pliability in the facial region will often cause asymmetry and an altered or diminished facial expression.

Surface area: In clinical practice, surface area is measured by planimetry. Planimetry is useful for calculating the wound size, but also for calculating the percentage of a scar that becomes hypertrophic, hypopigmentated, or the extent of scar contraction or expansion over time. Scars may contract in time, which regularly leads to scar contracture (Fig. 1 D). In these cases reconstructive surgery may be required. On the contrary, in linear scars expansion of the scar is frequently seen, which results in a broader scar and a less aesthetical result (Fig. 1 E). The extent of scar contraction or expansion is often used as an outcome parameter in research.

Although an increasing number of subjective and objective tools have become available, there is no general agreement as to the most appropriate tool(s) for scar evaluation [37]. In this chapter subjective scar assessment scales and objective scar as-

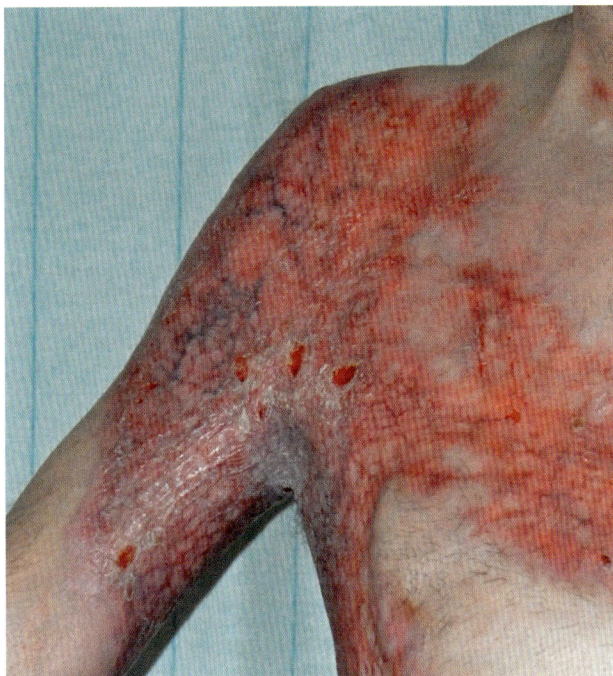

Fig. 1 D. Scar contracture after burn injury of the axilla with limited range of motion

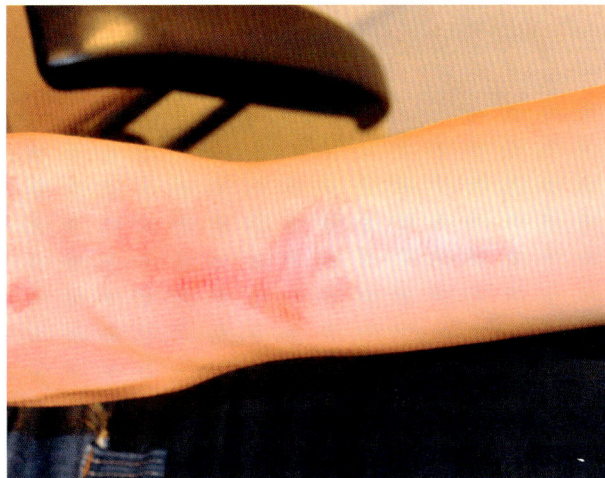

Fig. 1 E. Expansion of a linear scar on the upper arm

sessment tools are critically reviewed with respect to the concepts of internal consistency, level of agreement, reliability, validity, and feasibility.

Clinimetrical principles

Requirements for both subjective and objective measurement tools are *reliability, validity* and *feasibility*. Reliability refers to the reproducibility of measurements or ratings by observers [114]. An Intraclass Correlation Coefficient (ICC) higher than 0.7 is considered a minimum requirement for reliable results [91]. The validity refers to the exactness of the measurements or ratings [113], i. e. do they measure what we want to measure? A Pearson's Correlation Coefficient higher than 0.6 is considered as good, ranging from 0.3 to 0.6 as moderate, and lower than 0.3 as weak [3]. Feasibility of a measurement tool refers to its convenience, effectiveness, price and ease of use. It is hereby relevant to determine if the measurement tool can be used in a clinical or research setting.

Subjective measurement tools e. g. scar assessment scales can consist of either *nominal, ordinal,* or

categorical variables. *Nominal* scales assign items to groups or categories. No ordering of the items is implied and they do not provide quantitative information. (e. g. sex, race, etc.) In *ordinal* scales, the numbers assigned to objects represent the rank order (e. g. 1st, 2nd, 3rd, etc.) of the entities assessed. However, the interval between the numbers is not necessarily equal. *Categorical* scales are a nominal and ordinal scale combined into one. Combination can either be numerical (e. g. 1, 2, 3, etc.) or quantitative (e. g. normal skin, slightly hypertrophic, hypertrophic, keloid).

Clinimetrical parameters for scar assessment scales specifically are the *Cronbach's alpha* and *Cohen's Kappa or Weighted Kappa*. The Cronbach's alpha describes the internal consistency of a scale which generally gives an idea whether several items that propose to measure the same general construct, also produce similar scores. Results are considered good if the Cronbach's alpha ranges between 0.7 and 0.9. If the Cronbach's alpha is higher than 0.9 redundant items are included and a lower score than 0.7 means that no internal consistency has been reached [91]. The Cohen's Kappa or Weighted Kappa refers to the level of agreement between observers. The Cohen's Kappa is used in nominal scales and the Weighted Kappa is used for ordinal scales. Its cut off points are determined according to Landis et al: a Kappa above 0.6 is considered substantial and above 0.8 almost perfect [64].

Subjective scar assessment scales

Scar assessment scales are questionnaires that have been developed to give an overall impression of a scar. In general these scales are free of charge and easy to use which makes them very accessible in clinical practice. Ideally they should include the most important scar features described above. A drawback of assessment scales is its subjective nature. They are filled out by the observer or sometimes by the patient and are therefore susceptible to confounding factors. These factors may include (in)experience of an observer or patient and the psychological component, related to scarring which influences the judgment of the patient.

In the past decades, several attempts have been made to create an appropriate scale and mostly their origin is found in the assessment of burn scars. In 1988, Smith et al. were the first to show that *cosmetic disfigurement after burns* could be measured reliably [110]. Although this scale was far from perfect four raters were required to obtain reliable ratings, it inspired several authors to create a more suitable questionnaire for scars.

In 1990, Sullivan et al. introduced a new scar scale, which became known as the *Vancouver Scar Scale (VSS)* [116]. Again, this scale was designed to measure burn scars and included most scar parameters such as pigmentation, vascularity, pliability, and scar height (thickness). After being modified by Baryza et al. [9] for a better inter-observer reliability it became the most commonly used scale worldwide.

As stated by Sullivan et al., the VSS was still far from perfection and some problems were encountered. First, some important scar characteristics such as pain and itching were absent, since they concentrated on clinicians judgment rather than patient scores. Secondly, not all the variables in the VSS concerned ordinal data. The parameter pigmentation scored 0 for normal, 1 for hypopigmentation, 2 for mixed pigmentation and 3 for hyperpigmentation. Although the scale was originally designed to show the degree of a pathological condition it is often used to numerically indicate the absolute severity of a burn scar, with a high score indicating a worse scar. No evidence is found in literature that hypopigmentation should be considered a less severe condition than hyperpigmentation in scarring. In most cases the opinion will be guided by the patient's normal skin appearance: e. g. a hypopigmented scarred area is considered worse in dark skin compared to pale skin. Thirdly, not all variables add the same number to the score, while no evidence was provided why one parameter should add more or less to the score. Finally, two observers were required to obtain reliable data, which limits its clinical ease of use.

Beausang et al. proposed a new quantitative scale which is often referred to as the *Manchester Scar Assessment Proforma* or *Manchester Scar Scale* (MSS) [10]. It was considered to be more complete compared to the VSS and better suited for linear scars. Because it was difficult for observers to distinguish vascularization from pigmentation, they combined these two components by referring to 'color mismatching' with the ranking of none, slight, obvious and gross mismatch. Additionally, an overall global assessment was made using the Visual Analogue Scale (VAS). Still, the patients' component was lacking and multiple observers were necessary for the scale to have an acceptable reliability.

A scale by Yeong et al., named the *Seattle Scale*, was designed for clinical use and for photographic assessment. A drawback of this scale was that the parameter pigmentation was given a negative value when a scar was hypopigmentated, suggesting that less pigmentation could improve the appearance of the scar [136].

In 1998, Crowe et al. introduced the *Hamilton Scale* which was specially designed to evaluate photographs of scars. It was shown to have a 'substantial' to 'almost perfect' reliability and novice therapists were as reliable as scar experts in the use of this scale [23, 136].

One of the most recently developed and upcoming scar scales is the *Patient and Observer Scar Assessment Scale (POSAS)* [31]. It consists of an observer and a patient component and contains the most important scar parameters used in previous scar scales. The observers score vascularization, pigmentation, pliability, thickness and relief, while the patients score color, pliability, thickness, relief, itching and pain. All these parameters are scored in a 10-step scale making it possible to measure a mean score, even while using merely some of the components of the scale, needed for specific purposes. It was first tested on burn scars and also became useful for the evaluation of linear scars after modification by van de Kar et al. in 2005 [124]. Both the VSS and the POSAS were found to be valid. However, in a direct comparison the POSAS was shown to be more consistent, reliable and feasible than the VSS making it more useful for clinical purpose.

In the same year, a new scale using photograph analysis was introduced, named the *Matching Assessment of Scars and Photographs* (MAPS) [81]. This scale was a modification of the Seattle Scale and the negative scoring system persisted, making it impossible for the observer to add the different components and obtain an overall score. Nevertheless a good reliability was found, except from vascularization and it also showed that extensive training of the observers was not necessary.

Table 1 gives an overview of the above mentioned scar assessment scales.

Importance of different scar features on the general impression

Previous research has shown that the parameters color, thickness and relief influence the observers' general opinion of a burn scar the most [31]. The patients' opinion is predominantly influenced by itching and thickness of the scar. When testing the POSAS on the assessment of linear scars, it was shown that especially the parameters redness, pigmentation, relief, and contraction or expansion of the surface area influenced the observers' general opinion. Again, the patients' opinion was predominantly influenced by itching and thickness of the scar [124].

Objective measurement tools

Color

Color evaluation raises several practical problems, e. g. observers are not always able to make a good distinction between the two components vascularization and pigmentation. Also color-blinded observers will have a great difficulty in answering these questions in scar assessment scales. This underlines the importance of objective color measurement tools in scar evaluation, however, not all objective tools have this discriminative ability. At present, the most common objective method of measuring skin color is referred to as reflectance spectroscopy. Color is determined by measuring the intensity of light reflected from specific wavelengths. Within this principle, two different types of devices can be distinguished: the tristimulus reflectance colorimetry and the narrow-band spectrophotometry.

Tristimulus reflectance colorimetry was developed to objectively represent color in a manner the human eye perceives it. The level of light reflected through three broad wavelength filters is determined. In 1976, a color model based on human perception was established by the Commission Internationale de l'Eclairage (CIE) [132, 133]. Several devices integrated these values into their systems where any color can be described by three values: L*, the lightness; a*, the amount of green or red; and b*, the amount of yellow or blue. In practice the L* expresses the relative brightness of the color, a* the redness, and b* the pigmentation of the skin. Examples of tristimulus devices are the Colorwalk colorimeter (Photofolt, UMN Electronics, Indianapolis, IN), the Micro Color (DR Bruno Lange GmbH, Düsseldorf, Germany), the Labscan XE (Hunter Associates Inc., Texas, USA) and the Minolta Chromameter CR-200 and CR-300 (Minolta Camera Co., Ltd., Osaka, Japan).

The *Minolta Chromameter* is the most commonly used colorimeter for the color assessment of both normal and scarred skin [49, 89, 117, 126]. On normal skin, the device was shown to have an excellent intra-observer reliability for all three parameters (L*, a*, b*) with very low standard error of mean (SEM) values. It also showed a good to excellent inter-observer reliability, inter-instrument and day-to-day reliability and it can therefore be used by a single observer [125]. On scarred skin, the reliability was good for the three parameters and increased up to excellent when the measurement was performed by four observers. The measurement for redness correlated significantly but weakly with the POSAS. As far as pigmentation was concerned, an unacceptably low correlation was found compared to the pigmentation score of the VSS. It was stated by the authors that this lack of correlation might be related to the poor agreement of the observers in the assessment scale, especially with highly vascularized scars. It was hy-

Table 1. An overview of scar assessment scales and their relevant clinimetrical parameters

Scale (Authors + Ref)	Clinically or Photographs assessed & by Observer/ Patient	Included items	Observers used/ required	Tested on	Reliability		Validity
					Intra-observer	**Inter-observer**	
Cosmetic Disfigurement Scale [110]	Photographs & Observer	1. Irregularity 2. Thickness 3. Discolorisation 4. Overall clothed 5. Overall non-clothed	4	Burn scars	ICC: Irregularity: 0.89 Thickness: 0.91 Color: 0.85 Overall clothed: 0.98 Overall non-clothed: 0.94	ICC: (Averaged) Irregularity: 0.78 Thickness: 0.79 Color: 0.72 Overall clothed: 0.94 Overall non-clothed: 0.86	–
VSS [116]*	Clinically & Observer	1. Pigmentation 2. Vascularity 3. Pliability 4. Height	3	Burn scars	Not measured	Mean Kappa: each observer pair: 0.5 (± 0.1)	–
VSS with additional tool [9]	Clinically & Observer	1. Pigmentation 2. Vascularity 3. Pliability 4. Height	3	Burn scars	Not measured	Overall ICC: 0.81 Cohen's Kappa: Pigmentation: 0.61 Vascularity: 0.73 Pliability: 0.71 Height: 0.56	–
Seattle Scale [136]	Photographs & Observer	1. Surface 2. Border Height 3. Thickness 4. Color	8	Burn scars	Not measured	ICC: Surface: 0.94 Border Height: 0.95 Thickness: 0.90 Color: 0.85	–
Manchester Scar Scale [10]	Photographs & Observer	1. Color 2. Contour 3. Texture 4. Distortion	10	Surgical scars, hypertrophic scars, and keloid scars	Mean CV: 7.8% -14.8%	Overall correlation coefficient (Spearman's Rho): 0.87	Correlation with histology findings Contour: $R^2 = 0.62$ Texture: $R^2 = 0.69$
Hamilton Scale [23]	Photographs & Observer	1. Height 2. Irregularity (proportion of scar) 3. Vascularity 4. Color	2	Burn scars	Cohen's Kappa: Height: 0.75–0.79 Irregularity: 0.75–0.76 Vascularity: 0.66–0.72 Color: 0.72–0.90	Cohen's Kappa: Height: 0.82–0.84 Irregularity: 0.80–0.89 Vascularity: 0.73–0.78 Color: 0.80–0.72	–

Scale (Authors + Ref)	Clinically or Photographs assessed & by Observer/ Patient	Included items	Observers used/ required	Tested on	Reliability		Validity
					Intra-observer	Inter-observer	
Modified VSS [86]	Clinically & Observer	1. Pigmentation 2. Vascularity 3. Pliability 4. Height	3	Burns scars and Surgical scars	Not measured	ICC: Pigmentation: 0.20 Vascularity: 0.41 Pliability: 0.42 Height: 0.36	–
POSAS [31]**	Clinically & Observer and Patient	**Observer:** 1. Vascularity 2. Pigmentation 3. Thickness 4. Relief 5. Pliability **Patient:** 1. Pain 2. Itching 3. Color 4. Stiffness 5. Thickness 6. Irregularity	1	Burn scars	Internal consistency (Cronbach's alpha) Observer: 0.69 Patient: 0.76	ICC: Observer score: 0.73 (0.62–0.82)	Correlation observer scale with VSS Spearman's Rho = 0.89
MAPS [81]***	Photographs & Observer	1. Surface 2. Border Height 3. Thickness 4. Color 5. Pigmentation	3	Burn scars	ICC: Surface: 0.40 Border Height: 0.79 Thickness: 0.82 Color: 0.79	ICC: Surface: 0.25–0.38 Border Height: 0.63–0.70 Thickness: 0.60–0.74 Color: 0.5–0.71	–
Modified POSAS [124, 123]	Clinically & Observer and Patient	**Observer:** 1. Vascularity 2. Pigmentation 3. Thickness 4. Relief 5. Pliability 6. Surface area **Patient:** 1. Pain 2. Itching 3. Color 4. Stiffness 5. Thickness 6. Irregularity	1	Burn scars, Surgical scars	Internal consistency (Cronbach's alpha) Observer: 0.86 and 0.77 Patient: 0.90 and 0.74	ICC Observer: Vascularity: 0.81 and 0.62 Pigmentation: 0.71 and 0.73 Thickness: 0.72 and 0.39 Relief: 0.67 and 0.79 Pliability: 0.65 and 0.48 Surface area: 0.83 and -	– and correlation observer scale with VSS Spearman's Rho = 0.38

* VSS: Vancouver Scar Scale
** POSAS: Patient and Observer Scar Assessment Scale
*** MAPS: Matching Assessment of Scars and Photographs

pothesized that the vascularization of the scar could mask the pigmentation of the scar and this was confirmed by post-hoc analysis when the agreement and correlation improved at lower vascularized scars [30]. Although this device links to a computer, it performs relatively good in a clinical setting due to the connecting cable that gives the investigator an acceptable range of motion.

The *Labscan XE* is a full-scanning spectrophotometer that has been tested for its reliability and validity on scars. Although the inter-observer reliability for redness was only moderate, the results did seem to correlate well with the redness parameter of the VSS. The pigmentation measurements were more reliable, but a sufficient correlation with the pigmentation value b* could not be found. This device is also limited for clinical purposes because it is too big to be positioned correctly over body regions such as the neck, the back and the chest [72].

Narrow-band spectrophotometry devices were developed to measure skin or scar redness and pigmentation in the form of erythema and melanin. This method was first described by Diffey and Farr and is based on the differences in light absorption of red and green by haemoglobin and melanin [27, 28, 36]. These differences result in a certain intensity of reflected light which can be measured. Blood is colored red because haemoglobin absorbs much green light and reflects red light, while melanin is colored brown because it absorbs light of all wavelengths. The erythema index (E) is defined as $E = 100 \times \log$ (intensity of reflected red light/intensity of reflected green light) and the melanin index (M) is defined as: $M = 100 \times \log$ (1/intensity of reflected red light). The *DermaSpectrometer* (Cortex Technology, Hadsund, Denmark), the *Mexameter* (Courage and Khazaka, Cologne, Germany) and the *Erythema meter* (Dia-stron, Andover, United Kingdom) are examples of narrow-band reflectometers.

The *DermaSpectrometer* is a handheld tool, which makes it very feasible in general practice. It is equipped with a 6 mm diameter probe which is placed on the skin. After pressing the shutter button, the results are immediately displayed. The Derma Spectrometer was found to have a good reliability on normal and scarred skin, although a relatively high variation of day-to-day repeatability (8 %–22 %) was seen for the erythema index on normal skin [19, 30].

Oliveira et al. found a good correlation between the erythema and melanin values of the DermaSpectrometer with the VSS scores for respectively redness and pigmentation [92]. This was later confirmed by Draaijers et al. for redness (compared with the POSAS), but they failed to show an acceptable correlation with pigmentation [30].

The *Mexameter* has to be linked to a computer making it less suited for clinical purposes. However, the cable between the device and the probe gives the investigator an acceptable range of motion. The probe is equipped with 16 light-emitting diodes that send light at three defined wavelengths: 568 nm (green), 660 nm (red), 880 nm (infrared). The reflected light is measured through the above mentioned principle and is immediately displayed. Recent work by Nedelec et al. showed good intra- and inter-observer reliability values of the erythema and melanin index when using this device on normal and scarred skin [87, 88]. In addition, only a moderate correlation of the erythema index with the subscale vascularization of the modified VSS was found and there was a weak correlation of the melanin index with the pigmentation score [88].

The DermaSpectrometer and the Mexameter have been compared in vitro and in vivo on normal skin. The repeatability as well as the sensitivity of these two instruments was good. Both measurement devices were able to characterize skin color and to quantify small skin color changes [19]. On scarred skin, a comparison with the DermaSpectrometer has not been made.

Different types of tristimulus devices have been compared with narrow-band devices on normal skin [19, 109]. On scarred skin, Draaijers et al. compared the Minolta Chromameter with the DermaSpectrometer [30]. Although the Minolta gave the most reliable values, the DermaSpectrometer seemed to be more feasible in clinical practice and was therefore preferred.

In summary, the tristimulus colorimeter is capable of measuring all scar colors, whereas the narrow band reflectometers are designed for measuring the intensity of erythema and pigmentation. On scarred surface both types of devices seem reliable, but neither the tristimulus nor the narrow band devices seem able to perform measurements with an acceptable correlation with the gold standard. The DermaSpectrometer is the most feasible tool, but it has recently been withdrawn from the market. We conclude that there is no objective tool available for the analysis of scar color that measures redness and pigmentation in a reliable and valid way. Until further research is performed, the Minolta Chromameter and the Mexameter seem the best devices available for measuring scar color.

Thickness

When measuring thickness of a scar it is important to distinguish clinical thickness from histological thickness. Clinically, thickness is usually measured through comparing the height of the scar with the normal surrounding skin, while the histological thickness might differ because of bulky connective tissue, especially in immature scars.

A skin biopsy remains the gold standard to measure scar thickness but it is infrequently applied in the clinical setting because of its invasive character. Ultrasound has been shown to be reproducible and accurate in the determination of the thickness of normal and scarred skin [1, 87, 88, 119]. Today, in combination with the appropriate software, it is possible to create a three-dimensional image, including measurements of thickness, area, and volume of the scar tissue. This method is often used for the analysis of scar thickness after burns or surgical treatments [73, 90, 131]. The *Tissue Ultrasound Palpation System (TUPS)* (Biomedical Ultrasonic Solutions, Hong Kong) and the *Dermascan C* (Cortex Technology, Denmark) are frequently used devices.

The *TUPS* is a portable ultrasound machine which is connected to a probe that is equipped with an ultrasound transducer with both a transmitter and receiver at the tip. It was proven to have a high inter-observer and test-retest reliability, but it only seemed to correlate moderately with the VSS that was used to test its concurrent validity [66]. A phantom study by Du et al. showed that the TUPS was able to measure the volume of a scar with a 90 % accuracy [32].

The Dermascan C is a high-frequency (10–50 MHz), high resolution ultrasound scanner that captures and reproduces detailed images of the skin or scar. It is able to penetrate to a depth up to 15 millimeters, making it accessible for the measurements of

most common scars. A good inter-observer and excellent intra-observer reliability was found on scarred surfaces and measurements could also be reliably repeated the next week. The validity of the Dermascan C was tested and a statistically significant Spearman's Rho correlation of 0.41 and 0.50 was found between the total thickness of the instrument and the VSS subscale for height [88].

In 2007 a new scanning technique for accurate volume measurements of keloids was introduced [120]. The *Vivid 900* (Konica-Minolta, Milton Keynes, United Kingdom) is a non-contact scanning device that combines photography and laser technology for volume assessment using RapidForm 2004 3D reverse modelling software. This scanner is not portable and relatively expensive, making it less accessible for small centers. Although no reliability test was performed, the results seemed to correlate positively with the total score of the Manchester scar scale. Then again, whether a correlation of scar volume with a total scar score is desirable, remains debatable.

Magnetic Resonance Imaging (MRI) has been shown to accurately and reliably measure the thickness of normal skin [100]. This technique has not been applied for measuring scar thickness. Moreover, this method is very expensive and time consuming.

After reviewing the available evidence, ultrasound seems the first choice tool for measuring scar thickness. It is convenient in use and found to be accurate and reliable for the evaluation of scar thickness. Because the Dermascan C showed a slightly higher correlation with the VSS compared to TUPS, this device would be our first choice for this purpose.

Relief

Surface irregularities, also referred to as relief, can be measured by various measurement tools. A selection of the most important, non-invasive, objective measurement tools is reviewed below.

Most objective relief measurement methods measure the skin topography indirectly by using a negative replica of the skin [6, 50, 80, 102, 103]. SILFLO® silicon polymer (Flexico Developments Ltd., Hertfordshire, United Kingdom) is most widely used and previous studies have proven its reliability and reproducibility [70]. First, liquid silicone is placed onto the area of interest and mixed with a hardener in a fixed position. After the replica is hardened, which takes 1 minute to 24 hours, a negative print of the skin or scar is generated. To assess the relief, further investigation needs to be done on these replicas, which may include *Mechanical, Optical, Laser, Transparency or Interference Fringe Projection Profilometry.*

The *Mechanical Prolifometry* technique, which is also referred to as the stylus method, is a relief measuring method, which generates digitized data from a stylus that runs over a replica [57, 77, 122]. Relief can be measured up to several millimetres [70]. Even though Mechanical Profilometry has a high reliability, its feasibility is low, because of a long drying and measuring time of 24 hours and 8 minutes, respectively. In addition, it is uncertain whether this method would be suitable and reliable for measuring scar relief, since it has only been used to assess the depth of wrinkles, skin dryness, and atopic dermatitis in unscarred skin.

Optical Profilometry is a relief measuring method, which works by the detection of black and white reflections by light irradiation. This light irradiation is caused by differences in depth and angle of the replica. In a short time period, the image is processed by a high-resolution black and white video or CCD (Charge-Coupled Device) camera, which is projected on a computer and analyzed by using specialized software [21, 107]. This system is able to measure relief up to 6 mm [70], which makes it suitable to quantify scar relief. However, the Optical Profilometry method, which previously has shown good reliability on normal skin [21, 41], should first be tested on its reliability on scars before clinical use would be advocated.

Laser Profilometry is a relief measuring method, which is based on the principle of light amplification and reflection from a skin replica [84, 104]. After reflection of light from the replica, the laser is focused by a movable lens. These movements of the lens, which are proportional to the relief of the replica, are registered digitally and calculated by a specialized software program. This software program displays a three-dimensional picture, on which calculations such as the Fourier analysis can be performed [84]. The maximum vertical measuring range is 10 mm. Laser Profilometry is a very accurate and reliable method for relief measurements on normal skin [104]. However, reliability

for measurements of scars and validity have not been assessed. In addition, its feasibility is low because of a long measurement time (10 min–30 min), high costs, and complexity in use. Therefore, Laser Prolifometry is not recommended for use in a clinical setting, but may be used for research purposes.

Transparency Profilometry can be performed by using the Visiometer (Courage and Khazaka, Cologne, Germany) [26, 42, 43]. This measurement principle is based on light transmission through a thin replica of silicone of which the light absorption is known. The Visiometer measures reliably between a vertical range of 10 μm and 361 μm [26], but since relief in scars and relief of deeper wrinkles often exceeds 361 μm, this method will most likely not be useful for measurements of scar relief. Moreover, its validity has never been assessed.

Interferometry, also referred to as *Interference Fringe Projection Profilometry* (Breuckmann, Meersburg, Germany), consists of calculating a phase image from interference fringe image projection. The phase image gives access to the altitude at each point. By calculating the phase difference between the phase of the replica and that of the reference plane, the relief of the replica is obtained [2]. The Dermatop® system, and the Toposurf® software are used to generate the data. The Interferometry measurements showed good accuracy and reliability. Research showed that in the evaluation of micro- and macrorelief Interferometry was considered more feasible than the other four profilometry methods, which have been discussed above [62]. Since the vertical measurement range has not been mentioned it remains unclear whether it would be suitable for measurements of scar relief.

Besides indirect measurements of topography, which use skin replicas, skin topography can also be measured directly. The *PRIMOS (*Phases shift Rapid In vivo Measurement Of the Skin, GFMesstechnik GmbH, Teltow, Germany) is a non-contact measurement tool which assesses relief. It is able to measure skin relief with a vertical range up to 10 mm. First, a parallel digital stripe pattern is projected onto the skin and the reflected light is absorbed by a CCD-chip of a high-resolution camera. Subsequently, a digital three-dimensional image is achieved which is evaluated by use of a specialized software program [46]. The PRIMOS is a feasible measurement tool: generating the image and processing the data is an easy and short procedure compared to the measurement methods that analyze negative skin replicas. Currently the reliability and validity of the PRIMOS for scar relief measurements is being tested [11].

Relief measurement tools should be subdivided into tools, which are applicable on irregularities of normal skin and tools applicable on scar relief. Transparency Profilometry and Interferometry are able to precisely measure skin microrelief, which can be relevant for the evaluation of therapies for dermatological diseases or for the cosmetic industries. Mechanical, Optical, and Laser Profilometry could be more useful for quantifying macrorelief of scars. However, because of low feasibility these methods have a limited application in a clinical setting, but could be used for research purposes. The PRIMOS, which is a more feasible measurement tool, may very well be suitable for the quantification of scar relief in a clinical setting.

Elasticity

The mechanical qualities of the skin are well appreciated and studied. Experimental models identified the most important mechanical skin characteristics, which are tensile strength, ultimate extension, and stress-strain curves [130]. Tools that measure these mechanical qualities will be discussed by the following four subcategories, which are based on the type of load on the skin: suction, pressure, torsion, and tension. In Fig. 2 these types of load are visualized and explained.

Suction methods

The most frequently described elasticity measurement tool is the *Cutometer® Skin Elasticity Meter* 474 and 575, with its latest MPA 580 version (Courage and Khazaka Electronic GmbH, Cologne, Germany). During the measurement constant negative pressure is used for a short period, alternated with periods of normal pressure. This pressure is exerted over a small area of the skin, which ranges from 2 mm to 8 mm, depending on the diameter of the probe. The probe with a 6 mm aperture provides the most precise measurements of the dermal elasticity [7]. When

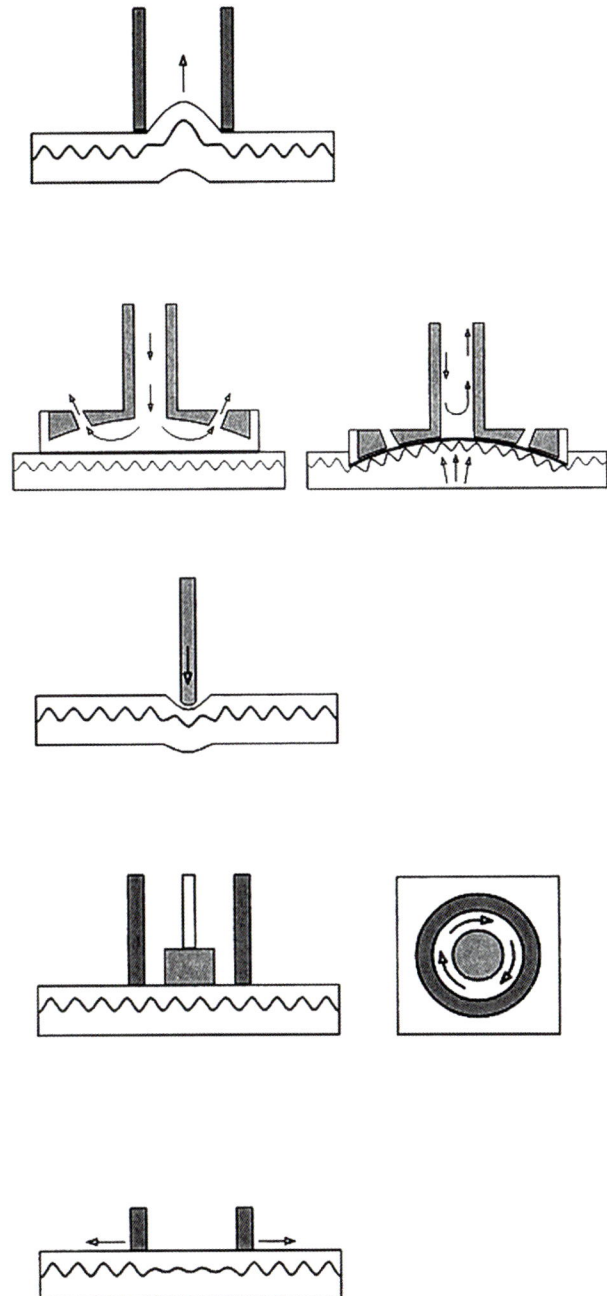

Fig. 2. Schematic drawings of the mechanisms based on the type of load on the skin: suction by the Cutometer and DermaLab *(above)*, pressure by the Pneumatonometer *(second from above)*, pressure by the Durometer *(center)*, torsion *(second from below)* by the Dermal Torque Meter, and tension by the Elastometer and Extensometer *(below)*. The working mechanism of the Pneumatonometer *(second from above)* is based on air that normally flows through the system *(left panel)*. This system is blocked at a certain pressure *(right panel)*

the Cutometer was tested on normal skin, reliable results were obtained [98]. In addition, the Cutometer was found to have a good reliability for measurements on both sclerodermal skin [34] and scars [29, 44]). Validity of the Cutometer has been assessed, which showed a weak to moderate correlation with the pliability score of the POSAS [29].

The *DermaLab®* (Cortex Technology, Hadsund, Denmark) [96], which has replaced the Dermaflex® [33, 95, 105, 106], measures the stress that is needed to achieve an elevation of the skin of 1.5 mm. Its measuring aperture is 10 mm, which is larger than the aperture of the Cutometer (2 mm-8 mm). Therefore, these devices measure different mechanical qualities of the skin: a smaller measuring aperture (Cutometer) predominantly measures qualities of the epidermis and the superficial dermis, whereas a larger measuring aperture (DermaLab) measures the dermis itself together with the sliding mobility of the junction between dermis and the layer of the subcutaneous fat [98]. Both measurement devices with a small and larger measuring aperture are of relevance in the scar evaluation. However, one should realize that dependent on this measuring aperture different mechanical qualities are measured. The reliability, validity, and feasibility of the DermaLab have been sparsely examined: only one report has shown that the DermaLab measures less accurately than the Dermaflex [96]. Therefore, before applying the DermaLab in the evaluation of scars more clinimetrical research needs to be performed.

Pressure methods

Tonometry is a measurement method which was originally developed to determine the intraocular pressure. Later, tonometry was used to quantify firmness and flexibility of skin and scars [55]. It is composed of an air flow system, a built-in sensor, and a membrane that makes contact with the skin surface. When applied to the skin, the amount of pressure that is needed to lock the system is measured. The measurement is displayed on a dial indicator. The *Cicatrometer, Pneumatonometer, Tissue Tonometer,* and *Durometer* are all tonometers which work by the same measurement technique. The *Cicatrometer* (University of California, San Diego, USA), is the first type of tonometer which has been used to assess

burn scars [55]. Subsequently, the *Pneumatonometer* (Medtronic Solan, Jacksonville, USA) was described and assessed on its validity: a moderate correlation with the pliability score of the VSS was shown in the measurement on burn scars [111]. Later the *Tissue Tonometer* (Flinders University Biomedical Engineering Department, Adelaide, Australia) was developed, which showed an excellent intra-observer reliability on burn scars [79]. The assessment of its validity showed a moderate correlation with the pliability score of the VSS [79].

The latest version of the Tonometer is called the *Durometer* (Rex Gauge Company Inc., Glenview, USA), which was originally designed to measure the hardness of material. Later, the durometer was used in the assessment of skin hardness in scleroderma [35], lipodermatosclerosis [101], and skin induration in venous diseases [67]. In multiple trials the Durometer was tested on sclerodermal skin with excellent reliability and good validity [60, 82, 108]. However, its reliability and validity for scars has not been investigated yet, but probably would be similar to the reliability and validity that has been found for the Tissue Tonometer and Pneumatonometer. The primary disadvantage of tonometry is that the measurement is influenced by the hardness of the underlying tissue. Therefore, it is less suitable for anatomical locations where bony structures are situated directly under the skin (i. e. the hand, fingers or face) [35].

Torsion methods

The *Dermal Torque Meter* (Dia-stron, Andover, United Kingdom) is a commercially available measurement tool that assesses elasticity via torsional force onto the skin [5, 39, 40]. It has a rotating flat disk which is placed in contact with the skin surface. This disk applies a rotational force along the plain of the skin surface. The rotational load is applied by a motor with controllable voltage and allows adjustment of the torque. A ring guard was constructed circumferentially to the disk leaving a strip of skin in between. The Dermal Torque Meter has been applied for the evaluation of normal skin [69] and burn scars [14], but no data on its reliability have been reported. Validity of measurements on normal skin has been evaluated, which showed a poor correlation with the Cutometer measurements [85]. Since reliability is unknown and torsion methods are not transferable to suction techniques, their suitability for scar assessment has yet to be determined.

Tension methods

The following measurement tools work by measuring the skin deformation, after tension is exerted in the horizontal plane of the skin. The *Elastometer* (Washington University, St. Louis, USA) is a hand-held measurement tool that has been developed for extension evaluation by distracting two loci of skin [8]. It has been used to measure normal skin and hypertrophic burn scars. Another measurement tool, which works by the same technique of skin extension is the *Extensometer* (University of Hong Kong, Hong Kong, China) [112]. A known rate of extension is applied to the skin via double-sided adhesive tape on two metal tabs. The skin extension related to the load intensity is displayed in a graph. The Extensometer has been used in the assessment of elasticity of normal skin and hypertrophic scars [18]. Unfortunately, reliability and validity of these type of measurement tools have not been examined.

In conclusion, we advise the Cutometer as the first choice for elasticity measurements, since this measurement tool is feasible and measures reliably, with a reasonable validity. Other possibilities could include Tonometry, which is both reliable and valid for measurements on scars. Unfortunately, Tonometry will be biased by the hardness of structures underneath the skin. Measurement tools that work by torsion and tension methods at present do not have a major role in the scar assessment armamentarium, because minimum requirements (reliability and validity) have not been investigated or have not been met.

Surface area: planimetry

The most simple and commonly used method of planimetry is tracing the scar or wound margins. In 1992, Bryant et al. described the *Transparent Acetate Wound Perimeter Tracing* (Labelon Projection Transparencies, Braintree, United Kingdom) [13, 16]. The wound is traced on a transparent grid paper and subsequently the observer counts the number of squares that fall within the tracing and calculates the area. This technique was found to be reliable,

valid, and feasible for quick wound assessment [38, 78, 121]. Beside tracing a wound or scar it is also possible to cut out this trace and use the *Weighing Method* (Transparency Film, Scotch 3M, St Paul, USA, and Gram-atic® Balance, Metler Instrument Corporation, Highstown, USA) [13], whereby the weight has a linear correlation with the surface area. This method was found to be reliable, but is less practical because the observer first needs to determine the mass/cm^2 and secondly needs a precise weighing scale. Moreover, tracing, cutting out this trace, and weighing could introduce extra variation into the measurements. Overall, cautiousness should be preserved in the tracing technique, since it appeared that the greatest source of error in wound tracings was in the tracings themselves rather than in the determination and calculation of the final wound area [13, 135].

More sophisticated surface area measurements can be done by *Computer Assisted Planimetry*. The wound or scar is traced on any kind of transparent sheet, followed by digitizing this sheet and analyzing the scanned sheet by a computer program. Various computer programs exist to determine the real area [4, 25, 54, 59]. Another example of computer assisted planimetry is tracing on a digital computerized tablet, e.g. a sonic digitizer or Visitrak (Smiths and Nephew, London, United Kingdom), which is a reliable way of area determination. However, these tablets can be very expensive and costs may rise up to several thousand dollars [20, 135]. Validity of computer assisted planimetry has not been reported to date.

Another frequently used and simple method of planimetry is photography. The use of photography has been applied in *Photogrammetry* and *Stereophotogrammetry*. In Photogrammetry, a calibrated grid is projected on the film image. The camera is held on a standard distance from the image of interest. In 1986, Bulstrode et al. found this technique to have an excellent reliability [17]. In 2004, van Zuijlen et al. found planimetry by photography (using a calibrated grid which is projected on the film image) to be valid and reliable, even more reliable than tracing on transparent sheets, except for extremely curved body parts [128]. Because difficulties remain in converting a three-dimensional image into a two-dimensional image, stereophotogrammetry has been developed. Stereophotogrammetry is Photogrammetry, which is extended by the use of two cameras. These cameras generate a more precise reconstruction of the area of interest. Stereophotogrammetry was found to be a reliable and valid measurement tool, which is more accurate than tracing or simple photography [45]. Although this tool measures very accurately, the use in clinical practice is limited because it is expensive, time-consuming and requires specialistic skills [54].

Eventually, in planimetry various more extensive imaging techniques can be used, such as *Ultrasound, Computed Tomography,* and *Magnetic Resonance Imaging* [51, 99, 134]. From these images, a three-dimensional computer reconstruction can be generated [134]. However, their applicability is limited by a low feasibility, very high costs, and potential inaccuracy because of movement of the area of interest. In addition, these measuring techniques have not been properly assessed on their reliability and validity.

In surface area measurements, two important problems must be taken into account: the first problem is that the borders of the wound or scar may become unclear, which may cause a broader variation in measured surface area. The second problem is that extremely curved body parts and areas with skin folds may influence the measurements that are done by the use of photography. In 2004 this was demonstrated by Van Zuijlen et al., who found that for extremely curved body parts planimetry by photography was less reliable than the tracing method [128]. Planimetry of circumferential wounds or scars may cause similar problems.

In summary, for surface area measurements we advocate the use of reliable, inexpensive, and uncomplicated methods which are clinically validated and can be applied without limitation.

Overall, we recommend the photographic technique as a standard evaluation method for wounds or scars which are not subjected to curved body parts and skin folds: digitized measurements show better results than manual tracing, because the greatest measurement errors lie in the manual tracing done by the observers [13, 135]. However, for extremely curved body parts, large surface areas, and locations, which are difficult to measure, the most feasible and advocated method would remain the manual tracing method, either on metric paper or on transparent sheets.

Table 2 gives an overview of the above mentioned scar assessment tools.

Conclusion

In the future decades, the role of reliable and valid scar assessment tools will become more prominent. In this chapter several measurement tools that may be considered for scar assessment are described.

In general, objective scar measurements are preferred over subjective scar assessment scales. However, subjective scar assessment scales performed by observers have several advantages. They are convenient, cheap, and give semi-quantitative information along several clinical parameters. Moreover, they can be performed in outpatient clinics, as they require little time to complete. On the other hand, several available assessment scales require more than one observer to obtain good reliability and to reduce the measuring error of a single observer.

It is debatable whether evaluation of all scar features (color, thickness, relief, pliability, and surface area) are necessary for a complete scar assessment scale. However, only after many years of experience with a certain scar assessment scale such lists may be shortened, because the relevance of parameters first needs to be evaluated for different scar categories in different patient groups.

Measuring devices provide objective parameters and make errors that are usually consistent and predictable. The best scar measuring devices in terms of reliability and validity are yet to be determined for many of the parameters that bear importance for research goals.

Furthermore, it should be taken into account whether the measurement tool can be used in a clinical setting, where the time element is highly important and anyone should be able to perform the measurement, or on the other hand, in a research setting, where more time is available and more specialized observers carry out the measurements.

In this chapter, we systematically discussed methods to access scar formation that are considered relevant to research involving scars. Surprisingly, only few scar assessment tools have been stud-

Table 2. An overview of scar assessment tools and their relevant clinimetrical parameters

	Inter-observer reliability normal skin	Inter-observer reliability scars	Validity scars	Price*	Clinical application
COLOR					
DermaSpectrom-eter	Redness: CV < 22 % Pigmentation: CV < 4 % ([19]	Redness: 1 obs: 0.72 4 obs: 0.91 Pigmentation: 1 obs: 0.94 4 obs: 0.98	Redness: 0.50[a] Pigmentation: 0.32[a] [30]	Not commercially available anymore	[48, 118] No scars
Labscan XE	Redness: 0.92 Pigmentation: 0.95–0.96 [72]	Redness: 0.50 Pigmentation: 0.88–0.99 [73]	Redness: 0.72[a] with VSS Pigmentation: 0.50–0.83[a] with VSS [73]	$ 26,455	–
Mexameter	Redness: 0.97 Pigmentation: 0.99 [88]	Redness: 0.82–0.97 Pigmentation: 0.95–0.98 [88]	Redness: 0.52–0.65[a] with VSS [88] Pigmentation: 0.37–0.50[a] with VSS [88]	$ 14,205	[71, 76, 83, 97] No scars
Minolta Chromameter CR-200	Redness: CV < 10 % Pigmentation: CV < 1 % [19]	Redness: 1 obs: 0.75 4 obs: 0.92 Pigmentation: 1 obs: 0.73–0.89 4 obs: 0.91–0.97	Redness: 0.42[a] with POSAS [30] Pigmentation: 0.23–0.24[a] with POSAS [30]	Not commercially available anymore	[90, 118]
Minolta Chromameter CR-300	Redness: 1 obs: 0.92 Pigmentation: 1 obs: 0.97–0.99 [126]	–	–	Not commercially available anymore	[58, 126]
THICKNESS					
Dermascan C	0.85 [88]	0.89–0.91 [88]	0.41–0.50[a] with height score VSS [88]	$ > 41,775	[68]
TUPS	–	0.84 [66]	0.34[b] with height score VSS [66] 0.42[b] with total score VSS [66]	$ 16,480	[73, 74]
Vivid 910 (volume)	–	–	0.63[b] with total score MSS [120]	$ 67,950	[56] No scars
RELIEF					
Mechanical Profilometry	CV < 0.5 % [57]	–	–	Unknown	[6] No scars
Optical Profilometry	CV < 3 % [41]	–	–	Unknown	–

	Inter-observer reliability normal skin	Inter-observer reliability scars	Validity scars	Price*	Clinical application
Laser Profilometry	–	–	–	Unknown	[104] No scars
Transparency Profilometry	Normal skin not assessed Metal plates: CV < 10 % [26]	–	–	Visiometer: $ 16,480	[42, 68] No scars
Interferometry	CV < 4 % [62]	–	–	$ 111,435	[63, 75] No scars
PRIMOS	0.74 [11]	0.82 [11]	0.53–0.70[b] with relief score POSAS [11]	$ 42,320	[46, 53]
ELASTICITY					
Cutometer	1 obs: 0.75–0.85 4 obs: 0.93–0.96 [29]	1 obs: 0.35–0.76 4 obs: 0.68–0.93 [29]	0.29–0.53[a] with pliability score POSAS [29]	$ 5,575	[24, 129]
Dermaflex	CV: 6.7–23.2 %	–	0.38–0.44[b] with DermaLab [96]	Not commercially available anymore	[94, 96] No scars
DermaLab	CV: 44.4–57.8 %	–	0.38–0.44[b] with Dermaflex [96]	$ 6,440	–
Tonometry	0.82–0.91 [82]	Sclerodermal skin: 0.95 [22]	0.57[c] with VSS [111] 0.442–0.457[b] with VSS [79]	$ 405–820	[22, 35, 79, 92, 111]
Dermal Torque meter	–	–	Poor[c] with Cutometer [85]	$ 14,690	[14, 85]
Elastometer	–	–	–	Not commercially available anymore	[8]
Extensometer	–	–	–	Not commercially available anymore	[18]
SURFACE AREA					
Transparent Acetate Wound Perimeter Tracing	0.48–0.88 [128]	–	Good[c] [128]	$ < 5	[61, 65, 121] No scars
Weighing method	–	–	–	$ 1,680–6,800	[13] No scars

	Inter-observer reliability normal skin	Inter-observer reliability scars	Validity scars	Price*	Clinical application
Computer Assisted Planimetry	–	–	–	Visitrak: not commercially available anymore	[47, 61, 115] No scars
Photogrammetry	0.72–0.93 [128]	–	Good[c] [128]	Unknown	[92] No scars
Stereophotogrammetry	–	0.98[b] [45] (wounds)	–	Unknown	[54] No scars

* = Prices based on the exchange rate of April 2010
Obs = Observer
CV = Coefficient of variation in % ((Highest value-Lowest value)/Lowest value) × 100
[a] = Spearman's Rho Correlation Coefficient
[b] = Pearson's Correlation Coefficient
[c] = Correlation coefficient unknown

ied sufficiently. Of course there is no need to perform the entire array of clinical analyses in a single study. The aim of a study must dictate the methodology and the preferred methods of evaluation.

References

[1] Alexander H, Miller DL (1979) Determining skin thickness with pulsed ultra sound. J Invest Dermatol 72(1): 17–19

[2] Altmeyer P, Erbler H, Kromer T, Duwe HP, Hoffmann K (1995) Interferometry: a new method for no-touch measurement of the surface and volume of ulcerous skin lesions. Acta Derm Venereol 75(3): 193–197

[3] Andresen EM (2000) Criteria for assessing the tools of disability outcomes research. Arch Phys Med Rehabil 81[12 Suppl 2]: S15–20

[4] Anthony D, Barnes E (1984) Pressure sores. One. Measuring pressure sores accurately. Nurs Times 80(36): 33–35

[5] Barbenel JC, Evans JH (1977) The time-dependent mechanical properties of skin. J Invest Dermatol 69(3): 318–320

[6] Barbenel JC, Makki S, Agache P (1980) The variability of skin surface contours. Ann Biomed Eng 8(2): 175–182

[7] Barel AO, Courage W, Clarys P (1995) Suction method for measurement of skin mechanical properties: the Cutometer®. Handbook of non-invasive methods and the skin. CRC Press Inc, Boca Raton, pp 335–340

[8] Bartell TH, Monafo WW, Mustoe TA (1988) A new instrument for serial measurements of elasticity in hypertrophic scar. J Burn Care Rehabil 9(6): 657–660

[9] Baryza MJ, Baryza GA (1995) The Vancouver Scar Scale: an administration tool and its interrater reliability. J Burn Care Rehabil 16(5): 535–538

[10] Beausang E, Floyd H, Dunn KW, Orton CI, Ferguson MW (1998) A new quantitative scale for clinical scar assessment. Plast Reconstr Surg 102(6): 1954–1961

[11] Bloemen MCT, van Gerven MS, van der Wal MBA, Verhaegen PDHM, Middelkoop E (2010) An objective measuring device for surface roughness in skin and scars. JAAD (in press)

[12] Bock O, Schmid-Ott G, Malewski P, Mrowietz U (2006) Quality of life of patients with keloid and hypertrophic scarring. Arch Dermatol Res 297(10): 433–438

[13] Bohannon RW, Pfaller BA (1983) Documentation of wound surface area from tracings of wound perimeters. Clinical report on three techniques. Phys Ther 63(10): 1622–1624

[14] Boyce ST, Supp AP, Wickett RR, Hoath SB, Warden GD (2000) Assessment with the dermal torque meter of skin pliability after treatment of burns with cultured skin substitutes. J Burn Care Rehabil 21(1 Pt 1): 55–63

[15] Brissett AE, Sherris DA (2001) Scar contractures, hypertrophic scars, and keloids. Facial Plast Surg 17(4): 263–272

[16] Bryant RA (1992) Acute and chronic wounds: nursing management CV Mosby, St. Louis

[17] Bulstrode CJ, Goode AW, Scott PJ (1986) Stereophotogrammetry for measuring rates of cutaneous healing: a comparison with conventional techniques. Clin Sci (Lond) 71(4): 437–443

[18] Clark JA, Cheng JC, Leung KS (1996) Mechanical properties of normal skin and hypertrophic scars. Burns 22(6): 443–446

[19] Clarys P, Alewaeters K, Lambrecht R, Barel AO (2000) Skin color measurements: comparison between three instruments: the Chromameter(R), the DermaSpectrometer(R) and the Mexameter(R). Skin Res Technol 6(4): 230–238

[20] Coleridge Smith PD, Scurr JH (1989) Direct method of measuring venous ulcers. Br J Surg 76(7): 689

[21] Corcuff P, De Rigal J, Leveque JL (1982) Image analysis of the cutaneous relief. Bioeng Skin Newslett 4: 16

[22] Corica GF, Wigger NC, Edgar DW, Wood FM, Carroll S (2006) Objective measurement of scarring by multiple assessors: is the tissue tonometer a reliable option? J Burn Care Res 27(4): 520–523

[23] Crowe JM, Simpson K, Johnson W, Allen J (1998) Reliability of photographic analysis in determining change in scar appearance. J Burn Care Rehabil 19(2): 183–186

[24] Cua AB, Wilhelm KP, Maibach HI (1990) Elastic properties of human skin: relation to age, sex, and anatomical region. Arch Dermatol Res 282(5): 283–288

[25] Cutler NR, George R, Seifert RD, Brunelle R, Sramek JJ, McNeill K, Boyd WM (1993) Comparison of quantitative methodologies to define chronic pressure ulcer measurements. Decubitus 6(6): 22–30

[26] De Paepe K, Lagarde JM, Gall Y, Roseeuw D, Rogiers V (2000) Microrelief of the skin using a light transmission method. Arch Dermatol Res 292(10): 500–510

[27] Diffey BL, Oliver RJ, Farr PM (1984) A portable instrument for quantifying erythema induced by ultraviolet radiation. Br J Dermatol 111(6): 663–672

[28] Diffey BL, Farr PM, Oakley AM (1987) Quantitative studies on UVA-induced erythema in human skin. Br J Dermatol 117(1): 57–66

[29] Draaijers LJ, Botman YA, Tempelman FR, Kreis RW, Middelkoop E, van Zuijlen PP (2004) Skin elasticity meter or subjective evaluation in scars: a reliability assessment. Burns 30(2): 109–114

[30] Draaijers LJ, Tempelman FR, Botman YA, Kreis RW, Middelkoop E, van Zuijlen PP (2004) Colour evaluation in scars: tristimulus colorimeter, narrow-band simple reflectance meter or subjective evaluation? Burns 30(2): 103–107

[31] Draaijers LJ, Tempelman FR, Botman YA, Tuinebreijer WE, Middelkoop E, Kreis RW, van Zuijlen PP (2004) The patient and observer scar assessment scale: a reliable and feasible tool for scar evaluation. Plast Reconstr Surg 113(7): 1960–1965; discussion 1966–1967

[32] Du YC, Lin CM, Chen YF, Chen CL, Chen T (2006) Implementation of a burn scar assessment system by ultrasound techniques. Conf Proc IEEE Eng Med Biol Soc 1: 2328–2331

[33] Elsner P, Wilhelm D, Maibach HI (1990) Mechanical properties of human forearm and vulvar skin. Br J Dermatol 122(5): 607–614

[34] Enomoto DN, Mekkes JR, Bossuyt PM, Hoekzema R, Bos JD (1996) Quantification of cutaneous sclerosis with a skin elasticity meter in patients with generalized scleroderma. J Am Acad Dermatol 35(3 Pt 1): 381–387

[35] Falanga V, Bucalo B (1993) Use of a durometer to assess skin hardness. J Am Acad Dermatol 29(1): 47–51

[36] Farr PM, Diffey BL (1984) Quantitative studies on cutaneous erythema induced by ultraviolet radiation. Br J Dermatol 111(6): 673–682

[37] Ferguson MW, Whitby DJ, Shah M, Armstrong J, Siebert JW, Longaker MT (1996) Scar formation: the spectral nature of fetal and adult wound repair. Plast Reconstr Surg 97(4): 854–860

[38] Ferrell BA, Artinian BM, Sessing D (1995) The Sessing scale for assessment of pressure ulcer healing. J Am Geriatr Soc 43(1): 37–40

[39] Finlay B (1970) Dynamic mechanical testing of human skin 'in vivo'. J Biomech 3(6): 557–568

[40] Finlay B (1971) The torsional characteristics of human skin in vivo. Biomed Eng 6(12): 567–573

[41] Fischer TW, Wigger-Alberti W, Elsner P (1999) Direct and non-direct measurement techniques for analysis of skin surface topography. Skin Pharmacol Appl Skin Physiol 12(1–2): 1–11

[42] Fluhr JW, Gehring W, Gloor M (1995) Analyse der Hautrauhigkeit bei Personen unterschiedlicher Altersgruppen mit dem Visiometer. Akt Dermatol 21: 151–156

[43] Fluhr JW, Bettinger J, Gloor M (1996) Skin Visiometer SV 400 zur Hautrauhigkeitsmessung: EDV-gestutzte Transmissions-Profilometrie. Kosmet Med 18: 42–47

[44] Fong SS, Hung LK, Cheng JC (1997) The cutometer and ultrasonography in the assessment of postburn hypertrophic scar–a preliminary study. Burns 23 [Suppl 1]: S12–18

[45] Frantz RA, Johnson DA (1992) Stereophotography and computerized image analysis: a three-dimensional method of measuring wound healing. Wounds 4: 58–64

[46] Friedman PM, Skover GR, Payonk G, Kauvar AN, Geronemus RG (2002) 3D in-vivo optical skin imaging for topographical quantitative assessment of non-ablative laser technology. Dermatol Surg 28(3): 199–204

[47] Gethin G, Cowman S (2006) Wound measurement comparing the use of acetate tracings and Visitrak digital planimetry. J Clin Nurs 15(4): 422–427

[48] Groth L, Serup J (1998) Cutaneous microdialysis in man: effects of needle insertion trauma and anaesthesia on skin perfusion, erythema and skin thickness. Acta Derm Venereol 78(1): 5–9

[49] Guarrera M, Brusati C, Rebora A (2001) Topical metronidazole does not abate UVB-induced erythema. Dermatology 203(2): 121–123

[50] Hatzis J (2004) The wrinkle and its measurement-a skin surface profilometric method. Micron 35(3): 201–219

[51] Hendrix RW, Calenoff L, Lederman RB, Nieman HL (1981) Radiology of pressure sores. Radiology 138(2): 351–356

[52] Herd AN, Hall PN, Widdowson P, Tanner NS (1987) Mesh grafts – an 18 month follow-up. Burns Incl Therm Inj 13(1): 57–61

[53] Jacobi U, Chen M, Frankowski G, Sinkgraven R, Hund M, Rzany B, Sterry W, Lademann J (2004) In vivo determination of skin surface topography using an optical 3D device. Skin Res Technol 10(4): 207–214

[54] Johnson M, Miller R (1996) Measuring healing in leg ulcers: practice considerations. Appl Nurs Res 9(4): 204–208

[55] Katz SM, Frank DH, Leopold GR, Wachtel TL (1985) Objective measurement of hypertrophic burn scar: a preliminary study of tonometry and ultrasonography. Ann Plast Surg 14(2): 121–127

[56] Kau CH, Cronin A, Durning P, Zhurov AI, Sandham A, Richmond S (2006) A new method for the 3D measurement of postoperative swelling following orthognathic surgery. Orthod Craniofac Res 9(1): 31–37

[57] Kautzky F, Dahm MW, Drosner M, Köhler LD (1995) Direct profilometry of the skin: Its reproducibility and variability. J Eur Acad Dermatol Venereol 5: 15–23

[58] Kim MS, Rodney WN, Cooper T, Kite C, Reece GP, Markey MK (2009) Towards quantifying the aesthetic outcomes of breast cancer treatment: comparison of clinical photography and colorimetry. J Eval Clin Pract 15(1): 20–31

[59] Kim NH, Wysocki AB, Bovik AC, Diller KR (1987) A microcomputer-based vision system for area measurement. Comput Biol Med 17(3): 173–183

[60] Kissin EY, Schiller AM, Gelbard RB, Anderson JJ, Falanga V, Simms RW, Korn JH, Merkel PA (2006) Durometry for the assessment of skin disease in systemic sclerosis. Arthritis Rheum 55(4): 603–609

[61] Lagan KM, Dusoir AE, McDonough SM, Baxter GD (2000) Wound measurement: the comparative reliability of direct versus photographic tracings analyzed by planimetry versus digitizing techniques. Arch Phys Med Rehabil 81(8): 1110–1116

[62] Lagarde JM, Rouvrais C, Black D, Diridollou S, Gall Y (2001) Skin topography measurement by interference fringe projection: a technical validation. Skin Res Technol 7(2): 112–121

[63] Lagarde JM, Rouvrais C, Black D (2005) Topography and anisotropy of the skin surface with ageing. Skin Res Technol 11(2): 110–119

[64] Landis JR, Koch GG (1977) The measurement of observer agreement for categorical data. Biometrics 33(1): 159–174

[65] Langemo DK, Melland H, Hanson D, Olson B, Hunter S, Henly SJ (1998) Two-dimensional wound measurement: comparison of 4 techniques. Adv Wound Care 11(7): 337–343

[66] Lau JC, Li-Tsang CW, Zheng YP (2005) Application of tissue ultrasound palpation system (TUPS) in objective scar evaluation. Burns 31(4): 445–452

[67] LeBlanc N, Falabella A, Murata H, Hasan A, Weiss E, Falanga V (1997) Durometer measurements of skin induration in venous disease. Dermatol Surg 23(4): 285–287

[68] Lee HK, Seo YK, Baek JH, Koh JS (2008) Comparison between ultrasonography (Dermascan C version 3) and transparency profilometry (Skin Visiometer SV600). Skin Res Technol 14(1): 8–12

[69] Leveque JL, de Rigal J, Agache PG, Monneur C (1980) Influence of ageing on the in vivo extensibility of human skin at a low stress. Arch Dermatol Res 269(2): 127–135

[70] Leveque JL (1999) EEMCO guidance for the assessment of skin topography. The European Expert Group on Efficacy Measurement of Cosmetics and other Topical Products. J Eur Acad Dermatol Venereol 12(2): 103–114

[71] Levy JL, Pons F, Agopian L, Besson R (2005) A double-blind controlled study of a nonhydroquinone bleaching cream in the treatment of melasma. J Cosmet Dermatol 4(4): 272–276

[72] Li-Tsang CW, Lau JC, Liu SK (2003) Validation of an objective scar pigmentation measurement by using a spectrocolorimeter. Burns 29(8): 779–784

[73] Li-Tsang CW, Lau JC, Chan CC (2005) Prevalence of hypertrophic scar formation and its characteristics among the Chinese population. Burns 31(5): 610–616

[74] Li-Tsang CW, Lau JC, Choi J, Chan CC, Jianan L (2006) A prospective randomized clinical trial to investigate the effect of silicone gel sheeting (Cica-Care) on post-traumatic hypertrophic scar among the Chinese population. Burns 32(6): 678–683

[75] Li L, Mac-Mary S, Marsaut D, Sainthillier JM, Nouveau S, Gharbi T, de Lacharriere O, Humbert P (2006) Age-related changes in skin topography and microcirculation. Arch Dermatol Res 297(9): 412–416

[76] Li YH, Chen JZ, Wei HC, Wu Y, Liu M, Xu YY, Dong GH, Chen HD (2008) Efficacy and safety of intense pulsed light in treatment of melasma in Chinese patients. Dermatol Surg 34(5): 693–700; discussion 700–691

[77] Linde YW, Bengtsson A, Loden M (1989) 'Dry' skin in atopic dermatitis. II. A surface profilometry study. Acta Derm Venereol 69(4): 315–319

[78] Liskay AM, Mion LC, Davis BR (1993) Comparison of two devices for wound measurement. Dermatol Nurs 5(6): 434, 437–441

[79] Lye I, Edgar DW, Wood FM, Carroll S (2006) Tissue tonometry is a simple, objective measure for pliability of burn scar: is it reliable? J Burn Care Res 27(1): 82–85

[80] Makki S, Barbenel JC, Agache P (1979) A quantitative method for the assessment of the microtopography of human skin. Acta Derm Venereol 59(4): 285–291

[81] Masters M, McMahon M, Svens B (2005) Reliability testing of a new scar assessment tool, Matching Assessment of Scars and Photographs (MAPS). J Burn Care Rehabil 26(3): 273–284

[82] Merkel PA, Silliman NP, Denton CP, Furst DE, Khanna D, Emery P, Hsu VM, Streisand JB, Polisson RP, Akesson A, Coppock J, van den Hoogen F, Herrick A, Mayes MD, Veale D, Seibold JR, Black CM, Korn JH (2008) Validity, reliability, and feasibility of durometer measurements of scleroderma skin disease in a multicenter treatment trial. Arthritis Rheum 59(5): 699–705

[83] Moon SJ, Kim DK, Chang JH, Kim CH, Kim HW, Park SY, Han SH, Lee JE, Yoo TH, Han DS, Kang SW (2009) The impact of dialysis modality on skin hyperpigmentation in haemodialysis patients. Nephrol Dial Transplant 24(9): 2803–2809

[84] Muller U (1995) Roughness (measured by profilometry: mechanical, optical and laser). In: Berardesca E, Elsner P, Wilhelm KP, Maibach HI (eds) Bioengineering of the skin: methods and instrumentation. CRC Press, Boca Raton, p 97

[85] Murray BC, Wickett RR (1997) Correlations between dermal torque meter, cutometer, and dermal phase meter measurements of human skin. Skin Res Tech 3: 101–106

[86] Nedelec B, Shankowsky HA, Tredget EE (2000) Rating the resolving hypertrophic scar: comparison of the Vancouver Scar Scale and scar volume. J Burn Care Rehabil 21(3): 205–212

[87] Nedelec B, Correa JA, Rachelska G, Armour A, LaSalle L (2008) Quantitative measurement of hypertrophic scar: interrater reliability and concurrent validity. J Burn Care Res 29(3): 501–511

[88] Nedelec B, Correa JA, Rachelska G, Armour A, LaSalle L (2008) Quantitative measurement of hypertrophic scar: intrarater reliability, sensitivity, and specificity. J Burn Care Res 29(3): 489–500

[89] Ngo K, Goldstein D, Neligan P, Gilbert R (2006) Colorimetric evaluation of facial skin and free flap donor sites in various ethnic populations. J Otolaryngol 35(4): 249–254

[90] Niessen FB, Spauwen PH, Robinson PH, Fidler V, Kon M (1998) The use of silicone occlusive sheeting (Sil-K) and silicone occlusive gel (Epiderm) in the prevention of hypertrophic scar formation. Plast Reconstr Surg 102(6): 1962–1972

[91] Nunnaly JC (1978) Psychometric theory, 2nd edn. McGraw-Hill, New York

[92] Oliveira GV, Chinkes D, Mitchell C, Oliveras G, Hawkins HK, Herndon DN (2005) Objective assessment of burn scar vascularity, erythema, pliability, thickness, and planimetry. Dermatol Surg 31(1): 48–58

[93] Peacock EE, Jr., Madden JW, Trier WC (1970) Biologic basis for the treatment of keloids and hypertrophic scars. South Med J 63(7): 755–760

[94] Pedersen L, Jemec GB (2006) Mechanical properties and barrier function of healthy human skin. Acta Derm Venereol 86(4): 308–311

[95] Pedersen LK, Jemec GB (1999) Plasticising effect of water and glycerin on human skin in vivo. J Dermatol Sci 19(1): 48–52

[96] Pedersen LK, Hansen B, Jemec GBE (2003) Mechanical properties of the skin: A comparison between two suction cup methods. Skin Res Tech 9: 111–115

[97] Pierard-Franchimont C, Pierard GE (2002) A double-blind placebo-controlled study of ketoconazole + desonide gel combination in the treatment of facial seborrheic dermatitis. Dermatology 204(4): 344–347

[98] Pierard GE, Nikkels-Tassoudji N, Pierard-Franchimont C (1995) Influence of the test area on the mechanical properties of skin. Dermatology 191(1): 9–15

[99] Powers PS, Sarkar S, Goldgof DB, Cruse CW, Tsap LV (1999) Scar assessment: current problems and future solutions. J Burn Care Rehabil 20(1 Pt 1): 54–60; discussion 53

[100] Richard S, Querleux B, Bittoun J, Jolivet O, Idy-Peretti I, de Lacharriere O, Leveque JL (1993) Characterization of the skin in vivo by high resolution magnetic resonance imaging: water behavior and age-related effects. J Invest Dermatol 100(5): 705–709

[101] Romanelli M, Falanga V (1995) Use of a durometer to measure the degree of skin induration in lipodermatosclerosis. J Am Acad Dermatol 32(2 Pt 1): 188–191

[102] Sampson J (1961) A method of replicating dry or moist surfaces for examination by light microscopy. Nature 191: 932–933

[103] Sarkany I (1962) A method for studying the microtopography of the skin. Br J Dermatol 74: 254–259

[104] Saur R, Schramm U, Steinhoff R, Wolff HH (1991) Structure analysis of the skin surface using computer-assisted laser profilometry. New method for the quantitative assessment of roughness structure of the skin. Hautarzt 42(8): 499–506

[105] Serup J, Northeved A (1985) Skin elasticity in localized scleroderma (morphoea). Introduction of a biaxial in vivo method for measurement of tensile distensibility, hysteresis, and resilient distension of diseased and normal skin. J Dermatol 12(1): 52–62

[106] Serup J, Northeved A (1985) Skin elasticity in psoriasis. In vivo measurement of tensile distensibility, hysteresis and resilient distension with a new method. Comparison with skin thickness as measured with high-frequency ultrasound. J Dermatol 12(4): 318–324

[107] Serup J, Keiding J, Fullerton A, Gnidecka M, Gnidecki R (1995) High-frequency ultrasound examination of skin: introduction and guide. In: Serup J, Jemec GBE (eds) Handbook of non-invasive methods and the skin. CRC Press, Boca Raton, pp 239–256

[108] Seyger MM, van den Hoogen FH, de Boo T, de Jong EM (1997) Reliability of two methods to assess morphea: skin scoring and the use of a durometer. J Am Acad Dermatol 37(5 Pt 1): 793–796

[109] Shriver MD, Parra EJ (2000) Comparison of narrow-band reflectance spectroscopy and tristimulus colorimetry for measurements of skin and hair color in persons of different biological ancestry. Am J Phys Anthropol 112(1): 17–27

[110] Smith GM, Tompkins DM, Bigelow ME, Antoon AY (1988) Burn-induced cosmetic disfigurement: can it be measured reliably? J Burn Care Rehabil 9(4): 371–375

[111] Spann K, Mileski WJ, Atiles L, Purdue G, Hunt J (1996) The 1996 Clinical Research award. Use of a pneumatonometer in burn scar assessment. J Burn Care Rehabil 17(6 Pt 1): 515–517

[112] Stark HL (1977) Directional variations in the extensibility of human skin. Br J Plast Surg 30(2): 105–114

[113] Streiner DL, Norman GR (2008) Validity. Health measurement scales, 4 th edn. Oxford University Press, Oxford, pp 247–276

[114] Streiner DL, Norman GR (2008) Reliability. Health measurement scales, 4 th edn. Oxford University Press, Oxford, pp 167–210

[115] Sugama J, Matsui Y, Sanada H, Konya C, Okuwa M, Kitagawa A (2007) A study of the efficiency and convenience of an advanced portable Wound Measurement System (VISITRAK). J Clin Nurs 16(7): 1265–1269

[116] Sullivan T, Smith J, Kermode J, McIver E, Courtemanche DJ (1990) Rating the burn scar. J Burn Care Rehabil 11(3): 256–260

[117] Swope VB, Supp AP, Cornelius JR, Babcock GF, Boyce ST (1997) Regulation of pigmentation in cultured skin substitutes by cytometric sorting of melanocytes and keratinocytes. J Invest Dermatol 109(3): 289–295

[118] Takiwaki H, Overgaard L, Serup J (1994) Comparison of narrow-band reflectance spectrophotometric and tristimulus colorimetric measurements of skin color. Twenty-three anatomical sites evaluated by the Dermaspectrometer and the Chroma Meter CR-200. Skin Pharmacol 7(4): 217–225

[119] Tan CY, Statham B, Marks R, Payne PA (1982) Skin thickness measurement by pulsed ultrasound: its reproducibility, validation and variability. Br J Dermatol 106(6): 657–667

[120] Taylor B, McGrouther DA, Bayat A (2007) Use of a non-contact 3D digitiser to measure the volume of keloid scars: a useful tool for scar assessment. J Plast Reconstr Aesthet Surg 60(1): 87–94

[121] Thomas AC, Wysocki AB (1990) The healing wound: a comparison of three clinically useful methods of measurement. Decubitus 3(1): 18–20, 24–25

[122] Tronnier H, Heinrich U (1991) Untersuchungen zur Messung der Hautoberfläche. Hautnah Derm 6: 80–86

[123] Truong PT, Lee JC, Soer B, Gaul CA, Olivotto IA (2007) Reliability and validity testing of the Patient and Observer Scar Assessment Scale in evaluating linear scars after breast cancer surgery. Plast Reconstr Surg 119(2): 487–494

[124] van de Kar AL, Corion LU, Smeulders MJ, Draaijers LJ, van der Horst CM, van Zuijlen PP (2005) Reliable and feasible evaluation of linear scars by the patient and observer scar assessment scale. Plast Reconstr Surg 116(2): 514–522

[125] Van den Kerckhove E, Staes F, Flour M, Stappaerts K, Boeckx W (2001) Reproducibility of repeated measurements on healthy skin with Minolta Chromameter CR-300. Skin Res Technol 7(1): 56–59

[126] Van den Kerckhove E, Stappaerts K, Fieuws S, Laperre J, Massage P, Flour M, Boeckx W (2005) The assessment of erythema and thickness on burn related scars during pressure garment therapy as a preventive measure for hypertrophic scarring. Burns 31(6): 696–702

[127] Van Loey NE, Bremer M, Faber AW, Middelkoop E, Nieuwenhuis MK (2008) Itching following burns: epidemiology and predictors. Br J Dermatol 158(1): 95–100

[128] van Zuijlen PP, Angeles AP, Suijker MH, Kreis RW, Middelkoop E (2004) Reliability and accuracy of techniques for surface area measurements of wounds and scars. Int J Low Extrem Wounds 3(1): 7–11

[129] Vloemans AF, Soesman AM, Suijker M, Kreis RW, Middelkoop E (2003) A randomised clinical trial comparing a hydrocolloid-derived dressing and glycerol preserved allograft skin in the management of partial thickness burns. Burns 29(7): 702–710

[130] Vogel HG (1994) Mechanical measurements of skin. Acta Derm Venereol [Suppl] (Stockh) 185: 39–43

[131] Wang GQ, Xia ZF (2009) Transplantation of epidermis of scar tissue on acellular dermal matrix. Burns 35(3): 352–355

[132] Weatherall IL, Coombs BD (1992) Skin color measurements in terms of CIELAB color space values. J Invest Dermatol 99(4): 468–473

[133] Westerhof W (1995) CIE colorimetry. In: Serup J, Jemec E (eds) Handbook of non-invasive methods and the skin. Taylor and Francis, Boca Raton (Florida)

[134] Wood FM, Currie K, Backm an B, Cena B (1996) Current difficulties and the possible future directions in scar assessment. Burns 22(6): 455–458

[135] Wysocki AB (1996) Wound measurement. Int J Dermatol 35(2): 82–91

[136] Yeong EK, Mann R, Engrav LH, Goldberg M, Cain V, Costa B, Moore M, Nakamura D, Lee J (1997) Improved burn scar assessment with use of a new scar-rating scale. J Burn Care Rehabil 18(4): 353–355; discussion 352

Correspondence: Paul P. M. van Zuijlen, Department of Plastic, Reconstructive, and Hand Surgery, Red Cross Hospital Beverwijk, Vondellaan 13, 1942 LE Beverwijk, The Netherlands, Tel: +31 031 251 265 785, Fax: +31 031 251 265 342, E-mail: paul.van.zuijlen@planet.nl

The future of wound documentation: three-dimensional, evidence-based, intuitive and thorough

Michael Giretzlehner[1], Lars-Peter Kamolz[2, 3], Johannes Dirnberger[1], Robert Owen[1]

[1] Johannes Kepler University Linz, RISC Software GmbH, Division of Medical Informatics, Hagenberg im Mühlkreis, Austria
[2] State Hospital Wiener Neustadt, Department of Surgery, Section of Plastic, Aesthetic and Reconstructive Surgery, Wiener Neustadt, Austria
[3] Medical University of Vienna, Department of Surgery, Division of Plastic and Reconstructive Surgery, Vienna, Austria

Wound management, which is based on wound diagnostic, will become more and more important and will develop even more towards evidence-based medicine. Evidence-based medicine is the current state of the art in clinical research. The data quality is very much dependent on the transparency of the treatment and its objective evaluation. An objectification requires comparable patients with comparable wounds as well as comparable documentation and quality of the documentation.

Requirements

The requirements for a modern wound documentation include much more than a traditional documentation. The best method to define the required features is to use the evidence-based literature and guidelines created by experts. One of these guidelines is called "Expertenstandard – Pflege von Menschen mit chronischen Wunden" [2], which was published in German language in 2008 by the Deutsches Netzwerk für Qualitätsentwicklung in der Pflege at the Fachhochschule Osnabrück, Germany. Another well-known work is an analysis of relevant literature called "Kriterien zur Wunddokumentation" [8] by the Hessisches Institut für Pflegeforschung. The following requirements for a wound documentation system are based on the relevant literature.

The traditional wound documentation on paper is no longer a valid alternative as the new requirements for an extensive wound documentation are too complex. Törnvall et al. confirmed a qualitative and quantitative advantage of an electronic wound documentation in a study on ulcers [10]. A digital documentation provides better availability and evaluability of the collected data, easier exchange of information and consultation of experts, easier access to resources and creation of new medical knowledge. This contributes remarkably to an improved quality in wound management. In particular the demand to make the existing data useful and easily accessible can only be met by a modern wound documentation. However, a computer-assisted documentation alone does not necessarily create scientifically useful data. To ensure an optimal basis for data evaluation, free text documentation needs to be avoided, and the documentation must be clearly structured. This allows clear recording of facts at defined places, as for example patient, condition or single examination. However, the given information might often be less extensive than in free text documents [5]. The quality of the data can be improved by the structured recording as well as by the common and uniform terminology.

As stated in "Expertenstandard" [2] and in Panfil's analysis of the relevant literature [8], the following special requirements must be met to ensure a modern and up-to-date wound documentation;

- Medical history (age of patient, wound history and wound anamnesis, social background, psychosocial situation and basic mood, attitude towards the condition, lifestyle, immune status, mobility, continence situation, blood flow, allergies, nutrition and fluid status, associated and metabolic diseases, surgeries, tumors, medication, pain, ...).
- Wound assessment (localization, wound dimension, wound bed, exudate/transudate, smell, wound edge, neighboring areas of the wound, pain, infection, ...)
- Wound duration and relapse number
- Therapy (compression therapy, pressure relief, movements and promotion of movements, pain therapy, therapy of wound smell and wound exudate, antiseptics, debridement, wound cleaning, wound dressings, management of malnutrition, dietary supplements, advising and education)
- General status of the patient
- Knowledge of the patients and their relatives
- Self-management of the patients and their relatives with regard to health care
- Individual schedule for measures that can be adjusted if necessary
- Documentation of the measures and their efficacy
- Result of a regularly carried out follow-up
- Traceability and verification of authors

A wound must not be regarded as an isolated problem. The general condition of the patient is also vital. To identify the general condition it is important to evaluate the background of the condition, general medical history, information about mobility and pain, other disorders and limitations, psychic condition etc. The success of a therapy can often only be determined after a long period of time. That is the reason why there is a demand for an objective wound documentation during the whole time of treatment, which can be made available to others afterwards.

Modern wound management requires multiprofessional and interdisciplinary co-operation of various professions. Thus a system is necessary, which can provide the relevant information clearly in due time and also over large geographical distances. As only the health care personnel that is directly involved in the dressing change can evaluate the status of the wound, it is essential to provide good photography material of the wound. Very often, a dressing

change has to be carried out fast, so details that might have remained unnoticed during dressing change can be reviewed on the digital pictures thus avoiding an unnecessary dressing change (i. e. only for the purpose of reviewing the wound).

To promote evidence-based medicine, it is necessary to make data from various institutions anonymous and to merge them in a central database. The merging of data from various sources is a great challenge as different institutions operate with different sorts of databases, have different conventions, time periods and different steps of data aggregation and include different errors. These kind of problems can be avoided already at the beginning if a single system to record the data is established and applied by all parties involved.

A well-known problem in medical research is that newly published knowledge is only very slowly integrated into the daily routine of medical practice. Dr. Günther Jonitz MD [6] states that knowledge is accumulated faster than medical practice progresses. Active proposals taken from relevant scientific publications by a computer-assisted system can have benefits when addressing this problem. The keyword that has appeared only recently is *evidence-based medicine*. David L. Sackett defines it as "the conscientious, explicit, and judicious use of current best evidence in making decisions about the care of individual patients." [9]. The practice of evidence-based medicine thus includes the need to find the best available, externally clinically relevant research results. The fundamental factor for such a knowledge-based assisting system for evidence-based medicine is an automated computer-assisted search for this best external clinical evidence in a database. Such an automated search system requires an extensive medical documenting system.

Existing systems

Despite Törnvall et al. stated that filling out papers in wound documentation has many shortcomings compared to a computer-assisted wound documentation, many institutions still use paper forms for the documentation and include them in the patient's file. Recent literature has shown that not all of the requirements for a successful wound documentation are met in clinical practice. Many systems show deficits in the record of a thorough medical history of the patient [4]. Advantages of a free text documentation are flexible terms, dynamic expressions and a more effective recording by dictation. However, it has serious shortcomings: due to the linguistic variety and the lack of structure, quality and completeness cannot be verified very easily or cannot be verified at all. Often, implicit information is assumed [5] and an evaluation beyond single patients is extremely difficult. Various solutions use given terms without stating their sources [4].

The Collins English Dictionary defines documentation as "the act of supplying with or using documents or references" [1]. The aim of any documentation is to make the documented facts available. In most cases, the focus of such documentations is the gathering of data itself instead of making existing data available. In some existing wound documentation systems it is not possible to evaluate the collected data statistically. Furthermore, only very few systems are able to gather data via mobile devices as for example laptops, tablet PCs or smartphones. Another shortcoming of the existing systems is that it is not possible to access evidence-based knowledge [4].

Research project Qutis 3D

Qutis 3D (www.qutis3d.com) is a research project, which is carried out by the division of medical informatics of the RISC Software GmbH in cooperation with an experienced team of physicians. The enterprise is part of the Johannes Kepler University Linz and the Upper Austrian Research GmbH. Since 2002 the project team has worked on the burn injury documentation system *BurnCase 3D* [3] (www.burncase.at), which is already internationally in use in clinical practice. Aim of the new project *Qutis 3D* is to make use of these experiences and to develop a software system, which will revolutionize the documentation, evaluation and therapeutical decisions in modern wound management.

An evidence-based background and an intensive cooperation within a research project according to the methods of action research [6] contribute to the development of a new wound documentation system, which will meet the requirements of medical documentation as well as the demands of all professionals involved. Action research according to Österle [7] connects deductive and empirical elements and is characterized by a synergy of practice and science in problem-solving. Science structures the problems and develops solutions for the practice. These proposed solutions are being tested and improved in practice in the form of prototypes.

Compared to other existing systems *Qutis 3D* improves the quality of data evaluation by structuring the characteristics and collecting predominantly qualitative characteristics with default specifications. To make the terminology transparent, the system provides an encyclopedia with terminology and charts including references to their source. The graphical interface allows to visualize these definitions easily and fast. This ensures that everyone involved can understand and interpret the information provided in the documentation system correctly.

To guarantee the completeness of the collected data, *Qutis 3D* offers an automatic reminding feature and a visual feedback of obligatory fields and their status. The users can see at a glance where they still need to fill in information (see Fig. 1).

As this is a medical documentation system, the traceability and verification of the authors is ensured by relevant mechanisms and audits in the database.

One of the crucial factors for the success of an electronic wound management system is its easy handling. The system should have a clearly-arranged and intuitive user interface that can be understood and operated easily. This is achieved by an adjustment to the application domain, which is carried out by the physicians of the research team. *Qutis 3D* uses a three-dimensional virtual body, which is adjusted to the real patient (physical parameters as for example height and weight). The documentation of wound areas or therapy steps can be carried out by drawings on the virtual body (see Fig. 2).

Information about wound, dressings, clinical findings, documents and an extensive photo documentation are positioned directly on the virtual patient. The different colors of the pins represent different objects. In the example shown in Fig. 2, both photos (blue pin) and wound swabs (red pin) were documented at a certain time. By locally documenting swabs and the like wound infection and complications can be consistently documented and under-

Fig. 1. *Qutis 3D* entry form with completeness check

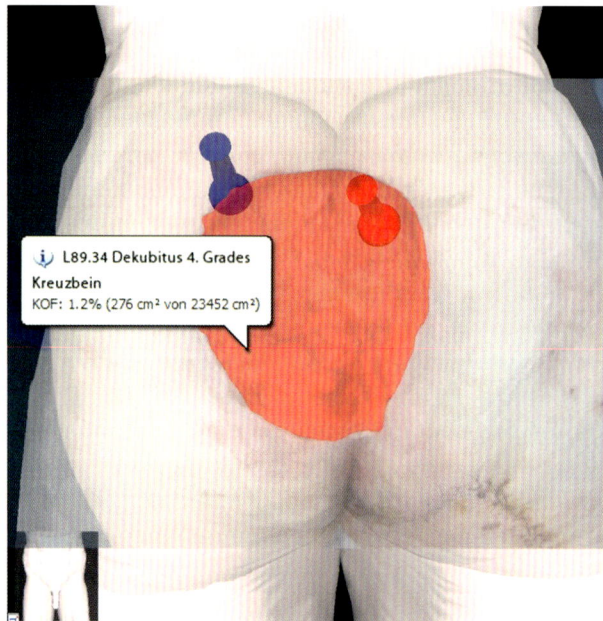

Fig. 2. Three-dimensional patient with wound and allocated information objects as digital photographs (blue pin) and wound swabs (red pin)

stood. *Qutis 3D* is a product of a multi-professional co-operation and thus provides a common terminology and illustrates the overall condition of the pa-

tient. It is network-compatible and can provide information also across long distances. Even in case that the health care team changes, a dressing change can be avoided because there is sufficient information available. This is a benefit for the patient (less pain, shorter healing time, etc.) as well as for the health care institution as the use of dressings and medication can be reduced.

Furthermore, *Qutis 3D* provides a complete photo archive, which allows a three-dimensional localization. The photos are positioned directly on the virtual three-dimensional patient and are thus easier accessible. Photos of wounds are two-dimensional but can be transferred by projection to the three-dimensional model (see Fig. 3)

In this projection the three-dimensional character of the wound is preserved (see Fig. 4). This ensures an objective and quantitative evaluation of the wound. The number of dressing changes is reduced and the patient suffers less as there is no direct contact with the wound. The three-dimensional recording facilitates an automatic localization and survey. The information stored in the three-dimensional patient model provides medical codes as for example ICD and OPS. *Qutis 3D* allows for a complete wound monitoring and thus an evaluation of the possible

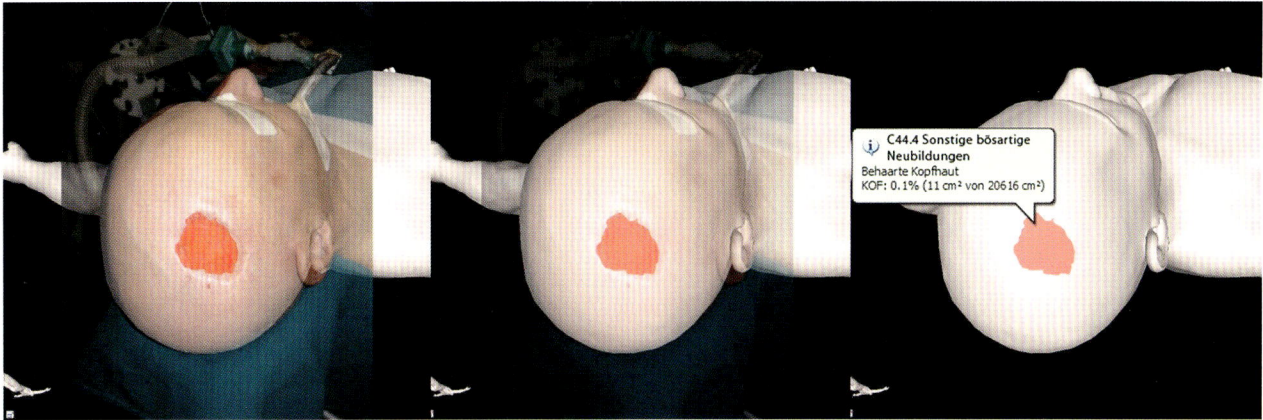

Fig. 3. Semi-transparent transition and transmission of wound information

success of a therapy. There is a chronological as well as an aggregated illustration of the history of each wound with according digital photographs.

To make the data stored in *Qutis 3D* accessible, the system has an analysis tool, through which the data can be extracted from the database, aggregated and prepared for further evaluation without special database knowledge. *Qutis 3D* contains a data acquisition tool for studies and expert systems. Data about wound management can be compared and evaluated across single institutions, which serves as basis for data-mining activities.

One of the focuses in the development of *Qutis 3D* was the implementation of reliable knowledge. The standardized wound documentation established with *Qutis 3D* and the possibility to compare the case data can contribute to an effective training of machine learning systems. The aim is to detect specific characteristics in the data and to make proposals concerning medical treatment alternatives. Applying this technique should generate knowledge from the given data, which can help physicians in their daily practice.

Recorded patient data can be transferred electronically. An additional opinion can thus be considered within a very short period of time. The advising physician can gain a good overview because of the three-dimensional patient model and the well structured display of information in *Qutis 3D*.

As most of the physicians have a smartphone, it will be reasonable to make use of the existing hardware. The research team has already gained experi-

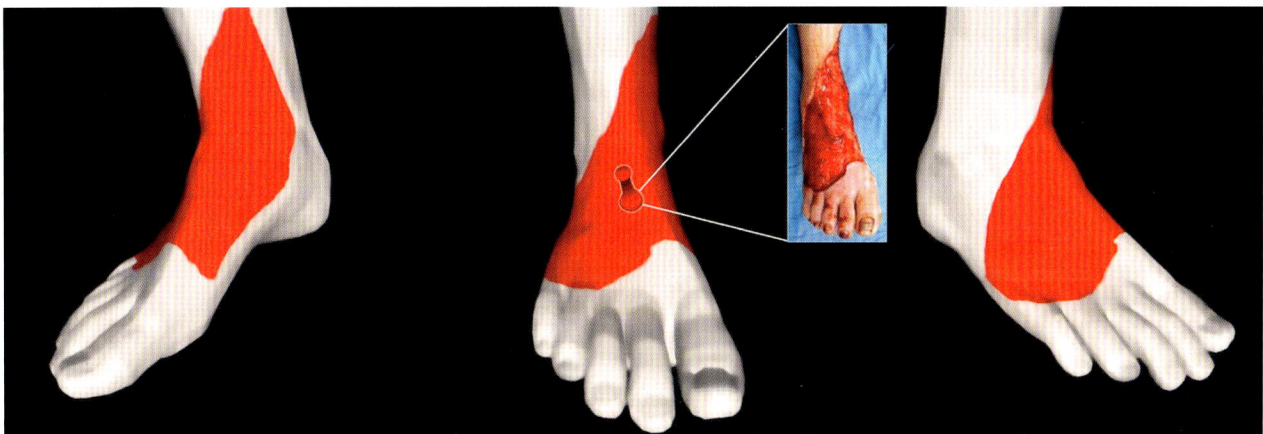

Fig. 4. The three-dimensionality is preserved in the documentation

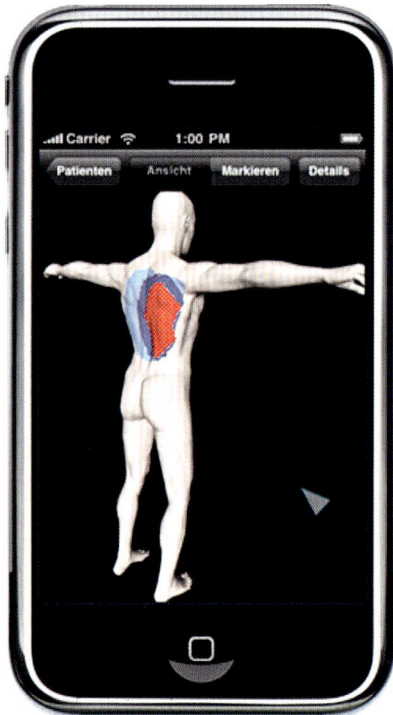

Fig. 5. Mobile version of the burn injury documentation system BurnCase 3D

ence in the implementation of burn injury documentation systems into mobile platforms (see Fig. 5). A mobile version for the platform iPhone OS™ (iPod, iPhone, iPad) by Apple™ will also be developed for the documentation system *Qutis 3D*.

Conclusion

Various systems meet most of the required demands for a wound documentation system. However they have shortcomings in recording the data objectively and well-structured, in applying not precisely defined terminology and in making the collected data accessible.

The aim of the research project *Qutis 3D* is to solve these problems and to provide the highest possible data quality. This can be achieved by a very well-structured data recording and by an objective determination of wound dimension and localization. Furthermore, the system will promote evidence-based medicine and provide the relevant information for the attending physician fast and easily accessible.

References

[1] Collins English Dictionary, Harper Collins Publishers, 2009

[2] DNQP (Deutsches Netzwerk für Qualitätssicherung in der Pflege e.V.): Expertenstandard Pflege von Menschen mit chronischen Wunden, Fachhochschule Osnabrück

[3] Haller HL, Dirnberger J, Giretzlehner M, Rodemund C, Kamolz LP (2009) Understanding burns: Research project BurnCase 3D – Overcome the limits of existing methods in burns documentation. Burns 35: 311–317

[4] Hübner U, Flemming D, Schultz-Gödker (2009) Software zur digitalen Wunddokumentation: Marktübersicht und Bewertungskriterien. WundM 3 (6): 99–103

[5] Ingenerf J (2009) Computergestützte strukturierte Befundung am Beispiel der Wunddokumentation. WundM 3 (6): 104–108

[6] Kunz R, Ollenschläger G, Raspe HH (2007) Lehrbuch Evidenzbasierte Medizin in Klinik und Praxis. Deutscher Ärzte-Verlag, ISBN 3 769 105 389

[7] Österle T, Gutzwiller H (1992) Ein Beispiel für die Analyse und das System-Design. AIT Angewandte Informations Technik 2

[8] Panfil EM, Linde E, DGfW (Deutsche Gesellschaft für Wundheilung und Wundbehandlung e.V.) (2006) Kriterien zur Wunddokumentation – Literaturanalyse, Hessisches Institut für Pflegeforschung, Frankfurt

[9] Sackett DL, Rosenberg WMC, Gray JA, Haynes RB, Richardson WS (1996) Evidence based medicine: what it is and what it isn't. Br Med J (BMJ) 312: 71–72

[10] Törnvall E, Wahren LK, Wilhelmsson S (2009) Advancing nursing documentation – An intervention study using patients with leg ulcer as an example. Int J Med Inform 78: 605–661

Correspondence: Lars-Peter Kamolz, M.D., Ph.D., M.Sc., Medical University of Vienna, Department of Surgery, Division of Plastic and Reconstructive Surgery, Vienna, Austria, E-mail: kamolz@plastchirurg.info

Evaluation of mimic function in patients with facial burns by use of the three-dimensional video-analysis

Maria Michaelidou, Manfred Frey

Division of Plastic and Reconstructive Surgery, Department of Surgery, Medical University of Vienna, Vienna, Austria

Objective evaluation of facial motion has always been a challenging task. Many grading systems have been developed through the years, but they have often been inconsistently reproducible and subjective or they have not been able to take into account the three-dimensional aspect of facial movements. Facial burns cause also a functional impairment apart from the visible deformity of facial characteristics and the anticipated consequences from an aesthetic and psychosocial standpoint. The loss of facial skin and the resulting scar formation after conservative treatment or after skin grafting lead to an altered facial expression both in repose and during facial animation.

The need for development of an accurate system for evaluation of facial motion became urgent as reconstructive surgery in facial palsy progressed. The most commonly employed system for evaluation of facial movements in this setting is still the House-Brackman scale in many centres, which was actually developed by otolaryngologists and primarily designed for the follow-up of Bell's palsy patients [10]. The scale, as such, serves as an approximate estimation of the overall state of palsy and thus, serves as a tool for the total assessment of the patient, without enabling, however, precise separate and detailed information in regard to individual parts of the face. Moreover, the House-Brackman scale is not based on actual measurements and is therefore fraught with a considerable degree of subjectivity.

Similarly, the paresis score system suggested by Stennert [16, 17] is also based on the subjective opinion of the examiner on whether each of the ten points constituting the system applies to the patient or not. Moreover, the paralyzed side is evaluated on its own without consideration of the contralateral healthy side. This leads sometimes to a faulty score of paresis, for instance when the statement upon the presence or not of a nasolabial sulcus must be marked as negative at a single patient and thereby increase the score of paresis although at this patient a nasolabial fold may not even be present at the healthy side, as in the case of young patients. Moreover, an ignoring of the contralateral healthy side in the estimation of the extent of the paresis leads to a neglect of individual patterns of smile, a problem that is best reflected when it comes to the points eight and nine of the system.

Johnson et al. described in 1994 [1, 11, 12] a quantitative method known as the maximum static response assay of facial motion for the evaluation of the success of functional free muscle transplantation in patients with chronic facial paralysis. Although the attempt to express the extent of paralysis in numbers and, thus, objectify the postoperative outcome was a well justified one, still this method was actually projecting a three-dimensional motion into a two-dimensional distance. Gross et al. [9] showed in 1996, however, that projecting 3D into 2D data leads to loss of accuracy of measurement because three-dimensional amplitudes are significantly larger than the two-dimensional amplitudes.

First attempts to overcome the limitation of two-dimensionality of the existing evaluation systems were yielded with success in 1992, when Frey et al. introduced a new documentation system for facial movements as a basis for the International Registry for Neuromuscular Reconstruction in the face [3,18]. The system, called VICON, enabled for the first time a three-dimensional motion analysis based on the measurement of movements of standardized static and dynamic points in the face during standardized mimic activities. Although this system was very useful for research purposes, it was too complicated for daily clinical application.

In 1994 an electronic instrument, called faciometer®, was introduced by Frey et al. in order to measure excursions of facial landmarks during animation after reconstruction in case of facial palsy [13]. The faciometer® consisted of calipers connected to a digital display, which showed the distance between the tips of the callipers [13].

Due to significant advances in computer technology, particularly in the field of image analysis, it became possible to achieve a three-dimensional analysis of a two-dimensional video taken during the course of a facial movement. This new system was completed and installed for the first time in the Laboratory for Movement and Image Analysis at the Division of Plastic and Reconstructive Surgery, Department of Surgery, Medical School of Vienna in January of 1998 [4]. Since then, the evaluation of all patients treated for facial paralysis at the above mentioned institution, was performed by use of of this system, which has become the standard tool for the preoperative documentation, for the planning of the treatment and for the postoperative monitoring and evaluation of the operative outcome.

The system consists of three main components (Fig. 1):
▶ The data acquisition system which includes the following:
  • a sample mirror system, consisting of two special mirrors arranged under a constant sharp angle and a comfortable seat placed underneath of them so that the patient's head is positioned between the two mirrors in a way that complete images of the patient's face can be

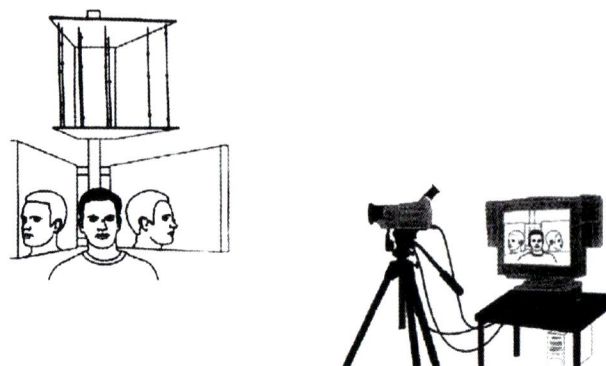

Fig. 1. Schema of the three-dimensional video-analysis system [4]

obtained and all marked points are seen by the camera in both mirrors at the same time,
  • a calibration grid, which is essential for the definition of the three-dimensional space prior to every recording session.
  • a digital video camera (Sony DCR-CX700E®) for the recording of the films,
  • a computer station, where the recorded sequences are transferred using DV Manager® 1.7 (FAST Multimedia mInc.,Wsoodville, WA, USA) and edited by a program of analysis.
▶ The data analyzing system with the following components:
  • the Ulead®5-Video Editor software (Ulead Systems Inc., Torrance, CA, USA) for selection of the most suitable sequences which were then cut from the others and edited through the
  • Facialis® software (Laboratory of Biomechanics of the Swiss Federal Institute of Technology, Zurich, Switzerland).
▶ The data visualization system: a specially designed program for presenting the data processed through the Facialis® software, called FaciShow® (Laboratory of Biomechanics of the Swiss Federal Institute of Technology, Zurich, Switzerland). The program enables the demonstration of landmarks both in two- and in three-dimensional perspective for every single movement as well as the demonstration of excursions of landmarks at each phase of the animation (Fig. 2). Additionally, the whole video clip for each and every movement can be reviewed or the picture of the patient's face both in repose and in the endpoint of every movement can be seen.

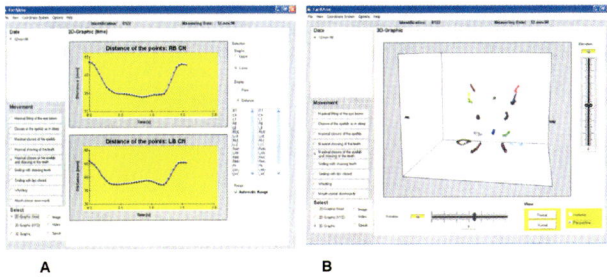

Fig. 2. FaciShow®: (A) graphical two-dimensional representation of the distances between landmarks of the face and (B) visualization of the movement of each landmark during the whole course of motion in a three-dimensional perspective [8]

The procedure of data acquisition follows a standard pattern which has been described by Frey et al. Extensively [4–6, 8] and is cited here in summarized form.

A selection of eighteen standard reproducible anatomical landmarks on the face, of which three are static and fifteen are dynamic (Table 1 and Fig. 3), are marked on the patient's face. A permanent marker is used to place a 2 mm black dot at each of the dynamic landmarks. The static points are marked with a plastic light ball 5 mm in diameter. All markings, except the points central nose and philtrum, are made on both sides of the face.

Each patient is videotaped under standard conditions. All recordings are made in the same room, in the same chair and by the same examiner. Light from four 1000 W Halogen Photo- optic lamps (Osram,

Table 1. Abbreviations of the standardized facial landmarks [4]

Abbreviations of the standardized facial landmarks [4]	
Central nose	CN
Left ala of the nose	LAN
Left brow	LB
Left lower eyelid	LLE
Left mouth corner	LMC
Left midlateral point of the lower lip	LML
Left midlateral point of the upper lip	LMU
Left tragus	LT
Left upper eyelid	LUE
Philthrum	PH
Right ala of the nose	RAN
Right brow	RB
Right lower eyelid	RLE
Right mouth corner	RMC
Right midlateral point of the lower lip	RML
Right midlateral point of the upper lip	RMU
Right tragus	RT
Right upper eyelid	RUE

Munich, Germany) is used to generate uniform, symmetrical and standardized lighting.

The patient sits relaxed and upright in a normal chair without head support, eyes looking forward into the camera, which is positioned 5 m away. After the patient has been positioned in the calibrated measurement field, a series of nine standardized facial animations are performed in a sequential order after a verbal signal.

Three repetitions of each set of facial animations are digitally collected through a video camera in real time with a sampling rate of 25 pictures per second and transferred to a computer, where the most suitable video sequence out of the three is edited and saved as video (.avi) and image (.uis) files. The selected data is then analyzed by the means of Facialis software [4] (Laboratory for Biomechanics, Swiss federal Institute of Technology, Zurich, Switzerland), which calculates the 3D coordinates of landmarks on the face. The processed data can then be visualized by the FaciShow software [4] (Laboratory for Biomechanics, Swiss federal Institute of Technology, Zurich, Switzerland). Two-dimensional (2D) and

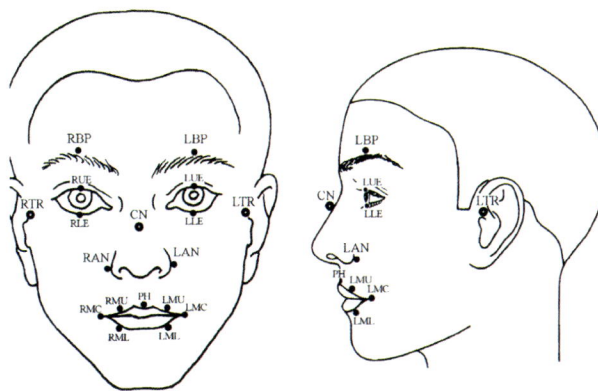

Fig. 3. The locations of the static and dynamic landmarks on the face in frontal and lateral view [3]

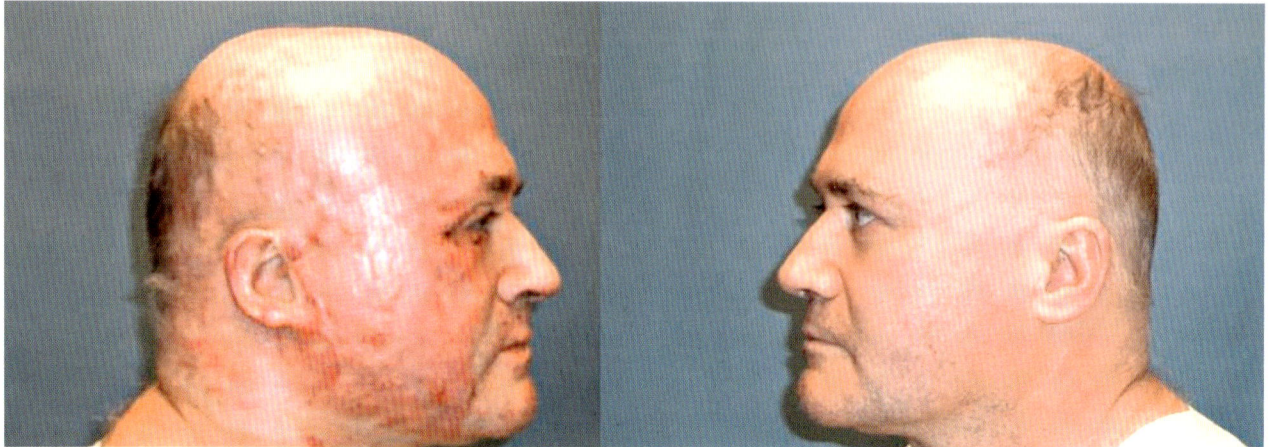

Fig. 4. Male patient with facial burn scars of the right hemiface from a lateral point of view [2]

three-dimensional (3D) trajectories of each landmark during movement can be presented.

This procedure is performed in every patient before every operative step and 6, 12, 18 and 24 months after surgery.

After having applied the system of three-dimensional video-analysis in order to evaluate results after reconstructive surgery in cases of facial palsy [7, 14, 15], we applied the system also in patients with facial burns that had been treated by excision and grafting with allogenous keratinocytes [2]. The results of facial analysis of these patients were compared with the values of healthy volunteers who had already been analysed in the same fashion in a previous study [8]. The burn patients showed on average smaller excursions of landmarks during facial ani-

mation and higher degree of static asymmetry than healthy volunteers. As in the case of healthy volunteers, the degree of asymmetry after animation of the face was smaller than in repose, i. e. static asymmetry was higher than dynamic asymmetry [2].

In Fig. 4 a male patient with facial burns is presented and the use of the three-dimensional system of video-analysis for quantification of the impact of the resulting scars on the static symmetry of the face and the facial motion is explained. In this patient the burn injury affects only the right hemiface (Fig. 5). The overall scar formation affecting the entire right hemiface leads to a lateral displacement of the mouth corner and a cranial displacement of the

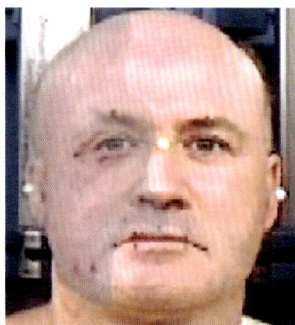

Fig. 5. The same patient as in Fig. 4 from a frontal point of view. The gray marking displays the extent of facial scar formation on the right hemiface [2]

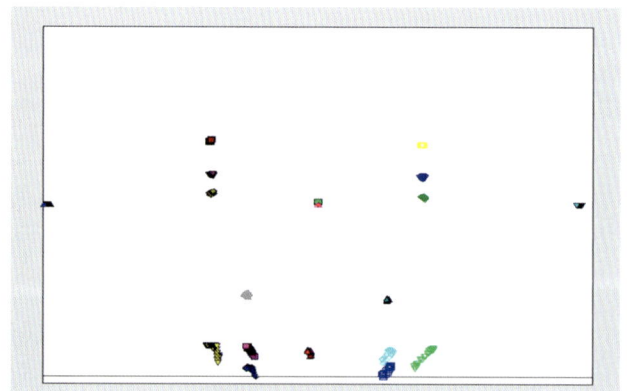

Fig. 6. Three-dimensional view of all static and dynamic points of the face of the patient in Figs. 4 and 5 during the motion "smiling with lips closed"

Table 2. Distance of the tragus to the mouth corner (TR-MC) and central nose point to the middle upper lip point (CN-MU) on the right and the left hemiface in repose and at the endpoint of motion [2]

	Right hemiface			Left hemiface			Asymmetry	
	Repose	Endpoint of motion	Amplitude	Repose	Endpoint of motion	Amplitude	Repose	Amplitude
TR-MC	100,50	94,64	5,86	101,45	93,54	7,91	0,95	2,05
CN-MU	64,46	63,10	1,36	66,79	64,50	2,29	2,33	0,93

middle upper lip point on the right side. Thus, there is a shortening of the distance of the mouth corner to the tragus and a shortening of the distance of the central nose point to the middle upper lip point on the right side of the face compared to the left one. As a consequence, the amplitude of motion of the mouth corner to the tragus and of the middle upper lip point to the central nose point is shorter on the right side of the face than on the left one. The three-dimensional video-analysis confirmed these observations (Table 2). In Fig. 6a three-dimensional view of all static and dynamic points of the face of this patient during the motion "smiling with lips closed" is displayed. A different course of motion of the corner of the mouth, the upper middle and lower middle lip point are observed on the right hemiface compared to the left one.

In future, we will consider the use of three-dimensional video-analysis in order to quantify the impact of facial scars and the impact of different concepts of treatment (conservative vs. operative treatment, reconstruction with keratinocytes vs. skin grafts vs. artificial agents such as Integra®, Matriderm®, Acticoat®) on the static symmetry of the face and on the facial motion.

References

[1] Bajaj-Luthra A, Müller T, Johnson PC (1997) Quantitative analysis of facial motion components: anatomic and nonanatomic motion in normal persons and in patients with complete facial paralysis. Plast Reconstr Surg 99: 1894

[2] Eggert S (2010) Quantitative Analyse der Gesichtsmotorik nach Verbrennungen mit dem System der Drei-Dimensionalen Video-Analyse. Doctoral Thesis, Medical University of Vienna, Austria, March 2010

[3] Frey M, Jenny A, Giovanoli P, Stüssi E (1994) Development of a New Documentation System for Facial Movements as a Basis for the International Registry for Neurovascular Reconstruction in the face. Plast Reconstr Surg 93: 1334–1349

[4] Frey M, Giovanoli P, Gerber H, Slameczka M, Stüssi E (1999) Three-dimensional video analysis of facial movements: a new method to assess the quantity and quality of the smile. Plast Reconstr Surg 104: 2032–2039

[5] Frey M (1999) Smile reconstruction using the gracilis muscle. Oper Techn Plast Reconstr Surg 6: 180–89

[6] Frey M, Giovanoli P (2002) The three-stage concept to optimize the results of microsurgical reanimation of the paralyzed face. Clin Plast Surg 29: 1–24

[7] Frey M, Michaelidou M, Tzou Ch.-H, Gerber H, Stüssi E, Mittlböck M (2008) Three-dimensional video analysis of the paralyzed face reanimated by cross-face nerve grafting and free gracilis muscle transplantation: quantification of the functional outcome. Plast Reconstr Surg 122(6): 1709–1722

[8] Giovanoli P, Tzou C-HJ, Ploner M, Frey M (2003) Three-dimensional video-analysis of facial movements in healthy volunteers. Br J Plast Surg 56: 644–652

[9] Gross MM, Trotman CA, Moffat KS (1996) A comparison of three-dimensional and two-dimensional analyses of facial motion. Angle Orthod 66: 189

[10] House JW (1983) Facial nerve grading systems. Laryngoscope 93: 1056–1069

[11] Johnson PC, Brown H, Kuzon WM, Balliet R, Garrison J, Campbell J (1994) Simultaneous quantification of facial movements: the maximal static response assay of facial nerve function. Ann Plast Surg 32: 171

[12] Johnson PJ, Bajaj-Luthra A, Llull R, Johnson PC (1997) Quantitative facial motion analysis after functional free muscle reanimation procedures. Plast Reconstr Surg 100: 1710

[13] Koller R, Kargül G, Giovanoli P, Meissl G, Frey M (2000) Quantification of functional results after facial burns by the faciometer®. Burns 26: 716–723

[14] Michaelidou M (2004) Comparison of surgical methods for reanimation of the paralyzed face by use of 3D-video-analysis. Doctoral Thesis, Medical University of Vienna, Austria, March 2004

[15] Michaelidou M, Tzou Ch.-H, Gerber H, Stüssi E, Mittlböck M, Frey M (2009) The combination of muscle transpositions and static procedures – a useful concept

for reconstruction in the paralyzed face of the patient with limited life expectancy or who is not a candidate for free muscle transfer. Plast Reconstr Surg 123(1): 121–129

[16] Stennert E, Limberg CH, Frentrup KP (1979) Paralysis and secondary defect score. In: Miehkle A, Stennert E, Chilla R (eds) New aspects in facial surgery. Clin Plast Surg 6: 458

[17] Stennert E, Limberg CH, Frentrup KP (1977) Parese- und Defektheilungs-Index. HNO 25: 238–245

[18] Stüssi E, Handschin S, Frey M (1992) Quantifizierung von Gesichtsasymmetrien. Eine Methode zur Objektivierung von Beeinträchtigungen der Gesichtsmotorik: eine Pilotstudie. Biomed Technik 37: 14–19

Correspondence: Maria Michaelidou, M. D., Division of Plastic and Reconstructive Surgery, Medical University of Vienna, Währinger Gürtel 18–20, 1090 Vienna, Austria, Tel: +43 1 40 400 6986, Fax: +43 1 40 400 6988, E-mail: maria.michaelidou@meduniwien.ac.at

Rehabilitation and scar management

Lars-Peter Kamolz[1, 2], Marc G. Jeschke[3]

[1] Medical University of Vienna, Department of Surgery, Division of Plastic and Reconstructive Surgery, Vienna, Austria
[2] State Hospital Wiener Neustadt, Department of Surgery, Section of Plastic, Aesthetic and Reconstructive Surgery, Wiener Neustadt, Austria
[3] Sunnybrook Health Sciences Centre, Ross Tilley Burn Centre, Toronto, Canada

Introduction

Survival was once the key parameter of success in managing serious burns, but due to improvements concerning burn care this has changed tremendously. Today, however, the aim of all treatment activities is the return of burn patients back into their private and social life under conditions, which allow independence and social sovereignty. This goal has extended the traditional role of the burn care team beyond wound closure.

Three broad aspects are involved in this effort: rehabilitation, reconstruction, and reintegration. Modern burn care may be divided into the following 4 general phases [1]:

▶ The first phase, initial evaluation and resuscitation, occurs on days 1–3 and requires an accurate fluid resuscitation and thorough evaluation for other injuries and co morbid conditions.
▶ The second phase, initial wound excision and biologic closure, includes the manoeuvre that changes the natural history of the disease. This is accomplished typically by a series of staged operations that are completed during the first few days after injury.
▶ The third phase, definitive wound closure, involves replacement of temporary wound covers with a definitive cover; there is also closure and acute reconstruction of areas with small surface area but high complexity, such as the face and hands.
▶ The final stage of care is rehabilitation, reconstruction, and reintegration. Although this begins during the resuscitation period, it becomes time-consuming and involved toward the end of the acute hospital stay.

Rehabilitation in the critically ill burn patient

Burn rehabilitation is undeniably difficult and time-consuming, but the time spent is worthwhile [2–6]. For every member of the burn team, rehabilitation must start from the time of injury on, but the final obtainable treatment goals and strategies can vary, depending on the patient's injury, age, and co morbidities.

In critically ill patients, the primary goals of rehabilitation are:

▶ Limitation of the loss of range of motion (ROM),
▶ Oedema reduction, and
▶ Prevention of predictable contractures.

If a body part is left immobile for a prolonged period of time, capsular contraction and shortening of tendon and muscle groups (which cross the joints) occur. Contractures often develop, if wounds are not closed promptly and adequately.

Several predictable contractures that occur in patients with burns can be prevented by a proper ROM, positioning, and splinting programs [1].

▶ Passive ROM is best performed twice daily, with the therapist taking all joints through a full ROM (Fig. 1). The therapist must be sensitive to the patient's pain, anxiety, wound status, extremity perfusion, and security of the patient's airway and vascular access.

▶ These procedures should be performed in coordination with the ICU staff. Attention to the security of endotracheal tubes, nasogastric tubes, and arterial and central venous catheters is paramount, as an unexpected loss can contribute to morbidity and mortality.

▶ Proper antideformity positioning minimizes shortening of tendons, collateral ligaments, and joint capsules; moreover, it reduces oedema formation.

▶ Inspect all splints at least daily for evidence of poor fitting or pressure injury.

Oedema reduction should be encouraged from admission on. The only body system that can actively remove excess fluid and debris from the interstitium is the lymphatic system. The principles of oedema reduction should be performed:

▶ Compression
▶ Movement
▶ Elevation or positioning of limbs
▶ Maximisation of lymphatic function

Beside the factors range of motion (ROM), oedema reduction, and prevention of predictable contractures, a long-term relationship has to be established with the patient and family members to ensure compliance with therapy goals and to increase the patient's morale for recovery. Moreover adequate pain control is important for long term compliance of the patient. The factors compliance and pain control will become even more important in the later phase of rehabilitation.

Rehabilitation in the recovering burn patient

As critical illness abates and wounds progressively close, the roles of the physical and occupational therapists (as well as the demands on the patient) expand and become more difficult. Patients become more aware of what has happened to them, and they can become fearful of the therapist and the associated potentially uncomfortable procedures.

▶ The principal components of burn therapy [2–6] that characterize this period include the following:
   • Continued passive ROM
   • Increasing active ROM and strengthening
   • Minimizing oedema
   • ADL training (activities of daily living) (Fig. 2)
   • Scar Management
   • Preparing for work or play or school

Long-term favourable outcome requires hard work during this period, but it is important for the ther-

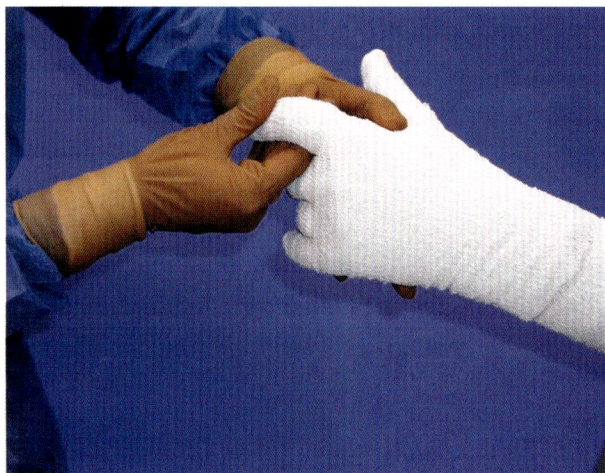

Fig. 1. Passive mobilisation

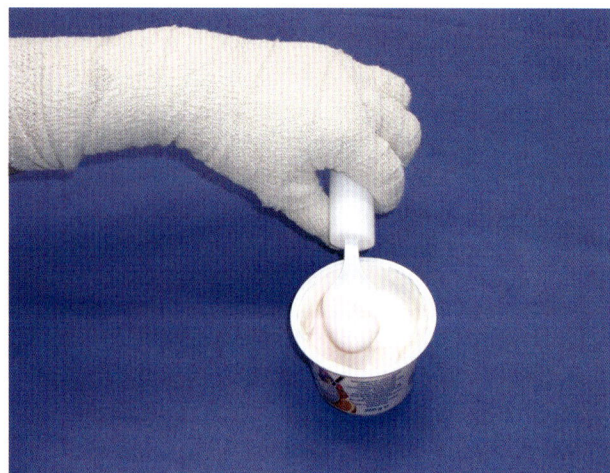

Fig. 2. ADL training

apist not to push too hard. An early program of passive ROM greatly facilitates successful retention of normal ROM during this period. Intraoperative ROM also can be useful; in coordination with the operating room team, passive ROM can be performed between induction of anaesthesia and preparation of the surgical site. Other manoeuvres that can be used to increase the patient's tolerance for passive ROM are the timing of the ROM session at the end of the dressing changes performed under pain medication.

▶ Burned and grafted extremities commonly have oedema that can contribute to joint stiffness. Reducing this oedema facilitates rehabilitation efforts.
  • In the early phase the use of self-adherent elastic will help to reduce digital oedema. Tubular elastic dressings, elastic wrap dressings, elevation, and retrograde massage also help reduce extremity oedema.
▶ As definitive wound closure nears and hospital discharge approaches, the focus of rehabilitation efforts becomes practical. Performance of ADL tasks and the impending return to play/school/work are important considerations.
  • Resisted ROM, isometric exercises, active strengthening, and gait training are important objectives.
  • When treating children, it is important to use developmentally appropriate play to facilitate rehabilitation goals.
▶ For many burn patients, the first 18 months after discharge are more difficult than the acute stay. The principal rehabilitation goals at this time include the following:
  • Progressive ROM and strengthening
  • Evaluation of evolving problem areas
  • Specific postoperative therapy after reconstructive operations
  • Scar management

Unfortunately, it is not uncommon for ROM and strength to be lost during the first months after discharge. The burn unit team should monitor the quality of outpatient rehabilitation services during routine clinic visits at the burn unit. If the patient is losing substantial ROM and strength due to inadequate therapy, readmission for focused rehabilitation efforts is appropriate and recommended.

Non-surgical scar management

The treatment of scars is a big challenging process and important part in the rehabilitation program. Scars can lead to emotional conflicts and psychosocial problems, but beside these aesthetic and emotional problems scars can cause also important functional restrictions and impairments. Due to the fact that the process of the hypertrophic scarring begins often after discharge and may last for several month and years, a need for special aftercare especially during the first 12–24 months is needed.

Although the process of the scar maturation is not fully understood yet, several approaches are propagated for non-surgical scar management.

Compression therapy

As early as possible compression therapy should be performed by use of special customized compression garments (Figs. 3 and 4). Compression therapy helps to provide functionally and aesthetically satisfying scars and reduces the need for surgical scar revisions. By use of compression good and satisfactory results can be achieved in 85 % of the patients suffering from hyperthrophic scars [7, 8], because as long as the scars are active, they can be influenced by compression. The exact mechanism of action is not cleared yet, but there is clear evidence that continuous pressure reduces the blood flow within the scar and thereby its activity. The metabolism of the scar is reduced and local ischemia and hypoxia is resulting in a reduced proliferation and activity of the fibroblasts and thereby of the collage synthesis [9]. Thereby excessive scaring is decreased [10].

Wounds, which heal within 14 to 21 days have a lower chance to develop hypertrophic scars, but if wound healing takes longer than 21 days, there is a higher chance to develop hypertrophic scars and a compression therapy is an absolutely must [10] for a period of several months (in children often also more than 2 years until the scars are mature) and should be worn 24 hours daily.

The optimum compression pressure, which should be exerted onto the scar, it is discussed still controversially [11–14]. A pressure of 10 mmHg is probably enough to reduce scars and a pressure more than 40 mmHg is possibly not good for the skin

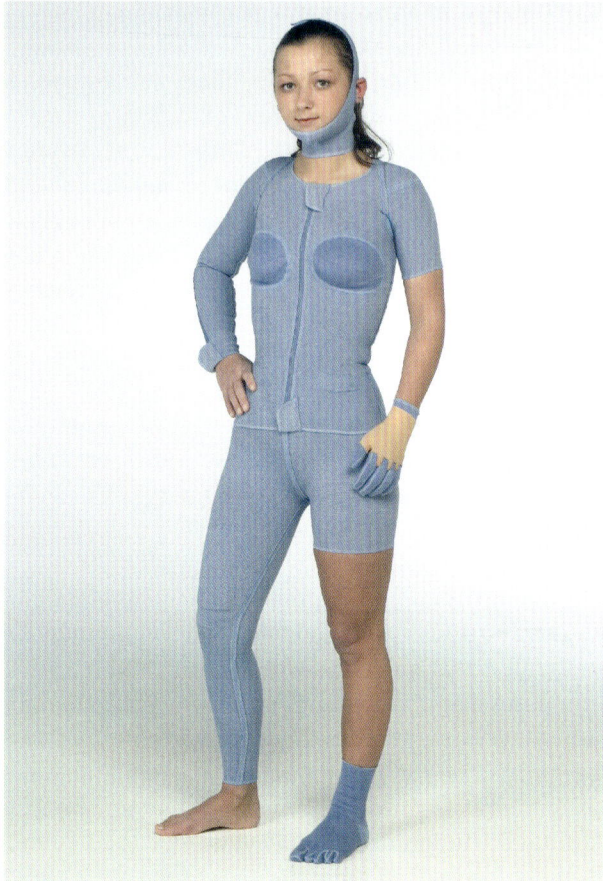

Fig. 3. Custom made compression garments

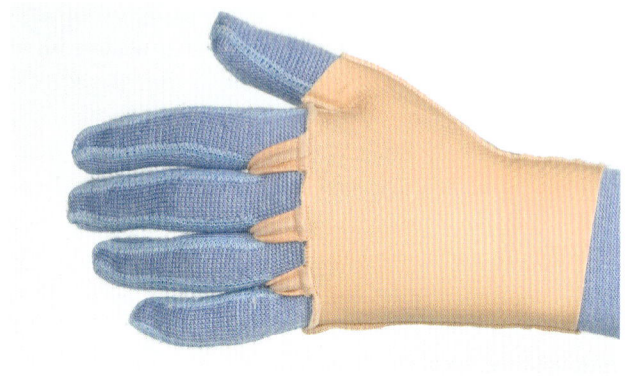

Fig. 4. Special compression gloves plus additional pressure for the web spaces

and can cause nerve irritations and pain. The compression pressure, which is generated with compression clothes, amount approx. 24–28 mmHg; this more or less identical with the capillary pressure, which amounts around 25 mmHg.

Pressure pads

Problems concerning compression therapy can occur in unfavourable localisations, above all in concave surfaces, as for example in the area of the sternum and the face. These are only hardly accessible to a suitable compression treatment. Mostly, a combination with special pads (pelotte), which can exert additional pressure, is useful. Pressure pads are made from different materials as for example from silicone gel, elastomeric and different plastic materials. The used material should be chosen depending on scar maturation and on the skin status of the pa-

tient. In general one begins with a soft, thin and elastic pad and exchanges this with the time for harder and stronger pressure-exercising pads.

Hydration and silicone

Silicone has been used with great success in order to reduce hypertrophic scars; hydration or the silicone related prevention of wound desiccation, appears to be the contributing mechanism. Hydration seems to inhibit the fibroblast related production of collagen and glycoaminoglycans. Silicone gel sheets can be worn 24 hours daily. Beside gel sheets [8] there are also silicone gels [7] available; they are normally applied twice a day after suture removal. Both, silicone sheets and gels seem to have positive influence on scare size and erythema reduction. The use is not limited to prophylactic scar treatment, but also for improving prexisting hypertrophic scars. The advantages of this kind of the scar treatment are the easy use and the quick improvement of the clinical symptoms.

Lubricants and solar exposition

Due to the functional impairment special skin care is needed after a burn injury. Hydration protects the skin against dryness. Special oils and creams, which do not irritate the skin, should be applied several times daily.

The patients should be cleared up thoroughly about the fact that the scars in the first year after a burn injury may be put out by no means to the direct sun. The danger of sunburn is very big and the scars will become probably darker in the sun. This discoloration is lasting and makes the scars even more remarkable. Solar-cream with a solar protection factor from at least 30 as well as adequate sun protection clothing is strictly recommended [15].

Creams/Salves

There is a great variety of creams for conservative scar management on the market; many of them are used, but few of them enjoy medical acceptance. A lot of these creams are Vitamin based or contain herbal extracts. Vitamin E, a lipid soluble antioxidant in skin has been used to reduce oxygen radicals, which alter collagen and glycosaminoglycan production. Topical Vitamin A has been used as a superficial resurfacing agent. Softening and flattening of scars are presented in the literature, but the use is not generally recommended. Other natural sources for scar improvements are on the market, but there efficacy is still under heavy discussion.

Scar massage

Massage is a very good treatment option in order to improve the mobility of joints in the case of rigid scars. Rigid scar ropes are thereby dissolved and the scar becomes softer, more elastic and more pliable. In the acute phase only a local pressure should be applied to the scar. Furthermore no special massage creams should be used in this early phase. If the skin tolerates friction, the scar can be manipulated by rotary and stroking movements under use of special oils and creams. It is recommended to carry out the massage at least twice daily. An electric massage device can be also used with additional heat application. Heat relaxes the tissue and raises the elasticity, so that the scars can be better mobilised. Here paraffin wax hydrotherapy and ultrasound are used with success. Conscientious scar massage can be effective in limited areas of scarring; it is also convenient, because it can be performed by family members.

Cortisone treatment

In the non-surgical scar management cortisone therapy has a firm place [16–19]; it is mainly used for the treatment of hypertrophic scars and keloids. The application of steroids can reduce collagen synthesis up to 60 % [18]. Moreover there is a significant reduction of glycosaminoglycan- and hyaluron acid synthesis by use of steroids. This leads to the decrease of the extracellular matrix and thereby to a scar reduction. Intralesioal injections are often performed every 4–6 weeks. They can be used alone or as an adjunct to other treatment modalities. It is often used in combination with compression and/or excision and postal-surgical radiatio [18]. The most frequent side effects are atrophy and hypopigmentation around the injection places [17].

Antimitotic drugs

A new intralesional scar treatment option is mainly based on antimiotic drugs such as beomycin and 5-fluorouracil (5-FU).

Verapamil

The intralesional injection of the calcium channel blocker Verapamil seems to be a new promising option for the treatment of hypertrophic scars and keloids. In a recent study Verapamil was injected into the wound edges directly after the scar and keloid excision [20–22].

Laser

Hypertrophic scars, keloids and mild to moderate acne scars may benefit from skin resurfacing procedures using the carbon dioxide (CO_2) laser and the Nd YAG laser [23, 24].

Radiotherapy

Nowadays the application of radiotherapy in the conservative scar treatment is critical because of its potential side effects and risks like radiodermatitis, ulceration and tissue atrophy, but there are also many reports available that this kind of treatment option is still useful and should be taken into account for scar treatment, especially after keloid excision [25].

Soft tissue augmentation

Atrophic and depressed scars may also benefit from filling procedures. There are different fillers available on the market. Collagen and collagen with fibroblasts are quite popular. Live cell transfer has been advocated as a long lasting solution for tissue augmentation. Lipotransfer has become popular for scar treatment, because it seems that fat cell transfer is not only able to improve volume and contour, but also to improve skin quality [26].

Conclusions

The ultimate goal of all burn care is the reintegration of the patient into society. A few years ago, the goal of the burn team was survival of the patient and discharge was the measurement of outcome. Ideally, patients return to their families, schoolmates, and communities as if the injury had never occurred. In order to achieve this, rehabilitation and reconstruction of the seriously burned patient became important parts of today's burn care.

References

[1] Sheridan RL. Burn Rehabilitation. http://emedicine. medscape. com/article/318 436-overview
[2] Robson MC, Smith DJ, Vander Zee AJ et al (1992) Making the burned hand functional. Clin Plast Surg 19(3): 663–671
[3] Harden NG, Luster SH (1991) Rehabilitation considerations in the care of the acute burn patient. Crit Care Nurs Clin North Am 3(2): 245–253
[4] Pessina MA, Ellis SM (1997) Burn management. Rehabilitation. Nurs Clin North Am 32(2): 365–374
[5] Trees DW, Ketelsen CA, Hobbs JA (2003) Use of a modified tilt table for preambulation strength training as an adjunct to burn rehabilitation: a case series. J Burn Care Rehabil 24(2): 97–103
[6] Staley M, Richard R (1994) Burn care and rehabilitation principles and practice. FA Davis, Philadelphia, Ch 14, pp 380–418
[7] Ahn ST, Monafo WW, Mustoe TA (1989) Topical silicone gel: a new treatment of hyperthrophic scar. Surgery 106: 781–787
[8] Katz BE (1995) Silicone gel sheeting in scar therapy. Cutis 56: 65–67
[9] Kischer CW (1992) The microvessels in hypertrophic scars, keloids and related lesions: a review. J Submicrosc Cytol Pathol 24: 281–296
[10] Mc Donald WS, Deitch EA (1987) Hypertrophic skin grafts in burn patients: a prospective analysis of variables. J Trauma 27: 147–150
[11] Cheng JC, Evans JH, Leung KS et al (1984) Pressure therapy in the treatment of post-burn hypertrophic scar – a critical look into its usefulness and fallacies by pressure monitoring. Burns Incl Therm Inj; 10: 154–163.Reid
[12] Giele HP, Liddiard K, Currie K et al (1997) Direct measurement of cutaneous pressures generated by pressure garments. Burns 23: 137–141
[13] Larson DL, Abston S, Willis B et al (1974) Contracture and scar formation in the burn patient. Clin Plast Surg 1: 653–656
[14] Robertson JC, Hodgson B, Druett JE et al (1980) Pressure therapy for hypertrophic scarring: preliminary communication. J R Soc Med 73: 348–354
[15] Huruitz S (1988) The sun and sunscreen protection: recommendations for children. J Dermatol Surg Oncol 14(6): 657–660
[16] Tang YW (1992) Intra- and postoperative steroid injection for keloids and hyperthrophic scars. Br J Plast Surg 45: 371–373
[17] Oikarinen A, Autio P (1991) New aspects of the mechanism of corticosteroid-induced dermal atrophy. Clin Exp Derm 16: 416–419
[18] Tang YW (1992) Intra- and postoperative steroid injection for keloids and hyperthrophic scars. Br J Plast Surg 45: 371–373
[19] Hirshowitz B, Lerner D, Moscona AR (1982) Treatment of keloid scars by combined cryosurgery and intralesional corticosteroids. Aesthetic Plast Surg 6: 153–158
[20] D'Andrea F, Brongo S, Ferraro G et al (2002) Prevention and treatment of keloids with intralesional verapamil. Dermatology 204: 60–62
[21] Lee RC, Doong H, Jellema AF (1994) The response of burn scars to intralesional verapamil: report of five cases. Arch Surg 129: 107–111
[22] Doong H, Dissanayake S, Gowrishankar TR et al (1996) The 1996 Lindberg Award: calcium antagonists alter cell shape and induce rocollagenase synthesis in keloid and normal human dermal fibroblasts. J Burn Care Rehabil 17: 497–514
[23] Alster TS, McMeekin TO (1996) Improvement of facial acne scars by the 585 nm flashlamp-pumped pulsed dye laser. J Am Acad Dermatol 35: 79–81
[24] Henderson DL, Cromwell TA, Mes LG (1984) Argon and carbon dioxid laser treatment of hypertrophic and keloid scars.Laser Surg Med 3: 271–277
[25] Kovalic JJ, Perez CA (1989) Radiation therapy following keloidectomy: a 20-year experience. Int J Radiat Oncol Biol Phys 17: 77–80
[26] Jeong JH (2010) Adipose stem cells and skin repair. Curr Stem Cell Res Ther 5(2): 137–40

Correspondence: Lars-Peter Kamolz, M.D., Ph.D., M.Sc., Medical University of Vienna, Department of Surgery, Division of Plastic and Reconstructive Surgery, Vienna, Austria, E-mail: kamolz@plastchirurg.info

Exercise

Karen J. Kowalske[1], Serina J. McEntire[2], Oscar E. Suman[2]

[1] Department of Physical Medicine and Rehabilitation, University of Texas Southwestern Medical Center, Dallas, TX, USA
[2] Shriners Hospitals for Children, and Department of Surgery, University of Texas Medical Branch, Galveston, TX, USA

Acute stage

The role of exercise in reversing the consequences of bed rest has been well documented. It is also clear that exercise after hospital discharge is critically important for facilitating physical functional and metabolic recovery following a major burn injury [14, 63]. The role of exercise during the critical care and acute care hospitalization following burn injury has not been fully described. The purpose of this section is to describe the importance of positioning, mobilization up out of bed, and aerobic exercise during the acute stage can be safely incorporated into the treatment plan following burn injury.

Exercise

It is well known that bedrest has detrimental effects yet it is the practice across the country for most patients in the intensive care unit to be sedated and on bedrest. This leads to many complications including atelectasis, pneumonia, hypovolemia, dampened carotid baroreceptor response, orthostatic hypotension, deep venous thrombosis and pulmonary embolism, constipation and ileus, hyperglycemia and insulin resistance, muscle atrophy and deconditioning, bone demineralization, joint contractures, and decubiti, depression and decreased functional capacity [12, 37]. Clearly these are not the optimal goals for our critically ill patients. A recent randomized trial showed that holding sedation combined with exercise, decreased days on the ventilator and the incidence of delirium and improved function and walking distance at hospital discharge [57].

How do we decide who can begin getting up out of bed? Timmerman and colleagues designed a specific decision tree that can be used as a guide. First the managing physician needs a thorough understanding of current medical condition, any medical co-morbidities, and the patients pre-morbid functional level. Obviously, the tolerance for sitting will be different between a geriatric patient and a teenager. Also, someone with pre-morbid tetraplegia or hemiparesis will be different than someone with no pre-morbid functional limitations. Other conditions like arthritis should also be taken into account [61].

The next consideration is the patient's cardiovascular reserve. At baseline the individuals heart rate should be less that 50 % of the age predicted maximum. This may be easier to achieve and perhaps less relevant now that many burn patients are treated with beta blockers during their acute care course. Blood pressure must be stable off of pressors. Close monitoring for orthostatic hypotension is essential as this is a common complication of bedrest. Ace wrapping the legs may help decrease this effect. A normal ECG without signs of ischemia or unstable arrhythmia is obvious. If a patient has had a recent MI, getting out of bed is still feasible but may need to proceed more slowly. Other cardiac contraindications include unstable angina, severe symptomatic aortic stenosis, decompensated CHF, acute myocarditis, or dissecting aneurysm [61].

Is there adequate respiratory reserve? In general, Oxygen saturation should be greater than 90 % on an inspired fraction of oxygen (FiO2) of less 60 %. Mechanical ventilation can not be high frequency oscillation. Other patient factors to be considered are hemoglobin greater than 7 without active bleeding, platelet count > 20,000, WBC stable and without an active acute metabolic compromising infection and blood glucose should be above 50 and less than 400. Patients should be afebrile and alert enough to participate and not significantly agitated. Neurologic complications include increased intracranial pressure, actively seizing or delirium tremors. Orthopedic limitations are unstable spine or fracture, severe osteoporosis or unstable boney metastasis [61]. Acute deep venous thrombosis can be managed with one day of bedrest and pulmonary embolism with 3 days.

Lastly, the burn community must address the issue of timing of getting up after a skin graft. Numerous studies have shown that ambulation is safe on the day of grafting for a lower leg burn. Obviously, these studies were done in otherwise healthy subjects with smaller burns. Losing precious skin graft in a patient with a large burn is to be avoided but is worth the trade off of additional ventilator days and a poorer outcome at hospital discharge?

There are many external factors that must be considered when mobilizing a crucially ill patient. Although tracheostomy is preferred, and endotracheal tube is not an absolute contraindication. Extra care must be taken to avoid dislodgement of the tube or trauma to vocal cords. Dialysis is not a contraindication but pragmatics suggests timing the activity around dialysis. Temporary pacemaker have fragile wiring, may be dislodged so are likely a contraindication to mobility [61]. The issue of lines is somewhat controversial. Central venous catheters and arterial lines are not a contraindication.

Lastly, the issue of staffing is critically important. Many burn units have had cut backs in therapy coverage. One component for future study is to show how this mobilization can decrease number of days on the ventilator or hospital complications which may justify the staffing essential for this activity even if it doesn't meet the traditional productivity criteria set for physical or occupational therapists.

Mobilization protocol

Complete bed rest orders for should be an exception and should be questioned if a legitimate reason not apparent. Once the above safety criteria have been reviewed, progressive mobility can begin.

Any patient immobile for more than 3 days will be deconditioned and will require orthostatic training for upright positioning. Patients ready to begin ventilator weaning are most likely ready for mobility. All patients should be turned every 2h while on bed rest with good documentation if turning is contraindicated or if the patient does not tolerate it.

All patients who can not actively participate in therapy should receive range of motion at least twice per day. Mechanically ventilated patients, should ave the head of the bed elevated > 30 degrees unless contraindicated.

Readiness for and progression of activity should be evaluated on each shift. If mobilization does not occur, reasons should be clearly documented. Progressive mobilization should occur 2–3 times a day unless patient meets exclusion criteria. Evaluate tolerance to activity and progress to the next step as tolerated

Progressive Mobility Proposal [68]:
1. Elevate HOB to 45 degrees.
2. Elevated HOB to 45 degrees plus legs in dependent position (partial chair position).
3. Elevated HOB to 65 degrees plus legs in full dependent position (full chair position).
4. Dangle with assistance once patient is conscious and following commands. Patient's feet should be touching the floor if possible. Support torso but encourage independence.
5. Stand patient at bedside with support once patient is able to lift his leg against gravity. Patient should bear weight.
6. Transfer to chair by pivoting or taking 1–2 small steps. Patient should sit up for 1–2 h
7. Walk with assistance. Use walker if needed.
8. Walk independently

Heterotopic ossification

Heterotopic ossification (HO) occurs in about 4 % of burn patients, the majority of which are critically ill [18, 29]. There is a significant debate on the factors that contribute to HO but it is most common in patients who are critically ill and have burns with persistent open wounds [18, 35]. There is certainly a contention that significant edema fluid, prolonged sedation and immobilization, as well as numerous missed therapy treatment sessions are also contributing factors [35]. Therefore, the burn team should emphasize keeping joints moving, avoiding over sedation and getting wound closure as quickly as safely feasible.

Positioning

Following burn injury, it is essential that the injured tissues be placed in a position of stretch [59]. Burned tissue has a tendency to shorten and leads to contracture which is the single most common complication following burn injury [56]. The classic description of positioning is well known in the burn community. This includes shoulder abduction, elbow extension, wrist neutral, and Metacarpal phalyngeal (MP) flexion with proximal interphalyngeal (PIP) and distal interphalyngeal (DIP) extension [52]. This decreases the edema in the hand avoids tension on any exposed extensor mechanisms and facilitates the return of MP flexion. Avoiding over abduction of the shoulders is critical to prevent stretch on the brachial plexus. Prolonged elbow flexion can produce ulnar nerve ischemia. Wrist flexion or extension may compromise the median nerve in the carpal tunnel. The lower limbs should be in slight hip abduction with rotation, knee extension and the ankles in neutral. The frog leg position can over stretch the peroneal nerve with resultant foot drop [28, 29]. The other key for positioning is to carefully monitoring for pressure points particularly on the occiput and heel. In conjunction with positioning, range of motion and prolonged stretch are essential for avoiding permanent contractures [38].

Edema following resuscitation can contribute to contracture formation particularly in the hands where significant edema with result in a hand position of MP hyperextension and PIP flexion [17]. This

edema can also cause microvascular ischemia with subsequent neuropathy. Appropriate positioning can be utilized to help limit edema and its consequences. This leads to the question of whether more patients should undergo escharotomy. One would think that we should do more escharotomies with a neuropathy rate of 12 % in major burn injury. The counter argument is that the majority of these neuropathies resolve over time without intervention [22].

We know exercise can reverse or attenuate the effects of bedrest and facilitates metabolic recovery in the late stages of burns. The above review, examines the evidence for safety and efficacy of beginning exercise for patients while they are in the ICU. This is combined with evidence for safely mobilizing individuals on the day of or the day after a skin graft. Leaving burn patients in bed for days, clearly impacts time on the ventilator and functional outcomes. Each individual member of the burn team should be challenged to speak up on the importance of exercise in providing the best possible care for our patients.

Outpatient stage

The purpose of this section is to describe a typical exercise rehabilitation program that can be implemented once a patient has been discharged from the acute unit and into outpatient care. The mode, duration, frequency and intensity of exercise are discussed. In addition, methods on the assessment of aerobic function and muscle function are described.

Exercise-background

Multiple physical and functional limitations are present post-burn and must be addressed in a long term rehabilitation program. Traditionally, standard physical and occupation therapy programs for burn injuries, concentrate on the return and maintenance of range of motion (ROM), scar reduction, and prevention of contractures [3, 58]. The major underlying factors that prohibit the patient with burns from becoming independent in self-care, home management, work duties, and leisure activities point to a limited ROM, loss of mobility, intolerance to standing or walking, pain, and decreased strength and endurance [11]. Indeed, ROM is reported to be the primary indicator for determining back to work status and impairment status [3]. However, despite participation in standard rehabilitation programs, the loss of LBM, muscle weakness, and diminished aerobic capacity persist [13, 16, 26] performed isokinetic testing of the ankle, wrist, and elbow in burned adults with normal ROM who complained of an inability to perform job related duties. Significant deficits in muscle strength and power were found. Despite normal ROM, these individuals were not ready to return to work and their complaints of difficulty with job related tasks were justified. Similarly, St-Pierre et al. [60] found that a 15–20 % decrement in muscle strength was present at approximately 35 months post-burn in adults with greater than 30 % TBSA burns compared to age matched controls.

Exercise has been demonstrated to be an essential component of the long term rehabilitation program post-burn. Exercise is reported to aid in controlling edema, decrease tendon adherence, joint stiffness, capsular shortening, muscle atrophy, and whole body deconditioning [25, 33, 53]. Also, exercise is reported to decrease the likelihood of additional surgical procedures needed to release burn scar contractures [10]. In addition, exercise training has been shown to maintain and improve LBM, augment the incorporation of amino acids into muscle proteins, increase muscle strength, increase walking distance by up to 50 %, and improve cardiopulmonary capacity [10, 14, 43].

However, published reports on the effects of exercise training in burn patients are limited. In adult burn patients, de Lateur et al. [16] demonstrated significant improvements in aerobic fitness following a 12 week treadmill exercise program. Matched controls, who only participated in a standard rehabilitation program, did not achieve the same gains in aerobic capacity as those in the training program. Suman et al. [66] have reported that a 12 week aerobic and resistance exercise program, in addition to a standard hospital rehabilitation program, results in significant improvements in physiologic function in children with severe burns (7–17 years of age and ≥ 40 % TBSA burned) compared to standard of care (SOC) alone. In this study, an isokinetic dynamometer test on the dominant leg extensors at a speed of 150°/sec was used to assess leg muscle strength.

Lean body mass was measured using dual-energy X-ray absorptiometry (DXA). In addition, peak oxygen consumption was measured during a standardized treadmill exercise test, and resting energy expenditure (REE) was measured after an 8–12 hour fast. All exercise testing was performed at 6 month post-burn and repeated 12 weeks later. Following the 12 week intervention, muscle strength increased 44 % in the exercise group compared to a 6 % increase in SOC group. Lean body mass increased approximately 6 % in the exercisers, but was unchanged in the SOC group. Aerobic capacity increased 23 % in the exercisers; but decreased 1.35 % in the non-exercisers. Resting energy expenditure was elevated in both groups at baseline, but increased an additional 15 % in the SOC group, while the REE of the exercise group was unchanged. In a similar population of children with burns, Suman et al. [64] also reported significant improvements in pulmonary function (MVV, FEV_1, and FVC), treadmill time, and aerobic capacity following a 12 week aerobic and resistance exercise training program. In burned children 2–6 years of age, Neugebauer et al. [47] reported significant improvements in both passive and active range of motion at the elbow and knee following a 12 week supplemental group music and movement program. Finally, McEntire et al. [40, 41] found that moderate intensity exercise at room temperature was safe for children with less than 75 % TBSA burns and did not result in hyperthermia or heat illness. Patients with burns who participate in regular physical exercise are also more likely to have the health related benefits of improved flexibility, balance, stamina, and strength, which are needed to return to an active and independent lifestyle [16].

Exercise prescription

Exercise-training may be prescribed for persons with severe burns once they have been discharged from the hospital and into an outpatient setting. In addition, it is expected that the physician in charge of the patient will have given the approval to participate in an exercise rehabilitation program or has even written the exercise prescription themselves. Exercise training is defined here as a "planned, structured and repetitive body movement done to improve or maintain one or more components of physical fitness" [21, 50, 69]. The exercise prescription describe in this chapter is based primarily on the outpatient exercise program that is implemented in severely burned children at Shriners Hospitals for Children in Galveston, Texas [66] and in some severely burned adults (unpublished data). This exercise program is supplemented with physical and occupational therapy. This program has been demonstrated to be beneficial in children 7–18 years old [63–66], but also in numerous adults with burns. The principles of designing exercise programs for children and adults with severe burns is based primarily on guidelines offered to healthy, non-burned children and adults [1, 21, 42, 48, 69].

An initial evaluation of risk factors and/or symptoms for chronic conditions concomitant to the burn should be performed prior to beginning exercise. Pre-existing conditions may include chronic cardiovascular, pulmonary, and metabolic diseases. The objective is to obtain the necessary information to provide a safe and effective exercise rehabilitation program. Subjective data should be obtained to characterize any limitations or problems that the patient may have. A history of pre-burn physical activity, current medical problems, symptoms, and limitations is valuable in designing an effective exercise program. Pain or weakness during ambulation, shortness of breath, or severe fatigue may adversely affect exercise tolerance. In addition, the medications that a patient is taking may impact their ability to exercise. Following this health screening, exercise testing should be performed to evaluate the patient's exercise or physical capacity.

Exercise testing

The objectives for exercise testing are multi-factorial. For cardiopulmonary testing, the primary objectives are to assess physical work capacity and aerobic fitness, observe cardiorespiratory and metabolic responses, determine the basis for exercise prescription, and assess changes in fitness due to exercise training. For muscular strength testing, the primary objectives include measurement of muscle strength (absolute and relative to body weight), measure antagonist/agonist muscle ratios, assess changes in body composition (lean mass, fat mass, and bone density), and to provide a basis for exercise prescription. Exercise testing should be conducted prior to the start of any exercise rehabilitation program and at the end of such program. Sometimes, if the program is of long duration, a mid-point evaluation can be done. It is important to consider the patient's developmental maturity when performing exercise testing and training. We recommend a chronological age of 7 years and older, although children as young as 3–4 years of age have been tested [54]. Though we briefly describe methods of exercise testing in patients with burns, the reader should also keep in mind that there exist numerous field tests and prediction formulas for the estimation of both cardiopulmonary and muscle fitness [23].

Peak oxygen consumption or aerobic exercise capacity

All patients should undergo a standardized exercise test. We use the treadmill exercise test and use the modified Bruce treadmill protocol. We must note that other treadmill protocols such as the "Ramp Protocol, can be used [39, 44–46]. In addition, if not possible for the patient to be tested on a treadmill, a cycle ergometer or arm ergometer can also be used to evaluate or assess the physical conditioning of the patient, before starting exercise rehabilitation or training program [34]. Heart rate can be easily obtained with monitors. Oxygen consumption (VO_2) should be measured if possible, but requires more expensive equipment that can perform breath-by-breath analysis is continuously made of inspired and expired gases, flow, and volume. The reader is referred to other publications for more detail in the methodology of assessing VO_2 [15, 34, 55]. For the Bruce protocol, speed and grade begin at 1.7 miles/hr and 0 %, respectively. Thereafter, the speed and level of incline are increased every 3 minutes. Patients are constantly encouraged to complete 3 minute stages and the test is terminated when peak volitional effort is achieved. Additional variable that can be collected during the test include blood pressure, Borg's rated perceived exertion (RPE) [7, 8], basic electrocardiogram (ECG), and spirometry. The peak VO_2 and peak heart rate can then be used to establish the intensity in which patients will exercise at during the exercise program.

Strength measurements

Isokinetic dynamometry strength testing can be performed to assess muscle function or to evaluate progress. If using the Biodex Isokinetic dynamometer, the test can be done on the dominant leg extensors and/or leg with burns. We recommend testing at various angular velocities, such as 180°/sec, 150°/sec, 120°/sec or 90°/sec; though we recommend 150°/sec based on our experience. For very young children (e. g. 7–10 years of age), a velocity of 180°/sec might be better, as the lower velocity of 90°/sec seems to be too difficult. The patients are seated and their position stabilized with a restraining strap over the mid-thigh, pelvis, and truck. All patients should be familiarized with the equipment before the actual test starts. We recommend that firstly, the procedure is demonstrated by the administrator of the test. Secondly, the test procedure is explained to the patients, and then, patients are allowed to practice the actual movement during three submaximal repetitions without load as warm-up. Thirdly, after the three submaximal warm-up repetitions, 10 maximum voluntary muscle contractions (full extension and flexion) can be performed consecutively without rest in between. The amount of repetitions and the number of times the sets of repetitions can be varied. For example, we recommend one set of 10 repetitions at each velocity, with a two minute rest interval between velocities. Values of peak torque, total work, and average power are calculated by the Biodex software system, and progress of muscle function can be monitored.

3 Repetition Maximum Test (3RM)

Typically, before starting a resistive training program, it is useful to determine a safe and also effective load for patients to use during workouts. To determine the amount of weight or load that can be used as baseline or starting loads, the *"Repetition Maximum"* method can be used. We recommend the 3 repetition maximum load (3RM). It is determined as follows: After an instruction period on correct weightlifting technique, the patient warms up with lever arm and bar (or wooden dowel) and is allowed to become familiar with the movement. After this, the patient lifts a weight that allows suc-cessful completion of 4 repetitions. If the fourth repetition is achieved successfully and with correct technique, a one-minute resting period should be allowed. After the resting period, a progressively increased amount of weight or load is instructed to be lifted at least four times. If the patient lifts a weight that allows successful completion of 3 repetitions, with the fourth repetition not being volitionally possible, due to fatigue or inability to maintain correct technique, the test is terminated and the amount of weight lifted from the successful set is recorded as their individual 3RM. We recommend the order of exercises to be from exercises that involve large muscle groups to ones that involve smaller muscle groups: bench press, leg press, shoulder press, leg extension, biceps curl, leg curl and triceps curl.

Lean body mass measurements

Lean body mass (LBM) measurements if possible should be made. We assess LBM using dual-energy X-ray absorptiometry (DXA). DXA with the appropriate software can measure the attenuation of two X-ray beams, one which is high energy and one which is low energy. These measurements are then compared with standard models of thickness used for bone and soft tissue. Subsequently, the calculated soft tissue is separated into LBM and fat mass. This is a great measurement to also assess progress of program and perhaps nutritional interventions. However, the DXA machine is expensive. It is not known if other methods to measure body composition such as underwater weighing or bio-impedance are applicable to patients with burns.

Additional testing

Major muscle and joint flexibility may be assessed using sit-and-reach or goniometry for ROM. Other tests may include gait analysis, balance, or reaction time. Sit-and-stand scores, timed walk/jog, and/or lifting exercises may be used to assess functional performance. The results of all evaluations should be used to identify problem areas, to write an exercise prescription, to design an exercise program, and to assess progress during and after an exercise program.

Table 1. Description of workouts

Aerobic Workout	
Intensity	70–85% of individual peak aerobic capacity ($VO2_{peak}$) or 50–85% of heart rate reserve (HRR). Heart rate and RPE measured at regular intervals.
Duration	20–40 minutes (excluding warm-up and cool-down); continuous or intervals of work to rest or easy to moderate
Frequency	3–5 days per week.
Mode	Treadmills, cycle ergometers, elliptical machines, arm ergometers, rowing machines. Sports such as soccer, basketball, and kickball.

Resistance Workout	
Exercise type	Multi-joint, assistance, and core exercises involving both the upper and lower body.
Weight/load lifted and repetitions	Weeks 1–2: 50–60% of 3RM for 12–15 reps; Weeks 3–6: 70–75% of 3RM for 8–10 reps, Weeks 7–12: 75–85% of 3RM for 8–12 reps.
Number of sets	2–3 sets.
Order of Exercises	Bench/chest press, leg press or squats, lat pulldown or row, leg extension, shoulder press, lunges, biceps curl, hamstring curl, triceps extension, toe raises, and core exercises (abdominals, back, or hip/gluteus). Larger muscles to smaller muscles.
Type of Exercises	10 basic resistance exercises using variable resistance machines, free weights, or resistance bands: 5 for upper body, 5 for lower body, plus 1–3 core exercises.
Rest period	Approximate 1–2 minutes between sets.
Frequency	3 days per week is recommended, but may do everyday if alternating upper vs lower body workouts. Need to account for type of aerobic workout.

Exercise programs

We provide here an example of our 12 week exercise rehabilitation program for individuals with severe burns (Table 1). This program is implemented at hospital discharge, but has also been successful if implemented at 6 months post-burn. We have also had success in implementing this program in patients up to 12 months post-burn. The results of our program have been published and the reader is referred to these for more details [47, 51, 64, 66, 67].

Aerobic training

Intensity

To improve aerobic fitness, the intensity of exercise should be between 65% and 95% of the peak heart or between 45% and 85% of the heart rate reserve (HRR) [32]. The heart rate reserve is the difference between the peak heart rate obtained during the maximal treadmill exercise test and resting heart rate. When it is not possible to perform a maximal treadmill exercise test, a simple method of estimating peak heart rate is to use the formula (220 minus age) [21]. This formula is more difficult to use in children, so we recommend that in children, rated perceived exertion (see below), together with the heart rate obtained during a maximal exercise capacity test be used.

The rating of perceived exertion (RPE) scale can also be used as a guideline for establishing exercise intensity [6–9]. RPE is a valuable indicator of exercise tolerance and intensity and is useful when it is impossible to obtain peak heart rate or if patients are on medications that affect heart rate, such as β-blockers. Currently, there are two commonly used RPE scales; the original or category scale, which rates exercise intensity on a scale of 6–20 and the revised or category-ratio scale of 0–10. The category-ratio scale has been reported to be better understood by patients, thus providing the tester with more valid information. An aerobic training effect and the threshold for the start of anaerobic training are achieved at a rating of "somewhat hard" to "hard", which equates to a category rating of 12–16 or a 4–5 on the category-ratio scale [20].

Another method of evaluating exercise intensity is the "Talk Test", or the point where speech first becomes difficult and approximates exercise intensity almost equivocally to the ventilator threshold. The patient should be advised to exercise at intensity where speech is comfortable. When speech becomes difficult, it is reported that one can assume that exercise intensity is consistently above ventilator threshold or above the desired intensity of exercise needed for general improvements in fitness [49]. Safety and effectiveness are equally important and the intensity should also be suitable to result in a long-term, active lifestyle.

Duration

The duration and intensity of an exercise session are closely linked. For burned patients, the duration of exercise should be 5–20 minutes during the first week and depends on the functional status and pain tolerance of the patient. The objective should be to perform 20–60 minutes of aerobic exercise. This can be done continuously or intermittently (intervals), with a minimum of 10 minute exercise bouts. Typically, exercise of 20–30 minutes, between 65–85 % VO_{2peak} or 40–50 % to 85 % of HRR (excluding warm-up and cool-down time) should induce health and fitness improvements [2, 71]. Burned patients with low aerobic capacity or endurance may benefit from an exercise program of 4–6, 5 minute bouts with rest periods between bouts. However, even intervals of one minute's worth of work and one minute rest for a total of 20 minutes, will confer benefits. The duration of the exercise bouts are progressively increased over time.

An aerobic exercise program should consist of a warm-up, endurance, and cool-down periods. The warm-up period should be approximately 5–10 minutes of low intensity exercises to increase body temperature and prepare the body for more strenuous work during the endurance phase. Stretching exercises were traditionally incorporated during the warm-up; however, recent evidence has shown stretching to be contraindicated at this point in the exercise session [5, 36]. Light aerobic exercise has

been demonstrated to be adequate for increasing flexibility prior to an exercise session [69]. For example, the warm-up may consist of slow, easy walking followed by moderately fast walk during the endurance phase. However, a moderate walk (3.5 mph) may be a warm-up speed for a patient that jogs at 5.5 mph during the endurance phase. Heart rate can be monitored to ensure that the warm-up activity is not too strenuous.

The objective of the endurance phase is to develop and improve cardiorespiratory or aerobic fitness. This phase should consist of 20–60 minutes of continuous or intermittent (minimum of 10 minute bouts accumulated throughout the day) aerobic exercise. The duration depends on the intensity of the activity. For example, moderate intensity exercise should be conducted for 30 minutes or more; while high intensity, vigorous exercise should train for at least 20 minutes or more [2]. Exercises during this phase should employ large muscle groups during rhythmic or dynamic exercises. Recreational activities or sports may be incorporated into this phase providing that they are of sufficient intensity, duration (minimum of 20 minutes), and are a complement to the endurance phase.

Following the endurance phase, a cool-down period of 2–5 minutes is recommended to gradually decrease HR and blood pressure toward resting values. These exercises should be lower intensity and may include slow walking or jogging or stretching exercises. The cool-down is important for reducing the possibility of a hypotensive event after exercise, as well as other cardiovascular complications [27].

Frequency

Optimal training frequency for improving aerobic capacity appears to be achieved with 3–5 exercise sessions per week. However, it has been reported that deconditioned persons can improve cardiorespiratory fitness with only 2 exercise sessions per week [2]. At 60–80 % of HRR or 70–85 % of peak aerobic capacity, 3–5 exercise sessions per week are sufficient to improve or maintain peak aerobic capacity. Patients with diminished aerobic capacities may benefit from multiple, short (5 days/week) exercise sessions. The number of sessions per week will vary depending on the patient's limitations and lifestyle.

Mode

The mode of exercise chosen should engage large muscle groups during rhythmic or dynamic exercise. Treadmill walking or running, cycling, elliptical trainer, or rowing are all examples of aerobic activities that engage large muscle groups and have been used during exercise in burned patients. Walking or jogging at a track or field is also appropriate. Swimming is also beneficial; however, closure of burn wounds must be ensured to minimize infection or contamination of others. Sports activities such as soccer, basketball, or tennis are also appropriate. However, care should be taken to avoid, hard or extreme physical contact. It is extremely important to prescribe exercises that are appropriate for the patients' physical and mental developmental maturity.

In burn patients, walking or cycling and even rowing are typically initially prescribed exercises. These activities are easy to tolerate, safe, intensity is easy to monitor, and the trainer can easily monitor the patient's progress during the first few weeks of the exercise program. Some patients may progress quickly through walking, jogging, and cycling programs due to the extent of the burn injury, personality, previous athletic experience, or psychosocial health. The risk of injury during high intensity or high impact exercises should be considered when prescribing exercise modalities; particularly in those with functional limitations, are overweight or obese, or novice exercisers. Cross training (participation in a variety of different exercise modes and intensities) is desirable to increase enjoyment, compliance, and to reduce repetitive orthopedic stresses. For children, play activity is also highly desirable and should be mixed with standard exercise training sessions.

Progression of exercise

The duration, intensity, and the transition to more difficult exercises should progress slowly to ensure the safety of the patient. This will decrease the potential for inducing excessive muscle soreness, causing new injuries, or aggravating pre-existing injuries. In addition, the patient should be educated to not move too quickly into demanding or challenging activities. For example, once the patient can walk 1–2 miles without fatigue or pain, then they may progress to a walk/jog or jogging program. The rate of progression depends on the patient's functional capacity, medical and health status, pain tolerance, location of burns, age, activity preferences and goals, and overall tolerance to the current level of training. For burn patients, the exercise prescription can be divided into three stages of progression: initial, improvement, and maintenance as described by Wallace and Kaminsky [69].

The initial stage should consist of light and moderate aerobic activities (50–60 % VO_{2peak} or 40–60 % HRR), which have a low potential for injury, muscle soreness, or pain. If the exercise is too hard or aggressive, adherence may be compromised. The amount of time spent in the initial stages varies. We recommend at least 4 weeks for initial conditioning. Exercise duration during this stage may begin with 15–20 minutes and progress to 30 minutes, at least 3 times per week. Deconditioned individuals should be allowed additional time to adapt at each conditioning stage. Age of the individual also needs to be considered, as conditioning may take longer in older or extremely deconditioned patients [2].

The goal of the improvement stage is to progressively increase the overall exercise stimulus to elicit significant improvements in aerobic fitness. This stage differs from the initial phase in that the patient is progressed at a more rapid rate. This stage usually lasts 4–5 months, during which time intensity is progressively increased within the upper half of the target range of 70–85 % VO_{2peak} or 50–85 % HRR. In our experience with a 12 week training program for burned children 7–18 years of age, some children are able to start the improvement phase after 3–4 weeks of initial conditioning. Duration is increased consistently every 2–3 weeks until participants are able to exercise at a moderate to vigorous intensity for 20–30 minutes continuously. Interval training is beneficial during this stage provided that the total time engaged in moderate to vigorous activity is at least 20 minutes.

Once the patient has achieved the objectives of the im provement stage, the long term maintenance of their cardiopulmonary fitness begins. At this time, the patient may not be interested in increasing the conditioning stimulus and further improvements may be minimal. However, continuing the workout routine will maintain their fitness level. Re-evaluation and establishment of new goals is recommended during this phase.

Resistance or strength training

Strength is defined as the ability to produce force, while the ability to produce force over an extended time period is defined as muscular endurance. Muscle strength and endurance play an important role in the ability to perform activities of daily living (ADL). Following a severe burn, extensive and prolonged losses of lean muscle mass occur. Therefore, resistance training, which increases LBM, should be part of a comprehensive exercise rehabilitation program for burned individuals [65, 66].

The principles for designing a resistance training program for burned individuals are similar to the aerobic training program outlined above. Strict rules and education of proper weightlifting technique, and safety should be enforced at all times to reduce the potential for injury or accidents. Breath holding should be avoided during lifting as it may increase blood pressure, which can be dangerous. Prior to beginning a resistance training program, strength testing (isokinetic or 3RM) and evaluation should be performed to identify problem areas, prescribe exercise workloads, and to track progress. Muscle strength tests are also valuable for determining return to work status [13].

Exercise type and order

Resistance training exercises can be divided into multi-joint, assistance, and core exercises. Multi-joint exercises involve one or more large muscle groups, such as chest, shoulder, back, or thigh. Assistance exercises are single-joint exercises that target smaller muscle groups, such as biceps, triceps, trapezius, and calves [70]. Core exercises are meant to strengthen and stabilize the spine, pelvis, and shoulder girdle and provide a solid foundation for the movements of the extremities [30, 31]. Eccentric exercises are not recommended for use in burn patients because they have a higher potential to cause delayed onset muscle soreness. Severe muscle soreness may discourage participation or adherence to exercise.

For deconditioned or untrained individuals, the order of exercises should be multi-joint or large muscle groups first, followed by assistance exercises [4, 19, 62] core exercises. In addition, alternating up-

per and lower body exercises allows more recovery time between exercises. In severely burned children, we have successfully implemented the following exercises into a resistance training program: bench or chest press, leg press or squat, lat pulldown or row, leg extension, shoulder press, lunges, biceps curl, hamstring curl, triceps extension, and toe raises. Core strengthening exercises follow and may include exercises such as crunches, back extensions, push-ups, plank exercises, bridging, bicycles, and hip and gluteus strength exercises. All types of equipment, including variable resistant machines, free weights, resistance bands, and medicine balls are acceptable for burned individuals to use during exercise. With children, it is important that the equipment used fits their size and may need to be adapted to support smaller body sizes.

Frequency

For severely burned individuals, we recommend 2–3 days per week of resistance training. Resistance training is often performed on alternate days as aerobic training, but can be combined into the same exercise session. If the patient desires to work out everyday using weights, we strongly recommend, splitting the days into routines for upper body and lower body. However, the type and intensity of aerobic workout needs to be accounted for as doing a lower body workout on one day, in addition to very high intensity aerobic workouts on two consecutive days, may be counterproductive.

Number of sets and repetitions

The current recommendations for resistance training include 1–3 sets of 8–15 repetitions using exercises that target all major muscle groups [70]. We recommend 8–15 repetitions at a light to moderate weight in children [66] and 8–15 repetitions of moderate to heavy weight intensity to improve muscle strength and endurance in burned adults. In children, we recommend the above sets and repetitions, but at light to moderate weight intensity. It may be possible to utilize heavy weight intensity in older children (i. e. 16, 17 year olds), but for general improvement of muscle strength, and function, we do not believe it is required.

Training load

If using the 3RM method to establish a load, we offer this example which is used in our 12 week hospital exercise program for patients with burns. During the first week of training, the individual is familiarized with the exercise and taught proper lifting form. The use of very light weights or a broomstick is recommended when individuals are learning new exercises. After the individual has mastered correct form, the weight should be set at 50–60 % of their 3RM for 12–15 repetitions for 1–2 weeks. The load can then be increased to 70–75 % of 3RM for 8–10 repetitions for 4–5 weeks. From weeks 7–12, the training intensity is increased to 75–85 % with 8–12 repetitions.

Rest periods

It is important to allow enough time between sets for the muscle to recover enough to be able to perform the next set of exercises with proper form. For 10–15 repetition sets, less than one minute of rest should be adequate, but up to 2 minutes is allowable. For recovery periods between resistive training sessions, we recommend at least one day of recovery period for a given muscle group.

Progressive overload

To continue to see improvements during the exercise program, it is important to monitor and record the individual's workout and weights lifted each session. Progressive overload may be achieved by increasing the weight, number of repetitions, or decreasing the rest periods. The 2-for-2-rule is ideal for use in deconditioned individuals or young children. This method states that once two or more repetitions can be performed above the repetition goal for two consecutive workouts for a specific exercise, then the weight should be increased for that exercise for the next training session [4]. The increase in the amount of weight for an exercise is dependent on the physical condition of the individual and the area of the body (upper or lower body). We recommend a 2–5 pound increase in weight for upper body exercises and a 5–10 pound increase for lower body exercises in severely burned individuals.

Special considerations

When working with children, it is very important that machines and exercises be adapted to their size, strength level, and maturity level. We have found that traditional machine weights are often too large for children, but can be modified to accommodate smaller statures using foam blocks, seat padding, etc to correctly position the child. Adaptive equipment, such as gloves, wrist or ankle weights, or elastic wraps is useful when working with patients with hand injuries or amputations. Resistance bands and medicine balls work well in deconditioned patients who do not have the strength needed to lift the minimum weight on a machine. Working with burned individuals often requires a bit of ingenuity, resourcefulness, and the ability to see outside the weight room when planning and adapting a resistance training program.

Goals for all patients should be set early in the exercise program. They should be evaluated regularly with the patient and adjusted as needed. The goals must be realistic and achievable. An intrinsic or extrinsic rewards system may be implemented to help the patient achieve their goals.

An exercise rehabilitation program should be supplemented with an outpatient physical and occupational therapy program. Exercise professionals must work together to avoid duplication of services, identify areas that need attention, and to provide the most comprehensive rehabilitation program for the individual patient.

Exercise should start early and as soon as possible after hospital discharge. The program should be structured and supervised by a trained professional. The ultimate goal of an exercise rehabilitation program should be to improve overall physical function. This program should be challenging, effective, safe, and fun. One must use common sense and follow established guidelines during programming. The exercise program should also teach and promote healthy lifestyle habits to ensure that patient's comply with the exercise program. The thought that "something is better than nothing" is correct, but safety should be the number one priority.

The American College of Sports Medicine (ACSM) has a manual with a list of absolute and relative contraindications to exercise and exercise testing for adults, children, and special populations [24]. Many of these contraindications will also apply to individuals with severe burns. This ACSM manual is a useful resource for information and one will find it helpful for use in exercise prescription and program design.

References

[1] Adams RB, Tribble GC, Tafel AC, Edlich RF (1990) Cardiovascular rehabilitation of patients with burns. J Burn Care Rehabil 11(3): 246–255

[2] American College of Sports Medicine Position Stand. The recommended quantity and quality of exercise for developing and maintaining cardiorespiratory and muscular fitness, and flexibility in healthy adults. (1998). Med Sci Sports Exerc 30(6): 975–991

[3] Association AM (1984) Guides to evaluation of permanent impairment, 2nd edn. American Medical Association, Chicago, IL

[4] Baechle TR, Groves BR (1998) Weight training: steps to success. Human Kinetics, Champaign, IL

[5] Behm DG, Button DC, Butt JC (2001) Factors affecting force loss with prolonged stretching. Can J Appl Physiol 26(3): 261–272

[6] Borg G (1982) Ratings of perceived exertion and heart rates during short-term cycle exercise and their use in a new cycling strength test. Int J Sports Med 3(3): 153–158

[7] Borg G, Hassmen P, Lagerstrom M (1987) Perceived exertion related to heart rate and blood lactate during arm and leg exercise. Eur J Appl Physiol Occup Physiol 56(6): 679–685

[8] Borg G, Linderholm H (1970) Exercise performance and perceived exertion in patients with coronary insufficiency, arterial hypertension and vasoregulatory asthenia. Acta Med Scand 187(1–2): 17–26

[9] Borg GA (1974) Perceived exertion. Exerc Sport Sci Rev 2: 131–153

[10] Celis MM, Suman OE, Huang TT, Yen P, Herndon DN (2003) Effect of a supervised exercise and physiotherapy program on surgical interventions in children with thermal injury. J Burn Care Rehabil 24(1): 57–61; discussion 56

[11] Cheng S, Rogers JC (1989) Changes in occupational role performance after a severe burn: a retrospective study. Am J Occup Ther 43(1): 17–24

[12] Convertino VA, Bloomfield SA, Greenleaf JE (1997) An overview of the issues: physiological effects of bed rest and restricted physical activity. Med Sci Sports Exerc 29(2): 187–190

[13] Cronan T, Hammond J, Ward CG (1990) The value of isokinetic exercise and testing in burn rehabilitation and determination of back-to-work status. J Burn Care Rehabil 11(3): 224–227

[14] Cucuzzo NA, Ferrando A, Herndon DN (2001) The effects of exercise programming vs traditional outpatient therapy in the rehabilitation of severely burned children. J Burn Care Rehabil 22(3): 214–220

[15] Davis J (1995) Direct determination of aerobic power. In: Maud PJ, Foster C (eds) Physiological assessment of human fitness. Human Kinetics, Champaign, IL, pp 9–17

[16] de Lateur BJ, Magyar-Russell G, Bresnick MG, Bernier FA, Ober MS, Krabak B J et al (2007) Augmented exercise in the treatment of deconditioning from major burn injury. Arch Phys Med Rehabil 88[12 Suppl 2]: S18–23

[17] Demling RH (2005) The burn edema process: current concepts. J Burn Care Rehabil 26(3): 207–227

[18] Elledge ES, Smith AA, McManus WF, Pruitt BA, Jr (1988) Heterotopic bone formation in burned patients. J Trauma 28(5): 684–687

[19] Fleck SJ, Kraemer WJ (1997) Designing resistance training programs. Human Kinetics, Champaign, IL

[20] Foster C, Florhaug JA, Franklin J, Gottschall L, Hrovatin LA, Parker S et al (2001) A new approach to monitoring exercise training. J Strength Cond Res 15(1): 109–115

[21] Franklin BA (2006) General principles of exercise prescription. In ACSM's guidelines for exercise testing and prescription. Lippincott Williams & Wilkins, Philadelphia, PA

[22] Gabriel V, Kowalske KJ, Holavanahalli RK (2009) Assessment of recovery from burn-related neuropathy by electrodiagnostic testing. J Burn Care Res 30(4): 668–674

[23] Guthrie J (2010a) Physical fitness testing and interpretation. In: Ehrman JK (ed) ACSM's resource manual for guidelines for exercise testing and prescription, 6th edn. Lippincott Williams & Wilkins, Philadelphia, PA, pp 308–319

[24] Guthrie J (2010b) Physical fitness testing and interpretation. In: Ehrman JK (ed) ACSM's resource manual for guidelines for exercise testing and prescription, 6th edn. Lippincott Williams & Wilkins, Philadelphia, PA, pp 310–315

[25] Harden NG, Luster SH (1991) Rehabilitation considerations in the care of the acute burn patient. Crit Care Nurs Clin North Am 3(2): 245–253

[26] Hart DW, Wolf SE, Mlcak R, Chinkes DL, Ramzy PI, Obeng MK et al (2000) Persistence of muscle catabolism after severe burn. Surgery 128(2): 312–319

[27] Haskell WL (1978) Cardiovascular complications during exercise training of cardiac patients. Circulation 57(5): 920–924

[28] Helm PA, Kevorkian CG, Lushbaugh M, Pullium G, Head MD, Cromes GF (1982) Burn injury: rehabilitation management in 1982. Arch Phys Med Rehabil 63(1): 6–16

[29] Higashimori H, Carlsen RC, Whetzel TP (2006) Early excision of a full-thickness burn prevents peripheral nerve conduction deficits in mice. Plast Reconstr Surg 117(1): 152–164

[30] Hodges PW, Richardson CA (1997a) Contraction of the abdominal muscles associated with movement of the lower limb. Phys Ther 77(2): 132–142; discussion 142–134

[31] Hodges PW, Richardson CA (1997b) Relationship between limb movement speed and associated contraction of the trunk muscles. Ergonomics 40(11): 1220–1230

[32] Howley ET (2001) Type of activity: resistance, aerobic and leisure versus occupational physical activity. Med Sci Sports Exerc 33[6 Suppl]: S364–369; discussion S419–320

[33] Humphrey CN, Richard RL, Staley MJ (1994) Soft tissue management and exercise. In: Richard RL, Staley M J (eds) Burn care and rehabiliation: principles and practice. F. A. Davis, Philadelphia, PA, pp 324–360

[34] Jones NL (1997) Approaches to clinical exercise testing. In: Clinical Exercise Testing, 4 th edn. W. B. Sunders Company, Philadelphia, pp 99–103

[35] Klein MB, Logsetty S, Costa B, Deters L, Rue TC, Carrougher GJ et al (2007) Extended time to wound closure is associated with increased risk of heterotopic ossification of the elbow. J Burn Care Res 28(3): 447–450

[36] Kokkonen J, Nelson AG, Cornwell A (1998) Acute muscle stretching inhibits maximal strength performance. Res Q Exerc Sport 69(4): 411–415

[37] Kortebein P, Ferrando A, Lombeida J, Wolfe R, Evans WJ (2007) Effect of 10 days of bed rest on skeletal muscle in healthy older adults. Jama 297(16): 1772–1774

[38] Kottke FJ, Pauley DL, Ptak RA (1966) The rationale for prolonged stretching for correction of shortening of connective tissue. Arch Phys Med Rehabil 47(6): 345–352

[39] Maeder M, Wolber T, Atefy R, Gadza M, Ammann P, Myers J et al (2005) Impact of the exercise mode on exercise capacity: bicycle testing revisited. Chest 128(4): 2804–2811

[40] McEntire SJ, Herndon DN, Sanford AP, Suman OE (2006) Thermoregulation during exercise in severely burned children. Pediatr Rehabil 9(1): 57–64

[41] McEntire SJ, Lee JO, Herndon DN, Suman OE (2009) Absence of exertional hyperthermia in a 17-year-old boy with severe burns. J Burn Care Res 30(4): 752–755

[42] Medicine, AAoPCoS (1990) Risks in distance running for children. Pediatrics 86(5): 799–800

[43] Mlcak RP, Desai MH, Robinson E, McCauley RL, Robson MC, Herndon DN (1993) Temperature changes during exercise stress testing in children with burns. J Burn Care Rehabil 14(4): 427–430

[44] Myers J (2003) A treadmill ramp protocol using simultaneous changes in speed and grade – a (ramp) step forward in exercise testing. Med Sci Sports Exerc 35(9): 1604

[45] Myers J, Buchanan N, Smith D, Neutel J, Bowes E, Walsh D et al (1992) Individualized ramp treadmill. Observations on a new protocol. Chest 101[5 Suppl]: 236S–241S

[46] Myers J, Buchanan N, Walsh D, Kraemer M, McAuley P, Hamilton-Wessler M et al (1991) Comparison of the ramp versus standard exercise protocols. J Am Coll Cardiol 17(6): 1334–1342

[47] Neugebauer CT, Serghiou M, Herndon DN, Suman OE (2008) Effects of a 12-week rehabilitation program with music & exercise groups on range of motion in young children with severe burns. J Burn Care Res 29(6): 939–948

[48] Pediatrics, T A A o (2001) Strength training by children and adolescents. Pediatrics 107(6): 1470–1472

[49] Persinger R, Foster C, Gibson M, Fater DC, Porcari JP (2004) Consistency of the talk test for exercise prescription. Med Sci Sports Exerc 36(9):1632–1636

[50] Physical Fitness Testing and Interpretation (2000) In: Franklin BA (ed) ACSM's guidelines for exercise testing and prescription. Lippincott Williams & Wilkins, Philadelphia, pp 68–90

[51] Przkora R, HerndonDN, Suman OE (2007) The effects of oxandrolone and exercise on muscle mass and function in children with severe burns. Pediatrics 119(1): e109–116

[52] Richard R, Baryza MJ, Carr JA, Dewey WS, Dougherty ME, Forbes-Duchart L et al (2009) Burn rehabilitation and research: proceedings of a consensus summit. J Burn Care Res 30(4): 543–573

[53] Richard RL, Staley MJ (1994) Burn patient evaluation and treatment planning. In: Richard RL, Staley MJ (eds) Burn care and rehabilitation: principles and practice. F. A. Davis, Philadelphia, PA, pp 201–220

[54] Rowland TW (1993) Aerobic exercise testing protocols. In: Rowland TW (ed) Pediatric laboratory exercise testing: clinical guidelines. Human Kinetics, Champaign, IL, pp 19–42

[55] Ruppel G (1986) Exercise testing. In: Raven EM (ed) Manual of pulmonary function testing, 4 th edn. C. V. Mosby Company, St. Louis, MO, pp 97–112

[56] Schneider JC, Holavanahalli R, Helm P, Goldstein R, Kowalske K (2006) Contractures in burn injury: defining the problem. J Burn Care Res 27(4): 508–514

[57] Schweickert WD, Pohlman MC, Pohlman AS, Nigos C, Pawlik AJ, Esbrook CL et al (2009) Early physical and occupational therapy in mechanically ventilated, critically ill patients: a randomised controlled trial. Lancet 373(9678): 1874–1882

[58] Simons M, King S, Edgar D (2003) Occupational therapy and physiotherapy for the patient with burns: principles and management guidelines. J Burn Care Rehabil 24(5): 323–335; discussion 322

[59] Smith K, Owens K (1985) Physical and occupational therapy burn unit protocol – benefits and uses. J Burn Care Rehabil 6(6): 506–508

[60] St-Pierre DM, Choiniere M, Forget R, Garrel DR (1998) Muscle strength in individuals with healed burns. Arch Phys Med Rehabil 79(2): 155–161

[61] Stiller K (2007) Safety issues that should be considered when mobilizing critically ill patients. Crit Care Clin 23(1): 35–53

[62] Stone MH, Wilson GD (1985) Resistive training and selected effects. Med Clin North Am 69(1): 109–122

[63] Suman OE, Herndon DN (2007) Effects of cessation of a structured and supervised exercise conditioning program on lean mass and muscle strength in severely burned children. Arch Phys Med Rehabil 88 [12 Suppl 2]: S24–29

[64] Suman OE, Mlcak RP, Herndon DN (2002) Effect of exercise training on pulmonary function in children with thermal injury. J Burn Care Rehabil 23(4): 288–293; discussion 287

[65] Suman OE, Mlcak RP, Herndon DN (2004) Effects of exogenous growth hormone on resting pulmonary function in children with thermal injury. J Burn Care Rehabil 25(3): 287–293

[66] Suman OE, Spies RJ, Celis MM, Mlcak RP, Herndon DN (2001) Effects of a 12-wk resistance exercise program on skeletal muscle strength in children with burn injuries. J Appl Physiol 91(3): 1168–1175

[67] Suman OE, Thomas SJ, Wilkins JP, Mlcak RP, Herndon DN (2003) Effect of exogenous growth hormone and exercise on lean mass and muscle function in children with burns. J Appl Physiol 94(6): 2273–2281

[68] Timmerman RA (2007) A mobility protocol for critically ill adults. Dimens Crit Care Nurs 26(5): 175–179; quiz 180–171

[69] Wallace J, Kaminsky LA (2006) Principles of cardiorespiratory endurance programming. In ACSM's resource manual for guidelines for exercise testing and prescription. Lippincott Williams & Wilkins, Philadelphia, PA, pp 336–349

[70] Weir JP, Cramer JT (2006) Principles of musculoskeletal exercise programming. In: Kaminsky LA (ed) ACSM's Resource manual for guidelines for exercise testing and prescription, 5 th edn. Lippincott Williams & Wilkins, Baltimore, MD, pp 350–365

[71] Welsch MA, Pollock ML, Brechue WF, Graves JE (1994) Using the exercise test to develop the exercise prescription in health and disease. Prim Care 21(3): 589–609

Correspondence: Karen J. Kowalske, MD, Department of Physical Medicine and Rehabilitation, University of Texas Southwestern Medical Center, 5323 Harry Hines Boulevard, Dallas, TX 75390-9055, USA, E-mail: karen.kowalske@utsouthwestern.edu

Burn reconstruction
(Principles and techniques)

Principles of burn reconstruction

Lars-Peter Kamolz[1, 2], David B. Lumenta[1]

[1] Medical University of Vienna, Department of Surgery, Division of Plastic and Reconstructive Surgery, Vienna, Austria
[2] State Hospital Wiener Neustadt, Department of Surgery, Section of Plastic, Aesthetic and Reconstructive Surgery, Wiener Neustadt, Austria

Due to extraordinary advances concerning the understanding of cellular and molecular processes in wound healing, wound care innovations and new developments concerning burn care have been made; burn care has improved to the extend that persons with burns frequently can survive. The trend in current treatment extends beyond the preservation of life; the ultimate goal is the return of burn victims, as full participants, back into their social and business life [1, 2].

A more aggressive approach in the acute phase has led to a higher survival rates on one side, but also to a higher number of patients, who will require reconstructive surgery on the other side. Successful reconstruction requires a profound understanding of skin anatomy and physiology, careful analysis of the defect and thoughtful considerations of different techniques suitable to execute the surgical plan [3].

From the reconstructive ladder to the reconstructive elevator

Based on concept of the reconstructive ladder by Mathes und Nahai new advances in the understanding of the anatomy, operative techniques, instrumentation, and surgical skills have led to the concept of the reconstructive elevator: complex procedures are no longer considered as last resort procedures only. In the quest to provide optimal form and func-

tion, it is currently accepted to jump several rungs of the ladder, due to the knowledge that some defects require more complex solutions. The goal of surgical reconstruction is restoration of preoperative function and appearance. The surgeon must reconstruct the defect with tissues that are missing and which allows defect coverage with tissues of similar contour, texture and color [4, 5].

The reconstructive clockwork

In clinical daily routine combinations of different techniques are often applied, in order to permit new reconstructive possibilities for the patient, but neither the reconstructive ladders of Mathes and Nahai in 1982 nor the reconstructive elevator permit a real combination of the different reconstructive procedures and techniques.

The image of interlocking wheels of a clockwork illustrate the integration of different reconstructive methods even more impressive than the conventional reconstructive ladder and elevator [6] (Fig. 1).

General principles

Hypertrophic scars and scar contraction with concomitant functional impairment are the most common problems that require correction or reconstruction. Choosing the right modality depends upon

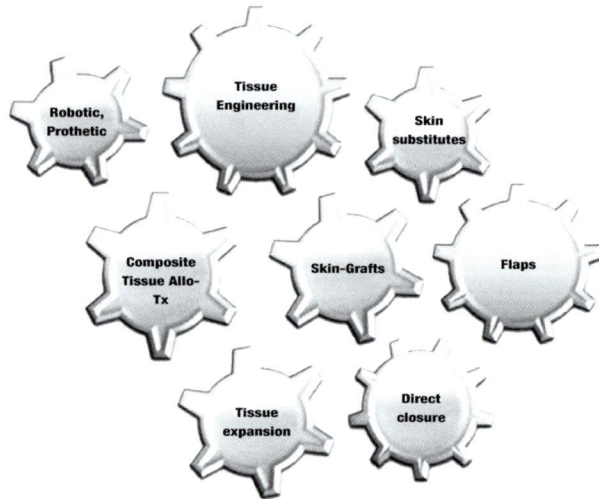

Fig. 1. The Reconstructive Clockwork: The interlocking wheels of a clockwork illustrates the integration of different reconstructive methods

several factors, e. g. the age or maturity of the scar. But also the knowledge of the healing properties of the patient (i. e. whether the patient has a tendency towards keloid or hypertrophic scarring) might help to decide on how aggressive or how conservative.

Objective assessment of deformities and functional impairment is of utmost importance for planning the right reconstructive procedure. Formulating a realistic plan to restore the functional problems requires analysis of the physical deformities and psychological disturbance of the patient. Psychiatric, psychosocial [7], and physiotherapeutic cares have to be continued while a surgical treatment plan is instituted.

Indication and timing of surgical intervention

For a surgeon, making a decision *how* to operate on a patient with burn deformities is quite simple. In contrast, deciding *when* to operate on a patient can be difficult. However, the basic principle is based on the following:
► restoring bodily deformities that impose functional difficulties must precede any surgical effort to restore the appearance.

In short, a surgeon's effort must be concentrated upon restoring the deformed bodily parts essential

for physical functions, if not for patient survival. In contrast, restoration of deformed regions in general, can be performed in a later phase.

It is postulated that attempts to correct burn deformities should be delayed for at least 1 to 2 years During this time needed for scar maturation an interim conservative treatment by using pressure garments and splinting is recommended to reduce scarring and to minimize joint contracture, because operating on an immature scar is technically more cumbersome and will lead to a higher number of complications. It is never too late to revise a scar, but conversely, it may be too early.

The techniques of reconstruction

There are several techniques routinely used to reconstruct deformities and to close defects related to the burn trauma.

Principally, they are:
► Excision techniques,
► Serial excision and tissue expansion,
► Skin grafting techniques with or without the use of dermal substitutes,
► Local skin flaps,
► Distant flaps,
► Allotransplantation,
► Tissue engineering,
► Robotics and prosthesis

Excision techniques

Excision with direct closure of the resultant wound is the simplest and the most direct approach in burn reconstruction. It is important to determine the amount of scar tissue that can be removed so that the resultant defect can be closed directly. A circumferential incision is made in the line previously marked and is carried out through the full thickness of the scar down to the subcutaneous layer. In case of a keloid, an intralesional excision might be better instead of an extralesional one in order to avoid recurrence. In order to minimize vascular supply interference along the wound edges, undermining of the scar edge should be kept to a minimum, whenever possible.

W-Plasty and geometric broken line closure

The *W-Plasty* [8, 9] is a series of connected, triangular advancement flaps mirrored along the length of each side of the scar, but aw-plasty, unlike a z-plasty does not result in an overall change in length of the scar, it makes the scar less conspicuous and it disrupts wound contracture with its irregular pattern. As with all other procedure, it is helpful to mark the planned design prior to the operation (Fig. 2).

The Geometric Broken Line Closure (GBLC) is a more sophisticated scar regularization technique than the W-plasty and requires more time to execute [10–13]; unlike the W-plasty's regularly irregular pattern, which results in a somewhat predictable scar pattern that can be followed by the observer's eye, the irregular irregularity of the GBLC allows maximum scar camouflage. This is acchieved by various combinations of triangles, rectangles, squares and semicircles in differing widths and lengths along the scar (Figs. 2, 3).

Serial excision and tissue expansion

The goal of surgical reconstruction is the restoration of preoperative function and appearance. The surgeon must reconstruct the defect with tissue of similar contour, texture and color. Surgical excision of scars relies upon recruitment of local tissue for closure of the resulting defect and thus adjacent skin will usually provide the best match for the defect. In areas where tissue laxity is poor or the resulting defect would be to big, tissue expansion and serial excision are useful techniques to overcome a lack of sufficient local tissue for closure. Tissue expansion allows large areas of burn scar to be resurfaced by providing tissue of similar texture and color to the defect. Moreover it is combined with the advantage of donor site morbidity reduction. Issues and disadvantages that need to be addressed are that the technique of pre-expansion requires additional office visits for serial expansion and at least one extra surgical procedure with potential for additional complications. A significant time period between 9 and 12 weeks for progressive tissue expansion is required. Tissue expanders are very versatile tools in reconstructive burn surgery, but still, careful patient selection, correct indications and realistic

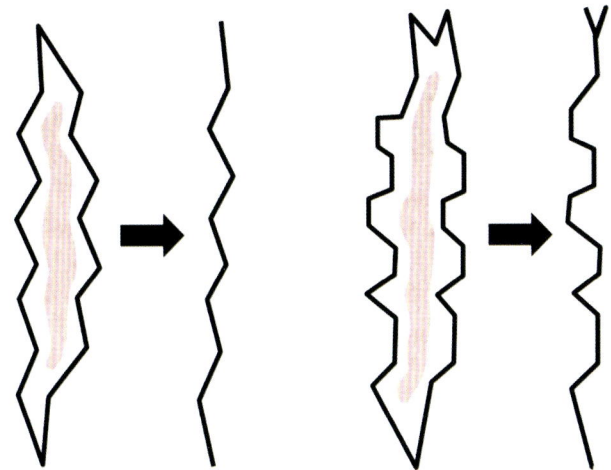

Fig. 2. W-Plasty (left) and Geometric Broken Line Closure (right); (Scar: pink)

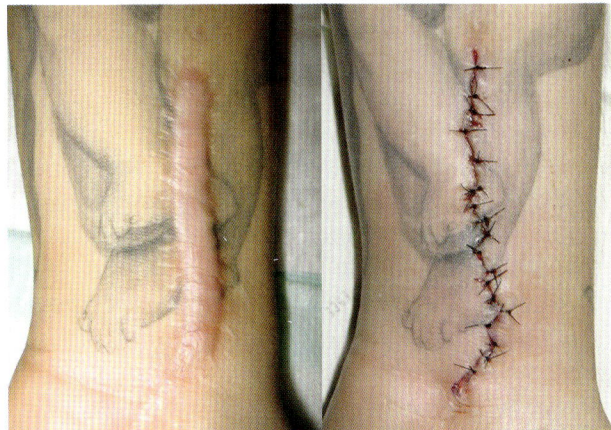

Fig. 3. Geometric Broken Line Closure: clinical example

treatment concepts, large experience and well- selected surgical techniques, precise instruction of the medical staff as well as detailed and continuous education of the patients are essential [14, 15].

Serial excisions involve the partial excision of the scar with consecutive advancement of adjacent skin. In a series of sequential procedures the area of a scar is completely excised. The number of procedures needed depends on the elasticity of the surrounding skin and the size of scar being excised. The primary disadvantage of this technique is the requirement for multiple operations. If more than two operations are needed, tissue expansion should be considered as an alternative treatment option.

Skin grafting techniques

Covering an open wound with a skin graft harvested at a various thickness is the conventional approach of wound closure. A skin graft including epidermis and dermis is defined as a full-thickness skin graft, and a piece of skin cut at a thickness varying between 8/1000 of an inch (0.196 mm) and 18/1000 of an inch (0.441 mm) is considered to be a partial- or a split-thickness skin graft. The thickness of a full-thickness skin graft is quite variable depending upon the harvest region.

In case of a full thickness skin graft a paper template may be made to determine the size of the skin graft needed to close a wound. The skin graft is laid down to the wound bed and is anchored in place by suturing or stapling the graft onto the wound bed. A continuous contact of the skin graft with the wound bed is essential to ensure an in-growth of a vascular network within 3–5 days and thereby for graft survival. A gauze or cotton bolster tied over a graft has been the traditional technique to anchor and to prevent fluid accumulating underneath a graft, if there is a flat and well vascularized wound bed. In regions, which are associated with a less good take rate (concave defects; regions, which are subject to repeated motion like joints) or in patients with co-morbidities, which may have an impact on graft healing, other techniques [16–18] instead of the bolstering technique, are used for skin graft fixation. The use of topical negative pressure or fibrin glue can lead to better skin graft healing [16] (Fig. 4).

The criteria for using skin grafts of various thicknesses are mainly based on:

▶ The use of a thin graft is more appropriate for closing wounds with unstable vascular supply, particularly if the skin graft donor site is scarce.
▶ Moreover the quality and the presence of dermis seem to have an influence on the extent of wound contraction. The extent of contraction, which is noted if a thin partial-thickness skin graft is used, is larger than using a full thickness graft. The presence of a sufficient dermal structure could reduce wound contracture.

Skin graft in combination with a dermal substitute – For the past several years, artificial dermal substitutes have been used in order to improve skin quality

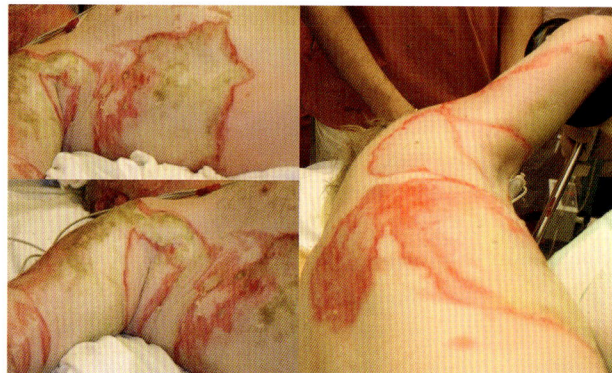

Fig. 4a. Dermal to full thickness burn

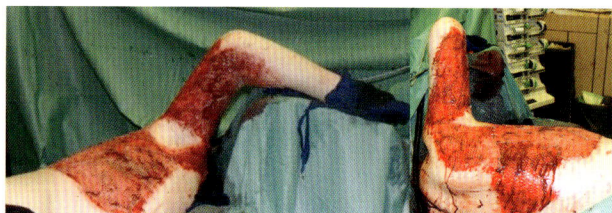

Fig. 4b. Tangential excision and grafting with 1:3 meshed skin graft

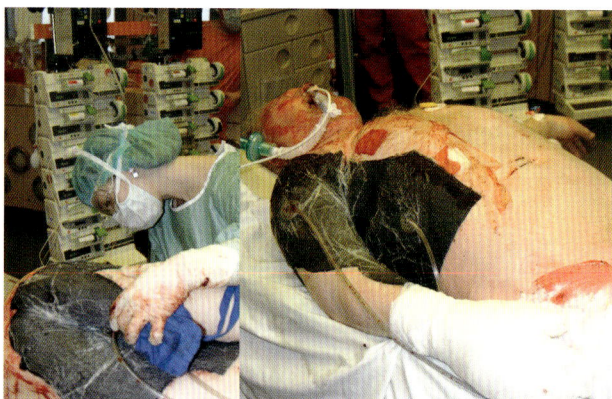

Fig. 4c. Skin graft fixation by use of V. A. C. for 5 days

e. g. Alloderm™, Integra™ [19]; these materials when implanted over an open wound, have been found to form a layer of close to normal dermis, thus providing a wound bed better for skin grafting and thereby better skin quality. However, the need for a staged approach to graft a wound using this technique is considered cumbersome. Matriderm™ is a new der-

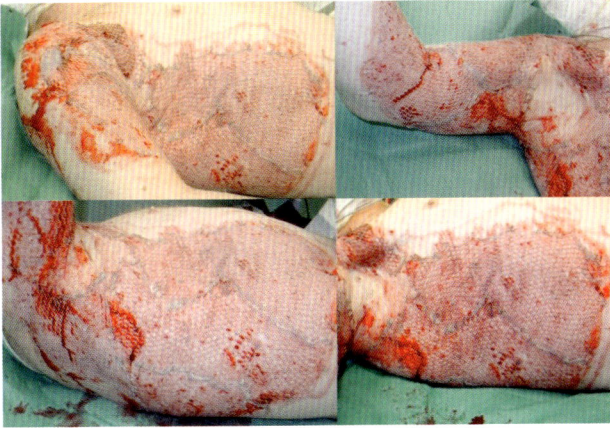

Fig. 4d. After removal of V. A. C. dressing: 100 % take rate of the skin grafts

mal matrix, which consists of collagen and elastin, and allows a single step reconstruction of dermis and epidermis in combination with a split thickness skin graft [20–22] (Fig. 5).

Local skin flaps

The approach using a segment of skin with its intrinsic structural components attached to cover a defect follows also the fundamental principle of reconstructive surgery to restore a destructed bodily part with a piece of like tissue. The recent technical innovation of incorporating a muscle and/or facial layer in the skin flap design, especially in a burned area, further expanded the scope of burn reconstruction as more burned tissues could be used for flap fabrication.

No single flap is optimal for every scar excision. Each individual scared area has to be analyzed for:
▶ Depth of the scar,
▶ Tissue involved and
▶ Availability of normal tissue for reconstruction.
Based on this, the ideal flap or the combination of flaps and techniques is chosen for reconstruction.

Often used skin flaps are the Z-plasty technique, the multiple Z-plasties, the ¾ Z-plasty technique.

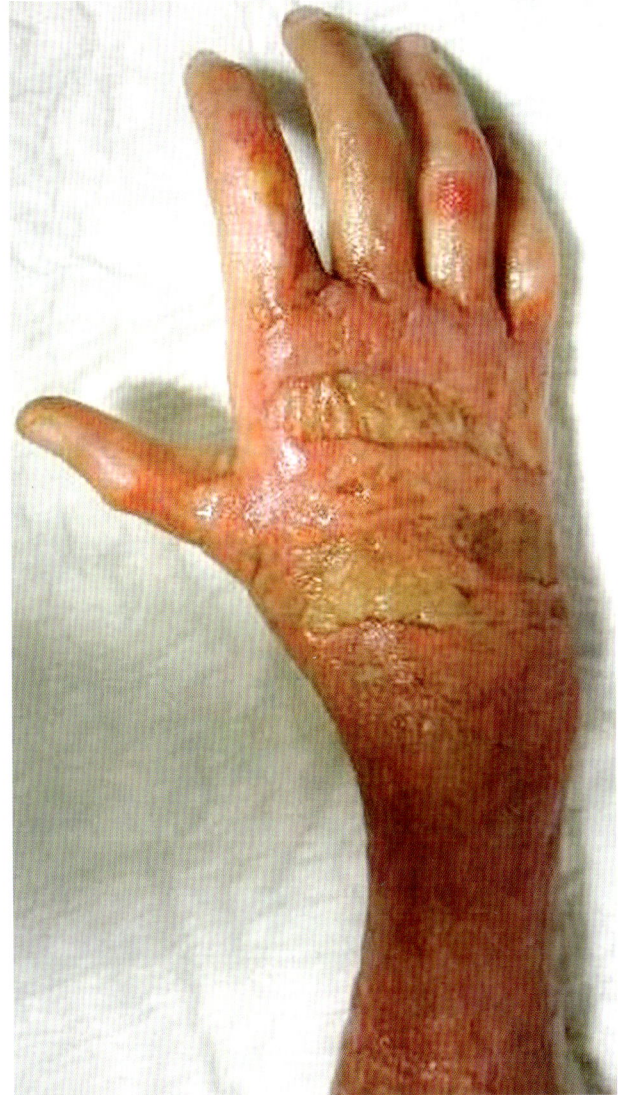

Fig. 5a. Hypertrophic and contracted scars (right hand)

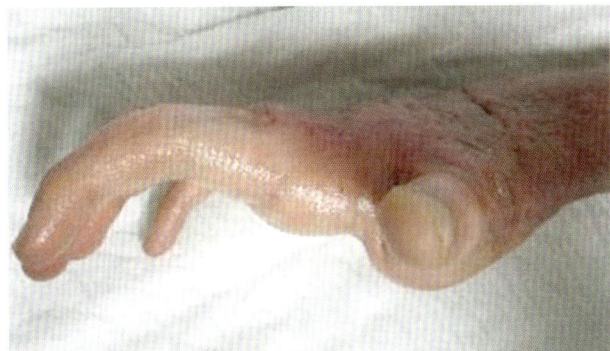

Fig. 5b. Hyperextension in the MCP joints

129

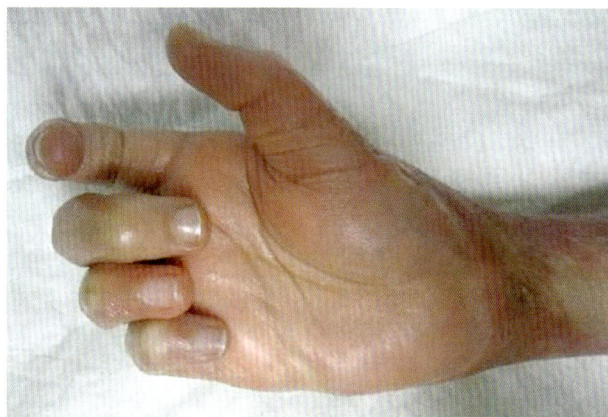

Fig. 5c. Flexion only possible in the PIP und DIP joints, hyperextensin in the MCP joints

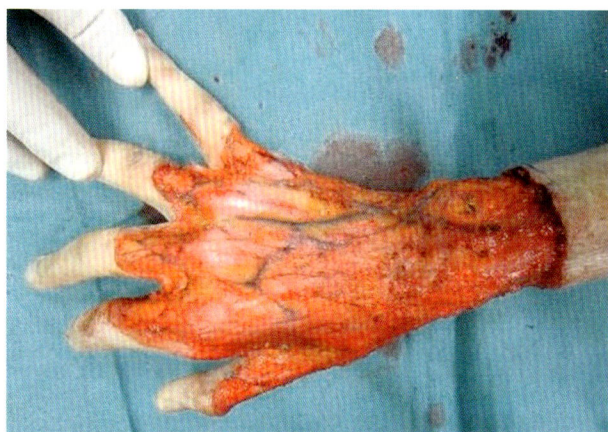

Fig. 5d. Complete excision of the hypertrophic and contracted scar plate

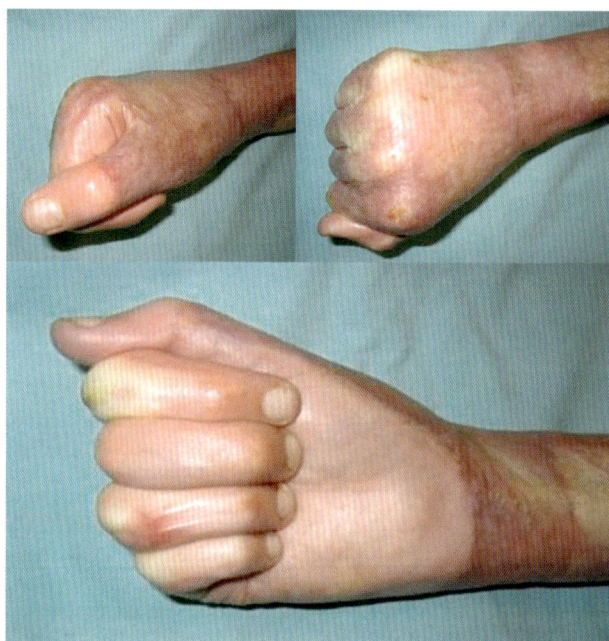

Fig. 5e. Early results obtained by use of Matriderm® and skin graft in a single step procedure (3 month postoperative)

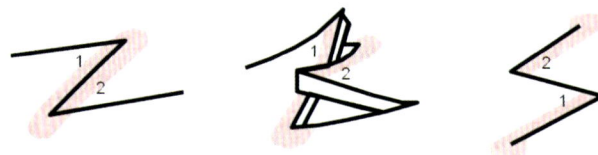

Fig. 6. Z-plasty (Scar: pink)

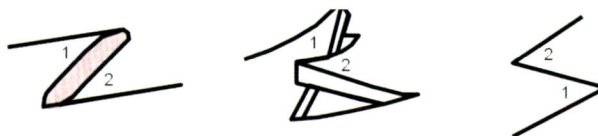

Fig. 7. Modified Z-Plasty (Scar: pink)

Z-plasty

There are 3 purposes to perform a Z-plasty:
▶ To lengthen a scar or to release a contracture
▶ To disperse a scar
▶ To realign a scar within a relaxed skin tension line.

The traditional Z-plasty consists of two constant features; first there are three incisions of equal length – two limbs and a central incision. Second there are two angles of equal degree – the limbs form 60 degree angles with the central incision (Fig. 6). Ideally the central incision should be placed along the axis of the scar; alternatively the scar itself may be completely excised with a fusiform defect acting as the central incision (Fig. 7).

Double opposing Z-plasty

Two Z-Plasty incisions placed immediately adjacent to one another as mirror images will produce an incision known as a double opposing Z-plasty (Figs. 8, 9) The advantage of this technique is that significant lengthening can be achieved in areas of limited skin availability. Ideal indication for this technique is the release of web space contractures (Fig. 10).

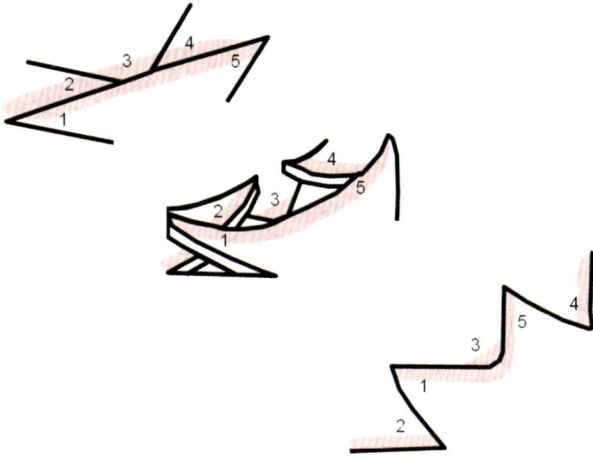

Fig. 8. Double opposing Z-plasty (Scar: pink)

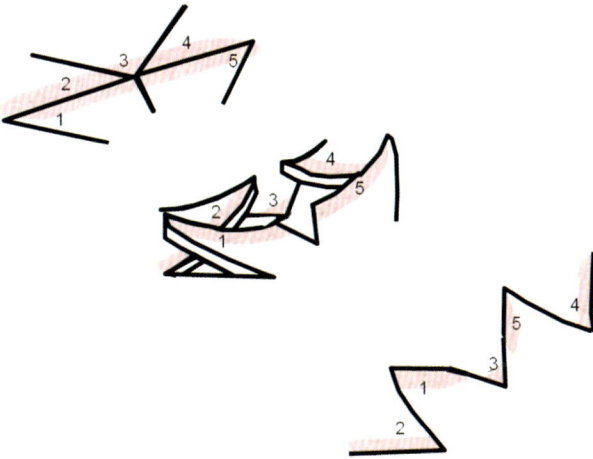

Fig. 9. Modified double opposing Z-plasty (Scar: pink)

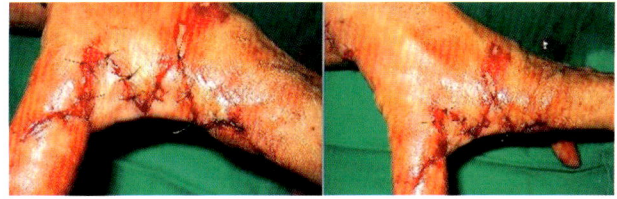

Fig. 10. Scar correction by use of a modified double opposing Z-plasty (1. Web space)

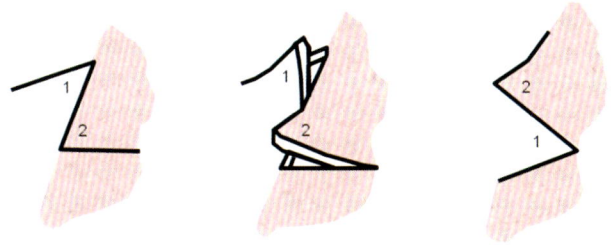

Fig. 11. ¾ Z-plasty or half-Z (Scar: pink)

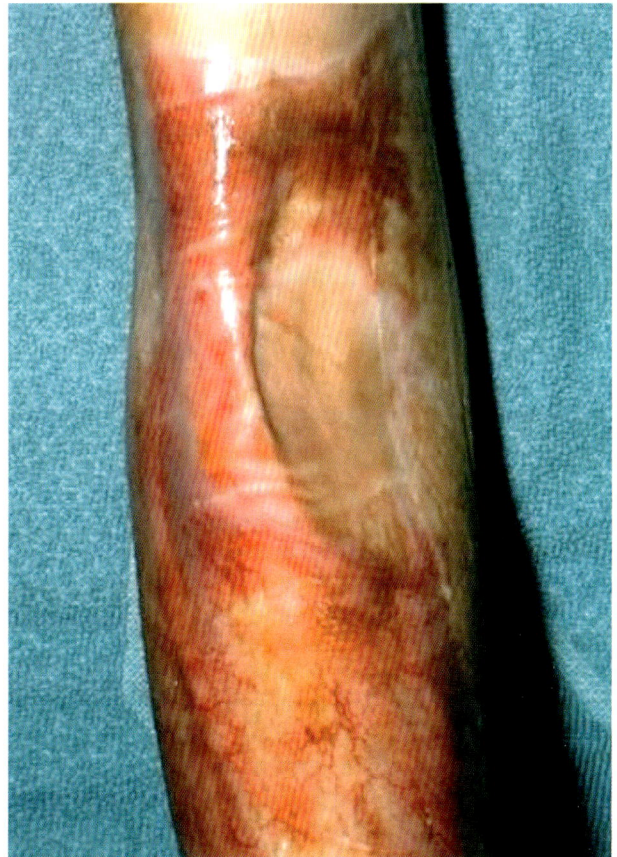

Fig. 12a. Scar contracture right cubita

The *¾ Z-plasty or half-Z* used to refer to a technique (Figs. 11, 12) with one limb incision being perpendicular to the central one. The incision is created on the scar side, which creates a fissure in the scar in which a triangular flap is introduced. The length gained on the scar side is directly proportional to the width of the triangular flap.

Despite its geometric advantage in flap design, fabricating a skin flap or skin flaps for reconstruction of burn deformities is not infrequently plagued with skin necrosis. Aberrant vascular supplies to the skin attributable to the original injury and/or surgical treatment could be the factor responsible for problems. In recent years, the use of a skin flap designed

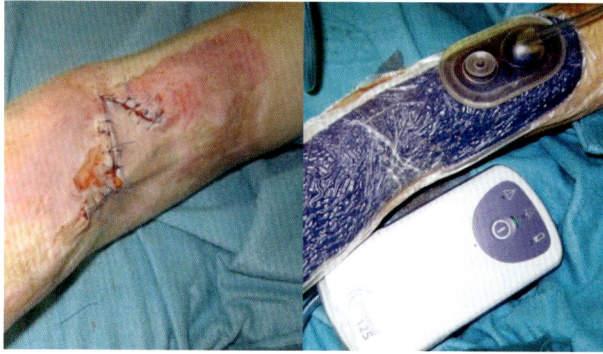

Fig. 12b. Correction by use of a ¾ Z-Plasty, Coverage with Prevena® for 6 days

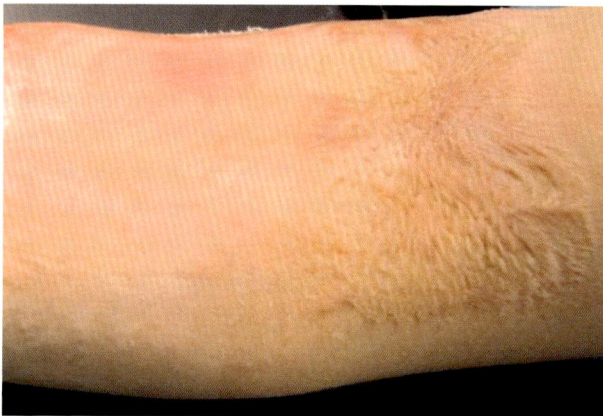

Fig. 13. Multiple Z-plasties (Scar: pink)

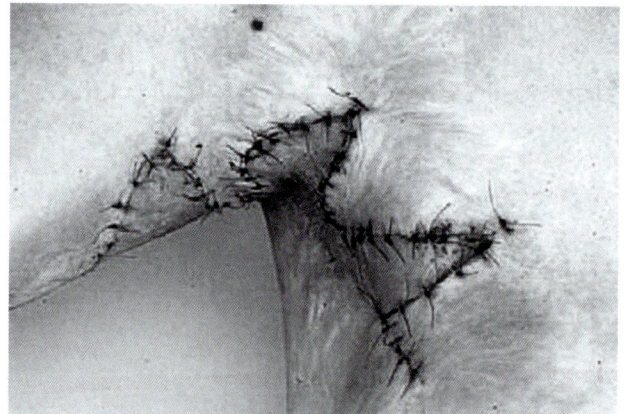

Fig. 12c. Long time result after correction by use of a ¾-Z-Plasty

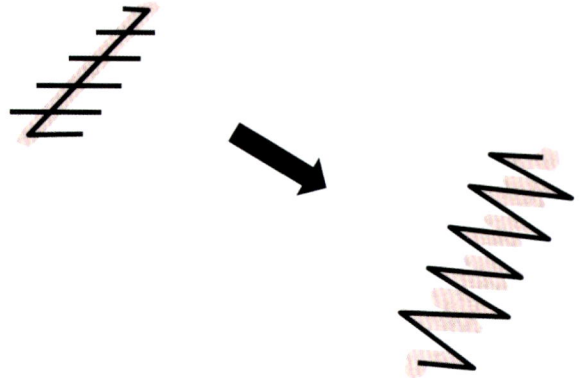

Fig. 14. Scar corrections by use of multiple Z-plasties (right axilla)

to include muscle or fascia underneath has further expanded the usefulness of conventional Z-plasty and the ¾ Z-plasty technique in burn reconstruction.

Musculocutaneous (MC) or fasciocutaneous (FC) flap technique

Inclusion of not only the skin but also the subcutaneous tissues and fascia and muscle is necessary to fabricate a skin flap to reconstruct a tissue defect in individuals with deep burn injuries. Which means, fabricating a flap in a burned area is possible, if the underlying muscle or the fascia is included in the design [23].

Moreover, multiple Z-plasties are often used for scar corrections (Figs. 13, 14).

Distant flaps

A distant flap involves a donor site, which is distant from the defect. The mode of transfer might be direct or microvascular. Direct flap, such as e.g. the forehead flap or the groin flap involve direct approximation of the recipient bed to the donor site. These flaps all require a second operation to divide the pedicle.

Free tissue transfer

The evolution of microsurgery and free tissue transfer has dramatically expanded the functional and aesthetic potential of reconstructive surgery. Due to microvascular anastomoses free transfer of single or compound tissues and replantation of amputated parts are possible. Moreover by using a free tissue transfer single step reconstructions are principally possible.

Perforator flaps

Based on the septocutaneous perforator vessels perforator flaps were developed. Song et al. described in 1984 [24] that the lateral femur region can serve not only as a skin harvest place, but also as the donor side for the "antero lateral thigh (ALT) flap" based on a long pedicle. Then Koshima and colleagues from Japan refined exemplarily the ALT-transfer subsequently. In 1989 Koshima introduced an abdominal skin and fat flap based on the inferior epigastric vessels and muscle perforators. Recently the theory of perforasomes is under evaluation: every perforator contains a unique vascula territory, the Perforasom [25]. This knowledge will lead to new useable pedicled and free flaps for reconstruction.

With the advent of microsurgical techniques, transplanting a composite tissue can be carried out with minimal morbidities. The regimen, in caring for burn victims, however, may be limited because of a paucity of donor materials. It is ironic that burn patients with suitable donor sites seldom require such an elaborate treatment, but those, who are in need of microsurgical tissue transplantation, are inevitably without appropriate donor sites because of extensive tissue destruction.

Composite tissue allo-transplantation

"Composite tissue allotransplantation" (CTA) of parts of the face, or forearms and upper extremities [26–29], is a young area of transplantation medicine. The first clinical results are promising in comparison to the first reports of organ transplantation, although the medium-term and long-term problems, for example tumor induction by the immunosuppression as well as chronic rejection have to be taken into account. This is not an unimportant fact, because CTA are normally not of vital importance. Nevertheless, for the affected persons, who must live in social isolation with exhausted reconstructive measures or prostheses, such operations may result a dramatic improvement concerning quality of life. However, it is important to mention, that currently only a selected small number of highly motivated patient are candidates for a CTA.

Regeneration – Tissue engineering

Tissue regeneration and tissue engineering has gained relevance for reconstructive surgery [30–32]. Recently, fat transplantation or lipo transfer is of utmost interest. Czerny transplanted in 1895 a lipoma for mamma reconstruction, and fat injection was described among other things by Eugene Holländer in 1910 within a patient with "progressive decrease of the fatty tissue". Erich Lexer dedicated in the first part of his book free fat transfers nearly 300 pages. In 2001 it was demonstrated that beside fat cells also "adipose-derived stem cells" (ADSC) beside other cell populations in the fatty tissue are usable for these purposes. The transplantation of ADSC was able to regenerate full-layered cartilage defects in the animal model [33]. The stem cell associated fat cell transplantation in patients with a radioderm has led to improved healing. Moreover, fat cell transplantation is not only able to improve volume and contour defects, but also skin quality [34–36]; thereby it seems that fat transfer will play an important part in burn reconstruction in the future.

Robotics/Prosthesis

If all reconstructive measures fail, myoelectric prostheses are a promising resort to go to. In recent years these have been improved tremendously by introducing targeted muscle transfers (TMR) to the armamentarium of reconstructive surgery [37, 38]. Modern myoelectric prostheses have multiple degrees of freedom that mandate a complex control system to provide dependable use for the patient. Extremity reconstruction in the 21st century will see many new avenues to replace the loss of a limb and reconstruct the loss of function. Both biological and technical advances will provide possibilities that may well open up therapies that have been unthinkable only a few years ago. Targeted muscle reinnervation together with the provision of a myoelectric prosthesis with several degrees of freedom is such an approach and will definitely be a solid stepping stone leading to new strategies in extremity rehabilitation and reconstruction.

Summary

The regimen of burn treatment has changed drastically over the past 50 years. The regimen of an early debridement and wound coverage, initially with biological dressings and later with autologous skin grafts, enhanced the survival rate. It is, however, ironic that this improvement in survival has caused an increase of patients, who will require reconstructive surgery.

Unsightly hypertrophic scar, scar contracture, affecting particularly the joint structures, and missing bodily parts are still the most common sequelae of burn injuries today.

The difficulty concerning burn reconstruction is largely due to a lack of adequate donor sites, but due to the improvements in reconstructive surgery better results are achievable. New areas like "composite tissue allotransplantation" of compound tissues like arms or parts of the face, prosthesis and also regenerative medicine with "tissue engineering" have already entered the clinical routine and will improve the final results obtained by burn reconstruction.

References

[1]   Williams FN, Herndon DN, Hawkins HK et al (2009) The leading causes of death after burn injury in a single pediatric burn center. Crit Care 13(6): 183

[2]   Kamolz LP (2010) Burns: learning from the past in order to be fit for the future. Crit Care 14(1): 106

[3]   Clark JM, Wang TD (2001) Local flaps in scar revision. Fac Plast Surg 4: 295–308

[4]   Mathes S, Nahai F (1982) Clinical application for muscle and musculocutaneous flaps. Mosby, St. Louis, p 3

[5]   Gottlieb LJ, Krieger LM (1994) From the reconstructive ladder to the reconstructive elevator. Plast Reconstr Surg 93(7): 1503–1504

[6]   Knobloch K, Vogt PM (2010) The reconstructive Sequence of the 21st Century- The reconstructive clockwork Chirurg 81: 441–446

[7]   Titscher A, Lumenta DB, Kamolz LP et al (2010) Emotional associations with skin: differences between burned and non-burned individuals. Burns 36(6): 759–763

[8]   Borges AF (1959) Improvement of antitension line scar by the "W-plastic" operation. Br J Plast Surg 6:12–29

[9]   McCarthy JG (1990) Introsuction to plastic surgery. In: Plastic Surgery. WB Saunders, Philadelphia, pp 1–68

[10]   Webster RD, Davidson TM, Smith RC (1977) Broken line scar revision. Clin Plast Surg 4: 263–274

[11]   Tardy ME, Thomas RJ, Pashow MS (1981) The Camouflage of cutaneous scars. Ear Nose Throat J 60:61–70

[12]   Alsarraf R, Murakami CS (1998) Geometric broken line closure. Fac Plast Surg Clin North Am 6: 163–166

[13]   Thomas JR (1989) Geometric broken-line closure. In: Thomas JR, Holt GR (eds) Facial scars: incision, revision and camouflage. CV Mosby, St. Louis, pp 160–167

[14]   Pallua N, von Heimburg D (2005) Pre-expanded ultrathin supraclavicular flaps for (full-) face reconstruction with reduced donor-site morbidity and without the need for microsurgery. Plast Reconstr Surg 115(7): 1837–1844

[15]   Bozkurt A, Groger A, O'Dey D et al (2008) Retrospective analysis of tissue expansion in reconstructive burn surgery: evaluation of complication rates. Burns 34(8): 1113–1118

[16]   Mittermayr R, Wassermann E, Thurnher M et al (2006) Skin graft fixation by slow clotting fibrin sealant applied as a thin layer. Burns 32(3): 305–311

[17]   Pallua N, Wolter T, Markowicz M (2010) Platelet-rich plasma in burns. Burns 36(1): 4–8

[18]   Roka J, Karle B, Andel H et al (2007) Use of V. A. C. Therapy in the surgical treatment of severe burns: the Viennese concept. Handchir Mikrochir Plast Chir 39(5): 322–327

[19]   Nguyen DQ, Potokar TS, Price P (2010) An objective long-term evaluation of Integra (a dermal skin substitute) and split thickness skin grafts, in acute burns and reconstructive surgery. Burns 36(1): 23–28

[20]   Haslik W, Kamolz LP, Nathschläger G et al (2007) First experiences with the collagen-elastin matrix Matriderm as a dermal substitute in severe burn injuries of the hand. Burns 33(3): 364–368

[21]   Haslik W, Kamolz LP, Manna F et al (2010) Management of full-thickness skin defects in the hand and wrist region: first long-term experiences with the dermal matrix Matriderm. J Plast Reconstr Aesthet Surg 63(2): 360–364

[22]   Bloemen MC, van Leeuwen MC, van Vucht NE et al (2010) Dermal substitution in acute burns and reconstructive surgery: a 12-year follow-up. Plast Reconstr Surg 125(5): 1450–1459

[23]   Huang T, Larson DL, Lewis SR (1975) Burned hands. Plast Reconstr Surg 56: 21–28

[24]   Song YG, Chen GZ, Song YL (1984) The free thigh flap: a new free flap concept based on the septocutaneous artery. Br J Plast Surg 37(2): 149–159

[25]   Saint-Cyr M, Wong C, Schaverien M, Mojallal A, Rohrich RJ (2009) The perforasome theory: vascular anatomy and clinical implications. Plast Reconstr Surg 124(5): 1529–44159

[26] Brandacher G, Ninkovic M, Piza-Katzer H et al (2009) The Innsbruck hand transplant program: Update at 8 years after the first transplant. Transplant Proc 41(2): 491–494

[27] Siemionow MZ, Zor F, Gordon CR (2010) Face, upper extremity, and concomitant transplantation: potential concerns and challenges ahead. Plast Reconstr Surg 126(1): 308–315

[28] Gordon CR, Siemionow M, Zins J (2009) Composite tissue allotransplantation: a proposed classification system based on relative complexity. Transplant Proc 41(2): 481–484

[29] Siemionow M, Gordon CR (2010) Overview of guidelines for establishing a face transplant program: a work in progress. Am J Transplant 10(5): 1290–1296

[30] Kamolz LP, Lumenta DB, Kitzinger HB, Frey M (2008) Tissue engineering for cutaneous wounds: An overview of current standards and possibilities. Eur Surg 40(1): 19–26

[31] Beier JP, Boos AM, Kamolz L et al (2010) Skin tissue engineering – from split skin to engineered skin grafts? Handchir Mikrochir Plast Chir 42: 342–353

[32] Mansbridge JN (2009) Tissue-engineered skin substitutes in regenerative medicine. Curr Opin Biotechnol 20(5): 563–567

[33] Dragoo JL, Carlson G, McCormick F et al (2007) Healing full-thickness cartilage defects using adipose-derived stem cells. Tissue Eng 13(7): 1615–1621

[34] Klinger M, Marazzi M, Vigo D, Torre M (2008) Fat injection for cases of severe burn outcomes: a new perspective of scar remodeling and reduction. Aesthetic Plast Surg 32(3): 465–469

[35] Mojallal A, Lequeux C, Shipkov C et al (2009) Improvement of skin quality after fat grafting: clinical observation and an animal study. Plast Reconstr Surg 124(3): 765–774

[36] Rennekampff HO, Reimers K, Gabka CJ et al (2010) Current perspective and limitations of autologous fat transplantation–"consensus meeting" of the German Society of Plastic, Reconstructive and Aesthetic Surgeons. Handchir Mikrochir Plast Chir 42(2): 137–142

[37] Aszmann OC, Dietl H, Frey M (2008) Selective nerve transfers to improve the control of myoelectrical arm prostheses. Handchir Mikrochir Plast Chir 40(1):60–65

[38] Hijjawi JB, Kuiken TA, Lipschutz RD, Miller LA, Stubblefield KA, Dumanian GA (2006) Improved myoelectric prosthesis control accomplished using multiple nerve transfers. Plast Reconstr Surg 118: 1573–1577

Correspondence: Lars-Peter Kamolz, M.D., Ph.D., M.Sc., Medical University of Vienna, Department of Surgery, Division of Plastic and Reconstructive Surgery, Vienna, Austria, E-mail: kamolz@plastchirurg.info

Tissue expanders in burn surgery

Norbert Pallua, Erhan Demir

Department of Plastic Surgery and Hand Surgery, Burn Center, University Hospital RWTH Aachen, Aachen University of Technology, Aachen, Germany

Part I
Introduction

Tissue expansion is based on a dynamic process of nature in which vital tissue responds to continuous mechanical stress load. The capability to gain or lose weight during pregnancy for instance demonstrates the skin ability to develop independently. Tissue expansion has a significant implication in different ethnic societies throughout the world. Enlarged lips of Ethiopian Mursi women or elongated necks of Padauang women attest the exotic aesthetics associated with tissue expansion [1]. Tissue expansion represents the medical application of this normal physiologic process for reconstructive purposes and has already provided to be a reliable principle in plastic and reconstructive surgery [2, 3].

Historical aspects

In 1905 the clinical use of tissue expansion gained significance when bone lengthening by distraction resulted in skin expansion [4]. However, the first clinical concept of tissue expansion was reported by Neumann in 1957 for the reconstruction of a traumatic ear defect with a post-auricular expanded skin flap to cover the cartilage framework of the ear [5]. Twenty years later skin expansion was re-introduced independently by Radovan and Austad [6, 7]. Ra-

dovan became the first surgeon to gain extensive experience in the use of silicone expanders, whereas Austad was the first to report his laboratory scientific experience prior to the subsequent clinical application. Primarily established for breast reconstruction, skin expansion represents one of the major developments in reconstructive surgery in recent years, particularly as a valuable approach for many problems in reconstructive burn surgery [8]. More recent surgical modifications advanced the basic concept of tissue expansion to preexpand flap donor regions or to prefabricate regional or microsurgical free flaps [9–15].

Biology of expanded tissue

Tissue expansion places an inflatable device beneath the skin flap, which is then expanded over a period of time. Basic studies confirmed that the increased surface area is the result of new regenerated tissue [16]. Experimental data on the biology of expanded skin in animal and human studies showed that the epidermis underwent significant thickening after 5 weeks to 5 months of expansion. The dermis and subcutaneous tissue, on the other hand, were significantly thinner after expansion. They found the greatest thinning over the dome of the expander and a gradually decrease toward the periphery [17–20]. Histologically, the most significant thinning occurred in the reticular dermis. These observed changes persisted two years. Expanded tissues two years after cessation of expansion had the same thickness as control tissues and had no remnant fibrous capsule [6, 21]. Additional increase in dermal collagen content with disruption of elastic fibers has been noted. The noticed dermal and subcutaneous collagen increase occurs with a constant ratio between collagen type I and III. Skin appendages are not affected by the expansion procedure [1].

Therefore some believe that much of the expanded skin represents stretch and reorganization of dermal collagen fibers rather than new skin created by mitosis. Austad postulated that tissue expansion causes a decrease in cell density in the basal layer of the skin and that cell density may regulate skin mitotic activity. A greater cell proliferation is a consequence of lower cell density, resulting in growth of additional skin [1]. The physiology of expansion by prolonged tissue expansion (PTE) is therefore considered not to be just a matter of skin stretching, but the formation of additional new skin, which has all the characteristics of the original tissue.

A significant increase in vascularity has been associated with soft tissue expansion. Experimental studies observed proliferation of blood vessels and numerous neovascular branches in expanded flaps [20, 22]. The measured blood flow after flap expansion was higher than contralateral non-expanded controls.

The ability of soft tissue to expand is based on several aspects. The skin has the constant ability to adapt, depending on the amount and distribution of structural proteins and tissue fluids. Collagen fibers become parallel with the stretching of tissue. Although elastin fibers are important for recoil after stretching, collagen fibers lengthen permanently [1].

Any expansion related muscle damage with fiber atrophy or degeneration dissolves after pressure relief with expander removal.

The process of tissue expansion not only affects adjacent tissue but also a number of cell types. On the molecular level a key-function in the mechanical intercellular signal transduction has been attributed to the proteinkinase C. In this context some growth factors, such as platelet-derived growth factor (PDGF), vascular-endothelial growth factor (VEGF), angiotensin II and transforming growth factor beta

(TGF-ß) have been reported to have important influence on cell proliferation and extracellular matrix production. TGF-ß can also enhance fibroblast proliferation [1, 22, 23].

In summary prolonged dynamic tissue expansion is a passive physical process with a metabolically active component [8].

Basic principles and techniques

Indications, patient selection and compliance

The appropriate patient selected for burn reconstructions with tissue expanders faces a difficult reconstructive challenge. The patients must be willing to subject themselves to a prolonged treatment concept. The patient must be able to emotionally deal with the temporary extreme deformity and the somewhat bizarre appearance of the expanded anatomic regions. This may require a thorough dialog with the patient and high individual compliance and motivation.

Indications for the use of expanders in burn reconstructions are instances, where there is not enough adjacent tissue to resurface or close a defect primarily or with a local flap. The same criteria used to select a suitable patient for a regional skin flap are applicable in the selection for tissue expanded skin or flap reconstruction. Ideally the patient should have no serious medical problems (e. g. diabetes, hypertension) and should not be a heavy smoker.

Tissue expansion allows large areas of burn scar to be resurfaced and provides tissue of similar texture and color to the defect to be covered combined with the advantage of reduced donor site morbidity. It is therefore indicated whenever defect repair by an alternative method such as a local, regional, or free flap may result in an unacceptable donor region or recipient site deformity [2, 11, 24, 25].

Issues and disadvantages that need to be addressed are that the technique of pre-expansion requires additional office visits for serial expansion and at least one extra surgical procedure with potential for additional complications. A significant time period between 9 and 12 weeks for progressive tissue expansion is required.

Expanders

Tissue expanders belong to the most frequently used implants in plastic and reconstructive surgery [26–28]. The most common used expanders are the different types and variations of Radovan expanders. Elliptical, rectangular, round, crescent type or custom made shapes with integrated or separate port systems are available. The various volumes range between 1cc and 1000cc. Expanders can be over inflated at least two times the stated maximum volume.

Expanders with an incorporated filling valve are designed in a way that the expander and injection port form a single unit. The port has a self-sealing membrane and is lined with metal or a thick polymer to prevent accidental puncture of the dome during injection of saline. The shapes include hemispheric, rectangular, crescent, and teardrop. Limitations are the size ranges between 50cc to 1000 cc, as this type of expander are not available as mini-expanders. The stiffness of the injection port causes an increased risk of skin erosion.

The third relevant expander groups are the self-inflating systems. They consist of a semi-permeable silicone membrane that surrounds a hydrogel-core (co-polymer based on methylmetacrylate and N-vinylpyrolidon) to create an osmotic gradient across the expander wall. The interior core of the expander is hypertonic relative to the extracellular water, causing a net influx of water into the expander. In burn reconstructions this type of expander is somewhat experimental [29].

Aspects in expander volume and shape selection

The three-dimensional expander geometry needs to match the expansion site and the design of the planned flap. The shape of the expander depends primarily on the site of expansion and the reconstruction needs. The use of a rectangular expander provides the most effective surface area gained when compared to the round or crescent types [30].

The selected expander size must be large enough to provide desired expansive forces necessary to achieve the sufficient tissue augmentation. One method of selecting the appropriate expander is based on the size of the expander base. The expander base and the defect width are helpful parameters

$$E = B + D$$

Expanded Area = Base size + Defect size

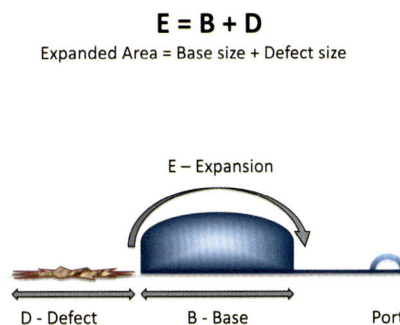

Fig. 1. Estimation of the expanded area, according to the base size and defect width

to estimate the required expansion (Fig. 1) [31]. While using a rectangular or crescent expander the appropriate size expander would be one in which the surface area of the expander base is 2.5 times as large as the defect to be closed. With round expanders, the diameter of the expander base should be 2.5 times as large as the defect [17]. Another method of expander selection is based on the circumference of the balloon portion of the expander. The expander must be of sufficient volume that the apical circumference of the dome of skin overlying the fully inflated expander is 2–3 times the defect width.

It is best to select the largest expander that can reasonable be placed beneath the donor region of expansion or to consider the use of two or more expanders to gain the needed tissue. Still, the proven safety of limited over inflation allows a margin of error in the initial choice of implant volume, and later permits to continue expansion if more tissue is required. The disadvantage of over inflation is the increased leakage from the injection port dome.

Surgical expander placement and expansion

The donor site is selected where tissues are most suitable (e. g. thickness, color, texture) to those of the anatomic region to be resurfaced with close proximity to the defect. The use of local tissue with the advantage of color and texture match with the recipient region is sometimes difficult or impossible to achieve in burned patients.

The incision for expander placement should be in a site well hidden or ideally perpendicular to the desired vector of expansion, to keep the forces of scar tension as low as possible. The incision can be incorporated into the scar area planned for reconstruction after expander removal, but should not potentially compromise the viability of advancement flaps during reconstruction. However, while using more then one expander it is crucial to respect appropriate distances between the expander pockets to prevent expander displacements with inefficient skin expansions.

The correct anatomic position while placing the expander is critical. In the face and neck it is usually beneath the subcutaneous fat or below the platysma in the neck. In the scalp, expander placement is in a subgaleal plane. While performing pre-expanded muscular flaps such as the pre-expanded trapezius flap the correct level of dissection while creating the expander pocket is submuscular. The dissected pocket needs to be large enough to fit the expander without any folding. The surgeon should make sure the implant is intact and functioning prior placement. The port system is placed subcutaneously in a more distant position approximately 5 cm away from the expander. Meticulous hemostasis is essential; suctions drains are placed to drain the wound. The implanted expander is inflated with 10 % of the end-volume to obliterate dead space and to aid with the hemostasis.

The procedure of serial ambulatory expansion is begun after completion of wound healing about 2–3 weeks postoperatively. During inflation aqua ad iniectabilia is instilled till tension of the overlying skin is noted or patients reports about discomfort. In a clinical observation the skin may blanch with pressure from the expander, but capillary refill should return to normal after pressure is withdrawn.

The process of expander inflation is continued on a weekly basis until the desired amount of volume and tissue needed is obtained (usually between 8 to 12 weeks). Meticulous documentation auf instilled volumes is important.

Expander explantation and management of the capsule

The second reconstructive step consists upon removal of the expander and local, regional or free flap reconstruction. Total capsule excision may create ultrathin and flexible flaps as desired in facial reconstructions [9, 32]. As an alternative it is useful to in-

cise the capsule or to remove the inner layers of the capsule to allow further lengthening of the expanded flap. Leaving the superficial layers of the capsule may prevent the compromise of the flap vasculature as the reported vascular proliferation occurs primarily at the junction of the capsule and the host tissue. Any surgical maneuver should be limited to the expander capsule, respectively [8].

Pre-expanded flaps

Since their introduction several pre-expanded flaps have been used in burn reconstructions. These include the lateral arm fasciocutaneous flap, the scapular/parascapular fasciocutaneous flap, radial forearm fasciocutaneous flap, the groin flap, the latissimus dorsi musculocutaneous flap, the trapezius muscle flap, the serratus anterior musculocutaneous flap, the tensor fascia lata flap or the supraclavicular island flap to name a few [9, 12, 13, 15, 33–35]. More recently methods of perforator-based tissue expansion for pre-expanded free cutaneous perforator flaps such as the anterior lateral thigh flap are becoming more common [36, 37].

Complications

Although the expansion related reconstructive procedure is based on a simple concept, this technique is associated with complications [38–43]. In studies providing data of all anatomical regions failure rates ranged up to 24 % [1, 44]. Appropriate patient selection and surgical experience may reduce the complication rates below 20 %.

Major complications are usually defined as those requiring expander removals. These complications may include tissue loss caused by overexpansion and induced ischemia, inadvertent flap thinning, fat necrosis, expander infection, expander exposure, implant failure and interference of the flap design due to incorrect incisions used to place the tissue expanders. This may occur secondary to trauma, flap erosion due to folds in the expander, aggressive expansion methods, or port placement over a bony prominence. If implant folding or flap ischemia secondary to overfilling of the expander is suspected, in an early stage, expander deflation and skin observation should be performed. If skin viability returns, the device can be slowly re-inflated in a later stage. In cases with skin necrosis or expander extrusion the implant needs to be removed. After surgical debridement the wound can be managed by conservative measures with broad-spectrum antibiotics and frequent wound dressings. Infections of the expander pocket may respond in some cases to antibiotics and partial implant deflation to minimize vascular compromise. If these procedures fail the implant should be removed, the pocket irrigated, drained and allowed to heal.

Minor complications are defined as seroma and drainage after expansion, poor compliance, intolerance of the injections to fill the expanders or alterations in the early preoperative plans secondary to incomplete coverage following expansion. Rates range between 17 % and 40 %, with a mean in the range of 20 % [1,44].

Part II:
Clinical applications of tissue expanders

Head and neck reconstruction

Alopecia reconstruction of the burned scalp

Deep scalp burns result in cicatrical alopecia in the long-term [1]. The treatment of these problems depends on the size, the particular location and the status of the remaining hear-bearing scalp. Burn alopecia is frequently noted in up to 32 % of the patient population. In addition a 2.2 % incidence of complications including scar alopecia, is due secondary to the use of the scalp donor site in burn patients [45, 46]. The reconstruction of scalp defects with serial excisions and rotational flaps may in some cases be not sufficient enough [25], therefore skin expansion and correction of alopecia using scalp rotational flaps has become the gold standard treatment.

McCauley classified burn alopecia in four types based on the pattern and the extent [1]. Patients with type I-A and I-B alopecia can be corrected with a single expansion. Patients with type I-C and I-D may achieve complete defect coverage with sequential expansion. Type II can be corrected with a single pre-expanded scalp flap. Patients classified as II-B, C or D may respond well to multiple expand-

Table 1. McCauley RL Classification of burn alopecia

Type I	Single alopecia segment
IA	Less than 25 % of hair-bearing scalp
IB	20–50 % of the hair-bearing scalp
IC	50–75 % of the hair-bearing scalp
ID	75 % of the hair bearing scalp
Type II	Multiple alopecia segments amendable to tissue expansion placement
Type III	Patchy burn alopecia not amendable to tissue expansion
Type IV	Total alopecia

ers. Unfortunately type III and IV patients are not good candidates for tissue expander procedures [1].

Multiple expanders (average volumes 200–400 cc) with distant injection ports are placed beneath the galea aponeurotica. Inflation of the expander begins two weeks postoperatively on a weekly basis. After an initial three week period with slow proceeding of the expansion due to galeal resistance or deformation of the external tabula in young patients adequate expansion can be accomplished in 8 to 10 weeks. The endpoint of expansion is until the distance across the expanded scalp is equal to the starting distance, plus the scalp width to be replaced. The second stage involves incision at the margin of the alopecia and expander removal. The bald scalp is excised only after advancing or transposing the expanded scalp to be sure sufficient tissue is available to close the proposed resection. If there is insufficient tissue to allow removal of the alopecia, tissue expanders can be replaced for further expansion. If there is adequate tissue, the capsule surrounding the expander is usually not excised. The wounds are closed in two layers, and suction drains are used.

Case sample: 11-year old boy with type II burn alopecia. Same patient with three implanted expanders and 2 years after scalp expansion and alopecia reconstruction (Figs. 2–4).

Eyelid reconstruction

The skin of the eyelids is best replaced by adjacent eyelid tissue, rather then skin grafts. In rare indications the ideal implant is a cigar-shaped, 1.2 cc silicone expander with an expansible anterior and rigid back wall to

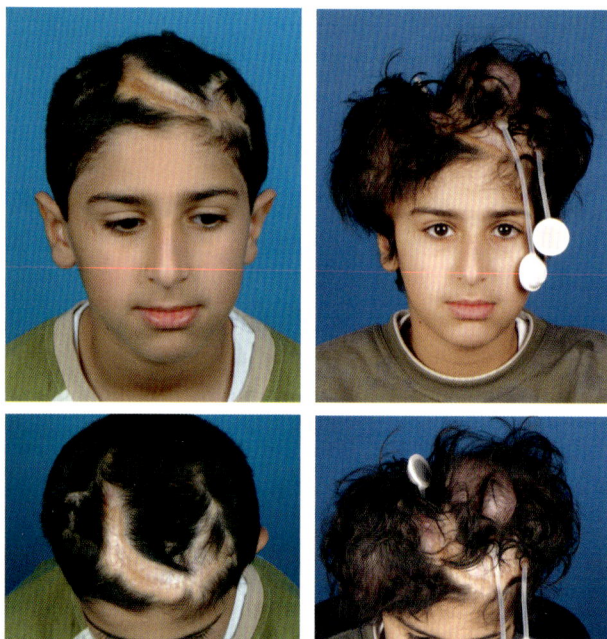

Fig. 2. 11-year old boy with type II Alopecia, multiple segments

Fig. 3. Implantation of 3 tissue expanders with external ports

prevent expansion and pressure on the globe. An oblique skin incision is made in the crow's feet lateral to the canthal region. The implant is placed in a subcutaneous pocket that extends from the medial to lateral canthus. The reservoir dome is placed in a remote pocket over the temporal region. After sufficient expansion the expanded skin will cover the lower lid defect.

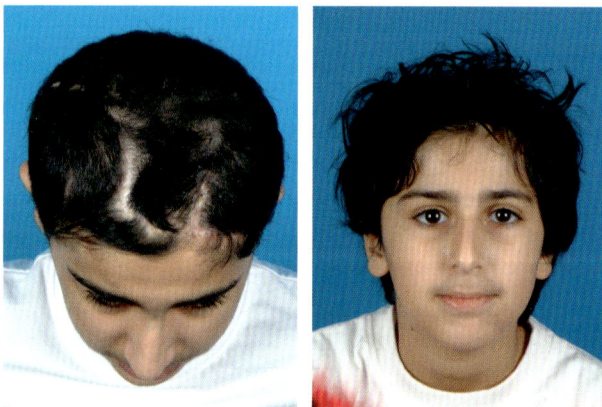

Fig. 4. Final result, 2 years post OP with short and long hair after burn scar excision and reconstruction with pre-expanded scalp flaps

Nose reconstruction

The total or partial reconstruction of the nose may require pre-expanded paramedian forehead flaps including the formation of the vestibular lining and columella. A careful staged plan with flap pre-lamination and pre-fabrication with previous placement of the cartilage framework prior reconstruction are the key to successful nose reconstruction with pre-expanded forehead flaps. A rectangular expander of 100 to 250 cc volume is placed through an incision behind the hairline in the subgaleal plane. The expansion of the forehead skin causes a desired thinning of the tissue to facilitate contouring to reconstruct the ala region.

Facial reconstruction

The implantation of expanders into the head and neck region to use randomized loco-regional flaps is an elegant procedure. Still, loco-regional flaps may have their limitations in facial reconstruction depending on the defect size. The pre-expanded ultrathin Supraclavicular Island flap is a useful option in facial resurfacing of hemifacial defects.

Generally to achieve satisfactory functional and aesthetic results, the texture, color and thickness of the flap need to be similar to those of the head and neck region. The primary indication for facial reconstruction after burns is scar reduction or improvement [8, 9, 47]. Preferable donor-sites in facial reconstruction are the supraclavicular area or the retroauricular area. As the retroauricular area is too small for large defects the cervicohumeral shoulder region is well suited [9, 47–49]. Controlled tissue expansion with expanders prior transfer to modify the donor-site and to increase the size of sensate thin pliable skin with good texture match create flaps to cover the whole aesthetic unit after complete scar resection [9, 35].

SIF flap

A random pattern flap of the supraclavicular region first described by Mutter in 1842 was modified after closer anatomic examination of the arterial blood supply of the shoulder region by Lamberty. The supraclavicular axial patterned flap was based on the supraclavicular artery arising from the superficial

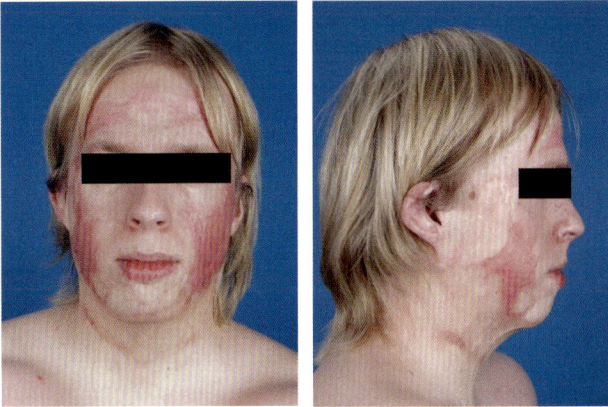

Fig. 5. Severe facial scarring following housefire

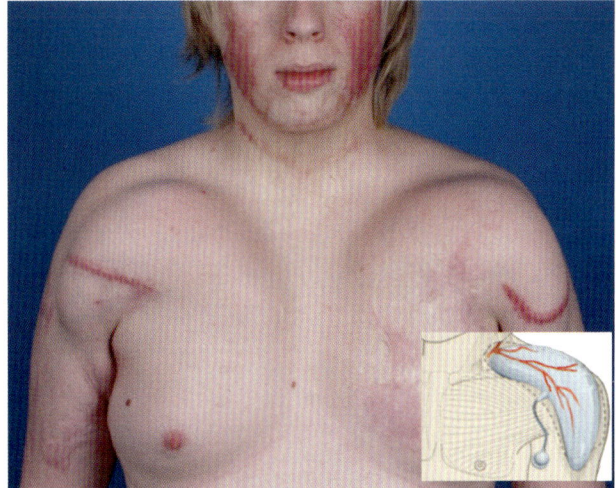

Fig. 6. Bilateral inflated crescent expanders in the angiosome of the Supraclavicular Island Flap

transverse cervical artery, beneath or lateral to the posterior part of the omohyoid muscle. The Supraclavicular Island Flap, after having identified the venous drainage of the angiosome, was first introduced to reconstruct mentosternal contractures, has been further optimized to expand the indications in facial reconstruction [49]. The technique of SIF flap pre-expansion with expanders in the anterior shoulder region increased the size of ultra-thin pliable skin with good texture match to cover the whole aesthetic unit of the face [9, 32].

Adequate planning and flap design needs to respect the aesthetic units of the facial area. In *hemifacial reconstruction* the entire scar area needs to be excised ranging from the nasolabial fold to the preauricular region, and from the inferior orbital rim and the temporal region to the mandibular rim. The defect sizes range between 12 × 16 up to 15 × 19 cm after complete excision with respect to the aesthetic unit [32].

The expander, previously inserted into the supraclavicular artery angiosome, will be carefully removed. After complete flap dissection the SIF flap is mobile on its vascular pedicle, allowing up to 180-degree angle of rotation on the vascular axis as required. To create an ultra-thin flap the expander capsule is partially removed taking care not to damage the flap vasculature. In facial reconstruction a lesser degree of flap rotation is required to reach the facial defect. The donor side defect of the anterior shoulder region will be closed directly in a double layer fashion after extensive undermining and preparation of two advancement flaps. A secondary procedure 3 weeks later to divide the pedicle will utilize the spare skin to perform small local flaps of the mental and cervical region.

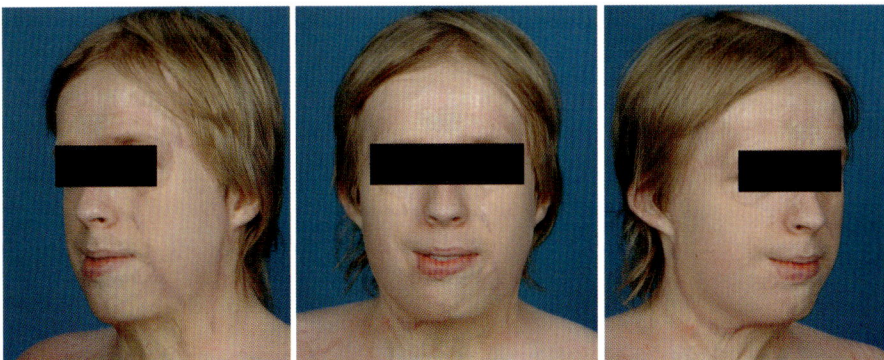

Fig. 7. Final outcome of facial reconstruction 6 years after bilateral pre-expanded Supraclavicular Island Flaps

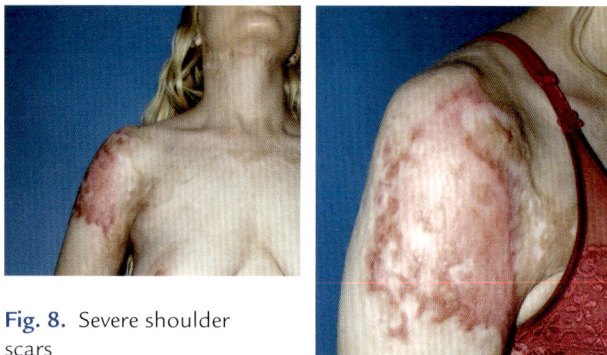

Fig. 8. Severe shoulder scars

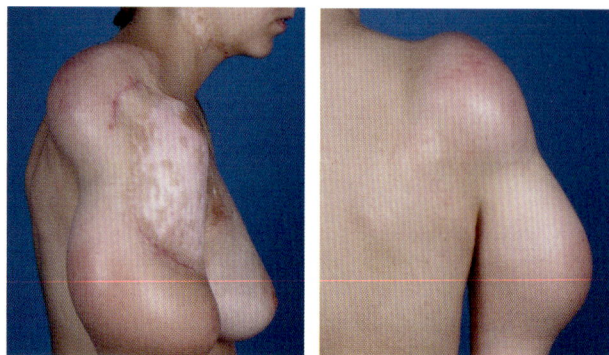

Fig. 9. Two implanted and inflated crescent expanders in the shoulder and uppert arm region (400cc)

Case sample: A 18 year patient recovering from 25 % TBSA full thickness flame injury in a house presented with heavy facial scarring following primary burn reconstruction with eschar excision and multiple skin grafting procedures (Fig. 5). A multistaged plan with bilateral pre-expanded SIF-reconstructions was scheduled. Consecutive bilateral expansion with 2 crescent type tissue expanders (Mentor Corporation, Irving, Texas, USA) of 700 cc each placed in the ventral shoulder regions has been carried out for 10 weeks (Fig. 6). The flap procedures were carried out 11 weeks after expander inflation with pre-expanded SIF-flaps on both sides. After bilateral pedicle division a pleasant color and texture match has been achieved. The final outcome 6 years after reconstruction is shown (Fig. 7).

Reconstruction of the trunk and extremities

All previously mentioned random pattern lipo- and fasciocutaneous flaps or musculocutaneous flaps

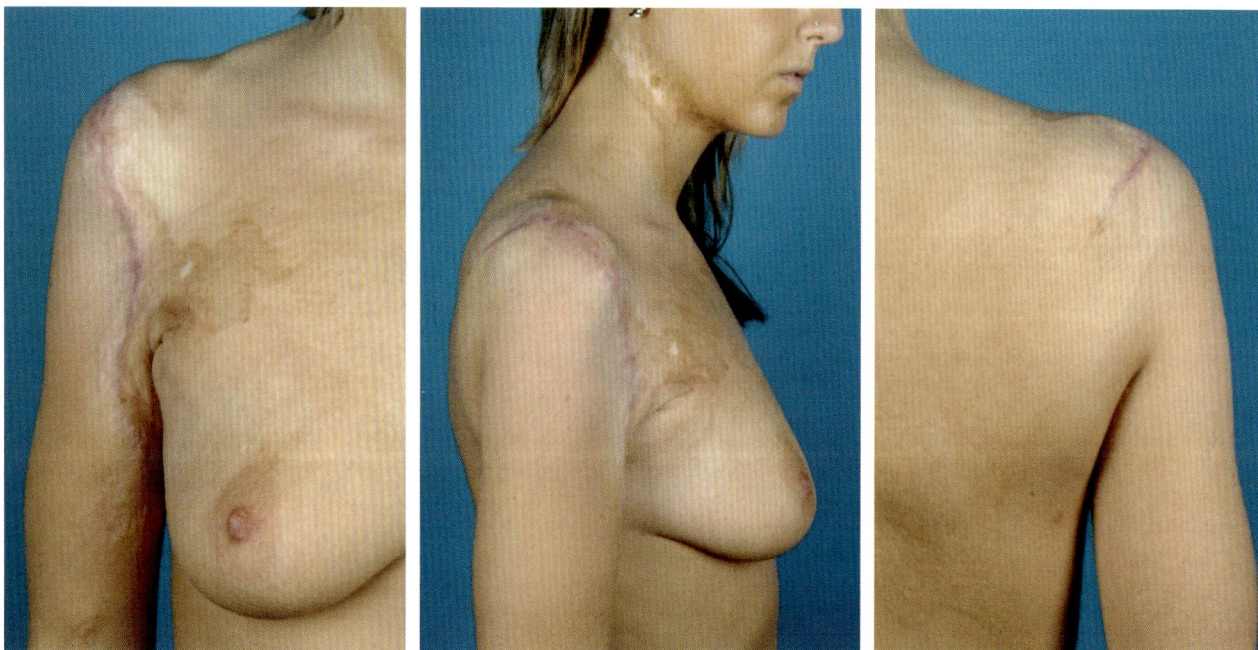

Fig. 10. Final outcome with pre-expanded locoregional flaps

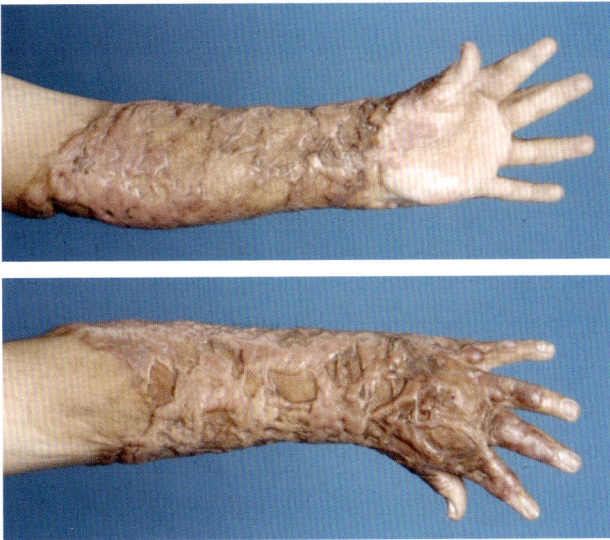

Fig. 11. Severe scarring of the left lower arm region

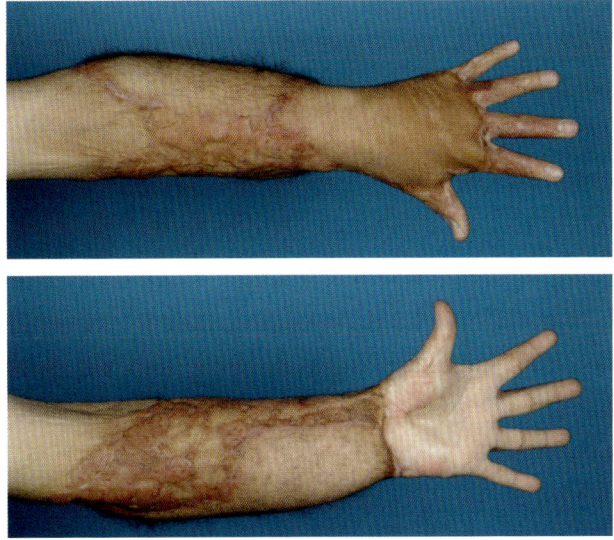

Fig. 13. Final outcome with pre-expanded parascapular flap

are useful in tissue expansion and reconstruction of the trunk and extremitites [8, 34, 47, 50, 51].

Case sample: Severe shoulder scars have been resurfaced following local skin expansion with two 400cc crescent type expanders. The final outcome illustrates acceptable scar reduction at the two year follow-up (Figs. 8–10).

Musculocutaneous flaps require expander placement below the dorsal muscle surface, whereas fasciocutaneous flaps should be placed direct underneath the deep fascia. The angiosomes of the body and their clinical use have been studied in detail. Most recent developments have increased the interest in perforator based expansion of angiosomes to create pre-expanded perforator flaps as needed. Vascularity and surface area resulting from tissue expansion allow the harvest of more healthy tissue beyond the anatomical angiosomes of local or regional flaps. The observed enhancements of perfusion rates in these flaps are attributed to a "delay phenomenon" in the distal parts of the flap. The meticulous preservation of the axial or segmental

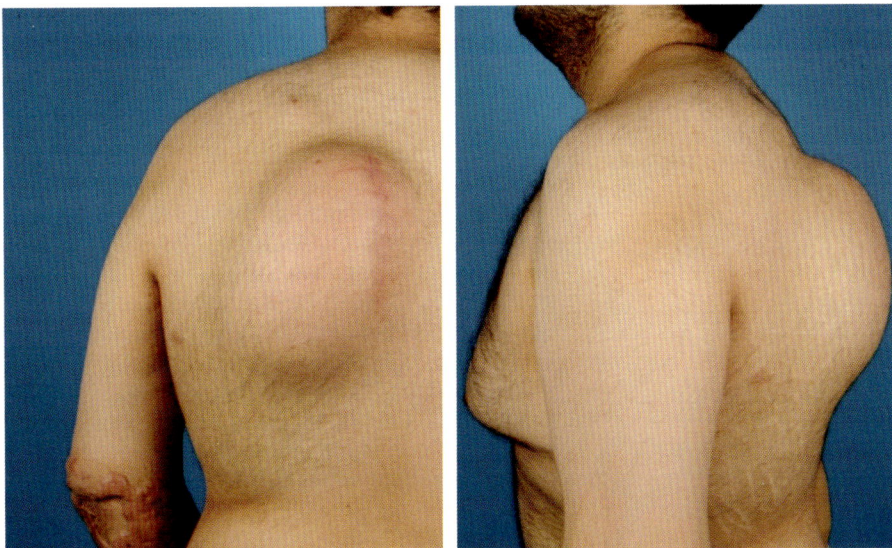

Fig. 12. Implanted rectangular expander for a microsurgical free pre-expanded parascapular flap

flap vasculature during expander implantation is critical [8].

Case sample: A pre-expanded parascapular flap has been worked out for a 25-year old patient with severe hypertrophic scarring of the left lower arm region following burns (Fig. 11). Ten weeks after implantation of a 700 cc rectangular expander of the left donor region a microsurgical free pre-expanded parascapular flap has been performed. The final outcome demonstrates sufficient defect coverage after scar excision (Fig. 12).

Summary

Tissue expanders are very versatile tools in reconstructive burn surgery. Still, careful patient selection, correct indications and realistic treatment concepts, large experience and well-selected surgical techniques, precise instruction of the medical staff as well as detailed and continuous education of the patients are essential. However, although afflicted with a broad range of possible complications, tissue expansion procedures remain a valuable and reliable technique for the reconstruction of burn patients suffering from extensive scarring.

References

[1] McCauley RL (2007) Correction of burn alopecia. In: Herndon DN (ed) Total burn care, 3rd edn. London, Saunders, pp 690–694

[2] Argenta LC (1984) Controlled tissue expansion in reconstructive surgery. Controlled tissue expansion in reconstructive surgery. Br J Plast Surg 37:520–529

[3] Hudson DA, Grob M (2005) Optimising results with tissue expansion: 10 simple rules for successful tissue expander insertion. Burns 31(1): 1–4

[4] Codivilla A (1905) On the means of lengthening, in the lower limbs, the muscles and tissues which are shortened through deformity. Am J Orthop Surg 2: 353–369

[5] Neumann CG (1957) The expansion of skin by progressive distension of a subcutaneous balloon. Plast Reconstr Surg 19: 124–130

[6] Austad ED (1988) Evolution of the concept of tissue excpansion. Facial Plast Surg 5: 277–279

[7] Radovan C (1984) Tissue expansion in soft-tissue reconstruction. Plast Reconstr Surg 74: 482–492

[8] Pallua N, O'Dey D (2006) II-7.1 Gewebeexpansion-Grundprinzipien und Funktion. In: Krupp S, Renne-

kampff S, Pallua N (Hrsg) Plastische Chirurgie. Ecomed, Landsberg, pp 1–14

[9] Pallua N, von Heimburg D (2005) Pre-expanded ultrathin supraclavicular flaps for (full-) face reconstruction with reduced donor-site morbidity and without the need for microsurgery. Plast Reconstr Surg 115(7): 1837–1844 [discussion 1837–1845]

[10] Acartürk TO, Glaser DP, Newton ED (2004) Reconstruction of difficult wounds with tissue-expanded free flaps. Ann Plast Surg 52: 493–499

[11] Teot L, Cherenfant E, Otman S, Giovannini UM (2000) Prefabricated vascularised supraclavicular flaps for face resurfacing after postburn scarring. Lancet 355: 1695–1696

[12] Hallock GG (1995) Preexpansion of free flap donor sites used in reconstruction after burn injury. J Burn Care Rehabil 16: 646–653

[13] Ninkovic M, Moser-Rumer A, Ninkovic, M, Ninkovic M, Spanio S, Rainer C et al (2004) Anterior neck reconstruction with pre-expanded free groin and scapular flaps. Plast Reconstr Surg 113: 61–68

[14] Abramson DL, Pribaz JJ, Orgill DP (1996) The use of free tissue transfer in burn reconstruction. J Burn Care Rehabil 17: 402–408

[15] Pribaz JJ, Fine N, Orgill DP (1999) Flap prefabrication in the head and neck: A 10 year-experience. Plast Reconstr Surg 103: 808–8020

[16] De Filippo RE, Atala A (2002) Stretch and growth. The molecular and physiologic influences of tissue expansion. Plast Reconstr Surg 109: 2450–2462

[17] Van Rappard JH, Sonnevald GJ, Borghouts JM (1988) Histologic changes in soft tissues due to tissue expansion (in animal studies and humans). Facial Plast Surg 5: 280–286

[18] Leighton WD, Russel RC, Marcus DE, Eriksson E, Suchy H, Zook EG (1988) Experimental pre-transfer expansion of free-flap donor sides: I. Flap viability and expansion characteristics. Plast Reconstr Surg 82: 69–75

[19] Leighton WD, Russel RC, Feller AM, Eriksson E, Mathur A, Zook EG (1988) Experimental pretransfer expansion of free flap donor sides: II Physiology, histology, and clinical correlation. Plast Reconstr Surg 82: 76–87

[20] Cherry GW, Austad E, Pasyk K, McClatchey K, Rohrich RJ (1983) Increased survivial and vascularity of random pattern skin flaps elevated in controlled, expanded skin. Plast Reconstr Surg 72: 680–687

[21] Pasyk KA, Argenta LC, Hassett C (1988) Quantitative analysis of the thickness of human skin and subcutaneous tissue following controlled expansion with a silicone implant. Plast Reconstr Surg 81: 516–523

[22] Lantieri LA, Martin-Garcia N, Wechsler J et al (1998) Vascular endothelial growth factor expression in expanded tissue: a possible mechanism of angiogenesis in tissue expansion. Plast Reconstr Surg 101: 392–398

[23] Takei T, Mills I, Katsuyuki A et al (1998) Molecular basis for tissue expansion: clinical implementation for the surgeon. Plast Reconstr Surg 102: 247–258

[24] Prasad JK, Bowden ML, Thomson PD (1991) A review of the reconstructive surgery needs of 3167 survivors of burn injury. Burns 17: 302–305

[25] Huang TT, Larson DL, Lewis SR (1977) Burn alopecia. Plast Reconstr Surg 60: 763–767

[26] Neligan PC, Peters WJ (1989) Advances in burn scar reconstruction: the use of tissue expansion. Ann Plast Surg 22(3): 203–210

[27] Cohen M, Marschall MA, Schafer ME (1988) Tissue expansion for the reconstruction of burn defects. J Trauma 28(2): 158–163

[28] Youm T, Margiotta M, Kasabian A, Karp N (1999) Complications of tissue expansion in a public hospital. Ann Plast Surg 42(4): 396–401 [discussion 392–401]

[29] Ronert MA, Hofheinz H, Manassa E, Asgarouladhi H, Olbrisch RR (2004) The beginning of a new area in tissue expansion: self-filling osmotic tissue expander: four year clinical experiemce. Plast Reconstr Surg 14: 1025–1031

[30] Hudson DA (2003) Maximising the use of tissue expanded flaps. Br J Plast Surg 56: 784–790

[31] Aachauer BM (1991) Burn reconstruction. Thieme, New York

[32] Pallua N, Demir E (2008) Postburn head and neck reconstruction in children with the fasciocutaneous supraclavicular artery island flap. Ann Plast Surg 60: 276–282

[33] Shenaq SM (1987) Pretransfer expansion of a sensate lateral arm free flap. Ann Plast Surg 19: 558–562

[34] Santanelli F, Grippaudo FR, Ziccardi P, Onesti MG (1997) The role of pre-expanded free flaps in revision of burn scarring. Burns 23: 620–625

[35] Furukawa H, Yamamoto Y, Kimura C, Igawa HH, Sugihara T (1998) Clinical application of expanded free flaps based on primary or secondary vascularization. Plast Reconstr Surg 102: 1532–1536

[36] Tsai FC (2003) A new method: perforator based tissue expansion for a preexpanded free cutaneous perforator flap. Burns 29: 845–848

[37] Tsai FC, Mardini S, Chen DJ, Yang JY, Hsieh MS (2006) The classification and treatment algorithm for postburn cervical contractures reconstructed with free flaps. Burns 32: 626–633

[38] Casanova D, Bali D, Bardot J, Legre R, Magalon G (2001) Tissue expansion of the lower limb: complications in a cohort of 103 cases. Br J Plast Surg 54(4): 310–316

[39] Cunha MS, Nakamoto HA, Herson MR, Faes JC, Gemperli R, Ferreira MC (2002) Tissue expander complications in plastic surgery: a 10-year experience. Rev Hosp Clin Fac Med Sao Paulo 57(3): 93–97

[40] Friedman RMIAJ, Rohrich RJ, Byrd HS, Hodges PL, Burns AJ, Hobar PC (1996) Risk factors for complications in pediatric tissue expansion. Plast Reconstr Surg 98(7): 1242–1246

[41] Gibstein LA, Abramson DL, Bartlett RA, Orgill DP, Upton J, Mulliken JB (1997) Tissue expansion in children: a retrospective study of complications. Ann Plast Surg 38(4): 358–364

[42] Governa M, Bonolani A, Beghini D, Barisoni D (1996) Skin expansion in burn sequelae: results and complications. Acta Chir Plast 38(4): 147–153

[43] Pisarski GP, Mertens D, Warden GD, Neale HW (1998) Tissue expander complications in the pediatric burn patient. Plast Reconstr Surg 102(4): 1008–1012

[44] Bozkurt A, Groger A, O'Dey D, Vogeler F, Piatkowski A, Fuchs PCh, Pallua N (2008) Retrospective analysis of tissue expansion in reconstructive burn surgery: evaluation of complication rates. Burns 34: 1113–1118

[45] Brou JA, Vu T, McCauley RL, Herndon DN, Desai MH, Rutan RL et al (1990) The scalp as a donor site: revisited. J Trauma 30: 579–581

[46] Barret JP, Dziewulski P, Wolf SE, Desai MH, Herndon DN (1999) Outcome of scalp donor sites in 450 consecutive pediatric burn patients. Plast Reconstr Surg 103: 1139–1142

[47] Achauer BM, VanderKam VM (2000) Burn reconstruction. In: Achauer BM, Eriksson E (eds) Plastic surgery indications operations outcomes. Mosby, St. Louis, MO, pp 425–446

[48] Aranmolate S, Atah AA (1989) Bilobed flap in the release of postburn mentosternal contracture. Plast Reconstr Surg 83: 356–361

[49] Pallua N, Machens HG, Rennekampff O, Becker M, Berger A (1997) The fasciocutaneous supraclavicular artery island flap for releasing postburn mentosternal contractures. Plast Reconstr Surg 99(7):1878–1884 [discussion 1876–1885]

[50] Manders EK, Oaks TE, Au VK, Wong RK, Furrey JA, Davis TS et al (1988) Soft-tissue expansion in the lower extremities. Plast Reconstr Surg 81(2):208–219

[51] Vogelin E, de Roche R, Luscher NJ (1995) Is soft tissue expansion in lower limb reconstruction a legitimate option? Br J Plast Surg 48(8): 579–582

Correspondence: Norbert Pallua, M. D., Ph. D., FEBOPRAS, Department of Plastic Surgery and Hand Surgery, Burn Center, University Hospital RWTH Aachen, Pauwelsstraße 30, 52074 Aachen, Germany, Tel. +49 241 80 89700, Fax +49 241 80 82 448, E-mail: npallua@ukaachen.de

Burn reconstruction:
Skin substitutes and tissue engineering

Raymund E. Horch, Volker J. Schmidt

Department of Plastic and Hand Surgery, University of Erlangen-Nürnberg Medical Center, Erlangen, Germany

Introduction

Skin, also known as the integument, is not only the largest laminar organ, but also the appropriate interface between the human organism and its environment. Beside other functions the skin represents the primary barrier of the immune system. Thus, an extensive skin loss due to thermal trauma represents in the majority of cases a life-threatening situation and demands particular requirements from the Plastic and Burn surgery to provide a sufficient skin substitution. Development and improvement of innovative strategies concerning skin expansion and Tissue Engineering have contributed to the fact that burns affecting more than 80 % of the body surface (TBS) are survivable today [110]. Although the application of cultured epidermis and compound cultured skin analogues is approved as a life-saving method today, the indications for this novel approach have become more differentiated. Beside historical aspects the present chapter gives insights into both the conventional techniques and the application forms of current cultured skin substitutes.

History of skin transplantation

Skin replacement by means of transplantation is one of the earliest approaches in the history of reconstructive surgery. Following Baronios early sheep skin experiments (1804) it was Bünger who reported for the first time about the transplantation of a full-thickness human skin graft [1]. In 1869 Reverdin has set the gold standard for skin replacement with his landmark publication about the transplantation of the patients own skin [2]. Nevertheless, Reverdin noticed a frequent loss of the small transplanted islands related to a strong wound secretion. During the following decades the full thickness skin graft practice according to Krause has become the most established technique. Meanwhile, insufficient integration into the healing wound and too little skin resources of the patients own body have driven investigators to find other approaches. In 1895 it was the German surgeon Mangoldt who described the clinical application scraped endothelial cells, which are considered to be the precursors of the recent kerationcyte-suspensions [6]. The so called "epithelial cell seeding" were epithelial cells or cell clusters harvested by scraping off superficial epithelium from a patients forearm with a surgical blade, that were grafted together with the exudated serum to various wounds. Based on this technique an additional approach was established later on whereby mechanical hackled skin particles were plunged into the granulation tissue [3]. Up to the present day this modified technique is still useful for the therapy of chronic or problematic wounds and for the treatment of perianal burns [109].

Large-scale skin transplantation was first mentioned by Ollier [4] and subsequently improved by

Thiersch. In this context he also designed the so called Thiersch knife, that allows to gain split-thickness skin grafts in a reliable manner via a tangential excision. Although the Thiersch knife enabled the release of large skin surfaces, it was still a challenge to provide an equal thickness for the entire skin graft, even for experienced surgeons. Especially at the edge regions, grafts exhibited often less homogenous and less aesthetic appearance. Encouraged by this disadvantage the search for new technologies led 1939 to the development of the dermatome according to Padgett-Hood [7]. The dermatome is nowadays usually driven by an electrical motor that represents down to present day the standard tool to gain skin grafts with the possibility to select the depth of the tissue to be excised.

Indication of skin grafting

In case of deep second-degree and third-degree burns a solitary conservative management fails to achieve an adequate functional and aesthetic result. Thus, surgical interventions are required whereby the early eschar debridement followed by a split-skin grafting (see below) is considered to be the gold standard [8, 9]. The choice of a respective skin substitute is also based upon the surgical procedure according to the depth of the eschar excision. For that reason a brief introduction in wound preparation before transplantation is outlined in the following (Fig.1).

Necrotomy

Since necrotic tissue after deep second-degree and third-degree burns represents a principal nidus for bacterial infection and a source for toxic cytokines, excision of necrotic areas improves the general patient state rapidly [10] and exposes a viable bed for skin grafting.

Until recently the most prevalent opinion concerning the ideal point of time for a nectotomy, was to do the procedure at the second to third day of therapy associated with a decline of interstitial oedema and a more stable patient state. However, today there is broad consensus that the eschar or necrosis debridement should start as soon as possible after stabilisation and that all the necrotic tissue should be excised during the following days in order to minimize vital threats due to toxins or bacterial infection [11]. Early tangential or epifascial excision of the burn eschar [12] is followed by a transplantation of either a split-thickness or a full thickness skin graft during the same intervention [8, 13]. This early approach has been shown to reduce inflammation, as well as the risks of infection, wound sepsis, and multiorgan failure [117]. Furthermore

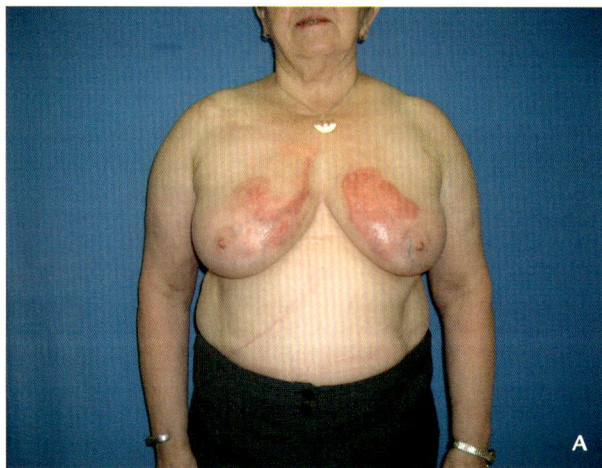

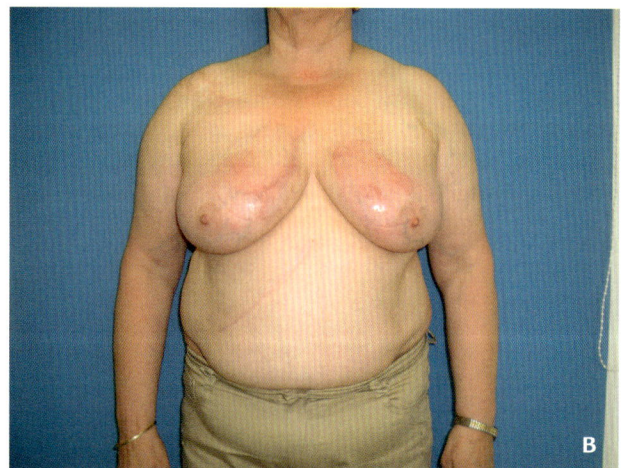

Fig. 1. Superficially burned skin (level IIa) depicted shortly after injury (A) and two months later (B). Up to a burn level of IIa a restitutio ad integrum take place without the need of surgical interventions

the length of hospitalization is reduced among patients who underwent early excision.

Methods of skin grafting

As a current standard wound surfaces are covered by means of full thickness or expanded respectively non-expanded split skin autografts after necrotomy [8, 13]. Although tangential excision induces usually a well bleeding wound basis due to opening of the capillary bed, it is especially this environment that maintains a rapid and secure nutritive junction between the graft and the subsurface [14, 15]. Responsible for a solid adhesion of the transplant is the formation of a strong interplanar fibrin bridge which is fixed between the elastin parts of the skin graft and the wound ground elastin [16]. This modest linkage allows the sprouting of capillaries and bridges the time until more differentiated adhesion structures arise.

Split and full thickness skin grafts

Skin grafts are distinguishable according to their dermal proportion into split thickness or split skin grafts and into full-thickness skin grafts. The latter occurs when the skin is excised under preservation of the complete dermis [17] (Fig. 2).

The typical split skin graft has a thickness between 0.20 and 0.45 mm. The sectional plane is located in a manner that not only the avasculare tissue but also parts of the microcirluation are cut and thus transferred to the lesion. The dermal appendage which is located in deeper cutaneous layers remains at the excision site after transplantation and serves as a source for the reepithelisation of the extraction site. An impressive reepithelisation occurs when the skull is used as a donor, because the high density of hair follicles accelerates the regeneration thus leading to an early restitutio ad integrum. Due to this shortened period of recovery the skull represents an area, which can be used immediately up to six times as a donor [18]. However, full thickness skin explanation sites are lacking for recovering dermal structures. Wound healing initiated from migrating keratinocytes of the surrounding intact tissue is only of limited extend whereby it is obligatory to close the extraction defect primarily.

Standard methods

Autologous full thickness skin grafts

The autologous full thickness skin graft is still considered to be the gold standard and is most commonly used for areas, which do not bleed extensively after excision and provide an opportunity for compression [19]. As the strong dermal component prevents an excessive scare formation the full thickness graft represents the best choice for aesthetic and

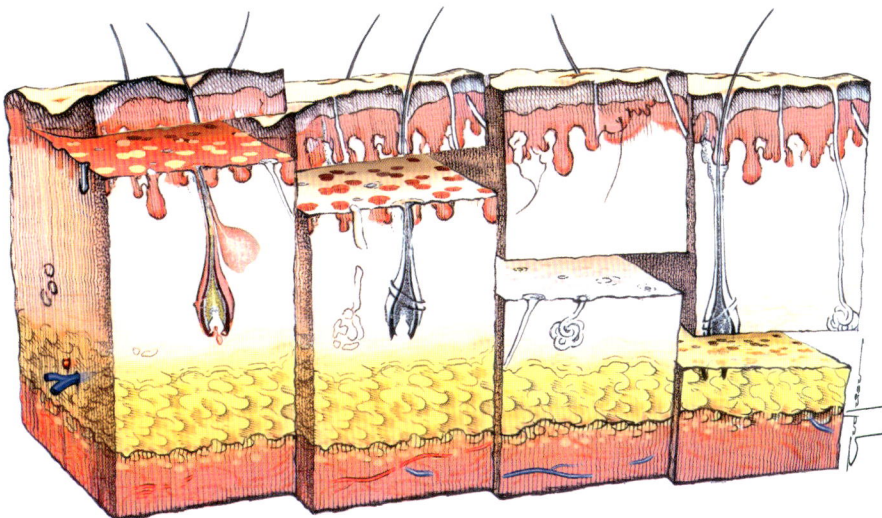

Fig. 2. Different skin grafts depicted according their thickness during excision. Graft thickness increases from thin split skin (0,2 mm, left-hand) to the full thickness skin grafts, which contain all skin layers (right-hand)

functional demands, especially for grafting of burned areas that involve the face, the hands or regions of large joints. Due to the limited amount solitary full thickness skin grafting is only suitable for burns which affect a minor percentage of the body surface.

Autologous meshed-split thickness skin grafts

Reduction in the size of the skin-graft donor site can be realized by turning the split thickness skin graft into a "mesh graft". Due to a specific parallel arrangement of scissors on a role multiple small slits can be placed in the graft, allowing it to expand up to six times of the original area. The method is based on the tendency of keratinocytes to migrate into the intermediate spaces. In addition these so called "mesh slits" provide a drain for wound secretions, thus preventing the appearance of hematoma respectively seroma. Mesh grafts are of special importance if the burn is so extensive that the surface of donor sites is limited. The most common expansion ratios are 1:1,5 to 1:3 [14, 15, 20] (Fig. 3).

Meek technique

In 1958 Meek invented a dermatome which was able to cut harvested split skin into small squares of equal size [21]. Meanwhile the mesh technique was founded which was mostly preferred to Meeks invention because of its simpler handling. Beside rare published Chinese reports it was Kreis and his colleagues who modified the Meek technique to a simple method that allows to cut of split skin as well as to expand it up to a ratio of 1:6 on a special cork and silk carrier in one step [22]. Due to its practicability and attractive magnification factor this modified approach is currently well established in many burn centres and in case of extensive burns often favoured towards mesh grafts (Fig. 4).

Stamp technique

The stamp technique has a higher prevalence in asia and is based on split skin cut into large squares. Afterwards the quadratic skin pieces are positioned in an appropriate manner over the débrided area. Via a variation of the square size respectively the distance between the islands it is also possible to

achieve an expansion ratio up to 1:6 [23, 24]. The stamp technique was no longer of practical importance in Europe after the microskin technique combined with allogenic or xenogenic skin as a carrier was implemented.

Alternative methods

The surgical procedures discussed above are dependent upon the availability of intact donor skin. If the burn is so extensive (> 70 % of TBS) that there are minimal viable areas of donor skin, alternative methods should be used to enable a chance of survival. Insights into research and experiences with these alternative methods are discussed in the following.

Temporary allogenic and xenogenic skin grafts

Allogenic skin grafts

When there is a lack of sufficient donor skin allogenic skin transplants can be used as a temporary skin graft. Usually this skin is submitted to a rejection process. Due to the burn injury of the mainly immunocompetent organ skin the rejection starting from the recipient occurs usually with a delay of 1 to 2 weeks after application.

First experiences were collected with cryo-conserved skin, which was used to cover deep second degree burns [25] or areas, where autologous grafts had not been grown in [26]. An advantage of the cryo-conservation is a partially loss of the antigenicity [27].

Burns treated with cryo-conserved allogenic skin become germ-free and exhibit an epithelial migration tendency starting from the wound edge [28]. Hence it is a useful tool to bridge the time to the autologous transplantation. Cryo-conserved allogenic grafts were also used for the so called sandwich-technique (see below), where largely meshed autologous transplants were covered with less expansive meshed allogenic skin. Although this approach did not represent a durable solution it was able to prolong the period of the rejection occurrence up to three weeks [26]. To minimize the allogenic skin

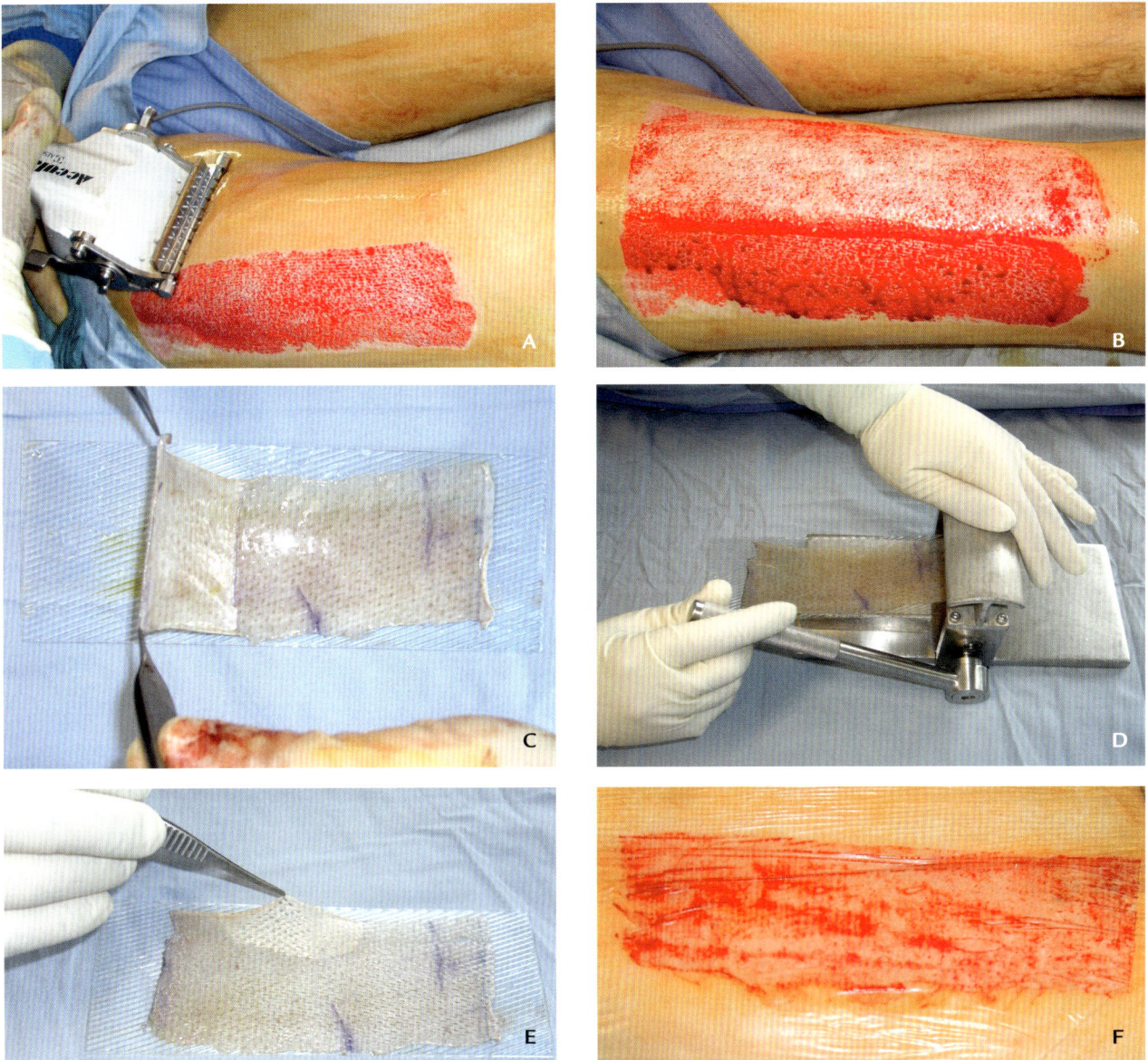

Fig. 3.
A) Excision of "thin" split skin (0,2 mm) using a battery driven dermatome.
B) Punctual bleedings of the superficial dermis after split skin removal.
C) Transfer of the split skin graft on a synthetic carrier with the dermis on top.
D) Split skin during meshing by means of a special dermatome.
E) Split skin graft after meshing (expansion ratio 1,5: 1) with the visible mesh net grid structure.
F) Foil bandage of the graft removal area guarantees an adequate wound milieu for the reepithelisation.
G) Split skin shortly after transplantation. Through the meshes wound secret can drain, thus preventing a diffusion barrier below the graft

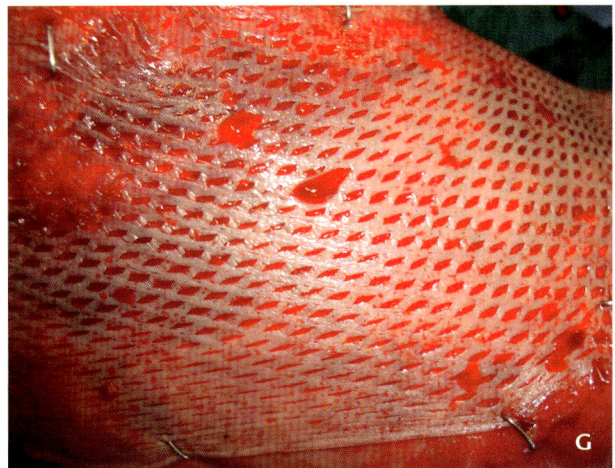

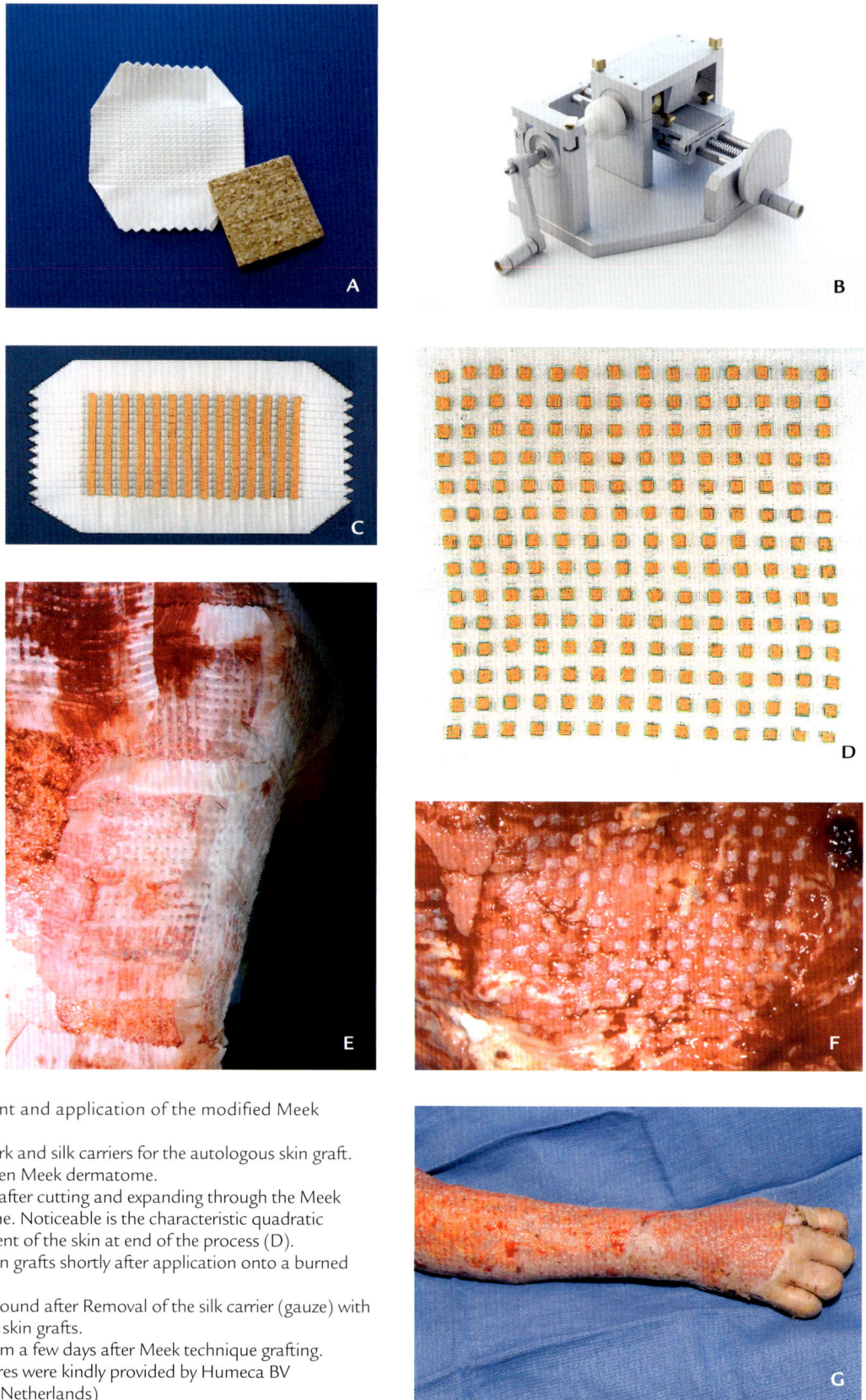

Fig. 4. Equipment and application of the modified Meek technique.
A)   Special cork and silk carriers for the autologous skin graft.
B)   Hand driven Meek dermatome.
C+D) Skin graft after cutting and expanding through the Meek dermatome. Noticeable is the characteristic quadratic arrangement of the skin at end of the process (D).
E)   Square skin grafts shortly after application onto a burned shoulder.
F)   Wound ground after Removal of the silk carrier (gauze) with remaining skin grafts.
G)   Burned Arm a few days after Meek technique grafting.
* Displayed Pictures were kindly provided by Humeca BV (Enschede, The Netherlands)

antigenicity among others a graft-conservation with 98 % glycerine was developed [26], whereby the cellular plasma was replaced by glycerine without affecting the tissue structure. Glycerinised allografts are well suited for the sandwich technique expressed by a high epithelialisation rate [29, 111].

Allogenic grafts mostly serve as a temporary cover when there is insufficient donor skin available. These grafts are usually attached with sutures or staples to the surrounding tissue after slitting at stated intervals with a scalpel to guarantee a draining of the secretions.

Until the rejection occurs allogenic grafts have the same beneficial properties as autologous ones including the ability to reduce inflammation, fluid loss as well as the risk of infection, wound sepsis, and multiorgan failure.

Up to the present day there are just a few cases known whereby selected immunosuppression has achieved a durable integration of the allogenic graft into the wound ground [30, 31]. Usually the antigenic potency of the epidermis is responsible for the rejection. In theory the dermal elements might survive, however selective y-chromosamtic methods for detection cannot prove the appearance of allogenic cells in all cases [30, 31]. Exposure to UV-light and the use of glucocorticoids can induce an inactivation of Langerhans-cells within the graft in order to delay the duration up to the allograft rejection [34]. Due to immunosuppression the interaction between Langerhans-cells and class-II-antigens of graft keratinocytes is diminished [35–38]. In this case cyclosporine is a suitable agent because of its sufficient inhibition of the keratinocyte DNA-synthesis without adverse effects for the vitality of the transplant [30, 39, 40].

Xenogenic skin grafts

Since the mid-1950s the use of pig skin has become famous for temporary grafting of large burns especially in china. There it was used particularly in combination with the so called "intermingled"-technique.

The nutritive maintenance of the xenogenic grafts occurs mainly due to diffusion [41] because an initial revascularisation disappears after a short period and is rapidly replaced by collagen structures [42]. In countries, that do not perform allogenic

grafting because of ethic concerns, xenogenic transplants are still an important tool for temporary wound covering. From South America comparable good results are also reported with frog or snake skin used as transplants.

Mixed skin grafts

The Chinese method: Intermingled-grafting

The intermingled grafting method is based on the migrative properties of epidermal cells. On a large sheet of homo- or heterologous skin islands of autologous skin are inserted into pre-punched holes at certain distances. The expansion ratio is dependent upon the distance and the size of the skin islands. Yang et al. selected a distance of 1 cm between their 0.25 qcm sized autologous islands which correlates with an expansion ratio of 1:4 [43, 44]. Bäumer and his group modified this method by raising the island size up to 1 qcm and by inserting the islands 3.5 cm away from each other, thus enhancing the expansion ratio up to 1:20 [45]. Despite its effectiveness the method is mostly restricted to the Far East primarily because of high personnel and manual requirements.

Autologous-allogenic intermingled grafts

The autologous-allogenic intermingled grafts technique was performed for the first time in the mid/ end 1950s to minimize the loss of blood during the allograft removal [46].

After transplantation the autologous epithelium grows concomitant to the recipient rejection from the placed islands rapidly in-between the allogenic dermis and the allogenic epidermis. This histopathomorphologic behaviour is called "sandwich phenomena" [44]. At the end of the process the desquaming allo-epidermis is replaced completely by the confluating neoepidermis. The allogenic dermis beneath the intact autoepidermis degenerates and is reabsorbed due to the immunogenic response [44, 111].

Autologous-xenogenic intermingled grafts

Intermingled grafts using xenogenic pig skin as a heterogenic donor show a similar outcome compared to autologous-allogenic intermingled grafts. After transplantation the xenogenic graft exhibits a vital character due to the plasma and tissue fluids of the underlying tissue that provide a nutritive environment [41]. Neocapillaries appear 2 to 4 days after transplantation within the heterogenic graft followed by an ingrowth of capillaries from the granulating wound ground on day 7–10 [47, 48]. The internal autologous transplants start to grow immediately leading to an undermining of the xeno-epidermis. The rejection of the pig skin dermis occurs either as an external or internal process [42]. The external rejection is associated with an infiltration of fibroblasts and inflammatory cells that degrade the heterogenic skin. The internal rejection describes the confluent and expansive growth of the autologous epithelium into the xenogenic corium. Rejection of the corium induces furthermore the desquamation of the xenogenic epidermis. During these processes the heterogenic connective tissue is infiltrated by a large number of capillaries, fibroblasts and lymphocytes. Finally the dermal collagen is degraded and partially reabsorbed.

"Sandwich"-technique

The term "Sandwich" describes the application of a wide meshed autologous split skin graft, which is covered either by a sparsely meshed (1:1,5), slit or untreated allogenic transplant. Knowing that the integration into the healing wound of wide meshed autologous skin grafts with expansion ratio up to 1:6 is rather weak because of the adverse relation between the gaps and the cell carrying grid like skin, this method improves the rate of the integration into the healing wound by means of a temporary coverage with allogenic skin. Thus, it is well suited for the treatment of severe burns with limited skin donor sites [10, 33, 49, 50] (Fig. 5).

Microskin grafts

According to microskin grafts thin split is harvested and mechanically reduced to small particles < 1 qmm (microskin grafts), which are placed onto the wound followed by a coverage with a homo- or heterlogous graft [54–57]. For this purpose the skin particles are distributed equally on a fat gauze using a NaCl water bath. The resulting pulp is topically applied to the wound ground. The microskin technique was developed and

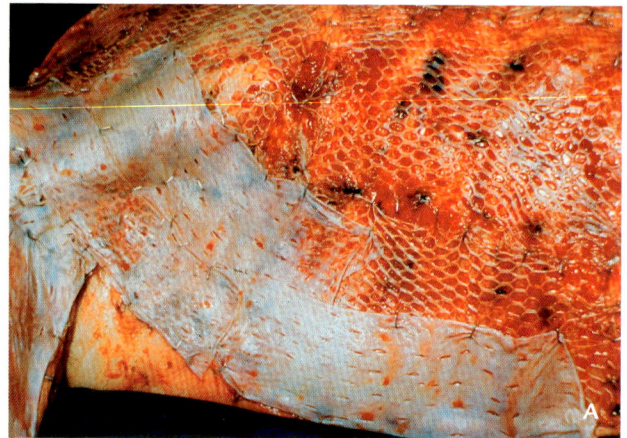

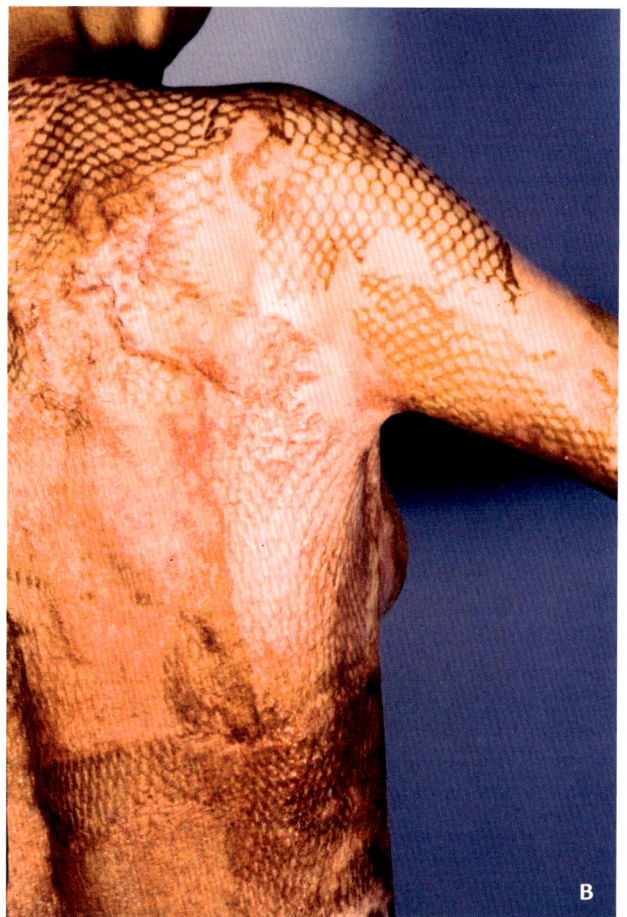

Fig. 5. Over transplantation of conservative external slit skin serves as a biological protector and enables the integration and healing of meshed skin grafts with large expansion ratios (e. g. 6:1 or 9:1).
A) Coverage of 3:1 and 6:1 mesh grafts with slit and glycerine-conserved allogenic skin.
B) Dark pigmented 6:1 and 3:1 expanded autologous split skin areas with the typical grid-like pattern after complete healing and rejection of the allograft

perfected in China, where it is today the first choice for the treatment of large burns in combination with an allogenic coverage instead of the transplantation of cultured keratinocytes. Besides the relatively easy handling the attainable expansion ratio up to 1:100 is one of the major benefits. Thereby, unburned areas are used economically offering satisfying results [55].

Buried chip graft technique

The effectiveness of conventional, meshed split skin is rather low in the critical perianal respectively perineal area because of the complex location und the usually heavily contaminated sore ground [51–53]. Therefore, in these areas the buried chip graft technique is particularly useful.

Within this method split skin taken from an unburned area is mechanically chopped into small pieces (1–2 qmm). Afterwards the particles are inserted obliquely (depth ~ 3–4 mm) and in rows (distance ~ 1 cm) into the wound ground, thus the gluteal skin's surface closes itself after a few weeks above the "seedlings" [3]. Usually a particle-free area is left within a radius of 5–6 cm around the anus. Due to their inoculation the small transplants are well protected against faecal contamination and mechanical cleaning activities. Even in the case of infection, the risk for destruction and a complete loss of the transplants is rather low [52, 110].

5–9 days after insertion first epithelial islands appear at the surface. Starting from their edges the epithelialisation runs concentrically leading to a closed epidermis. Histomorphological noticeable is a characteristic bell-shaped growth from the deep to the wound surface, which exhibits a regular epidermal layering [3].

Hand burns represent another sensitive field for skin grafting because of the particular anatomy. To preserve as much functional structures as possible (e. g. the sliding tissue) a spare and careful necrotomy is of special importance. The additional use of a VAC (vacuum-assisted closure) therapy has proved to be very effective in a lot of cases. Due to the negative pressure not only oedema reduction but also increased perfusion and formation of granulation tissue can be observed. Meanwhile it provides an adequate contact pressure for skin grafts, which is crucial because of the inconstant hand skin surface.

Furthermore the VAC therapy prevents the greatly feared dehydration of the tendon and its sliding tissue (Fig. 6).

Cultured epithelia and tissue engineering

In case of extensive burns the surgical standard methods described above are limited when the unburned skin is reduced to a minimum extent. A potential way out of this dilemma is the development and improvement of cultured skin substitutes as well as the integration of transplantable and resorbable biomaterials into the healing wound by means of tissue engineering. Aim of the former and recent efforts is the in vitro generation of tissues, which exhibit similar biomechanical and biochemical properties compared to the lost tissue and guaranty a permanent functional substitution. The first organ respectively layer of an organ that was ever generated in vitro and successfully transplanted in vivo, was the epidermis. This groundbreaking success paved the way for the treatment of extensive burns with an affected TBS > 80 % during the last 30 years. Today cultured autologous and allogenic skin substitutes are commercial available and used around the world [58–65].

Requirements

Demanded requirements to modern cultured skin grafts:
► Shortening of the culturing period for accelerated availability
► Sufficient quantity to decrease lethality after extensive burns
► Easy handling to reduce the operation time
► Reduction respectively prevention of bacterial infection due to an early restitutio ad integrum of large-scaled wound surfaces
► Economic consumption: Large amounts of transplants should be gained from a few autologous substrates
► Application of biomaterials should improve both the adhesion between cells and the wound ground as well as the functional and aesthetic results
► Time reduction of wound healing in order to decrease the period of therapy

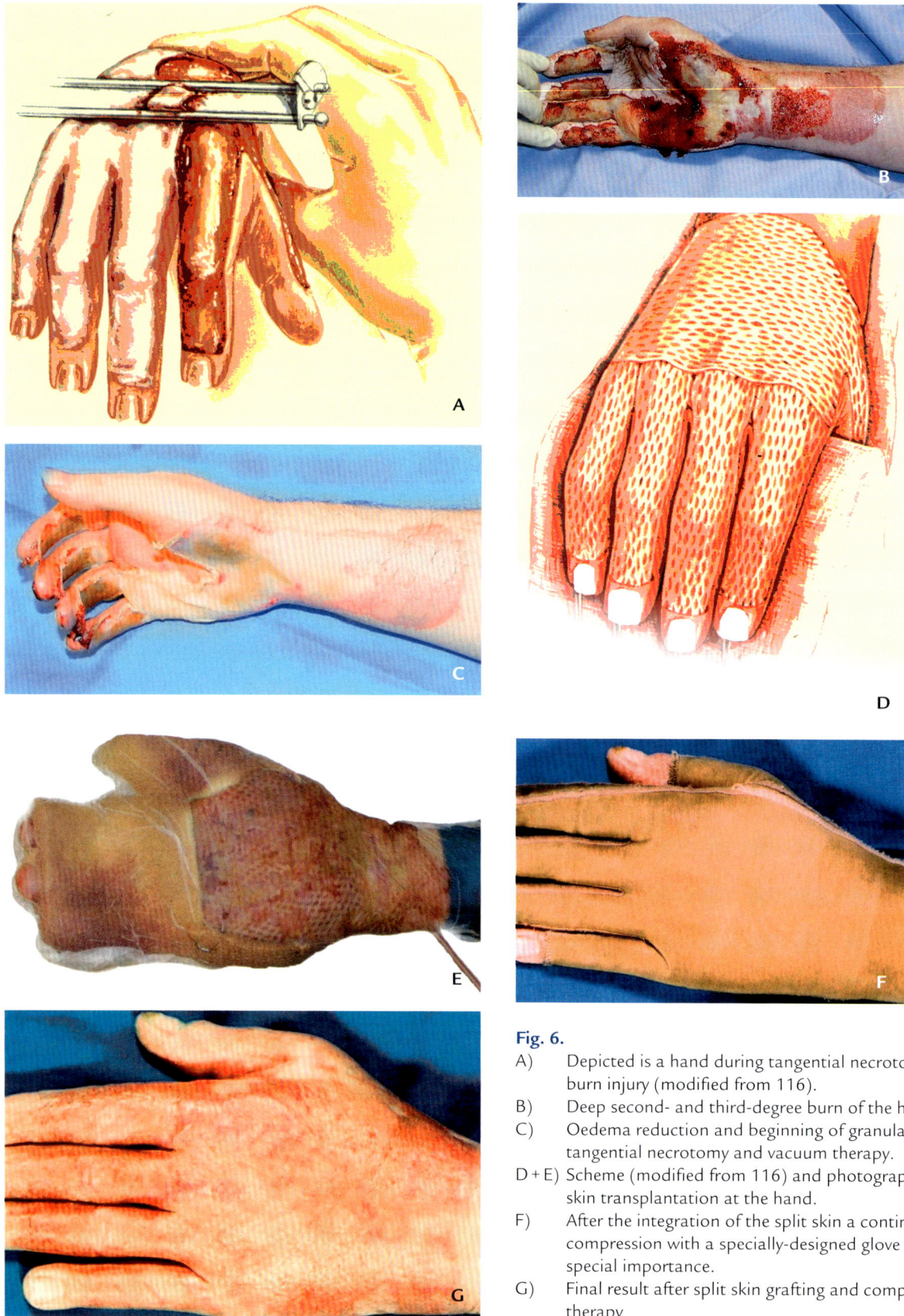

Fig. 6.

A)   Depicted is a hand during tangential necrotomy after burn injury (modified from 116).

B)   Deep second- and third-degree burn of the hand.

C)   Oedema reduction and beginning of granulation after tangential necrotomy and vacuum therapy.

D+E) Scheme (modified from 116) and photography of split skin transplantation at the hand.

F)   After the integration of the split skin a continuous compression with a specially-designed glove is of special importance.

G)   Final result after split skin grafting and compression therapy

Historical review

The beginnings of cell culturing go back to the 19th century. Since that time the culturing of skin has been an object of interest not at least because the therapeutic potential due to the substitution of destructed skin has been identified very soon. It was recognized, that explanted skin embedded into a culture medium exhibited an expansive growth starting from the peripheral edges.

According to the cell biology the cell culture can be distinguished into two forms: The explant and the dissociated culture assay.

Explant cultures

In 1899 Ljunggren kept human skin in a culture for the first time. He harvested small pieces of patient skin, transferred them for a longer time period into a special medium containing ascites and replanted them successfully to the donor [66]. Later on different investigators have observed that skin embedded into a suited medium exhibits a sprouting of epithelial and connective tissue cells [67–69]. The culture mediums used for these early assays were composed of physiological saline with or without glucose that were enriched with serum or ascites. The much later following additives of amino acids and peptides paved the way for the development of standardized mediums, which made it possible to compare results from different work groups [70].

Börnstein (1930) and Pinkus (1932) revealed in their experiments, that the epithelial sprouting is mainly based on the migration of keratinocytes within the explanted skin [71, 72]. A further landmark was the work of Medawar in 1941, who achieved an encymatic separation between dermis and epidermis due to the adding of trypsin. Furthermore, he revealed by means of clinical and microscopical studies, that elastic fibres from the basal membrane play an important role for the anchorage between the epidermis and the underlying tissue. In 1948 Medawar added fractionated explants to a continuously shaken culture and observed an overgrowth of the epidermal parts, which covered the dermal components after a few days [73]. Although the cell proliferation was abundant, this approach was still limited because the growth stopped while the dermis-coverage was finished. Following investigators were able to circumvent this contact inhibition by modifying the breeding medium and adding a particular agent. However, they also failed to suppress the fibroblastic overgrowth, which was the limiting factor for a therapeutic use of explant cultures [74].

In 1949 Lewis et al. figured out by means of cell dynamic studies using a time controlled film technique that keratinocytes own a peripheral lamellae-like membrane, which allow them to migrate [75].

In the 1960s culture techniques were perfected so that it was possible to gain epidermal growth without the limiting connective tissue factor which is associated with fibroblastic activity. It was shown that the sprouting neoepidermis in expant cultures exhibits a similar cell formation compared to the in vivo epidermis [76]. However, one failed to submit them into a subculture. These high density epithelial cell formations were primarily used for the dermatological research [77].

Several early investigators had recognized the therapeutic benefit of cultured skin for the treatment of burns and chronic wounds [69, 78, 79]. In 1948 it was the aforementioned anatomist Medawar, who was able to replant autologous cultured epidermis to the donor [80]. Moscana succeeded 1961 in transplanting a mixed dermal and epidermal cell suspension onto a wound surface [81].

The merit of the first well documented transplantation of keratinocytes is due to efforts of Karasek, who succeeded 1968 in transplanting primarily cultured autologous keratinocytes to rabbits [82]. Beside the evidence for a complete ingrowth of the cells he observed a histomorphological reformation of the cells to a fully functional epidermis. However, the neoepidermis degraded after a period of 6 weeks due to unknown circumstances. Several years later Freeman and his group continued Karasek's approach of generating transplantable epidermis from explant cultures [83]. They were able to increase the mitotic rate of isolated keratinocytes thus achieving a considerable augmentation of the cell mass [84]. In contrast to Freeman's work Rheinwald and Green presented in 1975 another approach to generate large amounts of keratinocytes based on a well-engineered system of subculturing [85, 86]. Their findings were a milestone on the way to therapeutically used keratinocytes cultures.

Dissociated cultures

After Medawar's invention of an encymatic separation between dermis and epidermis using trypsin [87] Billingham and Reynolds revealed in 1952 that trypsinized keratinocytes remain vital and are suitable for cell culturing [88].

In 1960 Cruickshank demonstrated the mitotic activity of cultured epithelial cells, thus enabling in vitro proliferation [91]. A further important step in the history of dissociated cultures was the development of fibroblast-free cultures due to Prunieras [92]. However keratinocytes in his setting exhibited a rapid differentiation with a tendency to poly-stratifications [93], hence a sufficient augmentation via replication was still impossible at this stage. A significant improvement in this context was the additional use of acid-precipitated collagen gel [94]. This setting increased the proliferation-rate of keratinocytes in a remarkable manner, plus enabling confluent growth and sub-culturing. Although the extraction rate has still been too small for a broad clinical use, it indicated the importance of the so called "feeder layer", that contains connective tissue elements, for a large production of keratinocytes. Especially the presence of radiated embryonic 3T3-fibroblasts achieved good results due to their ability to inhibit normal fibroblast growth while non-effecting the keratinocyte growth.

Finally the discovery of EGF (Epidermal Growth Factor) paved the way for the clinical implementation of cultured epidermis. By means of EGF epidermal proliferation could be induced without hormonal influence leading to a rapid and extensive growth of epidermal cell associations [96]. Thereby a transplantation of dissociated culture gained epidermis became possible [60, 97, 98].

Since the crucial studies of Green and others, who brought the therapeutic use of cultured epidermis into clinical praxis, several innovations improved the culturing technique. Among others it has been shown, that low potassium concentrations [99, 100] and the addition of trace elements [101, 102] have a positive impact upon the culture medium. Beneficial effects were also described after treatment with hydrocortisone, transferrin and insulin. Due to these modifications well-matched mediums arose over time, which enabled a proper proliferation of keratinocytes in absence of a feeder layer [103, 104]. These keratinocytes remained undifferentiated, grew in a monolayer-like manner and were suited for subculturing. By transferring these cells into a "normal" culture medium, enriched with fetal calf serum (FCS), differentiation as well as poly layer formation could be induced at a definite time.

Cultured skin substitutes

Although a large number of skin constructs is commercially available today (Table 1), only 3 techniques match to the former mentioned requirements for the treatment of extensive burns. The majority of available skin substitutes are not qualified for the acute therapy of severely burned patient according to their complex and prolonged production. However, these substitutes are rather aiming at the market of chronic wound therapy.

Cultured epidermal autografts – CEA

The transplantation of a cultured epidermal cuticle derived from autologous keratinocytes was the first clinical application of a bioartificial organ component with a lifesaving effect. Since then thousands of severely burned patients were treated and rescued by means of CEA worldwide. Nevertheless, the clinical use of CEAs is still discussed controversially. A major concern is the combination of high costs with uncertain healing rates, which may result in repeated transplantations [105, 106]. The estimated costs for 1 % successfully treated body surface with CEAs were approximately 13 000 US-$. The main reason for the transplant-loss, which occurs usually within the first days after transplantation (critical period) starting from the sensitive dermo-epidermal junction zone, is the liability of CEAs towards wound ground associated germs. Metaanalysis revealed that almost 50 % of the transplanted CEAs do not integrate into the wound ground, thus requiring further operations [107].

Applied cultured epidermal autografts usually contain 3 to 5 cell layers, hence not only the wound transfer but also the wound care within the first days after transplantation is rather difficult.

Until today a serious problem of CEAs is the insufficient adherence to the wound bed often combined

Table 1. Currently commercially available or marketed matrices and products for tissue engineered skin substitutes

Material	Brand Name	Manufacturer
collagen gel + cult. Allog. HuK + allog. HuFi	Apligraf™ (earlier name: Graftskin™)	Organogenesis, Inc., Canton, MA
cult. Autol HuK	Epicell™	Genzyme Biosurgery, Cambridge, MA
PGA/PLA + ECMP DAHF	Transcyte™	Advanced Tissue Sciences, LaJolla, CA
collagen GAG-polymer + silicone foil	Integra™	Integra LifeScience, Plainsborough, NJ
acellular dermis	AlloDerm™	Lifecell Corporation, Branchberg, NJ
acellular xenogenic dermis	Strattice™	KCI-Lifecell Corporation, Branchberg, NJ
HAM + cult. HuK	Laserskin™	Fidia Advanced Biopolymers, Padua, Italy
PGA/PLA + allog. HuFi	Dermagraft™	Advanced Tissue Sciences, LaJolla, CA
collagen + allog. HuFi + allog. HuK	Orcel™	Ortec International, Inc., New York, NY
fibrin sealant + cult. autol. HuK	Bioseed™	BioTissue Technologies, Freiburg, Germany
PEO/PBT + autol. HuFi + cult. autol. HuK	Polyactive™	HC Implants
HAM + HuFi	Hyalograft 3D™	Fidia Advanced Biopolymers, Padua, Italy
silicone + nylon mesh + collagen	Biobrane™	Dow Hickham/Bertek Pharmac., Sugar Land, Tx

ECMP = extracellular matrixproteins, DAHF= derived from allog. HuFi, GAG= glycosaminoglycan, PGA = polyglycolic acid (Dexon™), PLA = polylactic acid (Vicryl™), PEO = polyethylen oxide, PBT = polybutyliterephthalate, cult. = cultured; autol. = autologous, allog. = allogeneic, HuFi = human fibroblasts, HuK = human keratinocytes, HAM = microperforated Hyaluronic Acid Membrane (benzilic esters of hyaluronic acid = HYAFF-11®)

with blistering due to shear stress. An explanation for this phenomenon might be an incomplete formation of anchoring fibrils during culturing as well as an encymatic separation within the culturing bottles before transplantation [108]. In addition the lacking dermal component contributes to the development of bullae especially in case of third-degree burns. To solve this problem much effort was put into the development of dermal substitutes with varying compositions during the last years. Some of these substitutes are already used in the clinical praxis (Table 2).

Until an adequate amount of cultured epidermal autografts is available the temporary coverage with allogenic respectively xenogenic skin (see above) represents a lifesaving and well established opportunity [50, 109–113].

Cell suspensions

As mentioned introductorily in 1985 von Mangold performed a successful transplantation of scraped keratinocytes suspended in autologous wound serum [6]. However, even after the invention of the cell amplification via culturing this technique failed to prevail because of a lacking carrier substance.

Hunyadi et al. have been the first, who used fibrin glue as a suspension for trypsinized, non-cultured keratinocytes. By this means they succeeded in the therapy of chronic wounds [114]. As a member of the coagulation cascade fibrin is of special importance for the wound healing process. Beside its role as a carrier substance for keratinocyte suspensions fibrin is also useful to improve the adherence and healing of split skin grafts [115]. It was also shown, that fibrin glue does not affect the clonogenic properties as well as the growth and proliferation rate of epidermal cells. Especially in case of hardly manageable third-degree burns suspended keratinocytes embedded into fibrin glue exhibit good healing and take rates. In addition simultaneous covering with meshed allogenic skin grafts can be useful to increase the biostability by preventing a washing away effect of the cells after lysis of the fibrin clot. Moreover this "biologic bandage" protects the cells against dehydration. After a brief initial revascularisation the allogenic skin is rejected 12 to 14 days after transplantation.

Table 2. Summary of possible skin substitute techniques utilizing cultured human keratinocytes with regard to the various possible designs that are currently used or experimentally developed

I. AUTOLOGOUS CULTURED HUMAN KERATINOCYTES

1. Autologous epidermal sheet transplants ("sheet grafts" = gold standard)

2. In-vitro cultured and constructed dermo-epidermal autologous transplants:

  2.1. Keratinocytes on a collagen gel + fibroblasts

  2.2. Keratinocyte sheets + Kollagen-Glycosaminoglycane-Membrane + Fibroblasts

  2.3. Keratinocyte sheets on a layer of fibrin-gel

  2.4. Keratinocyte sheets on cell free pig dermis

  2.5. Keratinocyte sheets on cell free human dermis

  2.6. Keratinocytes on bovine or equine collagen matrices

  2.7. Keratinocyte sheets on micro-perforated hyaluronic acid membranes

  2.8. Keratinocyte sheets on collagen + Chondroitin-6-sulfate with silicon membrane coverage (living skin equivalent)

3. Combination of allogenic dermis (in vivo) with epidermal sheets

4. non-confluent keratinocyte suspensions

  as a spray suspended in saline solutions

  as spray or clots suspended in a fibrin matrix

  4.1. exclusively

  4.2. in clinical combination with fresh or preserved allogenic skin

  4.4. as non confluent keratinocyte monolayers on equine or bovine collagen matrices or on top of hyaluronic acid membranes

  4.6. in combination with collagen coated nylon on silicone backing

  4.7. dissociated keratinocytes without cell culture

  4.8. Outer root sheath cells (from plucked hair follicles) cultured or without culture

5. Three dimensional cell cluster cultures (spherocytes)

  5.1. Cultured on microspheres as carrier systems (experimentally on: dextrane, collagen, hyaluronic acid)

  5.2. Cell seeded microspheres + allografts/biomaterials

II. ALLOGENEIC KERATINOCYTES

Allogeneic Keratinocytes

  6.1. Keratinocyte-sheets – (as a temporary wound cover)

  6.2. Allogeneic keratinocyte suspensions (experimentally)

  6.3. Syngenic-allogeneic keratinocytes

In-vitro constructed dermo-epidermal composites/analogues

  6.4. Keratinocytes and Fibroblasts (collagen matrices)

Compared to CEAs the usage of cell suspensions is not only cheaper but also easier to handle and more quickly available.

Membrane cell transplants

The usage of bio-compatible membranes as a carrier for cultured cells for the coverage of burn wounds failed to prevail in the clinical practice. Although several constructs have shown good experimental results in vitro as well as in vivo, a further development remains questionable [49,50,89]. However a potential advantage of this method is especially an improved mechanical handling, thus simplifying the application of cultured cells.

Alloplastic and synthetic-biological carriers for cultured cells

The combination of cultured autologous keratinocytes with different alloplastic materials as dermal regeneration matrices has been investigated by different groups [76, 150]. In 1989 Yannas and Burke developed a skin equivalent by centrifuging trypsinized keratinocytes and fibroblasts in a collagen-glycosaminoglycan-matrix (C-GAG). This mixture was completely integrated into the healing wound after transplantation onto guinea pigs [150]. Despite these promising results, the technique failed to prevail among others due to the complex generating process.

A noticeable alternative is the usage of a bilaminare membrane (Integra®) containing a dermal component, which is covered by a silicone membrane as a temporary epidermal substitute [76]. Due to its porosity the dermal component allows the ingrowing of wound-grounded fibroblasts as well as the recapillarisation through sprouting vessels out of the wound, which has to be covered. During these processes there is a transformation of the substitute matrix through the incoming fibroblasts [104, 99]

with consecutive reconstitution of a vital dermal compound in vivo, which can be covered with thin split skin grafts or CEAs [76] after removal of the temporary artificial epidermis. Recent studies show, that the additional use of a vacuum sealing (VAC®) can shorten the time period until the healing of the dermal component is finished and improves significantly the take-rate.

Another approach is the transplantation of pre-confluent non contact-inhibited keratinocyte-monolayers embedded onto polymer-membranes or polyurethane (membrane-cell-constructs). These constructs are available after a short culture period and reconstitute the epidermis in vivo after application onto the excised burn wound (Fig. 8).

Summary

Cultured skin substitutes are nowadays a glimmer of hope for the recent and future treatment especially of high scaled burns. So far they can saves lives, but have to be improved to completely reach the quality of split thickness or full thickness skin grafts in the future. Until this goal is reached, mixed techniques,

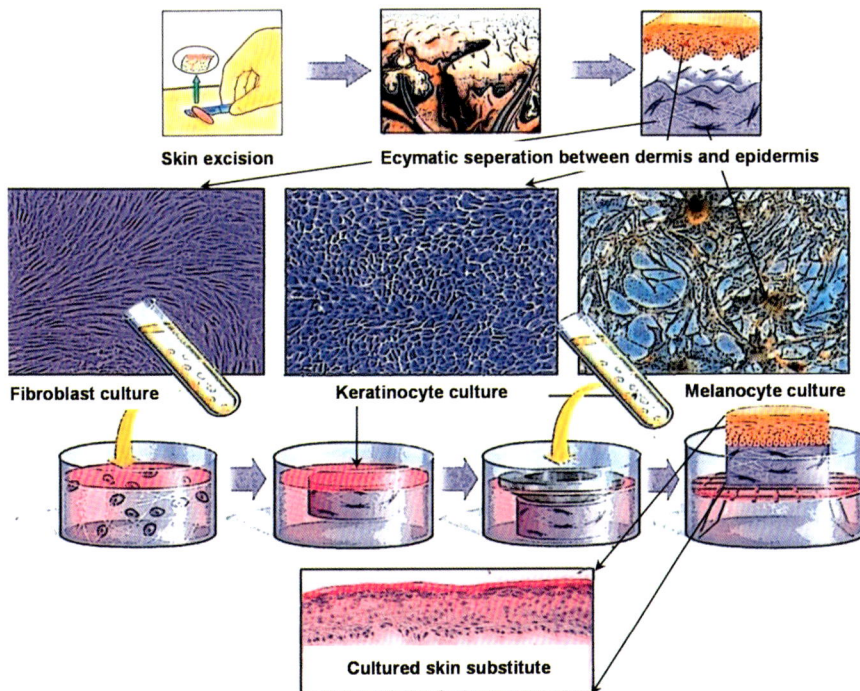

Fig. 7. Scheme of an ideal production process of tissue engineered skin substitutes. Subcultures of fibroblasts, keratinocytes and melanocytes are mixed and transplanted as a skin substitute. The depicted technique, which merges several components after subculturing to a skin like substitute, has since yet failed to prevail in the clinical practice due to several technical barriers

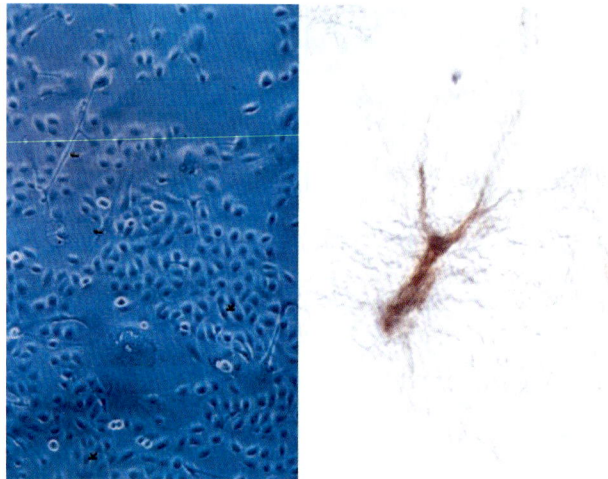

Fig. 8. Depicted is a subconfluent keratinocyte culture (left image) containing a few isolated fibroblasts. The right image displays melanocytes in a cell culture.
* These images are friendly provided by PD Dr. Jürgen Kopp (Hannover)

like temporary allogenic skin grafting combined with a one or second stage transplantation of autologous cultured skin substitutes, which already have achieved good clinical results, will be improved and used for the acute treatment of severe burned patients. In summary cell culture and tissue engineering support and improve the conventional techniques of burn therapy and might have the potential to replace them in the future.

References

[1]   Bünger C (1823) Gelungener Versuch einer Nasenbildung aus einem völlig getrennten Hautstück aus dem Beine. J Chir Augenheilkd 4: 569–573

[2]   Reverdin JL (1869) Greffe epidermique. Bulletin de la Societe Imperiale de Chirurgie de Paris 10: 511–4

[3]   Braun W (1920) Zur Technik der Hautpfropfung. Zentralb Chir 47: 1355–1361

[4]   Ollier L (1872) Sur le greffes cutanees ou autoplatiques. Bull Acad Med 1: 243–256

[5]   Thiersch C (1874) Ueber die feineren anatomischen Veränderungen bei Aufheilung von Haut auf Granulationen. Langenbecks Arch Klin Chir 17: 318–324

[6]   Mangoldt F (1895) Die Epithelsaat zum Verschluß einer großen Wundfläche. Med Wochenschr 21: 798–803

[7]   Mir Y, Mir L (1950) The gauze technique in skin grafting; a quick method in applying dermatome grafts. Plast Reconstr Surg 5(1): 91–96

[8]   Janzekovic Z (1970) A new concept in the early excision and immediate grafting of burns. J Trauma 10(12):1103–8

[9]   Fisher JC (1984) Skin – the ultimate solution for the burn wound. N Engl J Med 311(7): 466–467

[10] Alexander JW, MacMillan BG, Law E, Kittur DS (1981) Treatment of severe burns with widely meshed skin autograft and meshed skin allograft overlay. J Trauma. 21(6): 433–438

[11] Pallua N, Machens HG, Becker M, Berger A (1996) [Surgical prevention of post-traumatic infection by immediate necrectomy of burn wounds]. Langenbecks Arch Chir Suppl Kongressbd 113: 1144–1148

[12] Gabarro P (1943) A new method of grafting. Br Med J 1: 723

[13] Mac Millan B, Altemeier W (1962) Massive excision of the extensive burn. Research in Burns. Am Inst Biol Siences 9: 331

[14] Tanner JC, Jr, Vandeput J, Olley JF (1964) The mesh skin graft. Plast Reconstr Surg 34: 287–292

[15] Tanner JC, Jr, Shea PC, Jr, Bradley WH, Vandeput JJ (1969) Large-mesh skin grafts. Plast Reconstr Surg 44(5): 504–506

[16] Burleson R, Eiseman B (1972) Nature of the bond between partial-thickness skin and wound granulations. Surgery 72(2): 315–322

[17] Adams DC, Ramsey ML (2005) Grafts in dermatologic surgery: review and update on full- and split-thickness skin grafts, free cartilage grafts, and composite grafts. Dermatol Surg 31(8 Pt 2): 1055–1067

[18] Brou J, Vu T, McCauley RL, Herndon DN, Desai MH, Rutan RL et al (1990) The scalp as a donor site: revisited. J Trauma 30(5): 579–581

[19] Corps BV (1969) The effect of graft thickness, donor site and graft bed on graft shrinkage in the hooded rat. Br J Plast Surg 22(2): 125–133

[20] Smahel J, Ganzoni N (1972) The take of mesh graft in experiment. Acta Chir Plast 14(2): 90–100

[21] Meek CP (1958) Successful microdermagrafting using the Meek-Wall microdermatome. Am J Surg 96(4): 557–558

[22] Kreis RW, Mackie DP, Vloemans AW, Hermans RP, Hoekstra MJ (1993) Widely expanded postage stamp skin grafts using a modified Meek technique in combination with an allograft overlay. Burns 19(2):142–145

[23] Vandeput J, Tanner JC, Jr, Carlisle JD (1966) The ultra postage stamp skin graft. Plast Reconstr Surg 38(3): 252–254

[24] Chang LY, Yang JY (1998) Clinical experience of postage stamp autograft with porcine skin onlay dressing in extensive burns. Burns 24(3): 264–269

[25] Bondoc CC, Burke JF (1971) Clinical experience with viable frozen human skin and a frozen skin bank. Ann Surg 174(3): 371–382

[26] Kreis RW, Hoekstra MJ, Mackie DP, Vloemans AF, Hermans RP (1992) Historical appraisal of the use of skin allografts in the treatment of extensive full skin thickness burns at the Red Cross Hospital Burns Centre, Beverwijk, The Netherlands. Burns 18 [Suppl] 2: 19–22

[27] Abbott WM, Hembree JS (1970) Absence of antigenicity in freeze-dried skin allografts. Cryobiology 6(5):416–8

[28] Hermans RP (1983) The use of human allografts in the treatment of scalds in children. Panminerva Med 25(3): 155–156

[29] Kreis RW, Vloemans AF, Hoekstra MJ, Mackie DP, Hermans RP (1989) The use of non-viable glycerol-preserved cadaver skin combined with widely expanded autografts in the treatment of extensive third-degree burns. J Trauma 29(1): 51–54

[30] Achauer BM, Hewitt CW, Black KS, Martinez SE, Waxman KS, Ott RA et al (1986) Long-term skin allograft survival after short-term cyclosporin treatment in a patient with massive burns. Lancet 1(8471): 14–15

[31] Takiuchi I, Higuchi D, Sei Y, Nakajima T (1982) Histological identification of prolonged survival of a skin allograft on an extensively burned patient. Burns Incl Therm Inj 8(3): 164–167

[32] Hafemann B, Frese C, Kistler D, Hettich R (1989) Intermingled skin grafts with in vitro cultured keratinocytes – experiments with rats. Burns 15(4): 233–238

[33] Phillips A, Clarke J (1991) The use of intermingled autograft and parental allograft skin in the treatment of major burns in children. Br J Plast Surg 44: 608

[34] Alsbjörn B, SÝrensen B (1985) Grafting with epidermal Langerhans cell depressed cadaver split skin. Burns 11: 259

[35] Burke JF, May JW, Jr, Albright N, Quinby WC, Russell PS (1974) Temporary skin transplantation and immunosuppression for extensive burns. N Engl J Med 290(5): 269–271

[36] Burke JF, Quinby WC, Bondoc CC, Cosimi AB, Russell PS, Szyfelbein SK (1975) Immunosuppression and temporary skin transplantation in the treatment of massive third degree burns. Ann Surg 182(3): 183–197

[37] Hewitt CW, Black KS, Stenger JA, Go C, Achauer BM, Martin DC (1988) Comparison of kidney, composite tissue, and skin allograft survival in rats prolonged by donor blood and concomitant limited cyclosporine. Transplant Proc 20[3 Suppl 3]: 1110–1113

[38] Hewitt CW, Black KS, Harman JC, Beko KR, 2nd, Lee HS, Patel AP et al (1990) Partial tolerance in rat renal allograft recipients following multiple blood transfusions and concomitant cyclosporine. Transplantation 49(1): 194–198

[39] Frame JD, Sanders R, Goodacre TE, Morgan BD (1989) The fate of meshed allograft skin in burned patients using cyclosporin immunosuppression. Br J Plast Surg 42(1): 27–34

[40] Kanitakis J, Ramirez-Bosca A, Haftek M, Thivolet J (1990) Histological and ultrastructural effects of cyclosporin A on normal human skin xenografted on to nude mice. Virchows Arch A Pathol Anat Histopathol 416(6): 505–511

[41] Bromberg BE, Song IC, Mohn MP (1965) The use of pig skin as a temporary biological dressing. Plast Reconstr Surg 36: 80–90

[42] Ding YL, Pu SS, Wu DZ, Ma C, Pan ZL, Lu X et al (1983) Clinical and histological observations on the application of intermingled auto- and porcine-skin heterografts in third degree burns. Burns Incl Therm Inj 9(6): 381–386

[43] Min J, Yang GF (1981) [Clinical and histological observations on intermingled pig skin and auto-skin transplantation in burns (author's transl)]. Zhonghua Wai Ke Za Zhi 19(1): 43–45

[44] Yang ZJ (1981) Treatment of extensive third degree burns. A Chinese concept. Rev Med Chir Soc Med Nat Iasi 85(1): 69–74

[45] Baumer F, Henrich HA, Bonfig R, Kossen DJ, Romen W (1986) [Surgical treatment of 3d degree burns with mixed homologous/autologous and heterologous/autologous full-thickness skin grafts. Comparison of results with native and frozen homologous and heterologous tissues in animal experiments]. Zentralbl Chir 111(7): 426–430

[46] Jackson D (1954) A clinical study of the use of skin homografts for burns. Br J Plast Surg 7(1): 26–43

[47] Converse JM, Rapaport FT (1956) The vascularization of skin autografts and homografts; an experimental study in man. Ann Surg 143(3): 306–315

[48] Toranto IR, Sayler KE, Myers MB (1974) Vascularization of porcine skin heterografts. Plast Reconstr Surg 54(2): 195–200

[49] Herndon DN, Rutan RL (1992) Comparison of cultured epidermal autograft and massive excision with serial autografting plus homograft overlay. J Burn Care Rehabil 13(1): 154–157

[50] Horch R, Stark GB, Kopp J, Spilker G (1994) Cologne Burn Centre experiences with glycerol-preserved allogeneic skin: Part I: Clinical experiences and histological findings (overgraft and sandwich technique). Burns 20 [Suppl 1]: S23–26

[51] Sawada Y (1985) Survival of an extensively burned child following use of fragments of autograft skin overlain with meshed allograft skin. Burns Incl Therm Inj 11(6): 429–433

[52] Sawada Y (1989) Buried chip skin grafting for treatment of perianal burns. Burns Incl Therm Inj 15(1): 36–38

[53] Ming-Liang Z, Chang-Yeh W, Zhi-De C (1986) Microskin grafting II. Clinical report. Burns 12: 544

[54] Zhang ML, Chang ZD, Han X, Zhu M (1986) Microskin grafting. I. Animal experiments. Burns Incl Therm Inj 12(8): 540–543

[55] Zhang ML, Wang CY, Chang ZD, Cao DX, Han X (1986) Microskin grafting. II. Clinical report. Burns Incl Therm Inj 12(8): 544–548

[56] Lin SD, Lai CS, Chou CK, Tsai CW (1992) Microskin grafting of rabbit skin wounds with Biobrane overlay. Burns 18(5): 390–394

[57] Lin SD, Lai CS, Chou CK, Tsai CW, Wu KF, Chang CW (1992) Microskin autograft with pigskin xenograft overlay: a preliminary report of studies on patients. Burns 18(4): 321–325

[58] O'Conner N, Mulliken J, Banks-Schlegel S, Kehinde O, Green H (1981) Grafting of burns with cultured epithelium prepared from autologous epidermal cells. Lancet 1: 75–78

[59] Hefton JM, Madden MR, Finkelstein JL, Shires GT (1983) Grafting of burn patients with allografts of cultured epidermal cells. Lancet 2(8347): 428–430

[60] Gallico GG, 3rd, O'Connor NE, Compton CC, Kehinde O, Green H (1984) Permanent coverage of large burn wounds with autologous cultured human epithelium. N Engl J Med 311(7): 448–451

[61] Madden MR, Finkelstein JL, Staiano-Coico L, Goodwin CW, Shires GT, Nolan EE et al (1986) Grafting of cultured allogeneic epidermis on second- and third-degree burn wounds on 26 patients. J Trauma 26(11): 955–962

[62] Eldad A, Burt A, Clarke JA, Gusterson B (1987) Cultured epithelium as a skin substitute. Burns Incl Therm Inj 13(3): 173–180

[63] Teepe RG, Kreis RW, Hoekstra MJ, Ponec M (1987) [Permanent wound cover using cultured autologous epidermis transplants: a new treatment method for patients with severe burns]. Ned Tijdschr Geneeskd 131(22): 946–951

[64] Aubock J (1988) [Skin replacement with cultured keratinocytes]. Z Hautkr Jul 63(7): 565–567

[65] Aubock J, Irschick E, Romani N, Kompatscher P, Hopfl R, Herold M et al (1988) Rejection, after a slightly prolonged survival time, of Langerhans cell-free allogeneic cultured epidermis used for wound coverage in humans. Transplantation 45(4): 730–737

[66] Ljunggren C (1898) Von der Fähigkeit des Hautepithels ausserhalb des Organismus sein Leben zu behalten, mit Berücksichtigung der Transplantation. Dtsch Z Chir 47: 608–615

[67] Carrel A, Burrows M (1910) Cultivation of adult tissues and organs outside of the body. JAMA 55:1379–1381

[68] Hadda S (1912) Aus der chirurg. Abteilung des israelitischen Krankenhauses zu Breslau: Die Kultur lebender Körperzellen. Berl Klin Wschr 49: 11

[69] Kreibich K (1914) Aus der deutschen dermatologischen Klinik in Prag: Kultur erwachsener Haut auf festem Nährboden. Arch Dermatol Syph 120: 168–176

[70] Waymouth C (1965) Construction and use of synthetic media. In: Willmer E (ed) Cells and tissues in culture. Academic, London, p 99

[71] Börnstein K (1930) Über Gewebezüchtung menschlicher Haut. Klin Wschr 9: 1119

[72] Pinkus H (1932) Über Gewebekulturen menschlicher Epidermis. Arch Dermatol Syph 165: 53–85

[73] Medawar P (1948) The cultivation of adult mammalian skin epithelium in vitro. Q J Microsc Sci 89: 187

[74] Parshley MS, Simms HS (1950) Cultivation of adult skin epithelial cells (chicken and human) in vitro. Am J Anat 86(2): 163–189

[75] Lewis S, Pomerat C, Ezell D (1949) Human epidermal cell observed in tissue culture phase-contrast microscope. Anat Rec 104: 487

[76] Flaxman B, Harper R (1975) Primary cell culture for biochemical studies of human keratinocytes. Br J Dermatol 92: 305

[77] Flaxman BA, Harper RA (1975) Primary cell culture for biochemical studies of human keratinocytes. A method for production of very large numbers of cells without the necessity of subculturing techniques. Br J Dermatol 92(3): 305–309

[78] Blocker TG, Jr, Pomerat CM, Lewis SR (1950) Research opportunities with the use of cultures of living skin. Plast Reconstr Surg 5(4): 283–288

[79] Bassett CA, Evans VJ, Earle WR (1956) Characteristics and potentials of long term cultures of human skin. Plast Reconstr Surg 17(6): 421–429

[80] Medawar P (1948) Tests by tissue culture methods on the nature and immunity to transplanted skin. Q J Microsc Sci 89: 239

[81] Moscona A (1961) Rotation-mediated histogenetic aggregation of dissociated cells. A quantifiable approach to cell interactions in vitro. Exp Cell Res 22: 455–475

[82] Karasek MA (1968) Growth and differentiation of transplanted epithelial cell cultures. J Invest Dermatol 51(4): 247–252

[83] Igel HJ, Freeman AE, Boeckman CR, Kleinfeld KL (1974) A new method for covering large surface area wounds with autografts. II. Surgical application of tissue culture expanded rabbit-skin autografts. Arch Surg 108(5): 724–729

[84] Freeman AE, Igel HJ, Herrman BJ, Kleinfeld KL (1976) Growth and characterization of human skin epithelial cell cultures. In Vitro 12(5): 352–362

[85] Rheinwald JG, Green H (1975) Serial cultivation of strains of human epidermal keratinocytes: the formation of keratinizing colonies from single cells. Cell 6(3): 331–343

[86] Rheinwald JG, Green H (1975) Formation of a keratinizing epithelium in culture by a cloned cell line derived from a teratoma. Cell 6(3): 317–330

[87] Medawar P (1941) Sheets of pure epidermal epithelium from human skin. Nature 148: 783

[88] Billingham RE, Reynolds J (1952) Transplantation studies on sheets of pure epidermal epithelium and on epidermal cell suspensions. Br J Plast Surg 5(1): 25–36

[89] Perry VP, Evans VJ, Earle WR, Hyatt GW, Bedell WC (1956) Long-term tissue culture of human skin. Am J Hyg 63(1): 52–58

[90] Wheeler CE, Canby CM, Cawley EP (1957) Long-term tissue culture of epithelial-like cells from human skin. J Invest Dermatol 29(5): 383–91; discussion 91–92

[91] Cruickshank CN, Cooper JR, Hooper C (1960) The cultivation of cells from adult epidermis. J Invest Dermatol 34: 339–342

[92] Prunieras M, Mathivon MF, Leung TK, Gazzolo L (1965) [Euploid Culture of Adult Epidermal Cells in Monocellular Layers.]. Ann Inst Pasteur (Paris) 108: 149–165

[93] Constable H, Cooper JR, Cruickshank CN, Mann PR (1974) Keratinization in dispersed cell cultures of adult guinea-pig ear skin. Br J Dermatol 91(1): 39–48

[94] Karasek MA, Charlton ME (1971) Growth of post-embryonic skin epithelial cells on collagen gels. J Invest Dermatol 56(3): 205–210

[95] Cohen S (1962) Isolation of a mouse submaxillary gland protein accelerating incisor eruption and eyelid opening in the new-born animal. J Biol Chem 237: 1555–1562

[96] Cohen S (1965) The stimulation of epidermal proliferation by a specific protein (EGF). Dev Biol 12(3): 394–407

[97] Green H, Kehinde O, Thomas J (1979) Growth of cultured human epidermal cells into multiple epithelia suitable for grafting. Proc Natl Acad Sci USA 76(11): 5665–5668

[98] Cuono C, Langdon R, McGuire J (1986) Use of cultured epidermal autografts and dermal allografts as skin replacement after burn injury. Lancet 1(8490):1123–1124

[99] Hennings H, Michael D, Cheng C, Steinert P, Holbrook K, Yuspa SH (1980) Calcium regulation of growth and differentiation of mouse epidermal cells in culture. Cell 19(1): 245–254

[100] Yuspa SH, Koehler B, Kulesz-Martin M, Hennings H (1981) Clonal growth of mouse epidermal cells in medium with reduced calcium concentration. J Invest Dermatol 76(2): 144–146

[101] Barnes D, Sato G (1980) Methods for growth of cultured cells in serum-free medium. Anal Biochem 102(2): 255–270

[102] Shipley GD, Ham RG (1981) Improved medium and culture conditions for clonal growth with minimal serum protein and for enhanced serum-free survival of Swiss 3T3 cells. In Vitro 17(8): 656–670

[103] Tsao MC, Walthall BJ, Ham RG (1982) Clonal growth of normal human epidermal keratinocytes in a defined medium. J Cell Physiol 110(2): 219–229

[104] Wille JJ, Jr., Pittelkow MR, Shipley GD, Scott RE (1984) Integrated control of growth and differentiation of normal human prokeratinocytes cultured in serum-free medium: clonal analyses, growth kinetics, and cell cycle studies. J Cell Physiol 121(1): 31–44

[105] Kopp J, Jeschke MG, Bach AD, Kneser U, Horch RE (2004) Applied tissue engineering in the closure of severe burns and chronic wounds using cultured human autologous keratinocytes in a natural fibrin matrix. Cell Tissue Bank 5(2): 89–96

[106] Yasushi F, Koichi U, Yuka O, Kentaro K, Hiromichi M, Yoshimitsu K (2004) Treatment with autologous cultured dermal substitutes (CDS) for burn scar contracture in children. Wound Repair Regen 12: A11

[107] Freising C, Horch R (2001) Clinical results of cultivated keratinocyzes to treat burn injuries – a metaanalysis. In: Achauer B (ed) Cultured human keratinocytes and tissue engineered skin substitutes. Thieme, Stuttgart, pp 220–226

[108] Woodley DT, Peterson HD, Herzog SR, Stricklin GP, Burgeson RE, Briggaman RA et al (1988) Burn wounds resurfaced by cultured epidermal autografts show abnormal reconstitution of anchoring fibrils. Jama 259(17): 2566–2571

[109] Horch RE, Stark G, Spilker G (1994) Treatment of perianal burns with submerged skin particles. Zentralbl Chir 119: 722–725

[110] Horch RE, Corbei O, Formanek-Corbei B, Brand-Saberi B, Vanscheidt W, Stark G (1998) Reconstitution of basement membrane after ‚sandwich-technique' skin grafting for severe burns demonstrated by immunohistochemistry. J Burn Care Rehabil 19: 189–202

[111] Horch RE, Jeschke MG, Spilker G, Herndon DN, Kopp J (2005) Treatment of second degree facial burns with allografts – preliminary results. Burns 31(5): 597–602

[112] Munster AM, Smith-Meek M, Shalom A (2001) Acellular allograft dermal matrix: immediate or delayed epidermal coverage? Burns 27(2): 150–153

[113] Ronfard V, Rives JM, Neveux Y, Carsin H, Barrandon Y (2000) Long-term regeneration of human epidermis on third degree burns transplanted with autologous cultured epithelium grown on a fibrin matrix. Transplantation 70(11): 1588–1598

[114] Hunyadi J, Farkas B, Bertenyi C, Olah J, Dobozy A (1987) Keratinocyte grafting: covering of skin defects by separated autologous keratinocytes in a fibrin net. J Invest Dermatol 89(1): 119–120

[115] Altmeppen J, Hansen E, Bonnlander GL, Horch RE, Jeschke MG (2004) Composition and characteristics of an autologous thrombocyte gel. J Surg Res 117(2): 202–207

[116] Achauer BM (ed) (1991) Burn reconstruction. Thieme Medical publishers, New York

[117] Ong YS, Samuel M, Song C (2006) Metaanalysis of early excision of burns. Burns 32: 145–150

Correspondence: Raymund E. Horch M. D., Ph. D., Department of Plastic and Hand Surgery, University of Erlangen-Nürnberg Medical Center, 91054 Erlangen, Germany, E-mail: Raymund.Horch@uk-erlangen.de

Twelve year follow-up: a clinical study on dermal regeneration

Monica C. T. Bloemen[1,2], Paul P. M. van Zuijlen[1-4], Esther Middelkoop[1,2,5]

[1] Association of Dutch Burn Centers, Beverwijk, The Netherlands
[2] Burn Center, Red Cross Hospital, Beverwijk, The Netherlands
[3] Department of Plastic, Reconstructive and Hand Surgery, Red Cross Hospital, Beverwijk, The Netherlands
[4] Department of Plastic, Reconstructive and Hand Surgery, Academic Medical Center, Amsterdam, The Netherlands
[5] Department of Plastic, Reconstructive and Hand Surgery, VU University Medical Center, Amsterdam, The Netherlands

Introduction

Improved wound care has increased life expectancy in both patients with chronic and acute wounds. Nowadays, treatment is not only focused on patient survival; eventual patient outcome has also become more important. The long-term consequences of skin loss, e. g. scars that remain after burns or other trauma can be severe and cause physical and cosmetic problems. Therefore, therapies for improvement of scar quality is mandatory. The standard therapy for extensive full-thickness wounds is the application of an autologous skin graft. However, this treatment leads to poor skin quality and scar contractures. One of the causes of this poor skin quality, is the lack of dermis in the remaining scar. The dermal layer of the skin is responsible for pliability and mechanical resistance. Consequently, the lack of dermis predisposes to severe scarring.

In 1981, Yannas and Burke were the first to report on the development of an artificial dermis derived from bovine collagen [4]. Since then, research has focused on the use of dermal substitutes to improve the functional and cosmetic outcome. Dermal substitution in acute and reconstructive wounds is thought to lead to a better scar elasticity, mechanical stability and appearance. This could be due to the fact that the use of a dermal substitute results in the formation of a neodermis that is comparable with the normal dermis. It is hypothesized that dermal substitution serves as a support structure for the ingrowth of vessels and autologous fibroblasts [7, 8, 16, 21].

Multiple studies have investigated the use of dermal substitutes, such as Integra®, Apligraf®, Matriderm® and Alloderm®, in acute and reconstructive wounds [3, 12, 15–19, 23–25, 30–32]. Good results have been demonstrated, e. g. an increased scar elasticity and an improved cosmetic appearance [3, 12, 15–18, 23, 25, 31, 32]. The majority of these studies, however, only reported short term follow-up. To our knowledge, one study reported on the results of a study on dermal substitution with a follow-up longer than one or two years [25]. Sheridan et al. described a study on the use of Integra® in acute burns with a follow-up of up to ten years [25]. Good results were found for scar function and appearance in substituted scars. Unfortunately, only patients in who the artificial skin was successfully grafted were evaluated in follow-up, thus a selection bias might probably have occurred. In addition, the quality of substituted scars was only evaluated subjectively. Besides the above described study, little information is available on the long-term effectiveness of dermal substitutes. A clinical trial with a long-term follow-up can investigate long-term effectiveness of dermal substitution and show a long-lasting functional and cosmetic scar improvement. In addition, the need for reconstructive surgery and patient's quality of life can be investigated in long-term studies. This chap-

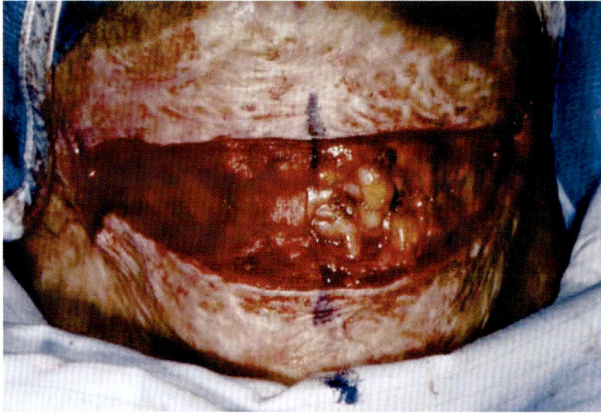

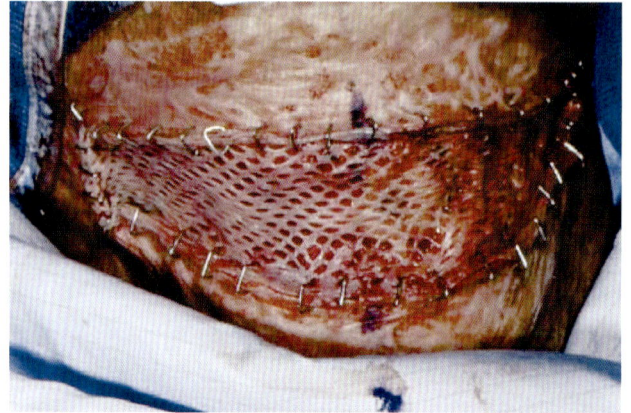

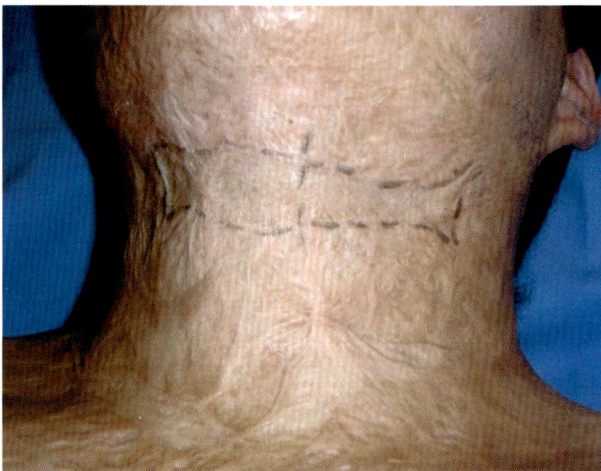

Fig. 1. Patient example of clinical application of the dermal substitute in a reconstructive burn wound and scar appearance 12 years post-operatively.
Upper left: Reconstructive wound in the neck with the substitute applied on the right side of the patient's wound (in the picture left).
Upper right: Reconstructive wound in the neck with an SSG applied on top of the substitute (patient's right side) and the wound (patient's left side).
Below: Scar appearance 11.6 years post-operatively is presented; substituted scar in the picture left, reference scar in the picture right

ter will focus on a study that was performed on the long-term effectiveness of a dermal substitute using objective and subjective criteria [1].

From 1996 to 1998, a controlled clinical trial was performed at the Burn Centre Beverwijk, The Netherlands in which effectiveness of a dermal substitute was investigated. Publications of this study reported on the graft survival and scar aspects three and 12 months post-operatively [27, 28]. Firstly, it was

shown that this dermal substitute could be successfully applied in a one-stage procedure. Secondly, in scar assessment three months post-operatively, the clinical effectiveness of this substitute was established by demonstrating a statistically significant increase of elasticity for reconstructive wounds [27]. Twelve months post-operatively, elasticity had improved in both scars and although the substituted scar was more elastic, the difference did not reach the level of statistical significance. Also, in a separate analysis of acute burn scars, it was seen that elasticity was higher in substituted scars treated with a large expansion graft [28]. Finally, in the follow-up 12 months post-operatively, substituted scars seemed smoother compared with reference scars [28].

The Vancouver Scar Scale (VSS) and the Cutometer were used to assess the scars at three and 12 months post-operatively. Since then, several additional measuring tools have been developed. First of all, an improved subjective assessment scale was developed, the Patient and Observer Scar Assessment Scale (POSAS), which was used in the follow-up 12 years post-surgery, instead of the VSS [11]. In addition, scar color and pigmentation were quantified with objective measuring tools and for the first time, the effect of dermal substitution on scar roughness was objectified [2, 13, 14, 22]. Summarizing, more scar aspects were investigated subjectively and objectively 12 years after application of the substitute.

Clinical trial

From 1996 to 1998, 62 burn patients were included in the controlled clinical trial. The use of a collagen-elastin matrix as dermal substitute was investigated in both reconstructive and acute burn wounds [27–29]. Patients were included if they were admitted to the Burn Centre and needed surgical treatment for their reconstructive and acute burn wounds. In all patients, a paired intra-individual comparison was made; one (part of the) wound was treated with the conventional split skin graft (SSG) and the other (part of the) wound was treated with the precursor of the dermal substitute, Matriderm® (Dr. Otto Suwelack Skin & Health Care AG, Billerbeck, Germany) and an SSG (Fig. 1). This substitute is a 1 mm-thick, highly porous membrane, composed of a native bovine type I, III and V collagen fiber template. The collagen fibers are coated with α-elastin hydrolysate derived from the bovine nuchal ligament in a concentration of 3 % weight-to-weight ratio (GfN-Herstellung von Naturextrakten GmbH, Wald-Michelbach, Germany). The substitute was treated with low-dosed γ-irradiation (approximately 1000 Gy) and stored at room temperature. Matrices were applied in a single-stage grafting procedure. During the operation, the experimental and reference treatment were allocated to anatomically related areas, therefore a right/left, superior/inferior or medial/lateral comparison was made to exclude any bias caused by selection of the surgeon.

After 12 years, all patients were addressed for a third follow-up. In total 46 of the initial 62 patients participated in this follow-up, consisting of patients with acute (26) and reconstructive burn wounds (26). Six patients were also included in the reconstructive group after being included in the burn wound category previously. The category of acute burn wounds consisted of 35 scar pairs which could be evaluated; in the reconstructive burn group 34 scar pairs were included in the follow-up. Table 1 demonstrates several patient characteristics of the study group. In each patient, the experimental scar (treated with the dermal substitute and a SSG) and the reference scar (treated with a SSG alone) were located with the use of a well-documented photographic archive and precise wound descriptions (Fig. 2). Consequently, scar elasticity, erythema,

Table 1. Patient characteristics

Acute	
Number of patients (n)	26
Number of scar pairs (n)	35
Male sex	15 (58%)
TBSA %	24.3 ± 14.7
Follow-up period in yrs	11.8 ± 0.4
Reconstructive	
Number of patients (n)	26
Number of scar pairs (n)	34
Male sex	16 (62%)
TBSA %	30.5 ± 17.6
Follow-up period in yrs	11.8 ± 2.1

TBSA   Total Body Surface Area

melanin and surface roughness were examined by means of different objective scar evaluation tools and scars were also evaluated subjectively.

Scar elasticity

Scar elasticity was measured with the Cutometer Skin Elasticity Meter (Courage and Khazaka GmbH, Germany) which has been established as a reliable and valid instrument for the evaluation of this scar aspect [9]. The Cutometer measures the vertical deformation of skin in millimeters during a controlled vacuum. The following elasticity parameters are provided (in millimeters): maximal skin extension, pliability, elasticity, retraction and visco-elasticity. In the analysis of all acute and reconstructive scars together, elasticity parameters in the substituted scars were similar to or higher than elasticity data in reference scars, although not statistically different. In the separate analysis of scars in the acute burn category, no differences in elasticity were seen between substituted and reference areas. In the reconstructive scars, all elasticity parameters were higher in substituted scars, although not statistically significant. Figure 3 shows the elasticity data 12-years post-operatively (student t-test). Figure 4 illustrates the improvement of elasticity of substituted areas compared to reference areas, on the short and long-term.

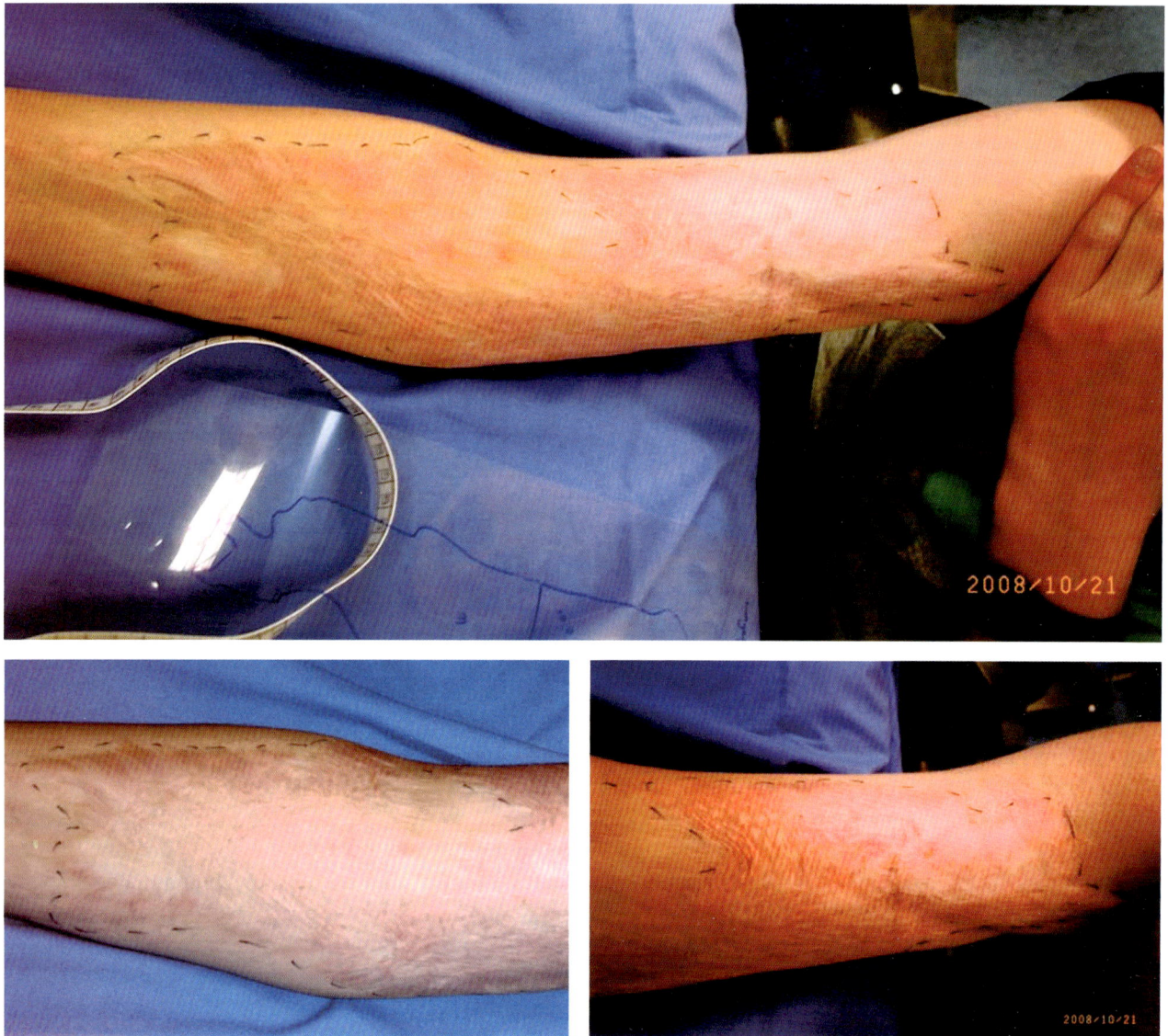

Fig. 2. Patient example of substituted and reference scar on arm with tracings of the previous assessment.
Substituted scar in picture left (distal scar of arm).
Reference scar in picture right (proximal scar of arm)

Scar erythema and melanin

Scar erythema and melanin were measured with the DermaSpectrometer (Cortex Technology, Denmark). This is a validated assessment tool, which emits light by means of diodes at two defined wavelengths: green light (568 nm) and red light (655 nm) [10]. Photodetectors measure the light reflected by the skin. As green light is absorbed by haemoglobin and red light is absorbed by melanin, an erythema and melanin index can be computed, based on the intensity of absorbed and reflected light. In the analysis of acute and reconstructive scars together and in the analysis of the acute burn group alone, no statistically significant differences in erythema and melanin were found between substituted and reference scars (student t-test, data not shown). In the reconstructive scars, a statistically significant difference was found between melanin of substituted and reference scars. In substituted scars, mel-

Elasticity 12 years post-operatively
in the acute burn group

(mm)

Extension   Pliability   Elasticity   Retraction   Visco-elasticity

Elasticity 12 years post-operatively
in the reconstructive burn group

(mm)

Extension   Pliability   Elasticity   Retraction   Visco-elasticity

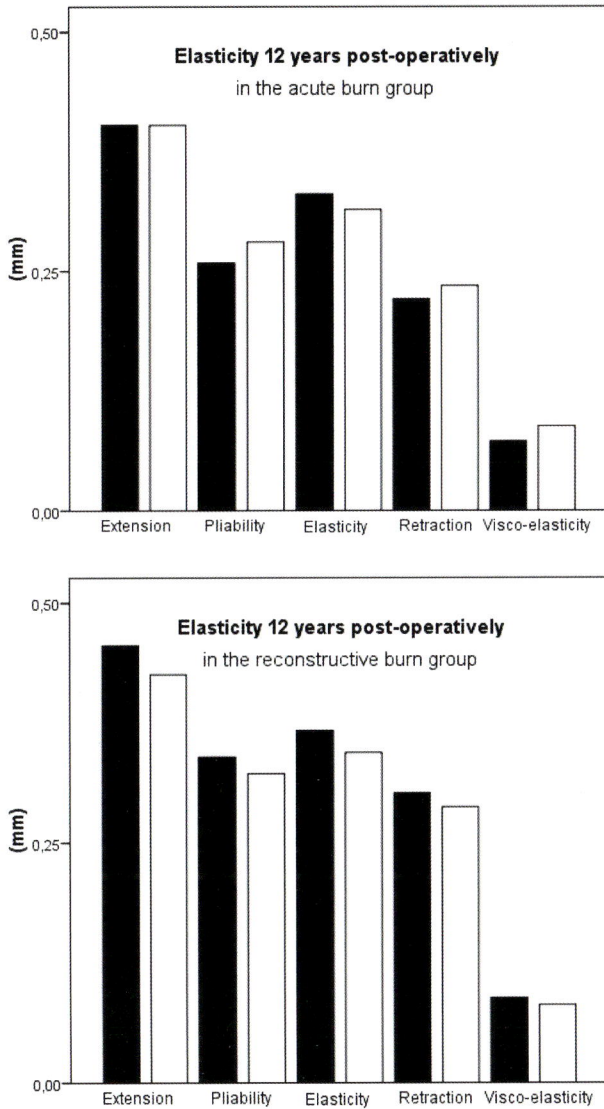

Fig. 3. Elasticity 12 years post-operatively. Different parameters of skin elasticity measured by the Cutometer in both scar groups. Black: substituted scar. White: reference scar

% increase in skin elasticity by dermal substitute

skin elasticity

3 months   12 months   12 years

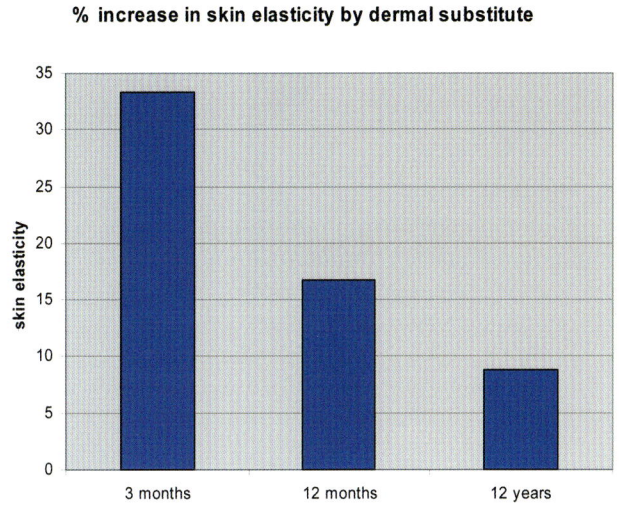

Fig. 4. Improvement in scar elasticity. Increase in elasticity of the substituted scar compared to the reference scar measured by the Cutometer in the reconstructive scar group (3 and 12 months, 12 years)

anin differed more from patient's normal skin compared to reference scars. However, this difference was only 5 % (substitute versus normal skin 1.05; reference versus normal skin 1.00, p < 0.010).

Scar surface roughness

In this study, the relevant parameter scar surface roughness was assessed objectively. Scar surface roughness was evaluated with the PRIMOS (GF-Messtechnik GmbH, Germany). This imaging system produces a three-dimensional image of the micro-topography of the skin and was proven to be reliable and valid in the assessment of surface roughness in scars [2, 13, 14, 20]. The system projects a parallel stripe pattern onto the skin and by means of elevation differences on the skin surface, a 3D image is achieved. Accordingly, images are digitized and the software reconstructs the data into several surface roughness parameters. In this study the parameters Sa, Sz and PC were used and are described as follows. Sa is the arithmetic mean of the surface roughness (μm), Sz is the mean of the five highest peaks and five deepest valleys from the measuring field (mm) and PC (Peak Count) demonstrates the number of peaks per unit length. In Fig. 5 the use of the PRIMOS is demonstrated in one of the patients. In the analysis of the acute and reconstructive scars together, Sa, Sz and PC were significantly lower (better) in substituted scars, indicating a smoother surface. In the scars of the acute burn category, the three roughness parameters were lower in substituted scars compared to the reference scars, although no statistically significant difference was seen. In the reconstructive scars, all roughness parameters showed lower scores in substituted areas compared to conventionally treated areas, of which Sz differed statistically significantly (Wilcoxon Signed-Rank test, Fig. 6 and Table 2).

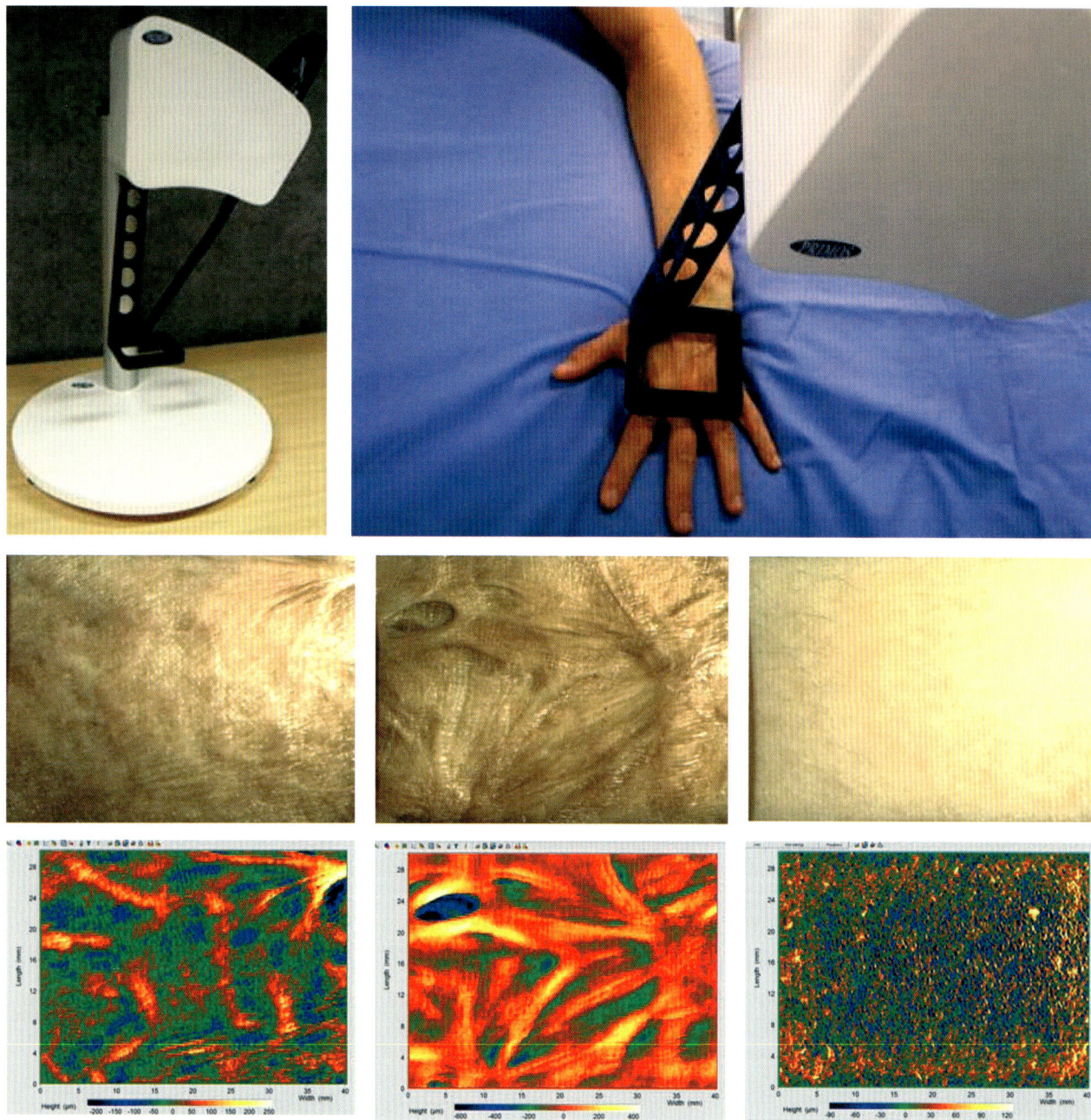

Fig. 5. Use of the PRIMOS in study patient.
Upper left: The PRIMOS as objective measurement tool of scar surface roughness.
Upper right: Use of the PRIMOS in the measurement of a scar on a hand.
Middle left: PRIMOS live picture of scar treated with a substitute and a split-skin graft (Substitute).
Middle center: PRIMOS live picture of scar treated with split-skin graft alone (Reference).
Middle right: PRIMOS live picture of normal skin.
Lower left: PRIMOS picture after filtering of scar treated with a substitute and a split-skin graft (Substitute).
Lower middle: PRIMOS picture after filtering of scar treated with split-skin graft alone (Reference).
Lower right: PRIMOS picture after filtering of normal skin.

Table 2. Results of surface roughness measurements   Wilcoxon Signed-Rank test

	Substitute	Reference	Normal skin	p-value
All scars ($n_{scar\ pairs}$ = 69)				
Sa	42.9	47.1	21.3	0.038*
Sz	558.8	682.0	297.5	0.015*
PC	30.0	39.4	15.2	0.022*
Acute ($n_{scar\ pairs}$ = 35)				
Sa	32.6	36.4	19.6	0.061
Sz	417.6	448.5	291.8	0.604
PC	25.3	34.1	16.3	0.083
Reconstructive ($n_{scar\ pairs}$ = 34)				
Sa	53.9	58.7	23.1	0.275
Sz	709.7	931.7	303.6	0.014*
PC	41.2	52.0	14.0	0.172

Substitute	Wound sites treated with the dermal substitute and a split-skin graft
Reference	Wound sites treated with a split-skin graft alone (control treatment)
CI	Confidence Interval
Sa	Arithmetic mean of the surface roughness (µm)
Sz	Mean of five highest peaks and five deepest valleys from the measuring field (mm)
PC	Peak Count, number of peaks
p-value	Substitute vs Reference
*	$p < 0.038$

Subjective scar evaluation

Lastly, all scars were evaluated subjectively with the POSAS. This is a validated tool which consists of two subscales: the patient and the observer scale [11, 26]. On a 10-point scale the patient gives his opinion on the parameters: color, thickness, surface roughness, pliability, itching and pain. The observer scale was first validated for the use in burn scars and contained five items: vascularization, pliability, pigmentation, thickness and relief [11]. Subsequently, the scale was validated for the use in linear scars as well and therefore, the item surface area was added to include aspects of contraction and scar widening [26]. The total observer score and the total patient score consist of adding the scores of the six items (range 6–60). A low score means a better scar quality: 1 is comparable to normal skin and a score of 10 reflects the worst imaginable scar or sensation. In addition to these items, the observer and the patient give a general opinion on the scar appearance (score 1–10, in which a score of 10 corresponds with the worst possible scar). The observer assessment was performed by three experienced researchers.

Twelve years post-operatively, subjective scores were low (good) for all evaluated scars; a mean score of 3.6 was the highest (worst) observer score. In the acute and reconstructive scars together, a significant difference in favor of the substituted scars was seen for the items pliability, pigmentation, thickness, relief, general score and the total score (data not shown). Substituted scars received lower (better) observer scores than the reference scars. In the separate analysis of scars in the acute burn group, a statistically significant difference was seen in favor of the substituted areas in all POSAS items, except for vascularization. In scars of the reconstructive category, observer scores for pliability, relief and the general score were significantly lower (better) for substituted areas (Table 3). Assessment by the patient demon-

Mean of the five highest peaks and five deepest valleys (Sz)

Mean of the five highest peaks and five deepest valleys (Sz)

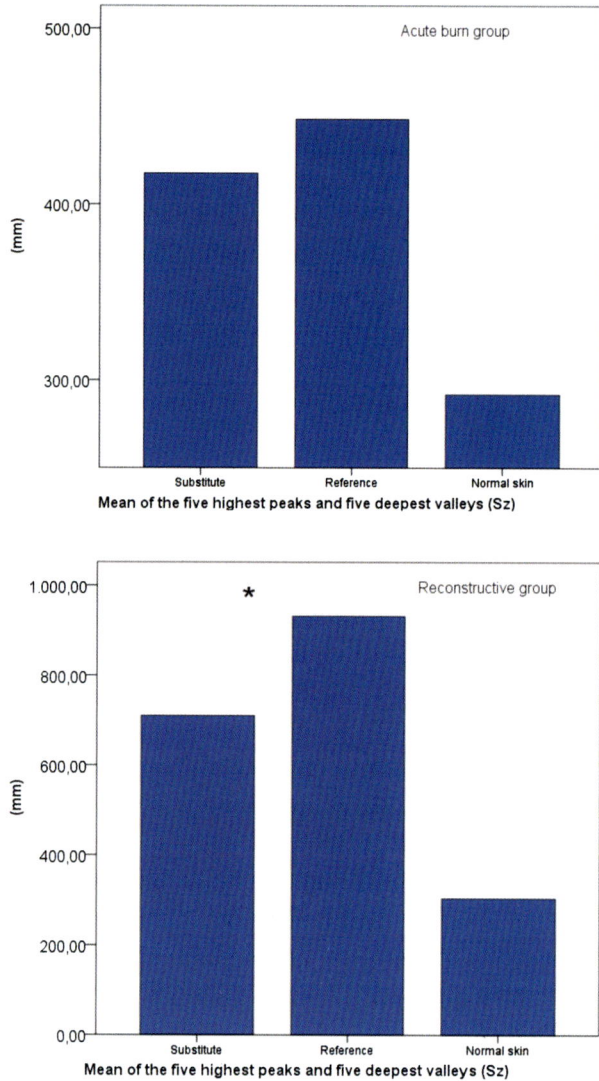

Fig. 6. Scar surface roughness in the acute and reconstructive group

Fig. 7. Elasticity and graft expansion. Elasticity of the acute burn scars measured by the Cutometer. The acute burn scars were divided into scars treated with a small graft expansion (mesh 1:1.5 and 1:2) and scars treated with a large graft expansion (mesh 1:3 and 1:4). Substitute: wound sites treated with the dermal substitute and a split-skin graft. Reference: wound sites treated with a split-skin graft alone (control treatment).

* p < 0.009

strated that substituted scars in the acute group received a lower (better) total score than the reference scars (substitute 3.2, reference 4.0, p = 0.034). In both groups, other POSAS items did not show significant differences (data not shown).

Substitution in combination with different graft expansions

All acute burn wounds in this study were treated with a split-skin graft, with or without a dermal substitute. For the skin grafts, different mesh expansions

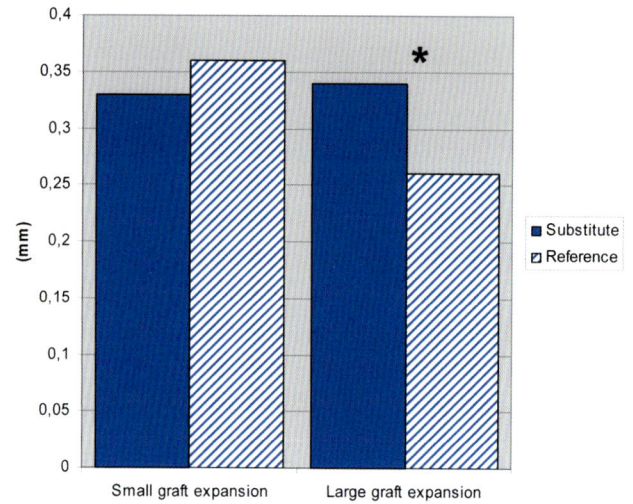

were used in each wound pair; small expansions (mesh 1:1.5 and 1:2) were applied in 20 wound pairs, and larger expansions (mesh 1:3 and 1:4) were used in 15 pairs. Twelve months post-operatively, an analysis was performed to investigate differences between these two groups. At that time, differences in elasticity between the large and small mesh expansion group were found.

In the analysis performed at 12 years post-operatively, significant differences were found for several elasticity parameters as well. The parameters pliability, retraction and visco-elasticity were significantly lower (indicating less pliable scars) in substituted scars compared to the reference scars, in the small expansion group. In the category treated with the larger expansions, significant differences for the elasticity parameters maximal skin extension, elasticity and retraction were found. Scars treated with the substitute showed higher scores of elasticity (i. e. more pliable) than the reference scars (Fig. 7). In this analysis, vascularization, pigmentation and surface roughness were not significantly different between substituted and reference scars. The subjective evalu-

Table 3. Results of observer scar assessment 12 years post-operatively

	Acute burn group			Reconstructive group		
	Substitute	Reference	p-value	Substitute	Reference	p-value
Vascularization	2.0	2.2	0.206	2.2	2.2	0.768
Pliability	2.5	3.0	0.023*	3.0	3.6	0.038*
Pigmentation	2.3	2.7	0.002*	2.6	2.6	0.661
Thickness	2.0	2.4	0.001*	2.3	2.5	0.129
Relief	2.3	3.1	< 0.001*	2.7	3.2	0.038*
Surface area	1.7	1.9	0.008*	2.4	2.5	0.496
Total score	12.8	15.0	< 0.001*	15.2	16.6	0.087

The mean scores of three experienced researchers of the observer scar assessment scale (O-SAS) are shown. In this scale, 1 is comparable to normal skin and a score of 10 reflects the worst imaginable scar.
* $p < 0.038$

ation showed significantly lower (better) scores for relief, surface area and the total score in substituted scars with a small expansion. In scars treated with a larger expansion, all POSAS items received significantly lower (better) scores in substituted scars, except for the item surface area (data not shown).

Discussion

In this chapter, the results of a long-term follow-up study on dermal substitution are presented. First long-term subjective and objective data are described in which the clinical effectiveness of a collagen-elastin matrix is shown 12 years after application. In contrast to the scar evaluation at three and 12 months post-operatively, an objective evaluation tool for surface roughness was used 12 years post-operatively. Short-term scar assessment had shown a smoother surface in substituted scars compared to reference scars (subjectively), for that reason, we expected a difference in roughness between substituted and reference scars [28]. In the analysis of the acute burn and reconstructive group together, all three surface roughness parameters were significantly better in the substituted scars, which implies a smoother surface of these scars (Fig. 6 and Table 2). In reconstructive scars, roughness parameter Sz was significantly lower in scars treated with the substitute. The larger number of patients in the analysis of all scars, could have resulted in statistically significant differences.

Results of the objective scar surface roughness support the clinical observation, as numerous substituted scars showed a reduced visibility of the mesh pattern. In addition, in the acute and the reconstructive substituted scars, a better score for relief was found, measured with the POSAS. This positive effect of dermal substitution could be of great value as an irregular scar surface can be cosmetically disturbing and long-lasting, despite scar maturation (Fig. 2). How can this effect of dermal substitution be explained? One hypothesis is that the dermal substitute replaces the dermis and bridges the interstices of the autograft. As a consequence, the hypertrophy, which appears in the interstices of the autograft, is less when a dermal substitute is applied. This could explain the smoother surface of the scar.

In several studies, an improvement of elasticity (often evaluated subjectively) was reported in scars treated with a dermal substitute, such as Matriderm® or Integra® [5, 6, 17, 23]. In preceding studies, Van Zuijlen et al had reported a significantly higher elasticity in substituted areas compared to reference areas in the reconstructive group, three months post-operatively [27]. In the scar assessment 12 months post-operatively, the absolute difference in elasticity between substituted and reference scars was the same, however, as both scars had improved, no statistically significant difference was found [28]. For this reason, no significant difference in elasticity was expected 12 years after application of the substitute. Nevertheless, similar to the results of 12 months post-operatively, scores were higher in the reconstructive scars treated with the substitute compared to reference scars. In addition, in the acute and the reconstructive substituted scars, a better score for pliability was found, measured with the POSAS. It appears that the application of a substitute in the early phase of wound healing contributed to a lasting higher elasticity. This gain in elasticity in the substituted scars, is highest shortly after surgery and remains present, even after 12 years (Fig. 4).

Wounds treated with a smaller skin graft expansion generally develop into scars with a higher scar quality compared to scars treated with a larger mesh expansion. Van Zuijlen et al reported that the effectiveness of the dermal substitute seemed to have a relation with the expansion of the overlying mesh graft [28]; a higher elasticity was found in acute burn scars treated with the substitute in combination with a largely expanded mesh graft (1:3 or 1:4) compared to the reference scars, after one year. Twelve years post-surgery, a higher elasticity was seen in the reference scars treated with a smaller expansion compared to the scars treated with the larger expansion. The substituted scars, however, showed almost the same elasticity when treated with large and small expansions (Fig. 7). Additionally, the elasticity of substituted scars treated with a larger expansion graft was significantly higher than non-substituted scars with the same expansion. In contrast to these results, the elasticity of substituted scars treated with a small graft expansion was lower than the reference scars. Dermal substitution appears to contribute to a higher elasticity, mainly in combination with a larger mesh expansion.

Besides the objective measurement tools, a subjective scar assessment tool was also used. The subjective scar data from this study are comparable with the results of other clinical studies on the use of dermal substitutes [3, 6, 17, 23, 28]. Three and 12 months after surgery, the subjective scar assessment using the VSS, showed no significant differences between scars treated with and without the dermal substitute. Twelve years after application, the POSAS was used for subjective scar evaluation, as this tool was found to be more reliable than the VSS. It was remarkable that subjective scores were relatively low (good) for all scars, probably due to prolonged scar maturation. Despite the results seen shortly after surgery, the appearance of substituted scars, 12 years post-surgery,

was found to be better than the reference scars; in both the reconstructive and the acute burn scars, significantly lower (better) scores were reported for the substituted scars in several POSAS items (Table 3). A shortcoming of the study was the impossibility to blind the observers, because no randomization procedure was applied and in each patient the substitute was applied on the right, superior or medial (side of the) wound. Therefore, a bias might have occurred.

Another disadvantage of this treatment allocation is that in patients with only one wound, two different therapies were used within the same wound. It is possible that treatments could have affected each other. Furthermore, after 12 years, some study areas were difficult to trace due to improvement of these areas. In several patients, it was therefore complicated to distinguish the substituted scar from the reference scar or even the surrounding skin or scar, especially when repeated corrective procedures were applied in that area. The scars were excluded if the original study areas could not be retraced or measured. Another limitation of the study, was the difficulty for some patients to assess their own scars. Patients with a high percentage total body surface area (TBSA) burned, found it complicated to give their opinion on a relatively small study area. Despite this, in the analysis of all scars, the total subjective patient score of substituted scars was lower compared to the reference scars, but not significantly different (substitute 18.2; reference 19.7; $p = 0.089$).

Conclusion

This chapter describes the first study that objectifies scar outcome after 12 years with the use of a collagen-elastin matrix in acute and reconstructive burn surgery. This dermal substitute showed clinical effectiveness by a significant increase of scar elasticity in the short term. Even after a period of twelve years, improved scar parameters in both acute and reconstructive substituted wounds were found. For the first time, scar surface roughness was objectified and it was shown that substituted areas were significantly smoother than areas treated with an SSG only. Another important finding was the increased elasticity in substituted scars treated with a largely expanded autograft. The results of this study indicate a long-lasting effect of dermal substitution on scar quality and it can be concluded that dermal substitutes play an important role in the treatment of full-thickness skin defects.

Acknowledgements

The original clinical trial was financially supported by grants from the Technology Foundation and the Dutch Organization for Scientific Research. The follow-up study was financially supported by the Dutch Burns Foundation.

References

[1] Bloemen MC, van Leeuwen MC, van Vucht NE, van Zuijlen PP, Middelkoop E (2010) Dermal substitution in acute burns and reconstructive surgery: a 12-year follow-up. Plast Reconstr Surg 125(5): 1450–1459

[2] Bloemen MCT, van Gerven MS, van der Wal MBA, Verhaegen PDHM, Middelkoop E (2011) An objective measuring device for surface roughness in skin and scars. J Am Acad Dermatol 64(4): 706–715

[3] Branski LK, Herndon DN, Pereira C, Mlcak RP, Celis MM, Lee JO, Sanford AP, Norbury WB, Zhang XJ, Jeschke MG (2007) Longitudinal assessment of Integra in primary burn management: a randomized pediatric clinical trial. Crit Care Med 35(11): 2615–2623

[4] Burke JF, Yannas IV, Quinby WC, Jr., Bondoc CC, Jung WK (1981) Successful use of a physiologically acceptable artificial skin in the treatment of extensive burn injury. Ann Surg 194(4): 413–428

[5] Clayman MA, Clayman SM, Mozingo DW (2006) The use of collagen-glycosaminoglycan copolymer (Integra) for the repair of hypertrophic scars and keloids. J Burn Care Res 27(3): 404–409

[6] Dantzer E, Queruel P, Salinier L, Palmier B, Quinot JF (2003) Dermal regeneration template for deep hand burns: clinical utility for both early grafting and reconstructive surgery. Br J Plast Surg 56(8): 764–774

[7] De Vries HJ, Mekkes JR, Middelkoop E, Hinrichs WL, Wildevuur CR, Westerhof W (1993) Dermal substitutes for full-thickness wounds in a one-stage grafting model. Wound Repair Regen 1(4): 244–252

[8] De Vries HJ, Middelkoop E, Mekkes JR, Dutrieux RP, Wildevuur CH, Westerhof H (1994) Dermal regeneration in native non-cross-linked collagen sponges with different extracellular matrix molecules. Wound Repair Regen 2(1): 37–47

[9] Draaijers LJ, Botman YA, Tempelman FR, Kreis RW, Middelkoop E, van Zuijlen PP (2004) Skin elasticity meter or subjective evaluation in scars: a reliability assessment. Burns 30(2): 109–114

[10] Draaijers LJ, Tempelman FR, Botman YA, Kreis RW, Middelkoop E, van Zuijlen PP (2004) Colour evaluation in scars: tristimulus colorimeter, narrow-band simple reflectance meter or subjective evaluation? Burns 30(2): 103–107

[11] Draaijers LJ, Tempelman FR, Botman YA, Tuinebreijer WE, Middelkoop E, Kreis RW, van Zuijlen PP (2004) The patient and observer scar assessment scale: a reliable and feasible tool for scar evaluation. Plast Reconstr Surg 113(7): 1960–5; discussion 6–7

[12] Eaglstein WH, Alvarez OM, Auletta M, Leffel D, Rogers GS, Zitelli JA, Norris JE, Thomas I, Irondo M, Fewkes J, Hardin-Young J, Duff RG, Sabolinski ML (1999) Acute excisional wounds treated with a tissue-engineered skin (Apligraf). Dermatol Surg 25(3): 195–201

[13] Friedman PM, Skover GR, Payonk G, Geronemus RG (2002) Quantitative evaluation of nonablative laser technology. Semin Cutan Med Surg 21(4): 266–273

[14] Friedman PM, Skover GR, Payonk G, Kauvar AN, Geronemus RG (2002) 3D in-vivo optical skin imaging for topographical quantitative assessment of non-ablative laser technology. Dermatol Surg 28(3): 199–204

[15] Hansbrough JF, Dore C, Hansbrough WB (1992) Clinical trials of a living dermal tissue replacement placed beneath meshed, split-thickness skin grafts on excised burn wounds. J Burn Care Rehabil 13(5): 519–529

[16] Haslik W, Kamolz LP, Nathschlager G, Andel H, Meissl G, Frey M (2007) First experiences with the collagen-elastin matrix Matriderm as a dermal substitute in severe burn injuries of the hand. Burns 33(3): 364–368

[17] Haslik W, Kamolz LP, Manna F, Hladik M, Rath T, Frey M (2010) Management of full-thickness skin defects in the hand and wrist region: first long-term experiences with the dermal matrix Matriderm. J Plast Reconstr Aesthet Surg 63(2): 360–364

[18] Heimbach D, Luterman A, Burke J, Cram A, Herndon D, Hunt J, Jordan M, McManus W, Solem L, Warden G et al (1988) Artificial dermis for major burns. A multicenter randomized clinical trial. Ann Surg 208(3): 313–320

[19] Heimbach DM, Warden GD, Luterman A, Jordan MH, Ozobia N, Ryan CM, Voigt DW, Hickerson WL, Saffle JR, DeClement FA, Sheridan RL, Dimick AR (2003) Multicenter postapproval clinical trial of Integra dermal regeneration template for burn treatment. J Burn Care Rehabil 24(1): 42–48

[20] Jacobi U, Chen M, Frankowski G, Sinkgraven R, Hund M, Rzany B, Sterry W, Lademann J (2004) In vivo determination of skin surface topography using an optical 3D device. Skin Res Technol 10(4): 207–214

[21] Lamme EN, de Vries HJ, van Veen H, Gabbiani G, Westerhof W, Middelkoop E (1996) Extracellular matrix characterization during healing of full-thickness wounds treated with a collagen/elastin dermal substi-

tute shows improved skin regeneration in pigs. J Histochem Cytochem 44(11): 1311–1322

[22] Oliveira GV, Chinkes D, Mitchell C, Oliveras G, Hawkins HK, Herndon DN (2005) Objective assessment of burn scar vascularity, erythema, pliability, thickness, and planimetry. Dermatol Surg 31(1): 48–58

[23] Ryssel H, Gazyakan E, Germann G, Ohlbauer M (2008) The use of MatriDerm in early excision and simultaneous autologous skin grafting in burns-a pilot study. Burns 34(1): 93–97

[24] Sheridan R, Choucair R, Donelan M, Lydon M, Petras L, Tompkins R (1998) Acellular allodermis in burns surgery: 1-year results of a pilot trial. J Burn Care Rehabil 19(6): 528–530

[25] Sheridan RL, Hegarty M, Tompkins RG, Burke JF (1994) Artificial skin in massive burns – results to ten years. Eur J Plast Surg 17: 91–93

[26] van de Kar AL, Corion LU, Smeulders MJ, Draaijers LJ, van der Horst CM, van Zuijlen PP (2005) Reliable and feasible evaluation of linear scars by the Patient and Observer Scar Assessment Scale. Plast Reconstr Surg 116(2): 514–522

[27] van Zuijlen PP, van Trier AJ, Vloemans JF, Groenevelt F, Kreis RW, Middelkoop E (2000) Graft survival and effectiveness of dermal substitution in burns and reconstructive surgery in a one-stage grafting model. Plast Reconstr Surg 106(3): 615–623

[28] van Zuijlen PP, Vloemans JF, van Trier AJ, Suijker MH, van Unen E, Groenevelt F, Kreis RW, Middelkoop E (2001) Dermal substitution in acute burns and reconstructive surgery: a subjective and objective long-term follow-up. Plast Reconstr Surg 108(7): 1938–1946

[29] van Zuijlen PP, Lamme EN, van Galen MJ, van Marle J, Kreis RW, Middelkoop E (2002) Long-term results of a clinical trial on dermal substitution. A light microscopy and Fourier analysis based evaluation. Burns 28(2): 151–160

[30] Wainwright D, Madden M, Luterman A, Hunt J, Monafo W, Heimbach D, Kagan R, Sittig K, Dimick A, Herndon D (1996) Clinical evaluation of an acellular allograft dermal matrix in full-thickness burns. J Burn Care Rehabil 17(2): 124–136

[31] Wainwright DJ (1995) Use of an acellular allograft dermal matrix (AlloDerm) in the management of full-thickness burns. Burns 21(4): 243–248

[32] Waymack P, Duff RG, Sabolinski M (2000) The effect of a tissue engineered bilayered living skin analog, over meshed split-thickness autografts on the healing of excised burn wounds. The Apligraf Burn Study Group. Burns 26(7): 609–619

Correspondence: E. Middelkoop, Association of Dutch Burn Centers, Postbus 1015q, 1940 EA Beverwijk, The Netherlands, Tel: +31031 251 275 500, Fax: +31031 251 216 059, E-mail: e.middelkoop@vumc.nl

Generation of adipose tissue based on tissue engineering: An overview

Maike Keck[1], David B. Lumenta[1], Lars-Peter Kamolz[1, 2]

[1] Medical University of Vienna, Department of Surgery, Division of Plastic and Reconstructive Surgery, Vienna, Austria
[2] State Hospital Wiener Neustadt, Department of Surgery, Section of Plastic, Aesthetic and Reconstructive Surgery, Wiener Neustadt, Austria

Introduction

Reconstruction of soft tissue is a very common scenario in plastic and reconstructive surgery. In 2008, 4.9 millions of patients had to undergo plastic reconstructive treatment in the USA, 3.8 of those in connection with tumor removal [1]. Apart from that, more than 12.8 millions of cosmetic surgeries were carried out including different forms of soft tissue augmentation with biologic and synthetic filling material and implants [1]. Shortcomings of the conventional plastic-surgical reconstruction of tissue defects i. e. transplanting autologous or allogenic tissue include donor site morbidity in autologous transplants and immunogenicity of allogenic transplants [27, 45, 46, 50]. In addition, the body's own resources are limited so availability is restricted.

Recently, autologous fat transplantation has again become increasingly popular although it has its shortcomings. Healing of grafted tissue depends on how many cells have the possibility to adhere to the vascular system. On the one hand this depends on the vascularity of the recipient site and on the other hand on the size of the grafted tissue. Thus a large tissue defect cannot be simply filled with fat cells, since the cells in the center of the defect would lack a sufficient adherence to the neighboring net of vessels. Other factors that influence the viability of the grafted cells in a negative way include how the fat is obtained, mechanic factors (suction, hypodermic needle, centrifugation) [4, 30, 51, 52] and the applied local anesthetics [32].

Patients with deep burns and eschar down to the fascia, congenital defects following trauma or tumor-resections might benefit from a decent soft tissue replacement treatment [33].

Research in tissue engineering has developed rapidly over the last years and offers alternative strategies for soft tissue augmentation, which might be superior to traditional surgical options. The conventional reparative approach is replaced by a regenerative approach.

"Tissue engineering" means to generate tissue. The principle is either to cultivate living cells outside of the target tissue to then implant them into the same organism (in vitro tissue engineering) or to insert a matrix into an organism to induce the generation of tissue and to restore the proper function of the tissue (in vivo tissue engineering). In both cases a synthetic or biological matrix serves as a scaffold for the desired tissue.

Successful tissue engineering is an interdisciplinary field and is only possible through cooperation of cell-biologists, biochemists, material scientists, engineers and medical scientists. A basic precondition is to understand the different components and their role in generating the target tissue.

For this purpose it is important to know exactly about the functions of adipose tissue and its physiological structure.

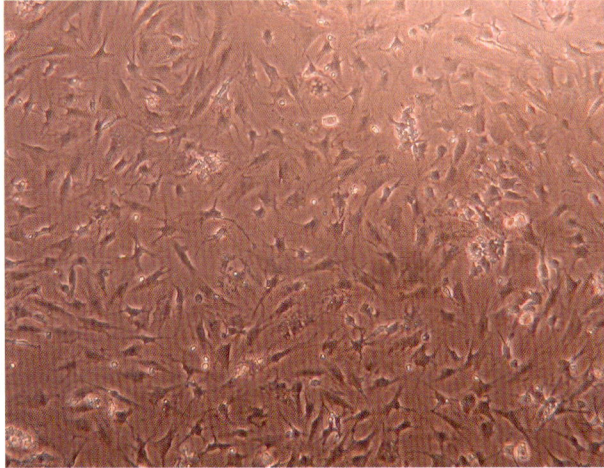

Fig. 1. Preadipocytes after isolation from human adipose tissue and induction. Contrary to ripe adipocytes these spindle-like cells are able to proliferate and differentiate and show a higher tolerance against ischemia. Some cells have already built fat vacuols

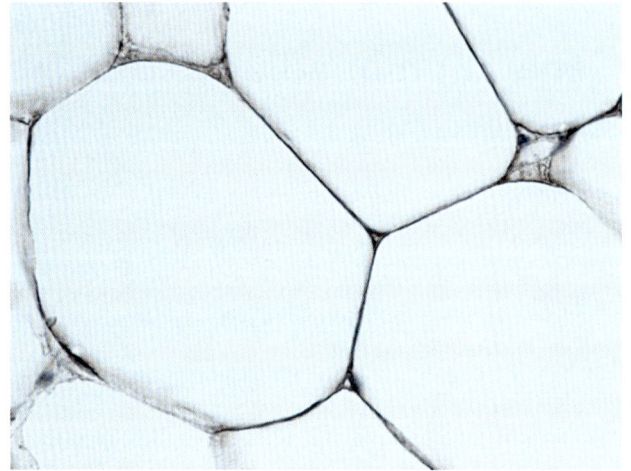

Fig. 2. Preadipocytes sit between ripe adipocytes in the adipose tissue

Physiology of the adipose tissue

Adipose tissue is a special kind of connective tissue that is mainly composed of lipoid cells, the so-called adipocytes. These cells adhere to one another due to collagen fibrils. 90 % of the cytoplasm of adipocytes consists of triglycerides. That is the reason why adipose tissue is the human body's biggest energy storage. Subcutaneous adipose tissue is also responsible for the shape of the human body and serves as structural fat, especially on palms and soles as a mechanic protection (padding). Since fat is a bad heat conductor it contributes to heat insulation in the body. Adipose tissue also fills the space between other kinds of tissue and helps to keep certain organs at their place [28]. Apart from these functions the adipose tissue is one of the most essential endocrinologic organs [60].

There are two different forms of adipose tissue: the white adipose tissue (WAT) whose cells contain a large central fat droplet and small peripheral fat droplets, and the brown adipose tissue (BAT) whose cells contain numerous fat droplets and numerous mitochondria and whose number of cytochromes is responsible for the brownish color of the tissue. During the first years of a human it helps maintain a stable body temperature. In adults nearly all of the adipose tissue is white tissue [28].

Other cells which can be found in adipose tissue are endothelial cells, fibroblasts, blood cells, muscle cells and preadipocytes. Due to their high level of differentiation, adipocytes have only a limited ability to proliferate. The preadipocytes, which sit among the adipocytes in adipose tissue, have an excellent ability to proliferate and differentiate [16] (Figs. 1 and 2). When undifferentiated, these spindle-like cells look similar to fibroblasts [40]. During differentiation to adipocytes, these cells adopt a round shape and in the course start producing vacuoles containing triglycerides [3, 41].

Approaches to generate adipose tissue

There is a vast number of different approaches to generate adipose tissue. The conventional approach is to seed a decent type of cells onto a matrix [42]. In the course the matrix will be either reshaped or reabsorbed. In the meantime the cells start to proliferate and finally differentiate to adipocytes. The success of tissue engineering can be influenced positively by modifying the environmental conditions e. g. by adding growth factors. Generally there are three components that play a major role in the generation of tissue:

1. Scaffold
2. Type of applied cells
3. Environmental conditions for tissue growth (e. g. growth factors)

In the conventional approaches to generate adipose tissue these three factors are constantly being modified.

Scaffolds

Numerous different matrices (Fig. 3) have already been tested in vitro and in vivo for their ability to generate tissue. There are synthetic materials as for example polyethyleneglycoldiacrylates (PEGDA) [2], polyglycolic acids (PGA) [18] and polytetrafluorethylene (PTFE) [35] and natural matrices as for example collagen derivates [21] and hyaluronic acid [25].

The advantage of synthetic scaffolds is that they can be produced uniformly under controlled conditions and that their chemical and physical properties can be modified according to specific needs [3, 5, 19]. The advantage of natural matrices is that they less often cause foreign body reactions.

Modifying the surface of the matrix should cause a better cell adhesion to the matrix. Molecules that support cell adhesion are for example RGD peptides (peptide sequence from amino acids arginine (R), glycine (G) and aspartic acid (D)) [17, 24, 42] and laminin and fibronectin binding peptides (YIGSR) [3, 39, 41].

Apart from their chemical composition, the mechanic properties of the scaffold also play a vital role. These should be as similar as possible to the target tissue. When generating adipose tissue in order to restore the original shape of the body, the matrix should be so flexible that it can assimilate to the present shape. Not only the shape but also the texture of the generated tissue should be as similar as possible to the adipose tissue. In an ideal case, the matrix sets the desired shape and finally reabsorbs completely while building the target tissue [5]. The shape of the matrices that have been used so far reaches from porous sponges and plates to polymeric cylinders.

The pore size of the scaffold also plays an important role. The pores of a matrix offer the cells a large surface to grow into and to proliferate. They need to be large enough to not inhibit the cells' proliferation

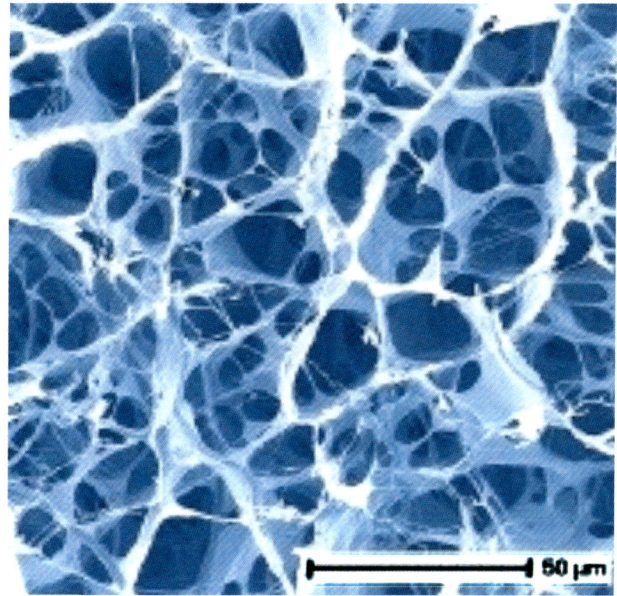

Fig. 3. Example of a matrix: Matriderm ® The matrix serves as a basic scaffold for cuiltivated cells. Apart from its chemical composition the mechanical properties of the matrix play an important role

and to offer enough space for the preadipocytes which will grow in size during differentiation [7, 12, 26, 57, 58].

They also need to supply a basic scaffold where cells can grow until they become a tight tissue (Fig. 4).

As the shape of the matrix determines the later application of the generated tissue, the idea of injectable matrices developed. In gel alone preadipocytes and adipocytes show only restricted performance since they lack an adequate surface for cell adhesion. For this reason Burg et al. developed microparticles which are surrounded by a hydrogel and thus can be injected. The microparticles supply the matrix to which the preadipocytes need to grow in. It could be shown that the different composition of these microparticles (including porous gelsponges, polyactidmatrices) influenced cell adhesion, gene expression and lipid formation of the preadipocytes [9]. In animal testing it could be shown too that the combination of microparticles and gel is suitable to generate adipose tissue [6].

Another method is the use of fragmented omentum. The omentum is a tissue that is well supplied with blood and mainly consists of fat cells and thus

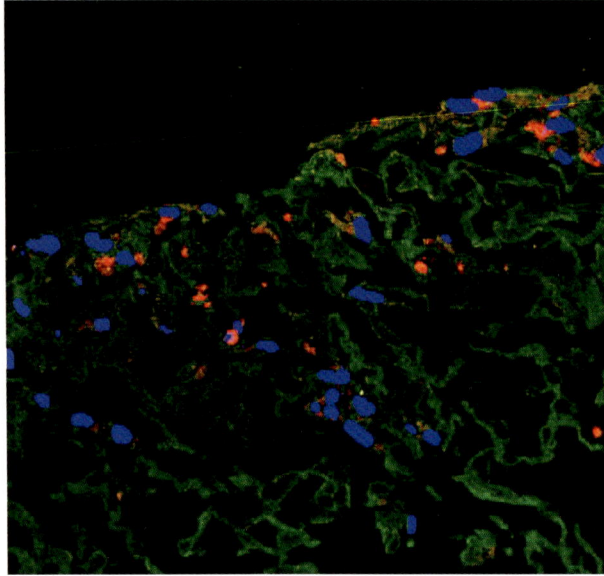

Fig. 4. Preadipocytes on a collagen matrix.
Immunofluorescence staining with DAPI (40,60 -diamidino-2-phenylindole) and preadipocytefactor-1-AK (Pref-1). Cores are blue, matrix green and the cystol of the preadipocytes red due to preadipocytefactor-1-AK. Image via konfocal lasermicroscope (40-fold enlargement)

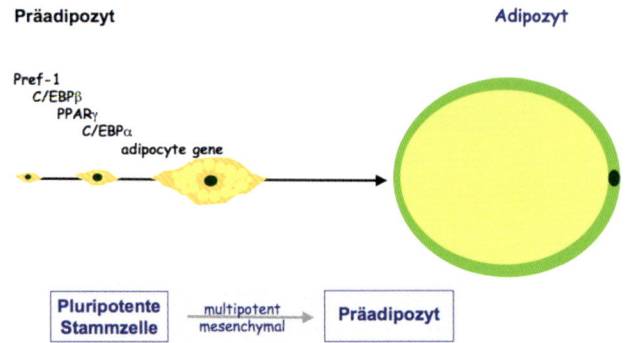

Fig. 5. Differentiation from preadipocyte to adipocyte

offers ideal conditions for tissue engineering. Masude et al. enriched fragmented omentum with preadipocytes and implanted it to mice. Results suggested that the omentum with preadipocytes could generate adipose tissue at the implantation site [38].

An entirely different approach to generate adipose tissue is to stimulate the migration of predipocytes to a certain site. In this approach cells are not supplied from outside but preadipocytes that already exist in the tissue are used to generate tissue. After injecting Matrigel in combination with basic fibroblast growth factor in mice, generation of fat pads could be observed at the injection site. This de novo adipogenesis is most likely due to the migration of preadipocytes and endothelial cells [31, 34, 53, 56].

Masuda et al. used photocured styrenated microspheres on a gelatine basis in combination with insulin and insulin-like growth factor to stimulate angiogenesis and adipogenesis [38]. After in vivo implantation generation of adipose tissue could be observed. Nevertheless, this method is still not sufficiently investigated and needs further optimizing.

Cells

Sort and origin of those cells that are being used for generating tissue comply with the structure that needs to be replaced. The cells need to show sufficient ability to proliferate and differentiate, need to be easily available and need to be obtained by rather simple techniques.

Preadipocytes

Preadiopcytes are ideal cells to cultivate adipose tissue. These multipotent stem cells from the adipogenetic cell line sit in the adipose tissue among ripe adipocytes and are – contrary to those – able to proliferate and differentiate (Fig. 5). They show a higher tolerance against ischemia than ripe fat cells do [58]. Preadipocytes are relatively easily available and can be easily harvested as they sit in subcutaneous depots. Preadipocytes can be harvested via liposuction or abdominal plastic, thus they are the kind of cells that are most commonly used in generating adipose tissue.

At present there is no clear distinction between preadipocytes and adult mesenchymal stem cells. The characteristic of preadipocytes is that they differentiate spontaneously towards adipocytes. They are not able to differentiate to other sorts of cells as for example chondrocytes or osteoblasts. Apart from that preadipocytes lose their ability to differentiate after some in vitro cycles. Despite of various promising research projects in this field it is still unknown if their ability to proliferate in vitro is sufficient to generate enough tissue for large soft tissue defects [11, 43].

Human embryonic stem cells

The reason for the huge scientific interest in stem cells is due to their ability to either split endlessly when in an undifferentiated state (potential to proliferate) or to differentiate into any type of cell of three blastodermic layers. According to how many different differentiated types of cells develop from one stem cell, the stem cells are called unipotent (ability to differentiate into one type of cell), multipotent (ability to differentiate into more types of cells of one blastodermic layer) or pluripotent (ability to differentiate into types of cells of more blastodermic layers) [46].

Basically, embryonic stem cells are distinguished from adult stem cells. Embryonic stem cells derive from the inner part of the blastocyst. Embryonic stem cells are omni- or totipotent thus can be used to develop any known form of basic tissue. After isolating the embryonic stem cells from the inner part of the blastocyst, the cells are cultivated on a culture medium. By adding embryonic mouse fibroblasts differentiation of the human embryonic stem cells will be inhibited. As soon as the human embryonic stem cells become adhesive they differentiate spontaneously. Being able to cultivate any type of tissue out of embryonic stem cells makes it possible to cultivate tissue that cannot be grafted and additionally can be used to test new medicaments.

Human embryonic stem cells are pluripotent stem cells and therefore have big potential in the field of tissue engineering.

There are still some problems to solve though before human embryonic stem cells can be used in a clinical setting. The use of human embryonic stem cells is also problematic from an ethical or religious point of view.

In Germany at present the isolation and usage of human embryonic germline cells for scientific purposes is only permitted when they are harvested from aborted or spontaneously aborted foetuses. Isolating human embryonic stem cells from in vitro fertilized blastocytes is prohibited in Germany. Since July 2002, however, it is possible to import and use human embryonic stem cell lines, which were cultivated before 01. 01. 2002, after applying for a special permission. For this purpose it must be granted that isolation of these stem cell lines was carried out in accordance with the legal situation in the original country [46].

That is the reason why in clinical settings there are only used autologous human stem cells [15, 23, 55, 62, 63].

Human adult stem cells

Contrary to embryonic stem cells, adult or mesenchymal stem cells derive from differentiated tissue of the postnatal organism. It could be observed that a pool of little differentiated cells stays in the postnatal organism, which spread to the organ tissue and seem to serve physiologic tissue generation. These multipotent stem cells are able to differentiate to adipocytes, fibroblasts, osteoblasts and chondroblasts for example. Thus these cells are also very promising for tissue engineering [8, 10, 20, 62, 63].

Adult stem cells can be isolated from bone marrow and adipose tissue. The bone marrow supplies for example haematopoetic stem cells which are probably the most popular group of mesenchymal stem cells. The bone marrow's mesenchymal stem cells sit in its stroma. Isolation and proliferation of the obtained stem cells is relatively easy. For the patient though obtaining bone marrow is an extremely unpleasant intervention [16].

Mesenchymal stem cells which have been harvested from adipose tissue show striking phenotypical and morphological similarities to stem cells obtained from bone marrow. They are also multipotent and have various mutual surface markers with the cells obtained from bone marrow.

Latest research showed that adipose tissue consists of 5000 adult mesenchymal stem cells per gram thus having the highest density of stem cells. Von Heimburg et al. showed that they were able to isolate considerably more mesenchymal stem cells from liposuctioned fat than from excised adipose tissue (350,000 cells per g adipose tissue) [57]. Other advantages are good availability and very simple harvesting via liposuction. Isolation of the cells from the adipose tissue happens through digestion supported by a collagen solution, repeated filtration and centrifugation. The cell fraction in the remaining cell pellet is subsequently cultivated and proliferation or differentiation is stimulated [13, 48, 49, 59]. It must be considered though that depending on age, sex and localisation, adipose tissue can show different endocrinologic activity, which can affect the proliferation and differentiation performance of the harvested stem cells [22, 54].

Growth factors

Applying decent growth factors can support the transformation of the cell-matrix construct to adipose tissue. There are two different methods of applying growth factors: in vitro and in vivo. In the in vitro method it is necessary to add certain growth factors as for example glucocorticoides and insulin to achieve a differentiation of the mesenchymal stem cells. In the in vivo method, applying them is only optional and might accelerate the transformation of the cell-matrix construct to adipose tissue. It could be shown that glucocorticoids, thyroid hormons, transforming growth factor β, epidermal growth factor and platelet-derived growth factor might have positive effects on the adipogenesis. In the in vitro method adding the aforementioned growth factors in a medium accelerates the differentiation of the preadipocytes into adipocytes. In the in vivo method they can have favorable effects on the transformation of the tissue constructs to ripe adipose tissue [14, 29, 31, 36, 61].

Apart from the adipogenesis, growth factors can be used to support angiogenesis. A decisive factor for the vitality of an ex vivo generated bioimplant is a rapid adhesion to the tissue net on the grafted site. To support the angiogenesis and to maintain a rapid vascularisation of the bioimplant, growth factors as for example VEGF can be used.

Conclusion

First research results in the field of regenerative medicine are very promising and are already applied in clinical practice. Regenerative medicine is a new dimension in the medical science and might be increasing the scope of conventional surgical methods. However, intensive research is still required to let these methods become part of the clinical day to day practice.

It is necessary to analyze and observe the risks of applying post natal stem cells (e. g. tumorgenity, infection vector). Concerning embryonic stem cells, ethical and religious questions should not be ignored.

References

[1] 2009 American Society of Plastic Surgeons Statistics. Available from: www.plasticsurgery.org

[2] Alhadlaq A, Tang M, Mao JJ (2005) Engineered adipose tissue from human mesenchymal stem cells maintains predefined shape and dimension: implications in soft tissue augmentation and reconstruction. Tissue Eng 11 (3–4): 556–566

[3] Beahm EK, Walton RL, Patrick Jr CW (2003) Progress in adipose tissue construct development. Clin Plast Surg 30 (4): 547–558

[4] Boschert MT, Beckert BW, Puckett ChL, Concannon MJ (2002) Analysis of lipocyte viability after liposuction. Plast Reconstr Surg 109: 761–765

[5] Burg KJ, Holder WD, Culberson CR, Beiler RJ, Greene KG, A. B. Loebsack AB et al (1999) Parameters affecting cellular adhesion to polylactide films. J Biomater Sci Polym Ed 10 (2): 147–161

[6] Burg KJ, Boland T (2003) Minimally invasive tissue engineering composites and cell printing. IEEE Eng Med Biol Mag 22 (5): 84–91

[7] Butterwith SC (1994) Molecular events in adipocyte development. Pharmacol Ther 61 (3): 399–411

[8] Cao Y, Sun Z, Liao L, Meng Y, Han Q, Zhao RC (2005) Human adipose tissue-derived stem cells differentiate into endothelial cells in vitro and improve postnatal neovascularization in vivo. Biochem Biophys Res Commun 332 (2): 370–379

[9] Cavin AN, Ellis SE, Burg KJL (2005) Adipocyte response to injectable breast tissue engineering scaffolds. In: Transactions of the 30 th annual meeting of the Society for Biomaterials, Memphis, TN

[10] Choi YS, Park SN, Suh H (2005) Adipose tissue engineering using mesenchymal stem cells attached to injectable PLGA spheres. Biomaterials 26 (29): 5855–5863

[11] Coleman SR, Saboeiro A (2007) Fat grafting to the breast revisited: safety and efficacy. Ann Plast Surg 119(3): 775–785

[12] Cornelius P, MacDougald OA, Lane MD (1994) Regulation of adipocyte development. Annu Rev Nutr 14: 99–129

[13] Cowan C, Shi Y, Aalami O et al (2004) Adipose-derived adult stromal cells heal critical-size mouse calvarial defects. Nat Biotechnol 22(5): 560–567

[14] Croissandeau G, Chretien M, Mbikay M (2002) Involvement of matrix metalloproteinases in the adipose conversion of 3T3-L1 preadipocytes, Biochem J 364 (Part 3): 739–746

[15] De Bari C, Dell Accio F, Luyten FP (2004) Failure of in vitro-differentiated mesenchymal stem cells from the synovial membrane to form ectopic stable cartilage in vivo. Arthritis Rheum 50: 142–150

[16] De Ugarte DA, Ashjian PH, Elbarbary A, Hedrick MH (2003) Future of fat as raw material for tissue regeneration, Ann Plast Surg 50 (2): 215–219

[17] Eiselt P, Yeh J, Latvala RK, Shea LD, Mooney DJ (2000) Porous carriers for biomedical applications based on alginate hydrogels. Biomaterials 21 (19): 1921–1927

[18] Fischbach C, Spruss T, Weiser B, Neubauer M, Becker C, Hacker M et al (2004) Generation of mature fat pads in vitro and in vivo utilizing 3-D long-term culture of 3T3-L1 preadipocytes. Exp Cell Res 300 (1): 54–64

[19] Fuchs JR, Nasseri BA, Vacanti JP (2001) Tissue engineering: a 21st century solution to surgical reconstruction. Ann Thorac Surg 72 (2): 577–591

[20] Gabbay JS, Heller JB, Mitchell SA, Zuk PA, Spoon DB, Wasson KL, Jarrahy R, Benhaim P, Bradley JP (2006) Osteogenic potentiation of human adipose-derived stem cells in a 3-dimensional matrix. Ann Plast Surg 57(1): 89–93

[21] Gentleman E, Nauman EA, Livesay GA, Dee KC (2006) Collagen composite biomaterials resist contraction while allowing development of adipocytic soft tissue in vitro. Tissue Eng 12 (6): 1639–1649

[22] Giorgino F, Laviola L, Eriksson JW (2005) Regional differences of insulin action in adipose tissue: insights from in vivo and in vitro studies. Acta Physiol Scand 183 (1): 13–30

[23] Goessler UR, Hörmann K, Riedel F (2005) Adult stem cells in plastic reconstructive surgery. Int J Mol Med 15: 899–905

[24] Halberstadt C, Austin C, Rowley J, Culberson C, Loebsack A, Wyatt S et al (2002) A hydrogel material for plastic and reconstructive applications injected into the subcutaneous space of a sheep. Tissue Eng 8 (2): 309–319

[25] Halbleib M, Skurk T de Luca C, von Heimburg D, Hauner H (2003) Tissue engineering of white adipose tissue using hyaluronic acid-based scaffolds. I: in vitro differentiation of human adipocyte precursor cells on scaffolds. Biomaterials 24 (18): 3125–3132

[26] Hemmrich K, von Heimburg D, Rendchen R, Di Bartolo C, Milella E, Pallua N (2005) Implantation of preadipocyte-loaded hyaluronic acid-based scaffolds into nude mice to evaluate potential for soft tissue engineering. Biomaterials 26 (34): 7025–7037

[27] Hurvitz KA, Kobayashi M, Evans GR (2006) Current options in head and neck reconstruction. Plast Reconstr Surg 118: 122e–133e

[28] Junqueira LC, Carneiro J, Gratzl M (2005) Fettgewebe In: Histologie. Springer, Berlin Heidelberg, S 75–80

[29] Katz AJ, Llull R, Hedrick MH, Futrell JW (1999) Emerging approaches to the tissue engineering of fat. Clin Plast Surg 26 (4): 587–603

[30] Kaufman MR, Bradley JP, Dickinson B et al (2007) Autologous fat transfer national consensus survey: trends in techniques for harvest, preparation, and application, and perception of short- and long-term results. Plast Reconstr Surg 119(1): 323–331

[31] Kawaguchi N, Toriyama K, Nicodemou-Lena E, Inou K, Torii S, Kitagawa Y (1998) De novo adipogenesis in mice at the site of injection of basement membrane and basic fibroblast growth factor. Proc Natl Acad Sci USA 95 (3): 1062–1066

[32] Keck M, Janke J, Ueberreiter K (2007) The influence of different local anaesthetics on the viability of preadipocytes. Handchir Mikrochir Plast Chir 39(3): 215–9

[33] Keck M, Haluza D, Burjak S, Eisenbock B, Kamolz L P, Frey M(2009) Cultivation of keratinocytes and preadipocytes on a collagen-elastin scaffold (Matriderm®): First results of an in vitro study. Eur Surg 41/4: 189–193

[34] Kimura Y, Ozeki M, Inamoto T, Tabata Y (2002) Time course of de novo adipogenesis in matrigel by gelatin microspheres incorporating basic fibroblast growth factor. Tissue Eng 8 (4): 603–613

[35] Kral JG, Crandall DL (1999) Development of a human adipocyte synthetic polymer scaffold. Plast Reconstr Surg 104 (6): 1732–1738

[36] Mandrup S, Lane MD (1997) Regulating adipogenesis. J Biol Chem 272(9): 5367–5370

[37] Masuda T, Furue M, Matsuda T (2004) Novel strategy for soft tissue augmentation based on transplantation of fragmented omentum and preadipocytes. Tissue Eng 10 (11–12): 1672–1683

[38] Masuda T, Furue M, Matsuda T (2004) Photocured, styrenated gelatin-based microspheres for de novo adipogenesis through corelease of basic fibroblast growth factor, insulin, and insulin-like growth factor I. Tissue Eng 10 (3–4): 523–535

[39] Patel PN, Gobin AS, West JL, Patrick Jr CW (2005) Poly(ethylene glycol) hydrogel system supports preadipocyte viability, adhesion, and proliferation. Tissue Eng 11 (9–10): 1498–1505

[40] Patrick CW, Mikos AG, McIntire LV (1998) Frontiers in tissue engineering, 1st edn. Pergamon, Oxford, UK and New York

[41] Patrick Jr CW (2000) Adipose tissue engineering: the future of breast and soft tissue reconstruction following tumor resection. Semin Surg Oncol 19 (3): 302–311

[42] Patrick Jr CW (2001) Tissue-engineering strategies for adipose tissue repair. Anat Rec 263 (4): 361–366

[43] Patrick CW Jr, Uthamanthil R, Beahm E, Frye C (2008) Animal models for adipose tissue engineering. Tissue Eng Part B Rev 14(2): 167–178

[44] Riedel F, Hormann K (2005) Plastic surgery of skin defects in the face – principles and perspectives. HNO 53: 1020–1036

[45] Riedel F, Reinhart Goessler U, Grupp S, Bran G, Hörmann K, Verse T (2006) Management of radiation-induced tracheocutaneous tissue defects by transplantation of an ear cartilage graft and deltopectoral flap. Auris Nasus Larynx 33(1): 79–84

[46] Riedel F, Goessler UR, Stern-Straeter J, Riedel K, Hörmann K (2008) Regenerative medicine in head and neck reconstructive surgery. HNO 56(3): 262–274

[47] Rowley JA, Madlambayan G, Mooney DJ (1999) Alginate hydrogels as synthetic extracellular matrix materials. Biomaterials 20 (1): 45–53

[48] Rubin JP, Bennett JM, Doctor JS, Tebbets BM, Marra KG (2007) Collagenous microbeads as a scaffold for tissue Engineering with adipose-derived stem cells. Plast Reconstr Surg 120(2): 414–424

[49] Schipper BM, Marra KG, Zhang W, Donnenberg AD, Rubin JP(2008) Regional anatomic and age effects on cell function of human adipose-derived stem cells. Ann Plast Surg 60(5): 583–544

[50] Shenaq SM, Yuksel E (2002) New research in breast reconstruction: adipose tissue engineering. Clin Plast Surg 29 (1): 111–125

[51] Shiffman MA, Mirrafati S (2001) Fat transfer techniques: The effect of harvest and transfer methods on adipocyte viability and review of the literature. Dermatol Surg 27(9): 819–826

[52] Smith P, Adams WP, Lipschitz, AH et al (2006) Autologous human fat grafting: effect of harvesting and preparation techniques on adipocyte graft survival. Plast Reconstr Surg 117(6): 1836–1844

[53] Tabata Y, Miyao M, Inamoto T, Ishii T, Hirano Y, Yamaoki Y, et al (2000) De novo formation of adipose tissue by controlled release of basic fibroblast growth factor. Tissue Eng 6(3): 279–289

[54] Tholpady SS, Llull R, Ogle RC, Rubin JP, Futrell JW, Katz AJ (2006) Adipose tissue: stem cells and beyond. Clin Plast Surg 33(1): 55–62

[55] Toma JG, Akhavan M, Fernandes KJ et al (2001) Isolation of multipotent adult stem cells from the dermis of mammalian skin. Nat Cell Biol 3: 778–784

[56] Toriyama K, Kawaguchi N, Kitoh J, Tajima R, Inou K, Kitagawa Y et al (2002) Endogenous adipocyte precursor cells for regenerative soft-tissue engineering. Tissue Eng 8(1): 157–165

[57] von Heimburg D, Serov G, Oepen T, Pallua N (2003) Fat tissue engineering. In: Ashammakhi N, Ferretti P (eds) Topics in Tissue Engineering. Chapter 8: 1–16

[58] Von Heimburg D, Kuberka M, Rendchen R, Hemmrich K, Rau G, Pallua N (2003) Preadipocyte-loaded collagen scaffolds with enlarged pore size for improved soft tissue engineering. Int J Artif Organs 26 (12): 1064–1076

[59] Wei Y, Hu Y, Lv R, Li D(2006) Regulation of adipose-derived adult stem cells differentiating into chondrocytes with the use of rhBMP-2. Cytotherapy 8(6): 570–579

[60] Wozniak SE, Gee LL, Wachtel MS, Frezza EE (2009) Adipose tissue: the new endocrine organ? A review article. Dig Dis Sci 54(9): 1847–1856

[61] Yuksel E, Weinfeld AB, Cleek R, Waugh JM, Jensen J, Boutros S et al (2000) De novo adipose tissue generation through long-term, local delivery of insulin and insulin-like growth factor-1 by PLGA/PEG microshperes in an in vivo rat model: a novel concept and capability. Plast Reconstr Surg 105: 1721–1729

[62] Zuk PA, Zhu M, Mizuno H et al (2001) Multilineage cells from human adipose tissue: implications for cell-based therapies. Tissue Eng 7: 211–228

[63] Zuk PA, Zhu M, Ashjian P, De Ugarte DA, Huang JI, Mizuno H et al (2002) Human adipose tissue is a source of multipotent stem cells. Mol Biol Cell 13 (12): 4279–4295

Correspondence: Lars-Peter Kamolz, M.D., Ph.D., M.Sc., Medical University of Vienna, Department of Surgery, Division of Plastic and Reconstructive Surgery, Vienna, Austria, E-mail: kamolz@plastchirurg.info

Burn reconstruction
(Specific regions)

Burn reconstruction: Neck region

Norbert Pallua, Erhan Demir

Department of Plastic Surgery and Hand Surgery, Burn Center, University Hospital RWTH Aachen,
Aachen University of Technology, Aachen, Germany

Part I – Basic principles

Introduction

The cervical region with its functional and anatomical design to achieve a maximum range of motion is of eminent importance. The anatomic prone interposition of the neck between the corpus and the head represents great challenges and opportunities. Therefore, the reconstructive surgeon is confronted with a unique set of problems compared with the rest of the body. The thin pliable neck is prone to contracture formation. It is important to emphasize that burn scar contractures of the neck region have an impact on facial deformities and may cause considerable problems especially in the developing period of young burn victims [1, 2].

The success in treatment requires sound surgical judgment, technical expertise in combination with a thorough understanding of the pathophysiology of the burn wound, scarring, neck contracture formation and the alteration of skin texture and pigmentation. Realistic expectations of both parts patients and surgeons are crucial to achieve and value successful treatment outcomes. Still, profound functional and aesthetic improvement of the neck region for this large group of challenging patients is possible [3].

The requirement of a well-functioning and extensive team in the approach to reconstructive head and neck surgery cannot be overemphasized [4]. Therefore, in addition to the plastic surgeon many disciplines such as skilled burn nursing, experienced occupational and physical therapy, and psychological and social support systems are required to successfully treat and care for patients with burns of the neck. The care of a patient from the onset of a major burn involving the head and neck to a successful reconstructive outcome requires skill, patience, determination, and enthusiasm from all who are involved [1].

Pathogenesis and associated problems of neck contractures

The skin of the neck is thin and pliable and highly flexible; it is prone to contracture formation following deep burns with tissue damage and scarring. While superficial second-degree burns usually heal without scars or pigment changes, still some completely epithelialized "medium-thickness" superficial burns may demonstrate long-term changes in skin texture and pigmentation. Deep second-degree burns in the neck region usually require surgical intervention with tangential excision and skin-grafting or the use of biological membranes (Biobrane® or Suprathel®). After the initial healing with wound closure and complete epithelialization these patients require careful management and monitoring, as they have the potential to develop severe late hypertrophic scars and contractures. Additional pre-

191

ventive perioperative measures after surgery include the immediate application of neck extension casts.

The pathologic process of wound contracture involves contraction of tissue by myofibroblasts until the limits of neck motion are reached. Wound contracture occurs during scar remodeling as collagen undergoes reorganization. The resulting distortion may be either extrinsic or intrinsic. Extrinsic contractures result from shrinking of adjacent tissues, whereas intrinsic contractures result from direct contracture of the affected region. Extrinsic contractures require release; intrinsic contractures require replacement of tissue.

Full-thickness injuries are usually excised and skin grafted. Any tension on the neck region may promote early hypertrophic scarring. Relief of neck tension requires either focal release with z-plasties or extensive adhesiolysis and defect coverage with flaps [1, 5].

At first signs or any tendency towards hypertrophic scarring and contracture formation of skin grafts, ancillary modalities such as compression garments or silicon pressure treatment need to be carried out.

Patients with neck contractures are confronted with several problems. Burn scar contractures not only affect neck movements but also face function as traction forces may pull the chin, cheeks and lower lip caudally or by tension through either normal or scarred cheek skin pulling down the lower eyelids. Increased tension in facial scars caused by burn contractures of the neck can create increases in the size, thickness and contracture of hypertrophic scars of the face.

In the developing child considerable problems, including flexion deformity with restricted extension, lateral flexion and rotation, aching of muscle and vertebral joints eventually with compensatory kyphosis posture, growth disturbances of the spine, incomplete oral occlusion with drooling of saliva, airway problems and dental imbalance with severe permanent damage due to neck contractures are well-documented [5, 6].

In addition to pure physical problems studies clearly indicate that children with extensive head and neck scarring from burns may have temporarily or permanently alterations in their process of psychological growth and development [7].

Evaluation and classification of burn related neck deformities

In 1958 Kirschbaum reported about Spina's classification of neck contractures into central, lateral or complete [8]. Later Achauer classified anterior neck contractures into mild, moderate, extensive and severe depending on the fraction of the anterior part of the neck involved in the contracting band [9].

A classification in three main groups of neck contractures (severe, moderate and mild) defined by the degree of involvement and functional deformity has been described by Remensnyder und Donelan in 2002 [5].

The classification proposed by Remensnyder und Donelan is very useful while reviewing and analyzing patients, as the degree of involvement and functional deformity is described very precisely by the abnormal joining up of various anatomical areas. During the assembly of an individual surgical treatment plan for mentosternal contractures, the Achau-

Table 1. Achauer classification of anterior neck contractures

Achauer classification of anterior neck contractures	
I – mild defect	Scar band which involves less than ⅓ of the anterior surface of the neck
II – moderate defect	More than ⅓ but less than ⅔ of the anterior surface involved
III – severe defect	Greater than ⅔ of the anterior surface of the neck
IV – extensive defect	A mentosternal adhesion

Table 2. Classification of cervical burn contractures by Remensnyder und Donelan (2002)

1. Severe neck contractures	
a.	Labio-sternal
b.	Mento-sternal
2. Moderate neck contractures	
a.	Cervico-sternal
b.	Heavy multiple bands
c.	Upper neck involvement exclusively
3. Mild neck contractures	
a.	Discrete linear bands
b.	Isolated cervical scars

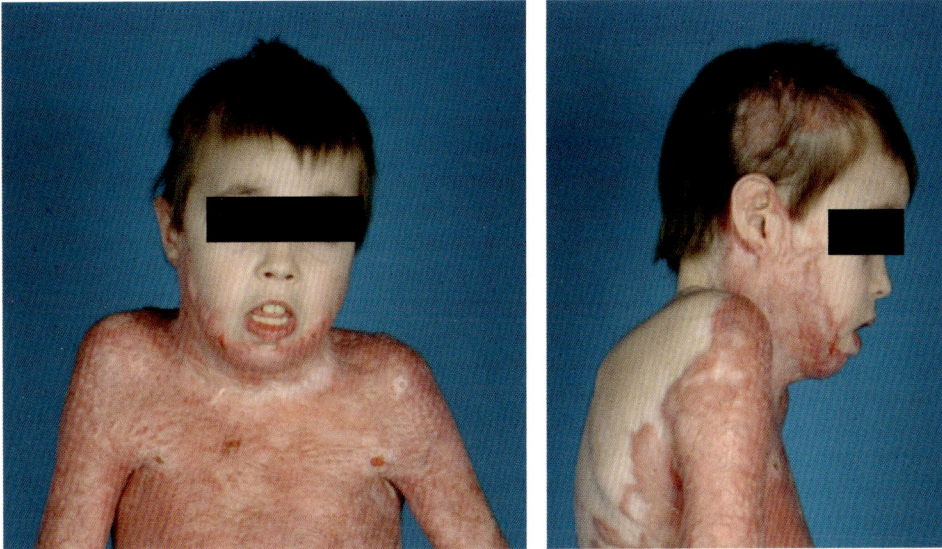

Fig. 1. Severe neck contracture

er classification describes the extent of the anterior neck defect after surgical release very well and is therefore of eminent practical use.

Case samples

Especially in the group with *severe neck contractures* the functional impairment is a very distressing problem, with the burn scar extending directly from the lower lip down to the sternum. The head is uncomfortably fixed in a caudal position to the chest with the mandible involved in all cases. The severe flexed position limits any head and neck movements to a certain degree. You may notice that these patients tend to walk around with their mouths constantly open to reduce the tension of the contracture (Fig. 1).

Moderate neck contractures cause discomfort and reduced neck movements with some degree of limitations in the lower facial features (Fig. 2).

Mild contractures with isolated scars create discomfort with a minor degree of tension on the lower face.

Prevention, non-surgical treatment modalities and adjunct surgical procedures

In the treatment of burn patients the development of hypertrophic scarring and contractures belong to the most common and frustrating problems. In the neck region due to the fact that the knowledge of the pathogenesis is still limited to some extent different techniques are used.

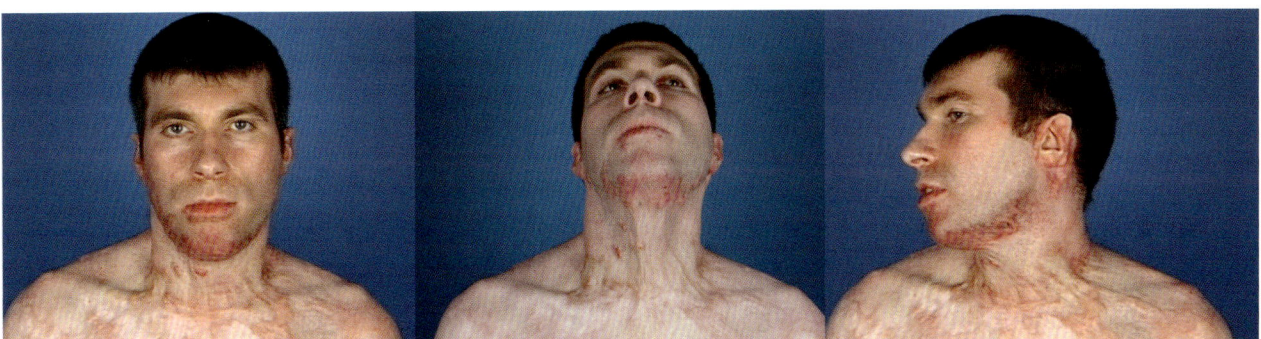

Fig. 2. Moderate neck contracture with multiple bands

Non-surgical management options include massage, hydrotherapy, ultrasound therapy or adhesive tapes. However, the two most commonly accepted non-invasive therapies without major side effects are topical silicone gel application and pressure therapy. Different studies have demonstrated that the silicone gel sheeting is a safe and effective option in the management of hypertrophic scars. Pressure therapy is essential in the treatment of neck burns and is recommended as a "first line therapy" even if scientific evidence of its efficacy is limited.

Useful *invasive strategies* such as laser therapy, radiotherapy, cryotherapy, high pressure steroid injections, application of cytokines such as TGF-ß or Interferon –Alpha-2b are most commonly used [10].

Part II – Surgical reconstruction of neck contractures

Indications

Neck contractures with functional and aesthetic deficits, drooling, dental deterioration, folliculitis, significant deformity and obstacle for intubation for general anesthesia are indications to reconstruct the neck region [11]. Severe neck flexion contractures on the acute phase often require early reconstruction to aid in airway management. Neck contractures should usually be managed prior to carrying out facial burn reconstruction. Due to the extrinsic contractile forces from the neck any facial deformity may adversely affect the maturation of facial scars [1].

Reconstructive options and guidelines

In comparison to burn injuries of the face with distorting features, proportions and expression, thermal injuries of the neck region result rather in functional impairments than aesthetic alterations. They require careful strategic planning in which different reconstructive options are analyzed and areas with distortion of neck features, displaced mobile structures and compression of soft tissue contours requiring reconstructive surgery are carefully prioritized [9]. However, major deformities of patients with various forms of neck contractures caused by burns may limit both neck and jaw mobility and may also influ-

ence and increase facial deformities. In order to achieve optimal correction of burned facial deformities of patients who have scarring of both the face and neck, it is necessary to correct the neck contracture first in order to attain the best possible result of successful facial reconstruction [5].

Ignoring these principles may result in iatrogenic failures and catastrophes during the process of reconstructive surgery of the head and neck following thermal injuries.

Many surgical approaches with varying success for the treatment of neck contractures or facial resurfacing following burns are favored including skin grafting, Z-plasties, a variety of local skin flaps with or without expansion, transferred regional flaps and microsurgical free flaps [11–14]. Generally, to achieve satisfactory functional and aesthetic results, the texture, color and thickness of the flap need to be similar to those of the original tissue [15]. Therefore, the technically most feasible operation is favored if functional and aesthetic results are good and postoperative risks for recurrence remain low.

Mild defects

Mild scar bands can generally be corrected by the use of local flaps or z-plasties. As vertical scars of the neck are likely to produce contractures, the vertical scar is converted to a transverse orientation.

Moderate defects

Local flaps are not useful to correct moderate neck contractures. One option is to consider tissue expansion: unscarred lateral aspects of the neck are expanded and afterwards the adjacent pre-expanded skin is brought into the area of contracture. The lateral skin can be stretched and transposed medially. The lack of hard tissue immediately underneath the expanded skin limits efficiency of expansion procedures in the neck region.

Skin grafting should be avoided if possible. There is a tendency for the transplanted skin to contract as the neck angle does not oppose shrinkage.

Severe and extensive defects

Severe contractures require regional flaps, any types of local flaps are not adequate.

Extensive (mentosternal adhesion) contractures require an extensive surgical release and flap coverage. The importance of an extensive, complete release cannot be overemphasized. The most common error is to do an inadequate release. All contracting bands regardless of the depth require release. This procedure may include strap muscles in depth and the midlateral neck in width. Defect coverage options include regional flaps such as the supraclavicular island flap (SIF-flap) or the trapezius flap as primary options; free flaps remain as second options [2, 17–21].

Skin grafts

Skin grafts after scar release are suitable, but there is a tendency for recurrence of contracture. Therefore, after extensive scar release and thorough hemostasis split thickness skin graft sheets (non-meshed) are placed in transversely oriented fashion. A pressure dressing with foam rubber sponges is applied. It is critical to immobilize the neck for 14 days with a custom made splint [9, 11]. A recurrence rate of 89 % without splinting in comparison to 17 % after splinting is reported [22]. However, skin grafts may work well, but they require the prolonged period of neck immobilization and pressure application, and are often not aesthetically pleasing.

Dermal regenerative templates

For the past several years artificial dermal substitutes have been developed from alloplastic or xenographic materials e. g. AlloDerm®, Integra® or Matriderm® [3, 23, 24].

Following full-thickness excision of scars and the release of contractures utilization of dermal substitutes or dermal regenerative templates such as Integra® or Matriderm® in combination with skin grafts demonstrated some promising results [23, 24].

Yannis and Burke initially described in 1980 the two-layered template composed of semipermeable silicone membrane and biodegradable collagen-glycosaminoglycan matrix [25]. The implanted material has been found to form a layer of parenchymal structures resembling dermis. In the second stage after skin grafting acceptable results of the neck region are possible [26, 27] (Figs. 3–6).

Another template is Matriderm® which contains non-crosslinked bovine collagen types I, III, V and elastine. It is available as 1 mm or 2 mm thick sheets. Good outcomes are recently reported after early excision and Matriderm® application with simultaneous autologous skin grafting in facial burns [24]. However, early experimental results revealed no major differences in engraftment rates or vascularization between Matriderm® and Integra® [23].

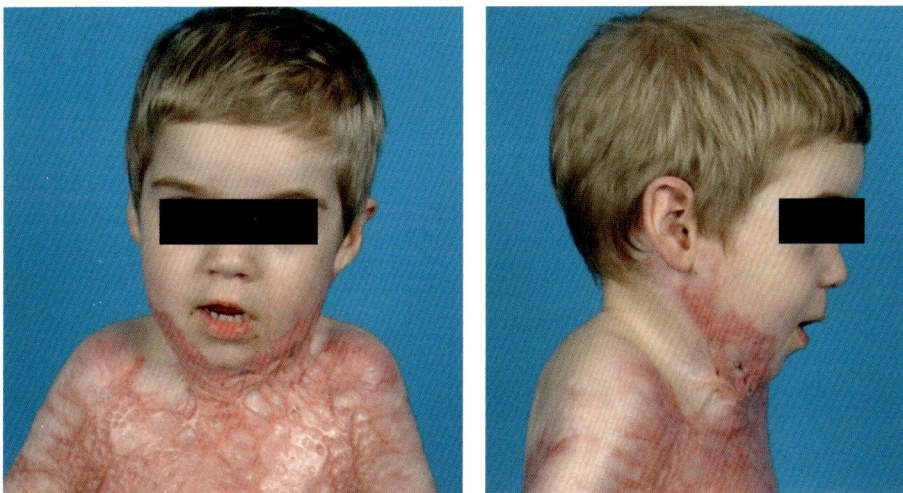

Fig. 3. Severe neck contracture, scheduled for scar release and Integra®-transplantation

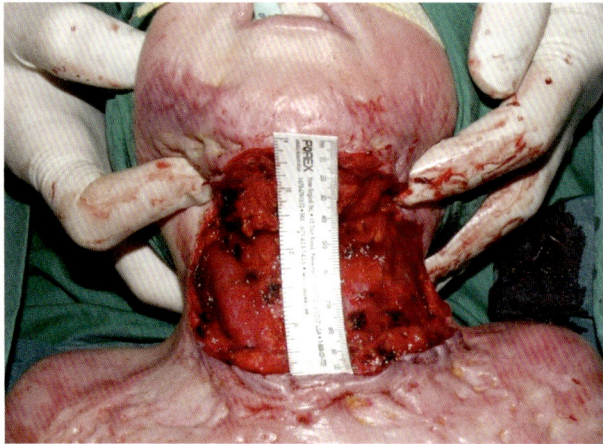

Fig. 4. Scar excision and release

Local flaps

Any type of local tissue without scars might become useful to restore smaller scar bands or contracture of the neck area after mobilization. Unfortunately, nearby tissue is often burnt and unavailable [28].

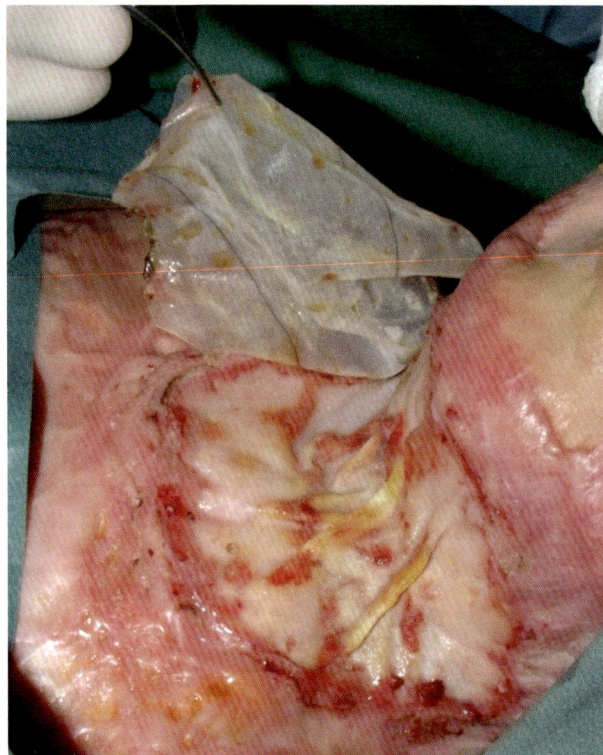

Fig. 5. Integra® transplantation

Any axial skin flap, z-plasty or w-plasty technique is based on the principle of mobilizing a full segment of skin without disturbance of their vascular supplies from an area adjacent to the region to be resurfaced. After scar excision and contracture release the local flaps are interposed in an opposite direction to release the vector of tension [3]. It might be very useful to include the platysma or cervical fascia underneath the transposed flap to secure vascular blood supply. Especially in severe cases with deep burns when z-plasties are performed to release tension bands without the possibility to resurface the neck region with uninjured skin, this technical modification of including muscle or fascia will enhance local flap survival rates.

Tissue expansion

The technique of tissue expansion is based on the dynamic nature in which the integument responds to constant mechanical stress load using an inflatable device system, such as an expander. The neck region is not the primary region for direct application of expanders, in comparison to pre-expanded regional or free flaps, which have a permanent place in the armamentarium of reconstructive burn surgery of the neck region. Tissue expanders should be used with caution in the head and neck region [1]. Stretching adjacent tissue in order to carry out scar excision may result in an increase in tension and can lead to iatrogenic contour changes. However, expansion of the skin and local flap coverage might be useful in smaller defects as tissue expansion offers the chance to replace unstable neck tissue with uninjured normal adjacent tissue. Larger defects usually require regional flaps from distant sites [1, 29–31].

Regional flaps

Extensive, and often recurrent neck flexion contracture with defects larger than two-thirds of the anterior neck require distant tissue and are usually not amenable to local flaps [9]. Regional flaps are the primary choice as they provide full-thickness skin and subcutaneous tissue, with improved aesthetics and superior resurfacing options compared to skin grafts without the need for microsurgery. Fasciocutaneous

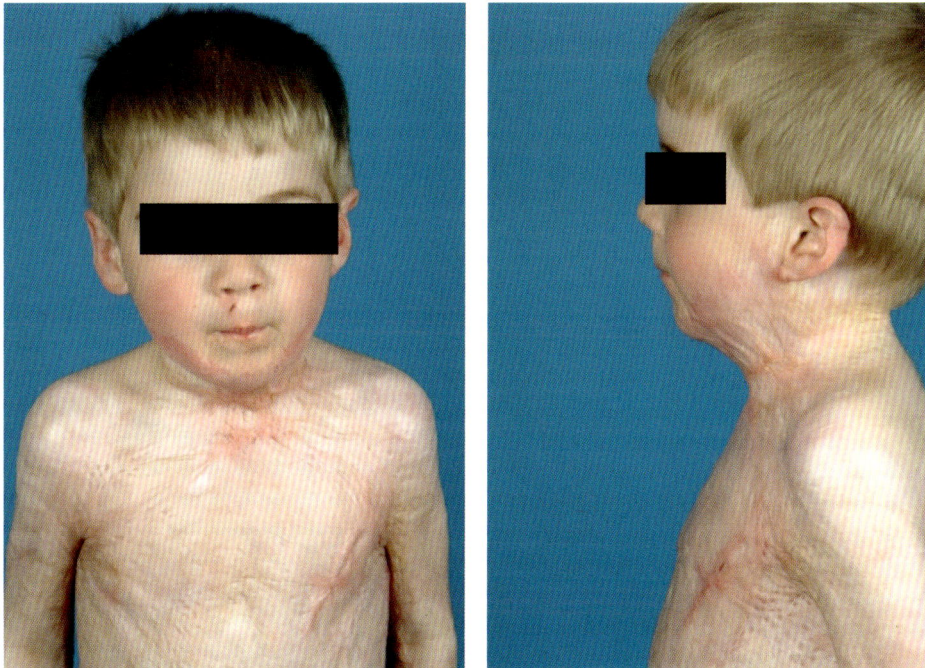

Fig. 6. Temporary sufficient outcome after full-thickness skin graft transplantation on Integra®

flaps are preferred as they are thin, elastic and easily contoured, leading to decreased bulk [2, 32]. Therefore, the first choice is the thin supraclavicular island flap with its good color and texture match of the anterior neck region followed by the myocutaneous trapezius flap or the dorsal scapular island flap if the angiosome of the SIF-flaps is scarred and unavailable [17, 33]. The pre-expansion of flaps allows their thinning and delay prior to transfer will enhance the safety in terms of tissue perfusion [16].

Supraclavicular Island flap (SIF)

A random pattern flap of the supraclavicular region first described by Mutter in 1842 was further modified after closer anatomic examination of the shoulder region angiosome by Lamberty [34, 35]. Anatomically, this supraclavicular axial patterned flap was based on the supraclavicular artery. In 1997 Pallua introduced the supraclavicular artery island flap (SIF) for the release of postburn mentosternal contractures [17]. Modifications have been added to optimize and expand indications in head and neck reconstruction [18]. Further modifications such as flap pre-expansion through tissue expansion resulted in ultra-thin SIF flaps [16].

Adequate planning and flap design needs to respect the aesthetic units of the neck. Mentosternal contractures require dissection up to the borders of the aesthetic units, until the neck is fully released. Deep scars such as collagen tension bands and plates of scar require special attention to create an optimal bed for the flaps and to release facial tensions. Due to the skin laxity a much larger defect than expected will occur after resection and release of severe neck contractures. The defect sizes after mentosternal scar excisions may reach dimensions of 12 cm × 21 cm up to 15 cm × 26 cm.

The supraclavicular vessels arise from the superficial transverse cervical artery, beneath or lateral to the posterior part of the omohyoid muscle. During the flap elevation from its lateral to its medial portion, skin and subcutaneous tissue are elevated en bloc with the axially running supraclavicular pedicle. In prefabricated flaps the tissue expander will be removed prior to flap preparation. After dissection of the medial portion the complete flap is mobile on its vascular pedicle, allowing up to a 180-degree angle of rotation on the vascular axis as required. In mentosternal contractures it is recommended to subcutaneously tunnel the isolated pedicles into the anterior cervical defect. The flap tissue will efficient-

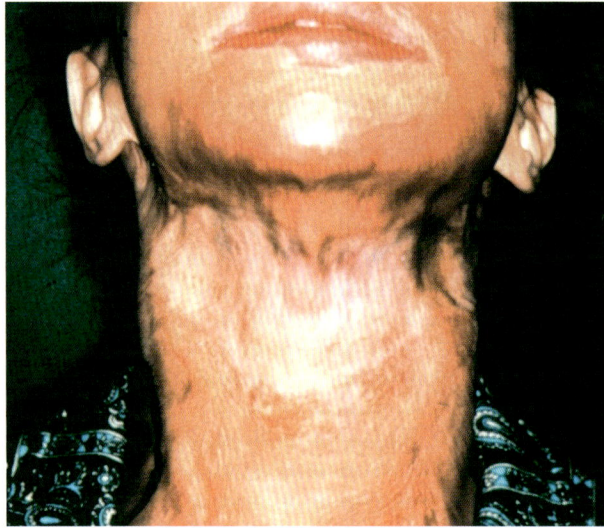

Fig. 7. Severe scarring with disfigured cervical and mental region. Scheduled for a Supraclavicular Island flap from the right donor region to restore the anterior neck region

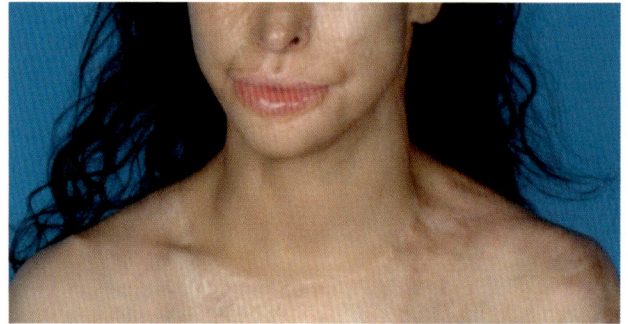

Fig. 9. Final outcome with good restoration of the anterior neck and mental region with bilateral pre-expanded Supraclavicular Island Flaps

ly cover the entire surface of the anterior neck region. The donor site defect will be closed directly in a double layer fashion after extensive undermining and preparation of 2 advancement flaps. A sterile

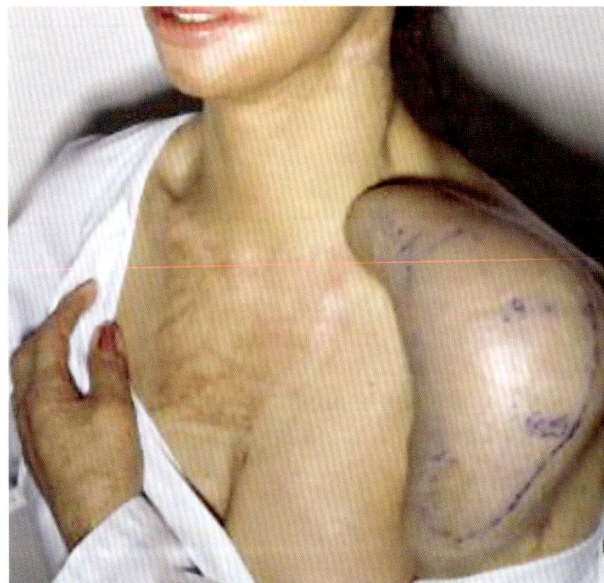

Fig. 8. Five years after successful mentosternal restoration with a Supraclavicular Island flap from the right shoulder region. She has been scheduled for a pre-expanded SIF- flap from the left side to resurface the mental region. Inflated crescent type expander with 700cc

soft dressing is placed on the wound together with a suited Philadelphia collar for 2 weeks [2, 16–18] (Figs. 7–9).

Trapezius muscle flap

The trapezius muscle flap is a useful myocutaneous flap to release contractures of the anterior and lateral neck. The trapezius muscle originates from the external occipital protuberance and the spinous processes of C7–T12. Fibers insert on the clavicle, the acromion and the scapular spine. Motor innervation is done by means of the spinal accessory nerve and ventral rami of the third and fourth cervical nerves. The trapezius muscle is vascularized through the trapezial branch of the occipital artery and the transverse cervical artery and its extension through the dorsal scapular artery. Based on these vessels superior, lateral and lower trapezius myocutanous flaps can be developed. The skin and subcutaneous tissue is supplied through cutaneous and musculocutanous perforators [36, 37].

The boundaries of the flap are the midline, the lateral muscle border of the trapezius and a keypoint approximately 5 cm to 10 cm below the scapula tip. After mentosternal contracture release the flap dissection is carried out to the level of the facial investment of the muscle including the fascia. The clavicle is the limit of the superior mobilization. The superior-medial aspect of the flap with the vascular pedicles, the dorsal scapular and the transverse cervical arteries, need to be handled with care to avoid injury to the vessels. The mobile longitudinal flap is trans-

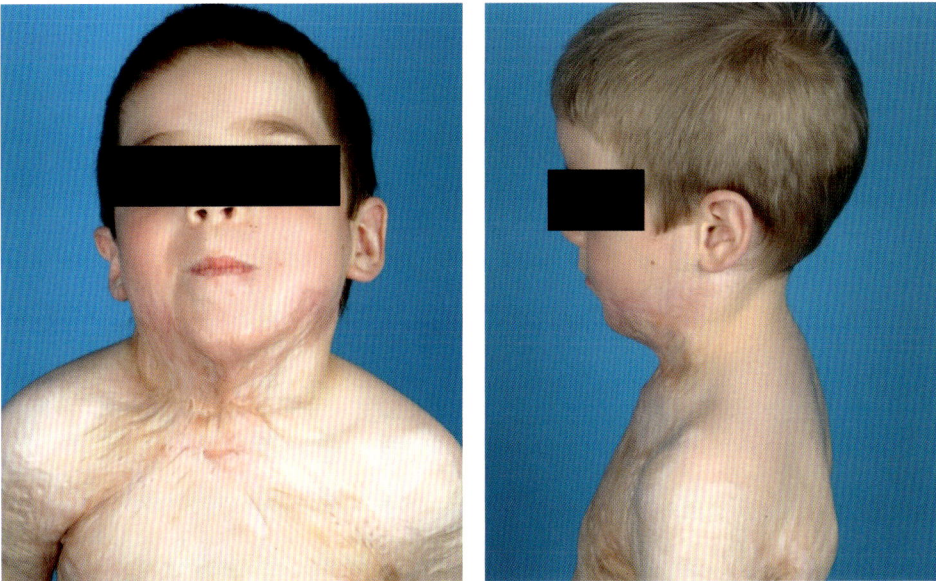

Fig. 10. Recurrence of mentosternal bands 2 years after initial surgery

posed anterior into the defect of the neck region and secured in two layers over two suction drains [37].

Further modifications with flap pre-expansion are possible to provide thin, large, and pliable tissue for the neck reconstruction [36]. The pre-expanded trapezius flap requires the insertion of a tissue expander below the trapezius muscle via a lateral incision in the first reconstructive stage. Two months later, after serial ambulatory expansion of the expander, the neck scar can be excised and the pre-expanded flap harvested and rotated anterior into the defect. Primary donor site closure is possible.

This procedure cannot be carried out without causing morbidity, even with muscle preserving techniques with skeletonization and tedious dissections of the proximal vascular pedicle. The muscle-sparing flap or its perforator alternative is the Dorsal Scapular Island flap utilizing the dorsal scapular arteries [33]. The Trapezius flap or the Dorsal Scapular island flap in anterior and lateral neck resurfacing belong to the most distant areas the flap can be harvested from, still we believe that mentosternal contracture release and defect closure with a trapezius muscle flap or the dorsal scapular island flap should remain in the armamentarium of reconstructive options for this anatomic region (Figs. 10–12).

Free flaps

Microsurgical transfer of free flaps is indicated whenever local or regional options are not available – it is usually not considered a first-line option in neck reconstruction. Published reports and series underline that the use of free flaps in the neck region is reserved for cases in which more conventional methods were considered to be less feasible. Still, the number of reports of successful utilization of free flaps in reconstruction of burns in the head and neck region has increased in the last years due to advances in free-tissue transfer and microsurgical techniques [12, 13, 38, 39]. Additional modifications such as flap prefabrication, prelamination, preexpansion, chimeric flaps and super-thin flaps have increased the quality of preexisting well established free flaps [15, 40–45]. These advances allow the use of thinner, customized flaps with better color and texture match of the head and neck region combined with low donor site morbidity [41]. Therefore, free flaps belong to the essential tools used in burn reconstruction of the neck region. Microsurgical free tissue transfer requires proper patient selection, long, complex staged operations with the need for revision procedures. Therefore, the surgeon and the patient must be flexible with realistic goals and expectations. Whenever regional options are unavailable, free flap reconstruction can be successfully applied.

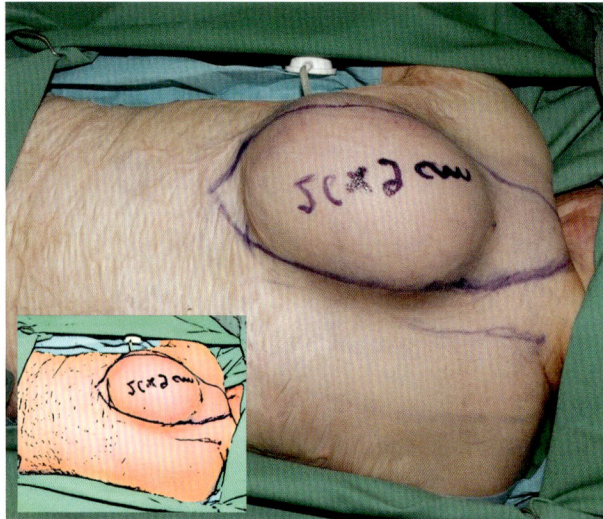

Fig. 11. Reoperative surgery with pre-expanded musculocutaneous trapezius flap. Inflated submuscular expander of the left donor region

In complex cases free flaps may be preferred to pedicled flaps to achieve the optimal functional and aesthetic result for the patient. The principle of the reconstructive ladder of Gillies may be transposed into a reconstructive elevator [15].

Among the well-established flaps the free fasciocutaneous scapular-parascapular flap and the groin flap are very versatile in the reconstruction of the anterior neck region [12, 13].

Perforator based free flaps are suitable as they provide thin, supple, large and well-vascularized tissue with low donor site morbidity. The anterolateral thigh perforator flap (ALT) and the thoracodorsal artery perforator flap (TDAP) are most commonly used [46, 47]. Especially the suprafascial dissection technique of ALT flaps provides a thin flap to improve the cervical contour.

Summary

The reconstruction of neck deformities is a difficult task. Careful selection of reconstructive tools and adequate timing of reconstructive procedures may achieve a functional and aesthetic restoration of the burn victim. Most recent technical innovations of pre-expanded, pre-fabricated or perforator flaps, to name a few, may overcome difficulties with the high functional and aesthetic requirements of the neck region. The pre-expanded ultrathin supraclavicular artery island flap for instance is a reliable and safe tool to resurface defects of the neck region after the release of cervical contractures following burns.

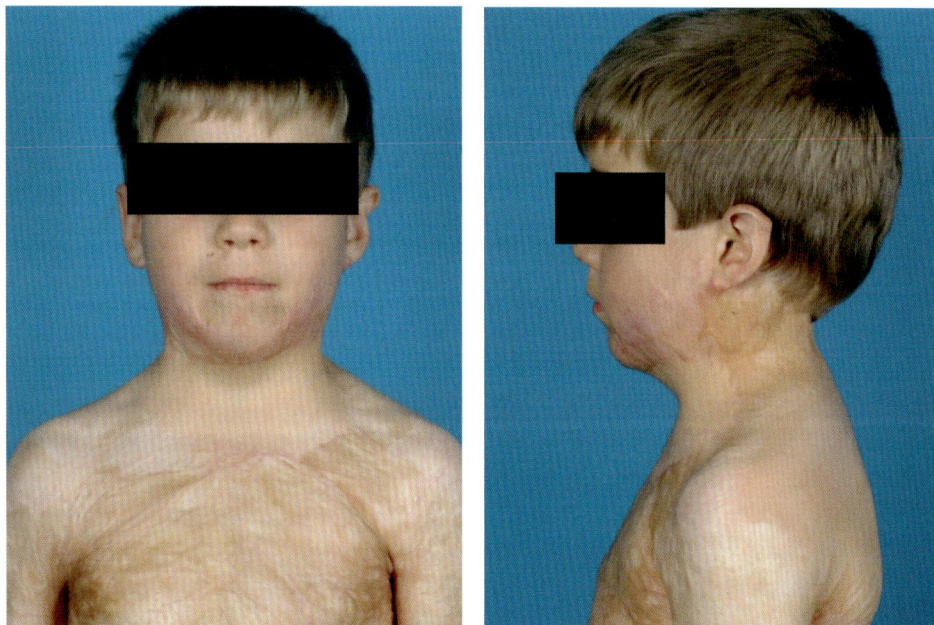

Fig.12. Final outcome with good mentosternal release

References

[1] Donelan MB (2007) Reconstruction of the head and neck. In: Herndon DN (ed) Total burn care, 3 edn. Saunders, London, pp 701–718

[2] Pallua N, Demir E (2008) Postburn head and neck reconstruction in children with the fasciocutaneous supraclavicular artery island flap. Ann Plast Surg 60: 276–282

[3] Huang T (2007) Overview of burn reconstruction. In: Herndon DN (ed) Total burn care, 3 edn. Saunders, London, pp 674–686

[4] Engrav L, Donelan MB (1997) Face burns: acute care and reconstruction. Oper Tech Plast Reconstr Surg 4: 53–85

[5] Remensnyder JP, Donelan MB (2002) Reconstruction of the head and neck. In: Herndon DN (ed) total burn care, 3 edn. Saunders, London, pp 656–689

[6] Fricke NB, Omnell L, Dutcher KD et al (1999) Skeletal and dental disturbances after facial burns and pressure garment use: a 4-year follow-up. J Burn Care Rehabil 20: 239–249

[7] Abdullah A, Blakeney P, Hunt R et al (1994) Visible scars and self-esteem in pediatric patients with burns. J Burn Care Rehabil 15: 164–168

[8] Kirschbaum S (1958) Mentosternal contracture: preferred treatment by acromial (charretera) flap. Plast Reconstr Surg 21: 131–138

[9] Achauer BM (1992) Reconstructing the burned face. Clin Plast Surg 19: 623–636

[10] Mustoe TA, Cooter TD, Gold MH, Hobbs FD, Ramelet AA, Shakespeare PG et al (2002) International clinical recommendations on scar management. Plast Reconstr Surg 100: 560

[11] Achauer BM, VanderKam VM (2000) Burn reconstruction. In: Achauer BM, Eriksson E (eds) Plastic surgery indications operations outcomes. Mosby, St. Louis, MO, pp 425–446

[12] Angrigiani C (1994) Aesthetic microsurgical reconstruction of anterior neck burn deformities. Plast Reconstr Surg 93: 507–518

[13] Ninkovic M, Moser-Rumer A, Ninkovic M et al (2004) Anterior neck reconstruction with pre-expanded free groin and scapular flaps. Plast Reconstr Surg 113: 61–68

[14] Cronin TD, Barrera A (1990) Deformities of the cervical region. In: McCarthy JG (ed) Plastic surgery, Vol. 3. Saunders, Philadelphia, pp 2057–2093

[15] Gillies, HD (1920) The tubed pedicle in plastic surgery. N. Y. Med J. 111:1

[16] Pallua N, von Heimburg D (2005) Pre-expanded ultrathin supraclavicular flaps for (full-) face reconstruction with reduced donor-site morbidity and without the need for microsurgery. Plast Reconstr Surg 115: 1837–1844

[17] Pallua N, Machens HG, Rennekampff O et al (1997) The fasciocutanous supraclavicular artery island flap for releasing postburn mentosternal contractures. Plast Reconstr Surg 99: 1878–1886

[18] Pallua N, Noah M (2000) The tunneled supraclavicular island flap: An optimized technique for head and neck reconstruction. Plast Reconstr Surg 105: 842–851

[19] Abramson DL, Pribaz JJ, Orgill DP (1996) The use of free tissue transfer in burn reconstruction. J Burn Care Rehabil 17: 402–408

[20] Aranmolate S, Atah AA (1989) Bilobed flap in the release of postburn mentosternal contracture. Plast Reconstr Surg 83: 356–361

[21] Motamed S, Davami B, Daghagheleh H (2004) Trapezius musculocutaneous flap in severe shoulder and neck burn. Burns 30(5): 476–480

[22] Waymack JP, Law E, Park R et al (1985) Acute upper airway obstruction in the postburn period. Arch Surg 120: 1042–1044

[23] Schneider J, Biedermann T, Widmer D, Montano I, Meuli M, Reichmann E, Schiestl C (2009) Matriderm versus Integra: a comparative experimental study. Burns 35: 51–57

[24] Atherton DD, Tang R, Jones I, Jawad M (2010) Early excision and application of matriderm with simultaneous autologous skin grafting in facial burns. Plast Reconstr Surg 125: 60e–61e

[25] Yannas IV, Burke JF (1980) Design of an artificial skin. I. Basic design principles. J Biomed Mater Res 14: 65–81

[26] Heimbach D, Luterman A, Burke J, Cram A, Herndon D, Hunt J, Jordan M, McManus W, Solem L, Warden G et al (1988) Artificial dermis for major burns. A multi-center randomized clinical trial. Ann Surg 208: 313–320

[27] Berger A, Tanzella U, Machens HG, Liebau J (2000) Administration of Integra on primary burn wounds and unstable secondary scars. Chirurg 71: 558–563

[28] Gahhos FN, Ariyan S, Cuono CB et al (1985) Burn wound excision and local flap closure. Ann Plast Surg 14: 535

[29] Neale HW, Kurtzmann LC, Goh KB et al (1993) Tissue expanders in the lower face and anterior neck in pediatric burn patients: limitations and pitfalls. Plast Reconstr Surg 91: 624–631

[30] LoGiudice J, Gosain AK (2003) Pediatric tissue expansion: indications and complications. J Craniofac Surg 14: 866–872

[31] Gibstein LA, Abramson DL, Bartlett RA et al (1997) Tissue expansion in children: a retrospective study of complications. Ann Plast Surg 38: 358–364

[32] Hallock GG (1992) The role of local faciocutanous flaps in total burn wound management. Plast Reconstr Surg 90: 629–635

[33] Angrigiani C, Grilli D, Karanas YL, Longaker MT, Sharma S (2003) The Dorsal Scapular Island flap: an alternative for head, neck and chest reconstruction. Plast Reconstr Surg 111: 67–78

[34] Mutter TD (1842) Cases of deformity from burns, relieved by operation. Am J Med Sci 4: 66

[35] Lamberty BG (1979) The supra-clavicular axial patterened flap. Br J Plast Surg 32: 207–212

[36] Ulrich D, Fuchs P, Pallua N (2008) Preexpanded vertical trapezius musculocutaneous flap for reconstruction of a severe neck contracture after burn injury. J Burn Care Res 29: 386–389

[37] Isenberg JS, Price G (1996) Longitudinal trapezius fasciocutaneous flap for the treatment of mentosternal burn scar contractures. Burns 22: 76–79

[38] Ohkubo E, Kobayashi S, Sekiguchi J et al (1991) Restoration of the anterior neck surface in the patient by free groin flap. Plast Reconstr Surg 87: 276–284

[39] Bootz F, Preyer S (1994) Microvascular tissue transplantation in plastic reconstruction of the external head-neck area. Laryngorhinootologie 73: 538–542

[40] Teot L, Cherenfant E, Otman S et al (2000) Prefabricated vascularised supraclavicular flaps for face resurfacing after postburn scarring. Lancet 355: 1695-1696

[41] Parrett BM, Pomahac B, Orgill DP, Pribaz JJ (2007) The role of free-tissue transfer for head and neck burn reconstruction. Plast Reconstr Surg 120: 1871–1878

[42] Pribaz JJ, Fine NA, Orgil DP (1999) Flap prefabrication in the head and neck: A 10 year experience. Plast Reconstr Surg 103: 808

[43] Hallock GG (1995) Preexpansion of free flap donor sites used in reconstruction after burn injury. J Burn Care Rehabil 16: 646

[44] Koshima I, Yamamoto H, Hosoda M et al (2005) Free combined composite flaps using the lateral circumflex femoral system for repair of massive defects of the head and neck regions: An introduction to the chimeric flap principle. Plast Reconstr Surg 58: 550

[45] Chin T, Ogawa R, Murakami M et al (2005) An Anatomical study and clinical cases of "super-thin flaps" with transverse cervical perforator. Br J Plast Surg 58: 550

[46] Mun GH, Jeon BJ, Lim SY, Hyon WS, Bang SI, Oh KS (2007) Reconstruction of postburn neck contractures using free thin thoracodorsal artery perforator flaps with cervicoplasty. Plast Reconstr Surg 120: 1524–1532

[47] Yang JY, Tsai FC, Chana JS, Chuang SS, Chang SY, Huang WC (2002) Use of free thin anterolateral thigh flaps combined with cervicoplasty for reconstruction of postburn anterior cervical contractures. Plast Reconstr Surg 110: 39–46

Correspondence: Norbert Pallua, M. D., Ph. D., FEBOPRAS Department of Plastic Surgery and Hand Surgery, Burn Center, University Hospital RWTH Aachen, Pauwelsstraße 30, 52074 Aachen, Germany, Tel: +49 241 80 89 700, Fax: +49 241 80 82 448, E-mail: npallua@ukaachen.de

Burn reconstruction: Eye region

Andreas Heckmann, Peter M. Vogt

Department of Plastic, Hand, and Reconstructive Surgery, Medizinische Hochschule Hannover, Hannover, Germany

Introduction

Facial burns occur in up to 30 % of thermal trauma patients admitted to burn units [1]. Eyelid and ocular involvement is relatively common [2], but the loss of an eye primarily from a thermal injury is rather rare [3]. Reasons therefore are mechanisms like protective movements of the head and arms to avoid the source of a burn, the blink reflex with the closure of the eye and the Bell phenomenon of the eyeball.

The lid is built-on of skin, the orbicularis muscle, the tarsus, lashes, meibomian glands, lid retractors, and tarsal conjunctiva. The lower eyelid is commonly described as a series of tissue layers (Figs. 1, 2):

▶ The anterior lamella is composed of the outer skin and orbicularis oculi muscle.
▶ The middle lamella consists of the orbital septum.
▶ The posterior lamella consists of the tarsus, the lower lid retractors, and the conjunctiva.

The goals of eyelid reconstruction are restoration of the lid lamellae, reconstitution of facial symmetry and provision of corneal protection. Inadequate reconstruction techniques may produce corneal exposure and sight-threatening keratopathy. Visual deprivation and amblyopia are rare but may also follow. Periocular skin is thin with no subcutaneous fat, resulting in deeper burns than a similar exposure to skin elsewhere. Eyelid burns (50–85 %) and

eyelid contractures (30–65 %) in burned people are more frequently than injuries to eyeball like conjunctival burns (3–11 %), corneal abrasions (7–22 %), corneal burns (5 %), corneal perforations (1–2 %) and cataracts (2 %) [1, 4]. A series of 143 burns patients with ocular injuries reported that 2 were left blind, 2 had impaired vision, and 3 underwent enucleation [5]. Mandatory in burns involving the eyelids is immediate consultation of the ophthalmologist and prophylactic ocular lubrication. Early surgical intervention is indicated if eyelid retraction causing corneal exposure occurs. But this often requires repeated procedures due to eyelid contraction. Secondary complications such as corneal ulceration, exposure keratopathy, secondary infection, and orbital compartment syndrome are potentially preventable by appropriate early and sustained management and are thought to be preventable. In further readings controversial meanings exist regarding the role of prophylactic ocular lubrication, excision and debridement of eschar, temporary suture and surgical tarsorrhaphy, timing of surgery for eyelid contraction, and the role of full and split-thickness skin grafts in eyelid reconstruction. For eyelid reconstruction each case needs an individual approach based on what defect exists and what skin is available. The lid surgeon needs a wide knowledge of the reconstructive principles and possibilities. The reconstruction of anterior lamellar has a significant risk of developing ectropion. Large de-

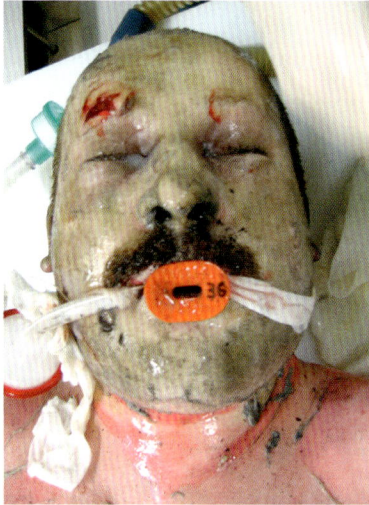

Fig. 1. Third degree burned face involving the eyelid region, directly after the damage, 45 year old male patient with burned 50 % of body surface area degree 2–3

fects may require different transposition flaps to achieve a good skin texture and color reconstruction. New autogenous and cadaveric materials for posterior lid reconstruction are known well meantime. They reduce donor site morbidity and surgical time, but they undergo contraction significantly after surgery. A new approach for entropion and symblepharon caused by conjunctival cicatricial changes is reached by amniotic membrane transplantation and may enhance the prognosis for patients.

Reconstruction of the eyelid region

Upper Eyelid and Anterior lamella of Lower Eyelid

Reconstruction of the anterior lamella of the upper eyelid can be done by:
1. Skin grafting
2. Local flaps
3. Free flaps (often used in combined damage of anterior and posterior lamella)

Reconstructive skin grafting (split-thickness or full-thickness skin graft) in the eyelid region

Both full-thickness skin grafts (FTSG) (most suitable harvested from post-auricular, supra-clavicular or

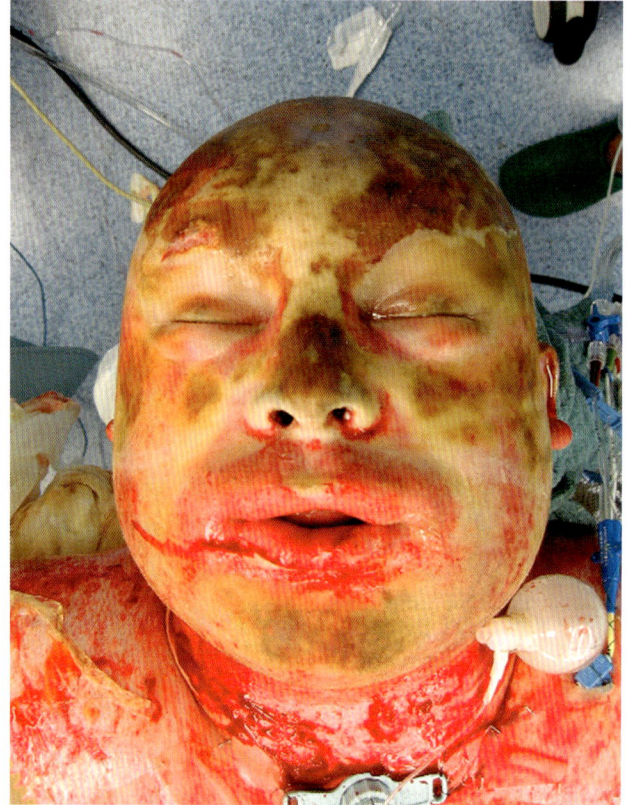

Fig. 2. Third degree burned face involving the eyelid region, seven days after damage

from the unburned contra lateral upper eyelid) and split-thickness skin grafts (STSG) (mostly harvested from the upper leg) are not ideal for eyelid burn reconstruction. In literature there are different reports concerning which method (FTSG or STSG) is the best for upper and lower eyelid reconstruction. Most authors use STSG (more mobility) for the upper eyelid and FTSG (less contraction tendency) for lower eyelid reconstruction. Some others prefer FTSG for both. Very thin, but full thickness skin grafts are often used grafts for reconstruction of both upper and lower eyelid. Both kinds of skin grafts have disadvantages and advantages in color-match, tendency to contraction, range of mobility, transplantation of root of hairs, developing ectropion and hyper pigmentation.

Wound contraction tendency is indirectly proportional to the amount of structurally dermal collagen. For this, FTSG (more dermis) should have fewer tendencies for contraction than STSG. In cases

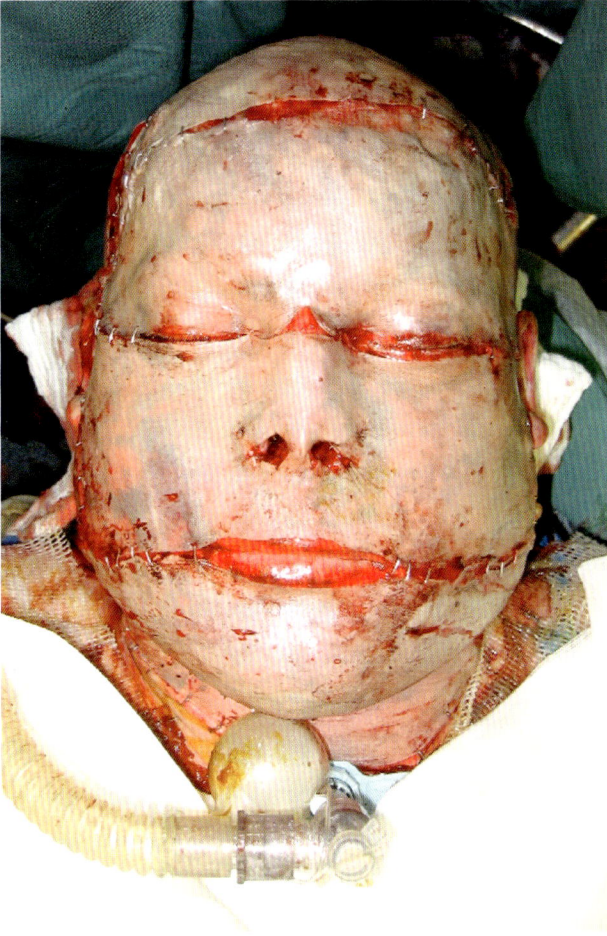

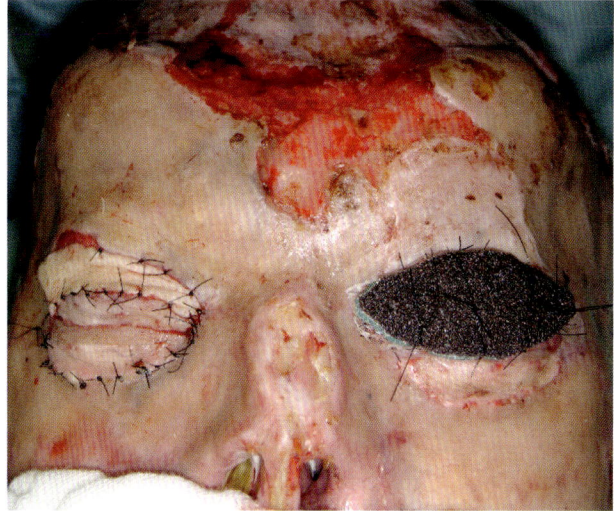

Fig. 4. Postoperative view after full thickness skin grafting of lower and upper eyelid because of skin contraction, left eye still covered with a bolster

Fig. 3. Postoperative view 3 days after split thickness skin grafting of the face region, first step in reconstruction of the face and eyelid region

of extensive burn damage with limited viable skin, FTSG is often reserved for later repair and STSG are used for first reconstruction [6, 7] (Figs. 3–5). Also STSG are used when FTSG-areas are not available. FTSG contracts less than STSG and does not compromise mobility or appearance too much. For a good color-match FTSG should be harvested from post-auricular, supra-clavicular or from the un-burned contra lateral upper eyelid and should be taken oversized because of contraction over time. If upper and lower eyelids require grafting it is best to perform grafting at separate sessions. This is to avoid insufficient skin being introduced to each and to maximize the stretched graft-bed for each eyelid. Some authors prefer first the upper and others the

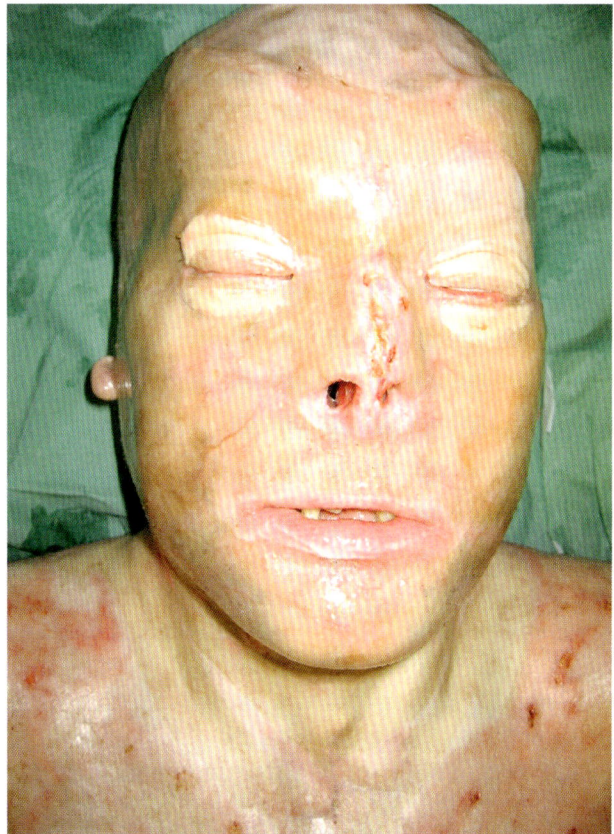

Fig. 5. Postoperative view 3 weeks after full thickness skin grafting of lower and upper eyelid

lower eyelid reconstruction. Maybe it should depend on the extent of the damage of the particular eyelid. The skin should be placed under tractioned wound-bed and padded for 5 days. The other eyelid can be reconstructed after sufficient skin grafting and healing 7 days later. Before skin transplantation to upper eyelid a skin crease incision is used at the lower border of the graft. For the lower eyelid a subciliary incision is preferred. For both upper and lower eyelids, the way of dissection should be canthus-to-canthus [8] and extend up to 2 cm beyond the lateral canthus, very slightly angulated upwards for lower eyelid incisions and well into the nose at the medial canthus [9, 10]. Dissection should be layered with a wide release and resection of all scar tissue because of later shrinking. Special attention should be placed to the preservation of Müllers muscle (if still present) and the levator aponeurosis. After this a thinned full-thickness graft could be fashioned to fit the recipient wound and a petrolatum gauze is placed over the graft and a bolster is tied in place for 5–7 days.

Reconstructive local flaps in the eyelid region

Local tissue flaps in the eyelid region include the skin pedicle flap with subcutaneous base, anterior and posterior lamellar advancement flaps, and more complex interpositional flaps for combined lid and cheek defects.

The possibilities of reconstructive flaps in the eyelid region in the treatment of burns and contracture are limited. Mostly the reason therefore is the lack of normal adjacent skin [7, 11]. Orbicularis oculi myocutaneous flaps are obviously indicated only in the rare circumstance where the upper eyelid is unaffected and available for harvesting. They have the advantage of additional support and possible lower eyelid suspension in the repair of lower eyelid burn-ectropion [12]. A destroyed tarsus because of severe burn damage complicates reconstruction possibilities because it normally stabilises skin grafts and flaps in their new position. The simple skin grafting of the posterior lamella is not a successful long lasting tool in reconstruction. This damage better needs a vascularised flap for reconstruction of the eyelid. Some possibilities are a tarsoconjuctival Hughes flap, a forehead periosteal flap or an island pedicle flap. If ambient skin is not damaged a local subcutaneous

based pedicled flap can be transposed into the defect after debridement. For this Tei et al. [13] described the advantage of using a subcutaneously based flap in lower lid reconstruction. They used for reconstructing of a lower lid defect a Hughes tarsoconjunctival flap in combination with a nasolabial skin transposition flap, with a deep subcutaneous base. A nasolabial flap results in an acceptable scar and provides a good color and texture match for the lower lid and the advantages of this approach over a cheek rotation flap, which also maintains its good blood supply, is a lower risk of ectropion, entropion, or inadvertent facial nerve damage, and that hair-bearing skin from the upper cheek is not brought medially. Large defects of the anterior lamella of the lower lid combined with burned cheek skin have a high risk for developing ectropion after reconstruction. They can be closed with a heteropalpebral skin flap from the unburned upper to the lower lid, and a temporomandibular and retroauricular transposition flap for closure of the cheek defect. This approach enables optimal color and texture matches [14].

Medial and Lateral Canthal Deformities after burn injury often result in displacement of the punctum and causing epiphora because of hypertrophic scars and vertical contracture [6, 8, 15]. Multiple Z-plasties or Mustarde's Jumping Man plasty may be good possibilities for correction of mild linear contractions on the medial canthus. Otherwise local transposition flaps or transplantation of skin after releasing the canthus are viable [15, 16]. Lateral epicanthal folds and scar bands can be corrected by a local transposition flap.

Spherical contraction due to full thickness skin burned eyelids (scar contracture, adhesion of eyelid margin) will lead to a minor function of the palpebral opening. The typical "round eye deformity" particularly resulting of skin contracture leads to lagophthalmos. The first step in reconstruction is the correction of the skin deficit of the eyelids. By incisional release including the whole horizontal opening length a reposition of the medial canthus is possible [9].

Reconstructive free flaps in the eyelid region

Myocutanous free flaps are often indicated in thermal fully damages of both eyelids and are combined with other reconstructive procedures when both the anterior and posterior lamella of the lower lid are burned. Thai et al. [17] report a patient with a unilateral complete defect of both upper and lower eyelids from a deep thermal injury with partial sclera burn (damage of anterior and posterior lamella). Local tissues were unavailable for donor sites due to the severe burn of the head and neck areas. They used a free-tissue transfer of the unburned dorsalis pedis flap (anastomosing with the superficial temporal vessels) as soft-tissue coverage for the outer lamella. The partially burned inner lamella was reconstructed by releasing and advancing the upper and lower conjunctiva. To preserve the natural inner lamella lining this can be achieved by advancing the conjunctival tissues from the conjunctival cul-de-sacs. Furthermore, it also serves as a vascularized bed for cartilage grafts for replacing a missing tarsal plate and providing support for the new eyelids. A conjunctivodacryocystorhinostomy was performed for lacrimal drainage. The dorsalis pedis flap's advantage as donor tissue is the thin and pliable nature of this flap. This coverage will only provide static support without active mobility of the reconstructed eyelids.

Posterior lamella

Reconstruction of the posterior lamella can be done by:
1. Nasal septal-, auricular- and hard palate cartilage
2. Bovine preserved sclera
3. Amniotic membrane transplants (AMT)
4. Dermis skin grafts
5. Conjunctival release

Posterior lamella can be reconstructed by using nasal septal-, auricular- and hard palate cartilage, bovine preserved sclera, amniotic membrane transplants and dermis skin grafts. In particular when more than 50 % of the lid has full-thickness burn damage a graft of stabilizing material is necessary. An allograft of preserved bovine sclera has the advantages of avoiding donor site morbidity and reducing surgical time. Fortunately allogeneic grafts for reconstruction of the posterior lamella of the lower lid are well tolerated without appearance of keratopathy in the interval between surgery and re-epithelialization at 3 months. Unfortunately, in several countries, the use of preserved sclera has fallen from favour due to the association with transmission of prion disease [18].

The use of autogenous dermis skin grafts has no risk of prion disease but leaves a little donor site defect. Therefore dermabrasio of preferably posterior auricular skin for complete absence of epidermal structures and keratin is performed and is used similar to a full-thickness skin graft [19]. Conjunctival epithelialization of the graft occurred within a month. Because of its tendency to contract the graft should be taken oversized. The advantage of autogenous dermis skin grafting includes low donor site morbidity and the availability of a material sufficiently supple to conform to the shape of the globe. Split-thickness dermal grafts or tenonplasty are procedures in large corneal and scleral defects without the possibility of reconstruction with conjunctival flaps [20]. After raising a superiorly hinged, thin epidermal flap the split-thickness dermal graft could be harvested from the thigh. A thin dermal graft may then be taken from the exposed dermal bed. The epidermis flap is then closed after being perforated. The graft is placed on the defect following a limbal peritomy, depending on the site of the defect with or without undermining of close-by conjunctiva. Postoperative thinning of the grafts may be needful

An alternative material to autogenous dermis without donor site morbidity is acellular allogenic human or porcine cadaveric dermis. This material has unfortunately a high tendency of contraction and shrinking (up to more than 70 % in comparison to hard palate mucosal cartilage grafts with only 15 %) and high costs [10, 38]. Because of this its application should be reconsidered well and should be used rather as a temporary spacer.

The structural arrangement of collagens and laminin in amniotic membrane transplants (AMT) is similar to that in conjunctiva. AMT acts as a scaffold for conjunctival re-epithelialization and restores the integrity of the corneal and conjunctival surfaces. Its advantages compared with buccal and labial mucous membrane grafting include no donor site morbidity, and no need for adjunctive irradiation or antimetabolite treatment for reducing shrinkage of an autogenous graft. AMT is an acellular nonimmunogenic material with stromal epithelial growth factors, antiangiogenic proteins, and antiinflammatory proteins.

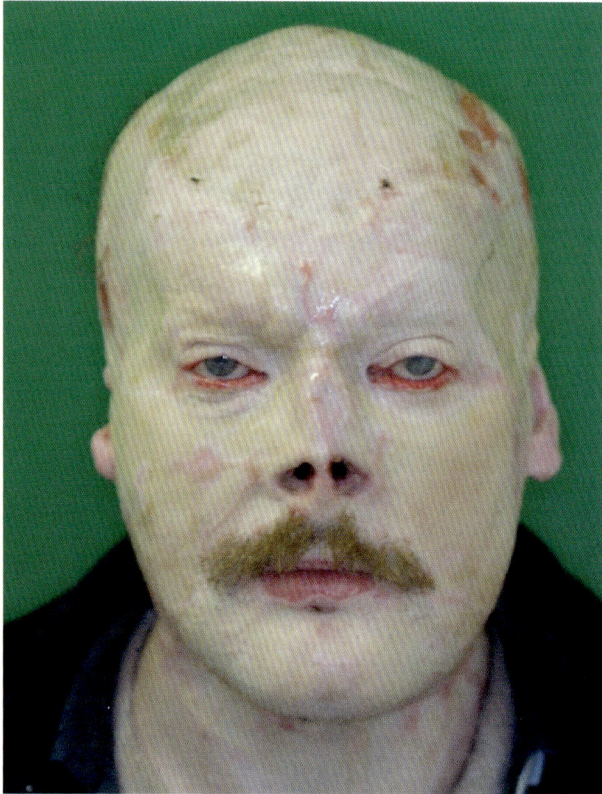

Fig. 6. 14 months after reconstruction face with split thickness skin grafts and upper and lower eyelid regions with full thickness skin grafts with scleral show and ectropion

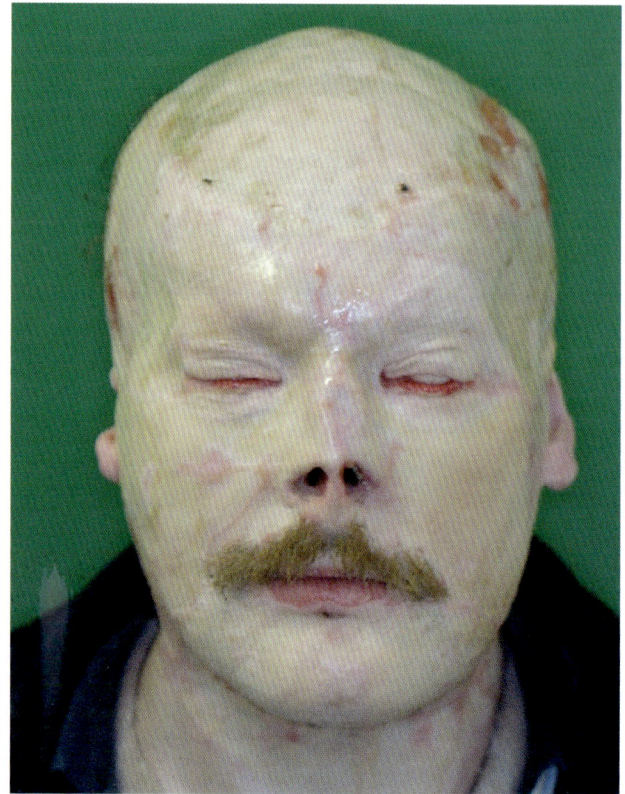

Fig. 7. 14 months after reconstruction face with split thickness skin grafts and upper and lower eyelid regions with full thickness skin grafts. Nearly fully eyelid closure

Scar management

Controlling burn scar contraction is a difficult task as usually in face burns. Compression with custom-made splints which are fitted inside a face mask or custom-fitted conformers is a common treatment. The patients have to be followed closely to see if the splint works effectively in preventing ectropion. If the eyeball is effectual covered it is acceptable to wait for scar maturation for definitive correction. Ectropion of the lower eyelid is the most appearing and feared problem after burn lid damage and unfortunately cannot been eliminated totally.

Retraction of upper eyelid and ectropion of lower eyelid

After early eyelid reconstruction combined with skin grafts appearance of progressive upper eyelid con-

traction and lower eyelid ectropion could be estimated (Figs. 6, 7).

In generally opposing forces in ectropion are levator function and scar contraction against gravity, edema, elasticity and orbicularis function in upper eye lid. In the lower eye lid tissue pliability, age (loss of elasticity), paralysis, gravity and lid scar contraction work against orbicularis function, tissue elasticity and tarsal rigidity [37].

The operative correction of entropion and retraction is one of the most important operations in the entire surgical rehabilitation of the facial burn and should be carried out before any other facial surgery [21], but early surgery has no evidence based advantage to reduce further reconstructive procedures required in the long-term. It has only been shown help reduce the risk of exposure keratopathy. Controversial is the time of debridement in deep eyelid burns. In general, eyelid burn debridement is performed later compared to burns elsewhere [6, 8]. Time of surgery is often at 2–3 weeks post injury. Then tissue destruction has become demarcated and eyelid contracture and lagophthalmos are present. Therefore fully, wide and overcorrecting releasing of the eyelids is essential. It is recommended that either the upper or lower eyelid should be reconstructed at one setting. The reason for this is the difficulty of doing an adequate and fully overcorrection of upper and lower eyelid release simultaneously. There is a big controversal in literature if the upper or the lower eyelid should be released first. It should be always individually decided due to the amount of damage of the particular lid and fear for the globe.

To avoid damage to the M. orbicularis oculi Huang [9] only excises the eschar. However, most of the authors consider a full debridement to receive a wound bed with a good blood supply and to prevent further wound contracture [22, 23]. If there are repeated problems with irritation of the eye and damage to the cornea the ectropion is released early in the post burn period. If there is no risk for the eye one can await scar maturation [24]. An important consideration is to eliminate extrinsic forces which cause entropion before correcting the eyelids. There could be a tight contraction over the face or neck which pulls on the eyelids and causes ectropion or retraction.

In summary generally the surgical release and skin grafting should be done delayed. If there is early appearing of lagophthalmos, corneal exposure, conjunctival injection or chemosis, the eyelids could be closed and secured with draw-string tarsorrhaphy sutures.

Surgical tarsorrhaphy

Surgical Tarsorrhaphy is discussed very controversy in facial burns and has largely been abandoned as routine practice. Tarsorrhaphy does not prevent wound contraction when there is cictricial ectropion present. Furthermore the basic principle of tissue replacement should be the better procedure [6, 21, 25]. This procedure seems to be ideal 2 weeks after burn accident when eyelid contracture occurs, overcoming any temporary suture tarsorrhaphy and producing ectropion. Suturing of the eyelids together may

be indicated in certain situations like following destruction of the eyelid margins if there is sufficient tissue remaining instead of the masquerade procedure [15]. also in combined grafting of upper and lower eyelid in cases where the tarsus is missing. A tarsorrhaphy combined with skin grafting may help reduce the need for further skin grafting or recurrent ectropion. As the risk for ectropion persists for months due to persistent eyelid shrinkage, a tarsorrhaphy would need to remain in place until facial scars mature [26].

Masquerade procedure

This is a temporary procedure of closing the eye for further reconstruction of the eyelids. It is used if there is severe damage of the eyelid and no viable or adjacent tissue is available. All necrotic tissue including muscle and eyelid margins get excised, then mobilizing and suturing together of a conjunctival flap from the remaining upper and lower eyelid to cover the anterior surface of the globe with the epithelial surface of conjunctiva. This is covered usually with a split thickness skin graft. Because of the poor vascularity of the wound bed a full-thickness graft will undergo necrosis. After 3 months the reconstructed lids get divided to create new eyelid margins. The globe has nearly normal coverage and the eyelid function is very good [7]. But we also could have appearance of slight eyelid eversion, followed by ptosis, stiffness and lagophthalmos.

If the upper and only the upper part of the lower eyelid need full reconstruction, advancing the M. levator palpabrae and covering with a full-thickness skin graft show good results after flap dividing with good function of the new eyelids [6].

Tenonplasty

In absence of nearby conjunctival flaps this alternative globe-preserving procedure involves dissection of the Tenon's layer and anterior advancement of Tenon's in a flap-like fashion and suturing to the globe at the limbus in order to provide a vascular supply and promote corneal epithelialisation [27]. The results nearly complete epithelialization of advanced Tenon's within 21 to 54 days [28] with prevention and healing of scleral ulceration.

Deformities of the eyebrows

A loss of the eyebrows is noticeable and defacing. A good cosmetic result could be achieved by temporal pedicle-flaps of hair bearing skin [8, 9]. The flap is outlined above an appropriate branch of the superficial temporal artery. Hair direction should correspond similar to the brow hair. The flap is then pedicled subcutaneous on the temporal artery and vein and transposed a little more medially than the normal eyebrow position because of tendency of contraction to the lateral side.

Hair transplantation is another good tool for correction after burn damage. Full-thickness composite skin graft of hair-bearing skin from the temporo-parietal region (because of the thinness of this regional skin) could be transplanted. A portion of the scalp should be taken that has the same general angle of hair follicles exiting the skin as the remainder of the eyebrow or the opposite eyebrow. While excising care must be taken to cut parallel to the hair follicles. Then they are positioned in the way that the hair can grow in the correct direction [29]. Due to the minor satisfactory vascularised wound bed they should be taken as 1 mm strips up to 5 mm grafts [8, 9]. Unfortunately there is loss of hair within 3 weeks but hair returns in the following 3 months with up to 70 % of surviving follicles [29]. Re-grafting is here often required.

The micrograft technique in hair transplantation shows good natural and long lasting results in eyebrow reconstruction. But this technique depends on a not too much scared wound bed and is very time consuming and may be repeated for a complete new eyebrow [30–32]. Using this technique or small grafts is useful in producing the correct angle of the eyebrow. McConnell and Neale prefer a pedicle island flap based on the superficial temporal artery especially for reconstruction in bushy male eyebrows. The vascular pedicle is tunnelled beneath the skin to the eyebrow. They recommend that free hair transplantation has marginal results due to the scarred recipient site [33].

The gender of the patient plays a big role in the choice of reconstruction. Male patients need more thick and bushy eyebrows and the flap procedure is more capable. In female patients permanent make up or eyebrow pencils can be an alternative methods to surgery [8, 9].

Horizontal eyelid shortening

Horizontal eyelid tightening is a possible procedure in ectropion after skin transplantation for eyelid reconstruction. The reconstructed eyelid has not the luxury blood supply like in normal circumstances so this is not a safe procedure in presence of severe burn induced progressive ischemic scarring.

Danger of necrosis if eyelid shortening is really required is less in the lower eyelid. To avoid central infarction the release should be at the lateral canthus maybe with a lateral tarsorrhaphy for a safer blood supply via an upper eyelid transconjunctival flap [7]. Normally an additional skin transplantation is essential.

Lower eyelid sling

For recurrent lower eyelid ectropion the use of lower eyelid fascial slings (fascia temporalis or fascia lata) have been reported [34]. It provides a vertical support and does not overcome contraction or tissue deficit, which requires release and tissue replacement. It is secured to the medial canthal tendon and to the lateral orbital rim and braces the lower lid margin [35].

Obstruction of canaliculi

A burn damage involving the puncta and canaliculi is infrequent. Meyer et al. recommend early punctal evaluation and daily dilatation if necessary during the first 10 days [36]. This may be a good opportunity to prevent early stenosis but is not practical for longer prophylaxis or for reconstruction.

References

[1]   Stern JD, Goldfarb IW, Slater H (1996) Ophthalmological complications as a manifestation of burn injury. Burns 22 (2): 135–136

[2]   Bouchard CS, Morno K, Jeffrey P et al (2001) Ocular complications of thermal injury: a 3-year retrospective. J Trauma 50 (1): 79–82

[3]   Spencer T, Hall HJA, Stawell RJ (2001) Ophthalmological sequelae of thermal burns over ten years at the Alfred Hospital. Ophthal Plast Reconstr Surg 18 (3): 196–201

[4]   Linhart GW (1978) Burn of the eyes and eyelids. Ann Ophthalmol 10: 999–1001

[5] Still JM, Law EJ, Belcher KE, Moses KC et al (1995) Experience with burns of the eyes and lids in a regional burn unit. J Burn Care Rehab 16: 248–252

[6] Marrone AC(1988) Thermal eyelid burns. In: Hornblass A, Haing CJ (eds) Oculoplastics, orbital and reconstructive surgery. Williams & Wilkins, Baltimore, MD, pp 433–437

[7] Mauriello JA Jr, Hollsten DA (2000) Cicatricial ectropion due to thermal burns of the eyelids. In: Mauriello JA (ed) Unfavourable results of eyelid and lacrimal surgery, prevention and management. Butterworth-Heinemann, Boston, pp 219–226, Chap 9

[8] Tsur H (1988) Eyelid burns. A general plastic surgeons's approach. In: Hornblass A, Haing CJ (eds) Oculoplastics, orbital and reconstructive surgery. Williams & Wilkins, Baltimore, MD, pp 448–454

[9] Huang TT, Blackwell SJ, Lewis S (1978) Burn injuries of the eyelids. Clinics Plastic Surg 5 (4): 571–581

[10] Sloan DF, Huang TT, Larson DL et al (1976) Reconstruction of eyelids and eyebrows in burned patients. Plast Reconstr Surg 58: 340–346

[11] Jackson DM, Roper-Hall MJ (1983) Preservation of sight after complete destruction of the eyelids by burning. Burns 7: 221–226

[12] Kostakoglu N, Ozcan G (1999) Orbicularis oculi myocutaneous flap in reconstruction of postburn lower eyelid ectropion. Burns 25: 553–557

[13] Tei TM, Larsen J (2003) Use of the subcutaneously based nasolabial flap in lower eyelid reconstruction. Br J Plast Surg 56: 420–423

[14] Zaccagna A, Raiteri E, Picciotto F (2003) Repair of a large surgical defect involving the lower lid, cheek, and temporal region. Dermatol Surg 29: 182–184

[15] Achauer BM, Adair SR (2000) Acute and reconstructive management of the burned eyelid. Clin Plast Surg 7: 87–95

[16] Tajima S, Aoyagi F (1977) Correcting post-traumatic lateral epicanthic folds. J Br Plast Surg 30: 200–201

[17] Thai KN, Billmire DA, Yakuboff Kevin P (1999) Total eyelid reconstruction with free dorsalis pedis flap after deep facial burn. Plast Reconstr Surg 104(4): 1048–1051

[18] Mehta JS, Franks WA (2002) The sclera, the prion and the ophthalmologist. Br J Ophthalmol 86: 587–592

[19] Brock WD, Bearden W, Tann T 3rd et al (2003) Autogenous dermis skin grafts in lower eyelid reconstruction. Ophthal Plast Reconstr Surg 19: 394–397

[20] Mauriello JA, Pokorny K (1993) Use of split-thickness dermal grafts to repair corneal and scleral defects – a study of 10 patients. Br J Ophthalmol 77: 327–331

[21] McIndoe AH (1983) Total reconstruction of the burned face. Br J Plastic Surg 36: 410–420

[22] Hollsten DA, White WL (1994) Management of periorbital burns. Semin Ophthalmol 9: 152–164

[23] Lille ST, Engrave LH, Caps MT et al (1999) Full-thickness grafting of acute eyelid burns should not be considered taboo. Plast Reconstr Surg 104 (3): 637–645

[24] Achauer BM (1991) Burn reconstruction. Thieme Medical Publishers, ISBN 0-86577-341-6, pp 40–51

[25] Frank DH, Wachtel T, Frank HA (1983) The early treatment and reconstruction of Eyelid burns. J Trauma 23: 874–877

[26] Malhotra R, Sheikh I, Dheansa B (2009) The management of eyelid burns. Surv Ophthalmol 54(3): 356–371

[27] White WL, Hollsten DA (1994) Burns of the ocular adenexa. Curr Opin Ophthalmol 5 (5): 74–77

[28] Kuckelkorn R, Redbrake C, Reim M (1997) Tenonplasty, a new surgical approach for the treatment of severe eye burns. Ophthalmic Surg Lasers 28 (2): 105–110

[29] McIndoe AH (1983) Total reconstruction of the burned face. Br J Plastic Surg 36: 410–420

[30] Choi YC (2000) Single-hair transplantation by Choi's procedure. Int J Cosmetic Surg Aesth Dermatol 2 (3): 187–194

[31] Goldman GD (2001) Eyebrow transplantation. Dermatologic Surg 27 (4): 352–354

[32] Wang J, Fan J (2004) Cicatricial eyebrow reconstruction with a dense-packing one to two hair grafting technique. Plast Reconstr Surg 114 (6): 1420–1426

[33] McConnel CM, Neale HW (1977) Eyebrow reconstruction in the burn patient. J Trauma 17: 362–366

[34] De la Torre J, Simpson RL, Tenenhaus M et al (2001) Using lower eyelid fascial slings for recalcitrant burn ectropion. Ann Plast Surg 46: 621–624

[35] Tyres AG, Collins JRO (2001) Colour atlas of ophthalmic plastic surgery, 2nd edn. Butterworth Heinemann, Edinburgh, UK, pp 118–121

[36] Meyer DR, Kersten RC, Kulwin DR et al (1995) Management of canalicular injury associated with eyelid burns. Arch Ophthalmol 113 (7): 900–903

[37] Bowers DG Jr (1976) Burn trauma of eyelids: Late reconstruction. Symposium on plastic surgery in the orbital region. In: Tessier P (ed). C. V. Mosby, St. Louis, pp 31–38

[38] Sullivan SA, Dailey RA (2003) Graft contraction: a comparison of acellular dermis versus hard palate mucosa in lower eyelid surgery. Ophthal Plast Reconstr Surg 19: 14–24

Correspondence: Peter M. Vogt M.D., Ph.D., Department of Plastic, Hand, and Reconstructive Surgery, Medizinische Hochschule Hannover, Carl-Neuberg-Straße 1, 30625 Hannover, Germany, E-mail: vogt.peter@mh-hannover.de

Reconstruction of the post burn ear

Andrew Burd

Division of Plastic, Reconstructive and Aesthetic Surgery, Department of Surgery, The Chinese University of Hong Kong, Prince of Wales Hospital, Hong Kong

Introduction

The reconstruction of the human ear is a considerable challenge for the Plastic Reconstructive and Aesthetic Surgeon. This challenge is considerably increased when the need for reconstruction is due to damage following burn injury. The external ear is conceptually simple; a sandwich of skin, cartilage and skin. However the construction of the ear; the curves, the folds, the shape and the placement give a complexity, a grace, an elegance that is impossible to fully reconstruct. In this chapter I will first describe the anatomy of the normal ear and then discuss the management of the acute ear burn. Prevention is always better than cure. When a patient does present, however, with an ear burn then an assessment of the damage and a risk/benefit analysis of potential reconstructions is essential. At the very outset it is important to listen carefully to the patient's concerns and their expectations. Where the expectations are unrealistic it is very important to sensitively address them as no reconstruction is going to be better than a failed reconstruction. 'Failure' being defined as not achieving the desired outcome.

The anatomy of the external ear (pinna)

Figure 1 shows a normal external ear. Viewed from the lateral aspect the helix forms a rim to the ear. The anti-helix is an elevation which is rostral and parallel to the helix and splits into two crura which bound the triangular fossa. The scapha is the groove or valley between the helix and anti-helix. The concha is the shell-like concavity rostral to the anti-helix and forms the posterior aspect of the external auditory meatus. Anterior to the external auditory meatus and projecting over it is the tragus. The caudal part of the pinna is the lobule.

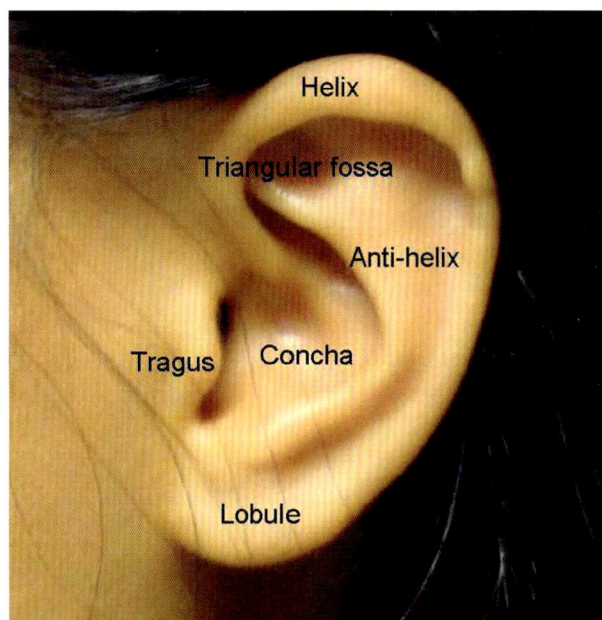

Fig. 1. The elegance of the human ear-anatomy

The arterial supply to the external ear is primarily the anterior auricular artery, a branch of the superficial temporal artery and the posterior auricular artery, a branch of the external carotid. The nerve supply comes from the aurical branches of the vagus and auricular temporal branches of the mandibular (V) nerve.

The position of the external ear

In Fig. 2 the grace and beauty of the anti-helix is apparent as an iconic 'ear maiden', right arm raised and surging forwards with fluid curves. It is the elegance of the natural ear that contributes to the considerable challenge of ear reconstruction post-burn. Another feature is the inner composition of the ear. Figure 3 shows the basic internal structure of the ear with the framework of elastic cartilage together with a padding of dense fibrous tissue overlaid with a closely adherent skin. Of particular interest is the external auditory canal which is skin lined and is made up of a fibroelastic cartilaginous tube. This can be easily distorted allowing for ear examination with an otoscope or can be permanently deformed by post burn scarring.

The 'normal' ear comes in a range of shapes and sizes with different degrees of protrusion and lobule attachment. Studies have looked at variations of ear positioning in different racial groups [10, 19]. There are no distinct racial features as far as the external structure of the ear is concerned and the relative position of the external ear is another global feature. The vertical position of the ear is shown in Fig. 4. It is the same height on the nose and when looking at the lateral aspect of the face the lower edge of the ear is at the level of the lateral ala base and the upper level of the pinna typically lies on the same level as the lateral extent of the eyebrow.

The ear can be considered to pivot around the external auditory meatus and the horizontal position of the central point of the upper margin of the external auditory meatus, the porion, lies in the same vertical axis as the vertex of the skull (Fig. 5).

The long axis of the ear is not vertical and the normal ear inclines backwards and the axis of recline is parallel to that of the line from tip to nasion of the nose (Fig. 6).

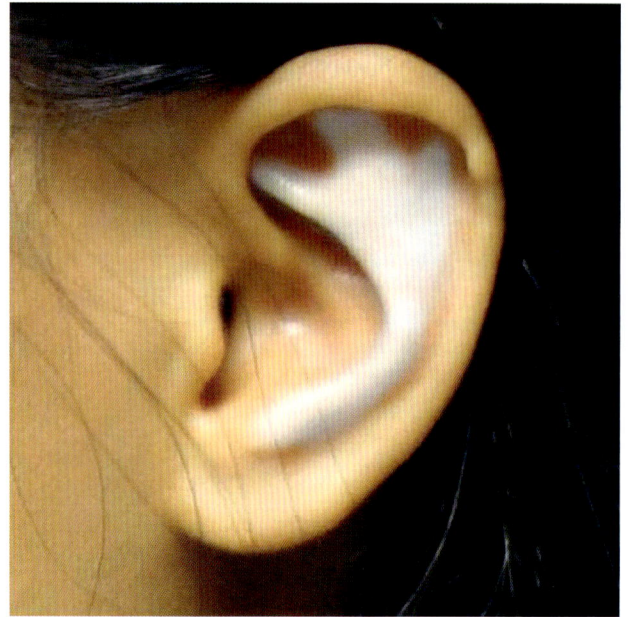

Fig. 2. The elegance of the human ear-imagery

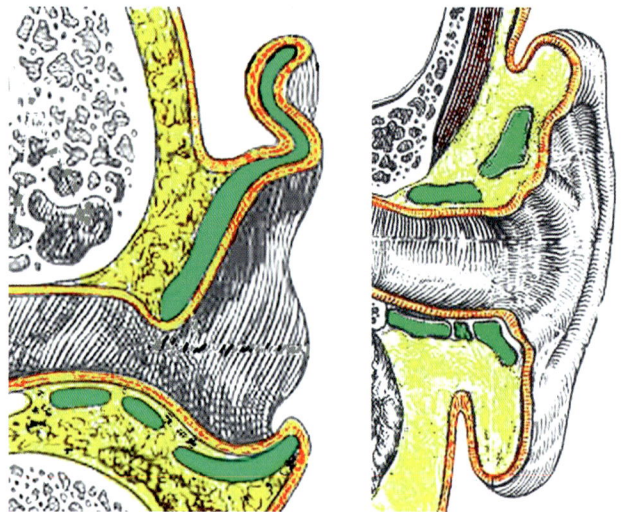

Fig. 3. The 'sandwich' with cartilage in green and fibrous connective tissue (yellow)

The influence of the position of the external ear on the overall aesthetics of the lateral view of the head and neck is illustrated by this patient who has sustained a unilateral facial burn (Fig. 7).

The scarring on the ear has caused the pinna to curl forwards losing the grace and 'flow' of the contralateral (normal) ear. In addition the right side of the face is scarred and there has been a contracture

Fig. 7. A unilateral facial burn resulting in malpositioning of the right ear

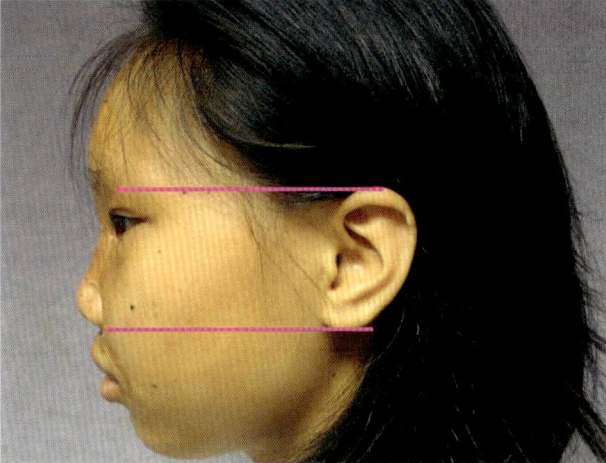

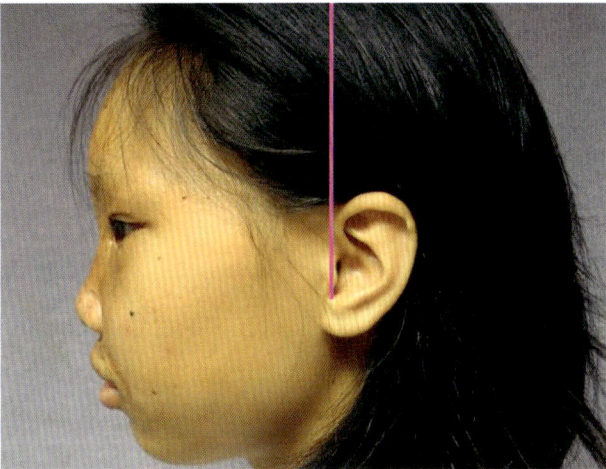

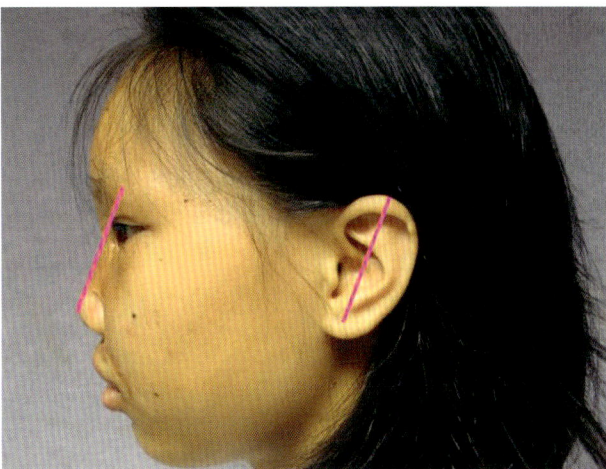

Figs. 4–6. The position of the normal ear

of the right cheek and neck which is distorting the position of the ear. The entire ear is pulled forwards and also downwards. This is possible due to the mo-

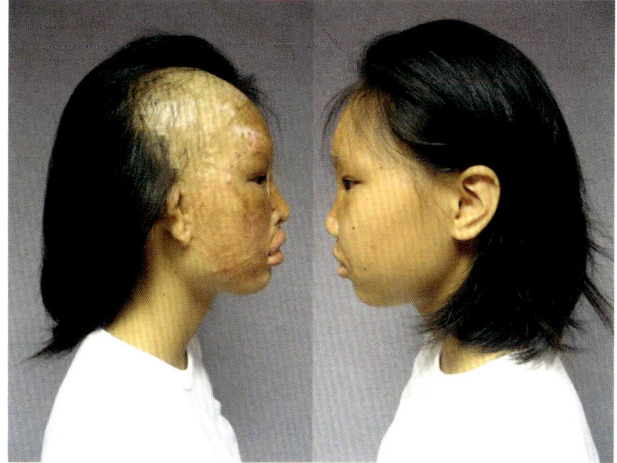

bility of the external auditory canal. Figure 8 shows a computer generated overlay of the right and left sides of the face which puts into perspective the two contrasting ear positions.

The ear can be adored with rings and jewels and is part of the overall aesthetics of the face but in general term the position of the ear is a more critical determinant of the aesthetic appreciation than the shape of the ear.

Management of the acute burn involving the ear

Burns of the Head and Neck will invariably involve the ears because of their exposed position. As in all burns there is a broad spectrum of severity of injury from small areas of superficial burn that heal quickly and leave no scarring through to the devastating destruction leading to complete loss of the ear and stenosis of the external auditory meatus.

In general the aims of acute management of ear burns involve recognition that injury has occurred; promotion of healing; prevention of infection and preservation of shape. It is an unfortunate observation that all too often with a complex major burn the priority of survival takes precedence over the attention to optimum care for the extremities. The ear is particularly vulnerable to secondary damage, from pressure and mal-position and it is essential to focus attention on appropriate dressing and bandaging techniques when dealing with the acute burn. Topical antibacterial cream can be used such as silver sulphadiazine; with plain or medicated paraffin gauze lightly packed into the concavities of the ear and the entire ear or ears dressed with shaped gamgee dressings to make 'ear-muffs'. It is very important to check that the upper pole of the ear is not folded over when the dressings are applied as this is one of the most common ear deformities found when patients are referred for late reconstruction (Fig. 9).

In the very severe head and neck burn there may be loss of vision as well as loss of the external ear. In such cases, the blind patient, hearing is a very important sensation to preserve as much as possible. The possibility of stenosis of the external auditory meatus must be prevented and the use of cut down Merocel® (Polyvinyl acetyl sponge) splints can be used to maintain patency.

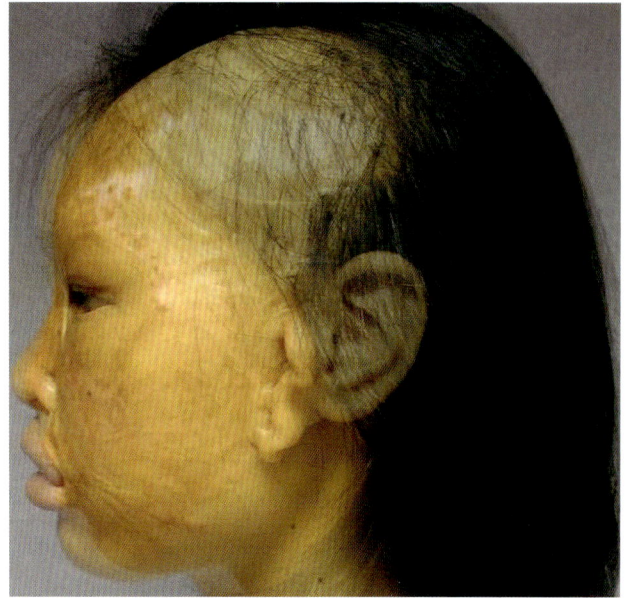

Fig. 8. An overlay of right and left lateral views to emphasis malposition

Post burn reconstruction

When a patient is being reviewed regarding problems related to the ear after a burn; the patient will focus on one, or a combination, of the following problems:
(1) Impaired hearing
(2) Abnormal scarring
(3) Loss of function
    a. Retention of glasses
    b. Inability to adorn with jewellery
(4) Deformity of the ear (without loss of tissue)
(5) Displacement of the ear due to surrounding scarring
(6) Loss of part or whole of the extend ear

Impaired hearing

Whilst this may be due to meatal stenosis there are other causes of unilateral or bilateral hearing impairment that could be completely unrelated to the burn injury. In view of this it is important to arrange for a baseline audiometric assessment to be made when the patient presents with such a concern. Other causes need to be excluded.

If the hearing impairment can be attributed to a physical blockage or distortion of the external audi-

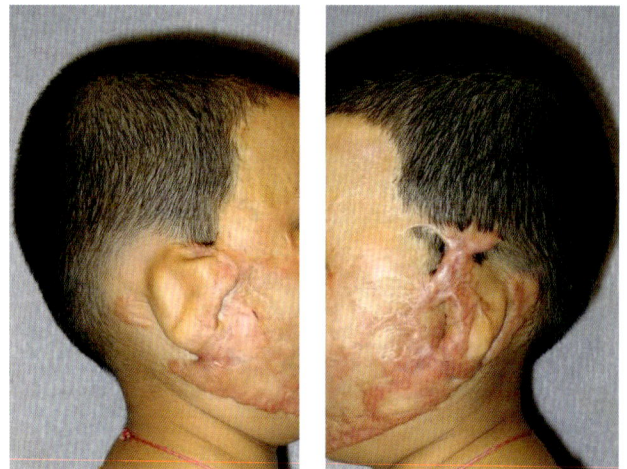

Fig. 9. The unfortunate consequences of suboptimal acute care

tory meatus then the cause and the nature of the distortion needs to be determined in order for the appropriate corrective procedure to be followed.

Again attention is focused on the composition of the external auditory canal which is a skin lined fibro-cartilaginous tube. Direct involvement of the skin by the original burn injury can result in scarring and a cicatricial stenosis. Another cause for deformity can be scarring of the skin adjacent to the ear causing a linear traction force on the external auditory meatus thus distorting it and causing it to become more like slit.

There are various descriptions on how this may be successfully achieved and one approach is a release and serial splintage [7]. Other methods described have involved interdigitating flaps of vestibule and nostril sill and ala margin skin as in the starplasty or double cross plasty [20, 22].

If the deformity is more like a slit due to a traction force then release of this force will be needed. The case illustrated shows a typical example of how this can be achieved by insetting a flap into an incisional (or excisional) defect created by the surgical release of the deforming scar tensions. The patient illustrated had been the victim of an acid assault and had developed extensive scarring of the mouth, nostrils, chin and neck and left ear. She was referred having had the acute burn treated and some initial reconstruction commenced but her specific concerns were the ectropion of the lower lip and the deformity of the left neck and the impaired hearing. A splint had been made to try and counteract the 'stenosis' of the EAM but on inspection it was the scarring in the neck that was causing the problem. To address both problems a bi-paddled antero-lateral thigh flap was raised. This actually proved to be anatomically interesting as the perforators came from two completely separate systems allowing the flaps to be placed some distance from each other whilst there was only one anastamosis to the recipient vessels (Fig. 10).

The two flaps were inset with the anterior paddle oriented horizontally to correct the lower lip ectropion. The posterior paddle was oriented vertically and was inset into the lateral neck defect left after an

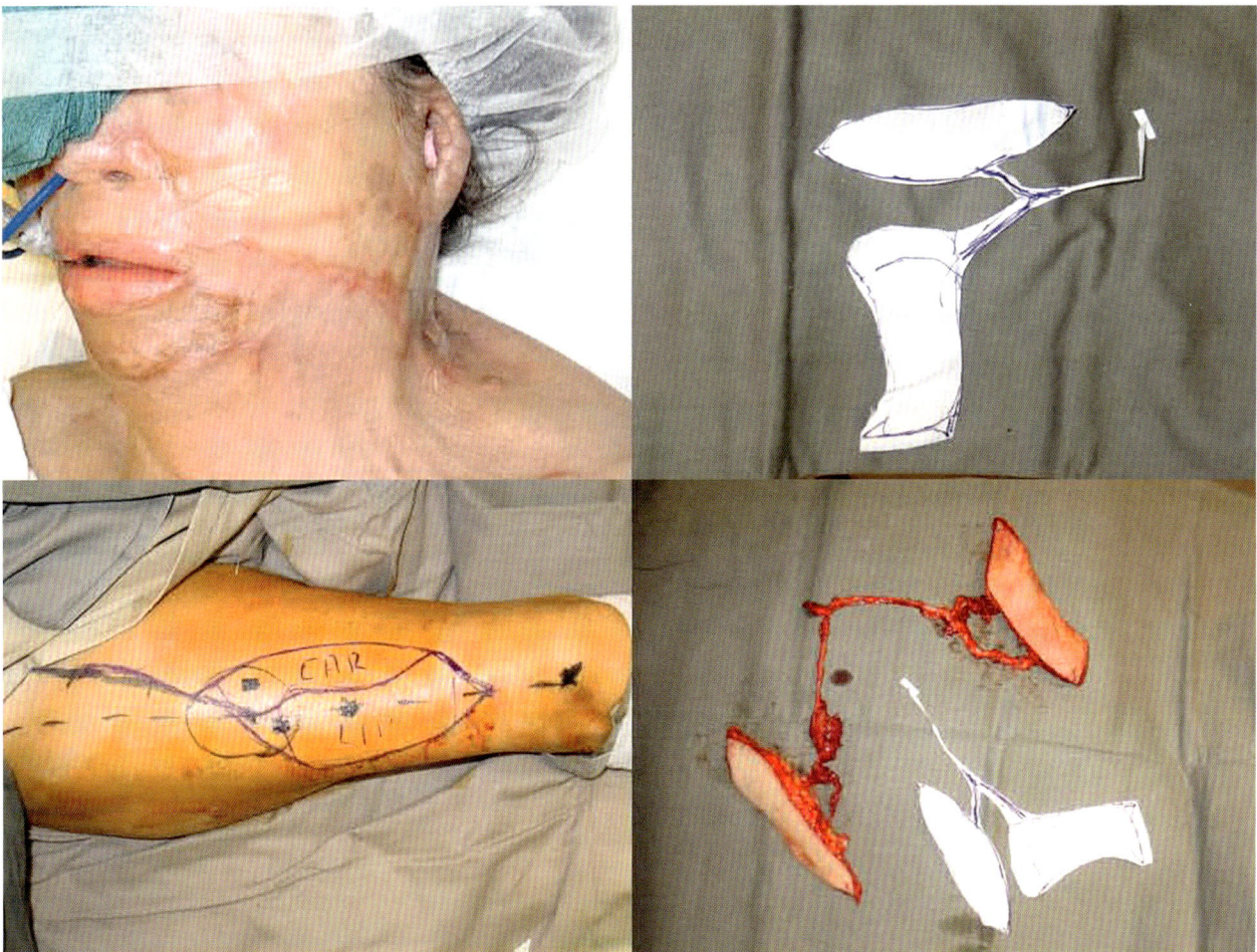

Fig. 10. An intra-operative series indicating the two flaps

incisional scar release. The upper tip of the flap was inset into the external audiotory meatal canal to release the cicatricial stenosis (Fig. 11).

Abnormal scarring

The exposed position of the ears means that they are frequently involved in burns of the head and neck region. Of course there will be many of these burns that are partial thickness and heal with dressings only. In many children and adults the healing of ear burns is relatively uneventful. There are a small number of patients, particularly children, who react very differently to the injury.

In certain patients there is an accumulation of excessive connective tissue which forms an abnormal scar. The two principle forms of abnormal scar are hypertrophic and keloid scars. These do appear to be two very different forms of scar [5]. A major clinical difference is that the hypertrophic scar appears to be associated with active tissue remodelling and the effect is that tensions are created within the skin surrounding the scar tending to cause a contracture of the scar area. This can be seen by the effects of the scar on the surrounding soft tissues, for example, the mouth or eyelids. When the hypertrophic scar is excised the resulting defect is always much larger than the area of excised scar. The keloid scar behaves very differently and is characterized more by an accumulation of connective tissue matrix which appears to grow into the surrounding tissues. The edge of the scar is often raised and rolled and when the scar is excised the resulting defect is usually the same size as the excised scar. There is another very important clinical difference between the keloid scar and the hypertrophic scar and that relates to the duration of the abnormal scarring. Typically a keloid scar will grow to a certain size and then remain at that size for a prolonged period of time. Indeed the keloid scar is generally taught not to involute. The hypertrophic scar in contrast is a self-limiting form of abnormal scarring and will mature albeit over the course of several years.

The two forms of scarring are rarely seen together in any patient group other than in post burn patients and particularly children. The reason for this is not clear and it is also clear that the pathology as well as the pathogenesis of the keloid scar, in par-

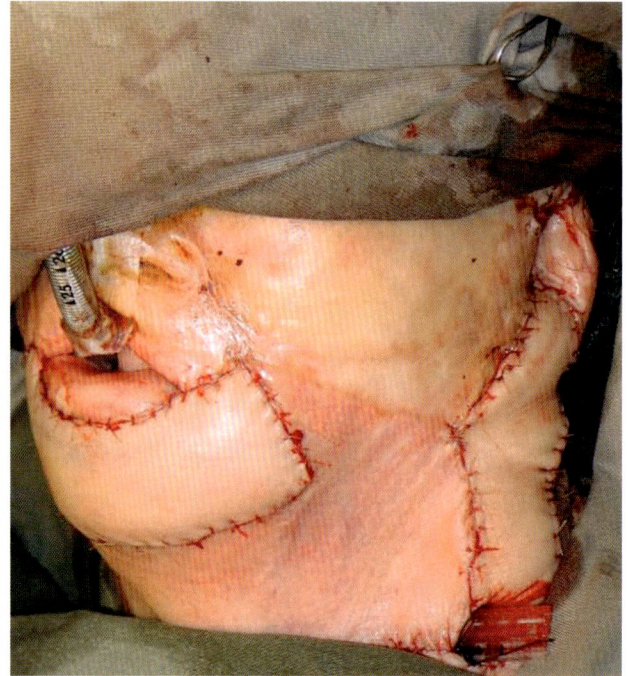

Fig. 11. Two flaps inset

ticular, is different in the burns patient when compared to keloid arising form other stimuli, such as acne or ear piercing. Our understanding of the nature of the evolution of the post-burn keloid scar remains rudimentary and it is possible that it does have a tendency to be more self-limiting than other types of keloid.

Figure 12 shows both right and left lateral views of a young boy who developed classical keloid type scarring of the upper helical ruin. The close-up view shows the massive raised, rolled accumulations of scar tissue (Fig. 13). The standard teaching is that if a keloid scar is excised then it ALWAYS recurs and also tends to be more aggressive. To prevent or reduce the incidence of recurrence it is always necessary to apply some adjuvant treatment in combination with the surgery. This may involve the application of cytotoxic agents to the post-excisional wound, the injection of steroids or exposure to irradiation. These approaches reduce the cellular response to further wounding and appear to have an immunosuppressive effect.

Our approach to the post burn keloid is rather different and the first case was detailed in a case report involving a large buttock and posterior thigh keloid [4]. Basically the keloid was showed flush with

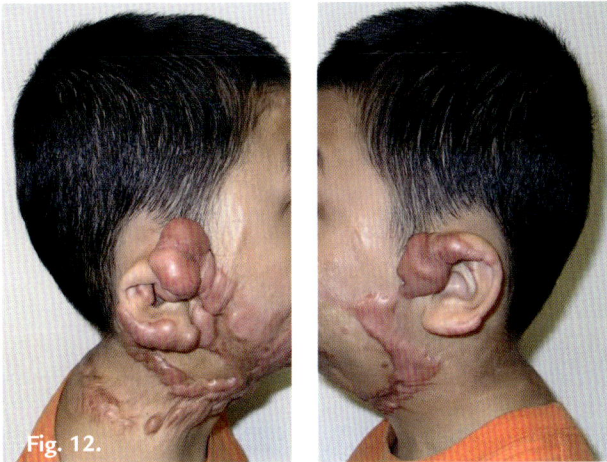

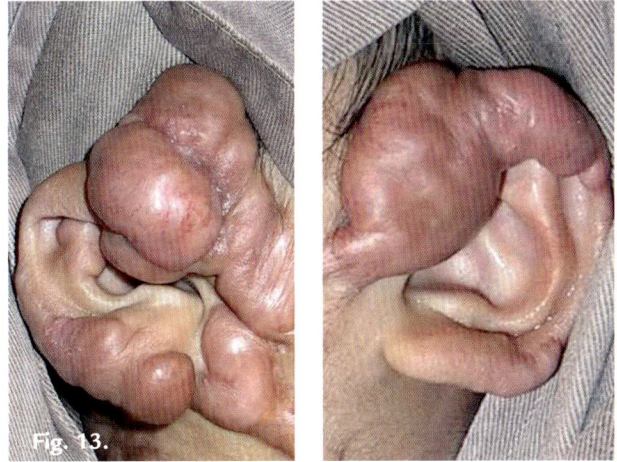

Figs. 12–13. Abnormal scarring with close-up view

the normal skin and cells cultured from a biopsy taken from a site of normal skin were applied as suspension with a concentration of 8.3×10^4 cells per cm^2. The cells were pipetted onto the excisional defect and 'fixed' in place by the subsequent application of Tisseel® fibrin glue. The glue was sprayed on gently taking care not to blow the liquid suspension off the wound. The wound was then allowed to dry and Mepitel was then applied. The healing of the wound is depicted in Fig. 14.

The upper two pictures show the post excisional wound at one week post cell spray. Of note as the 'excision' of the keloid was flush with the surface of the surrounding skin there is still keloid tissue in the wound bed. The lower two pictures show the wound dressed with gentian violet and complete healing occurred in three weeks. Figure 15 shows the appearance at six months post cell-spray. The scar is raised and red but subsides and when viewed three years post cell spray (the lower two pictures of Fig. 15). The scarring is all flat and mature. Again the underlying biological mechanisms at work remain unknown but in a series of five cases the response has been similar and persistent.

Loss of function

Apart from the function in association with the middle and inner ear for hearing, the external ear has a function for retaining ear mounted devices. These may simply be spectacles although there is an in-

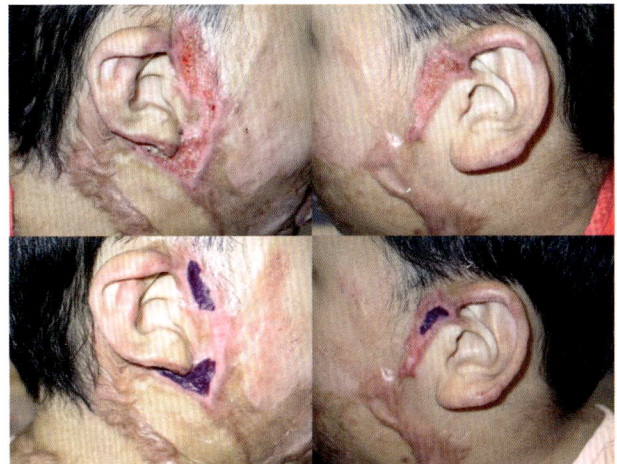

Fig. 14. Early post-operative views

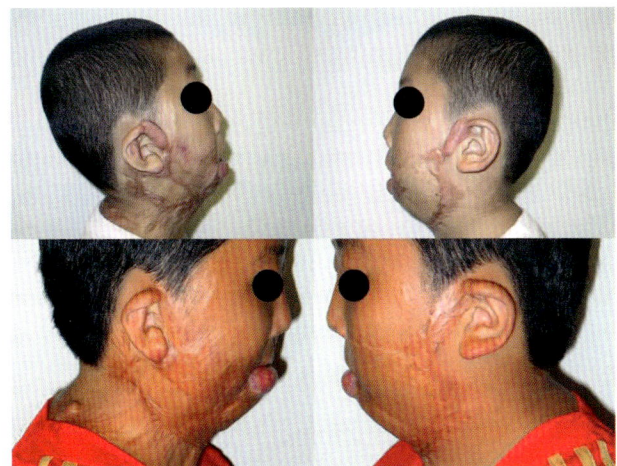

Fig. 15. Lateral views. It appears as if the scar trajectory has changed and whilst initially there is obvious scar growth this does resolve in twelve months

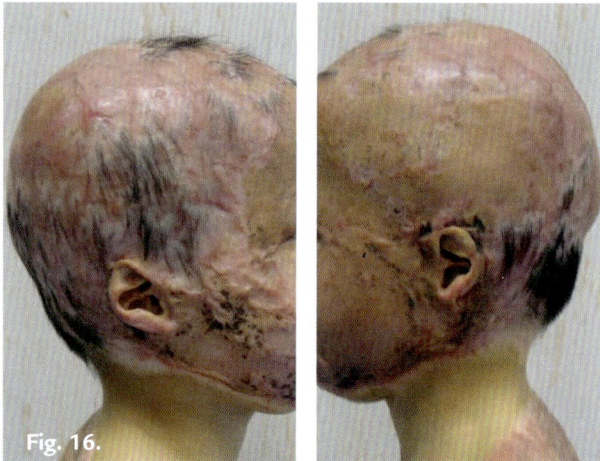

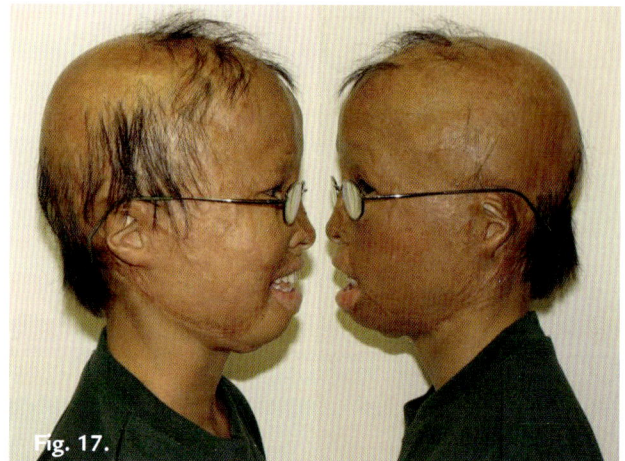

Figs. 16–17. Early and late views of bilateral ear burns which caused deformity but retained the function of supporting eyeglasses

creasing range of wireless free devices that can be attached to the ears. This retention function depends more upon the well defined upper pole of the ear with a retro-auricular sulcus. The other function is for the adornment of jewellery and this is typically applied to the lobe of the ear. Thus loss of the lobe can be a concern for some patients.

Figure 16 shows a patient who sustained 65% BSA burns in an injury involving a mosquito net [3]. The scalp was severely damaged and the external ears were deformed but the patient was not concerned about the ears as they retained their function of stabilizing his eye glasses (Fig. 17).

The interval between Figs. 16 and 17 was three years and in that time the patient had received multiple surgeries to improve the function of his hands. Another case shows the creation of a retro-auricular sulcus by elevating the cartilage together with a rim of scar approximately 8 mm wide and then inserting a split thickness graft secured with a tie over dressing (Fig. 18).

The appearance is shown two years later and the sulcus has been maintained although some graft contracture has distorted the upper pole of the ear, and the superior sulcus has not been satisfactorily defined.

Deformity of the ear without loss of tissue

This is a preventable but unfortunately all too common complication of inadequate primary treatment of ear burns. The deformity is a consequence

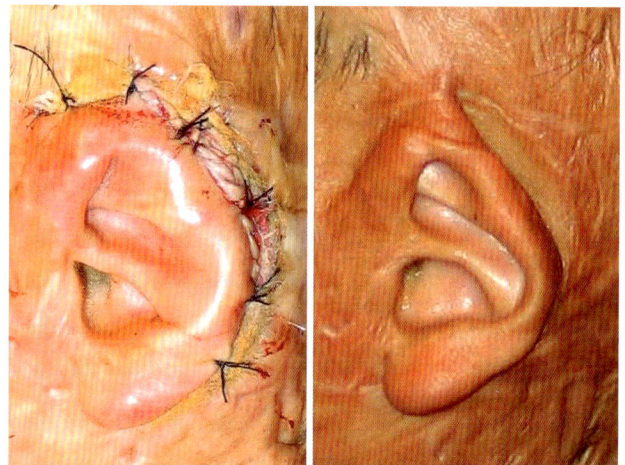

Fig. 18. Both this and the previous patient suffered from Mosquito net related burns.

These cause deep burns of head and neck and hands. The patient was happy with a very limited procedure

of dressings that are either inappropriately applied or not checked. The ear becomes folded forwards and the helical rim becomes attached to the pre-auricular skin or scar tissue. Where the attachment occurs there will inevitably be an accumulation of scar tissue and when releasing the anteriorly displaced ear the helical rim will appear as a secondary deformity.

There will also be a defect in the pre-auricular region that was the site of the attachment. This defect can often be conveniently closed using a superiorly based flap of post-auricular skin. The ear thus formed lacks the helical definition of the normal ear but is acceptable to most patients.

Examples of this type of reconstruction are shown in Figs. 9 and 19–20. Figure 9 is the deformity at presentation. The entire cartilaginous framework is present but the ear has been folded anteriorly and scarring is maintaining the deformity. When the scar is released there is a significant loss of skin that prevents a direct closure of the defect in the pre-auricular area and on the helical rim. A superiorly based post-auricular flap can be used to close the defect. Although the resulting ear does not have the aesthetic impact of the natural ear the return to a normal position and a grossly normal ear has produced a result that is acceptable to the patient.

Of interest in this case is the keloid-like scar nodule that is arising from the anterior aspect of the ear. The follow up two years after the surgery shows a result that is acceptable to the patient. Of interest is that the keloid like scar has matured and is no longer visible suggesting atypical keloid behaviour.

Displacement of the ear due to surrounding scarring

It is quite fascinating how the human brain processes information with regard to facial features. With regard to the ear the extent and nature of a de-

formity of shape is secondary to an appreciation of an abnormal position. The external ear is joined to the skull by a deformable cartilaginous tube lined by skin and surrounded by fibro-fatty tissue. Scarring of the neck and/or the cheek can cause the ear to be pulled down and/or anteriorly. The extent and nature of the scarring will determine the extent and nature of the deformity and in turn the extent of the defect created as the ear is returned to its original position.

In the neck which is a highly flexible part of the body a substantial and permanent release is most often achieved by the use of flaps. These have the shared advantages of requiring no post-operative immobilization or splinting and there will be no subsequent contracture.

The cheek is not so dynamic in its movement and full-thickness, or thick split-thickness grafts or the use of tissue engineered material specifically Integra dermal regeneration template can achieve satisfactory closure of the defect left after excision of the scar causing the positional deformity.

The series of pictures in Fig. 21 show the excision of the right facial scar of the patient with unilateral facial scarring shown in Fig. 7. The defect is resurfaced with a sheet of full thickness skin graft. The three pictures at the bottom of Fig. 21 show the situation before the surgery and the immediate and four year post-reconstruction appearance. Figure 22 show

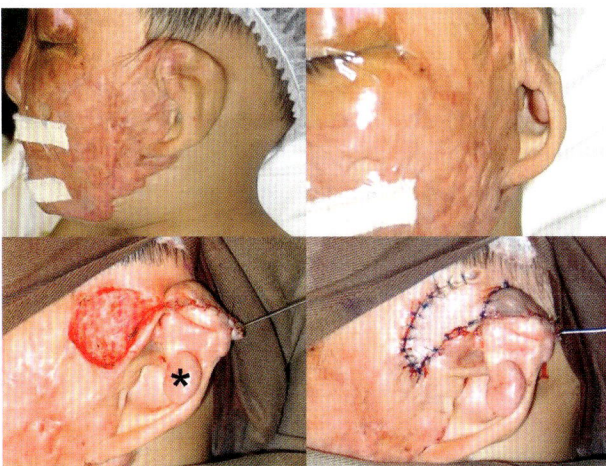

Fig. 19. Another case using the superiorly based post-aurical flap. A 'keloid' nodule is present on the anterior surface of the ear (*)

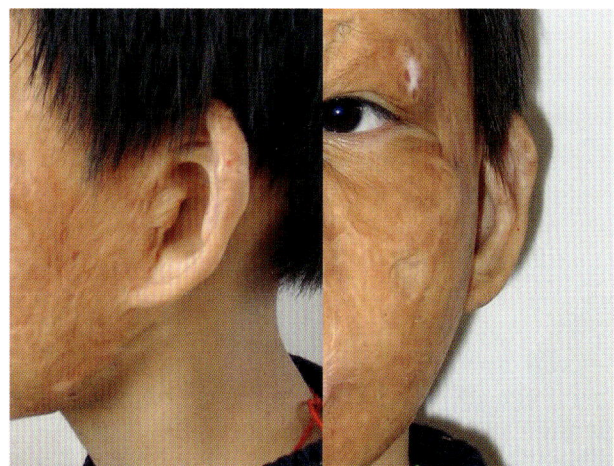

Fig. 20. Two years later the ear shape is acceptable and the 'keloid' nodule has gone

computer composites of the pre and post surgery to show the change in ear position and also a composite of the right and left sides which underlines the importance of ear position in the overall aesthetics of the face.

Loss of part or whole of the external ear

There is a major difference in reconstructing the ear after congenital absence and reconstructing an ear after traumatic loss and in particular burns. The difference relates to working with skin on the one hand and scar tissue on the other. Skin is a much more versatile reconstructive medium and the quantity can always be increased by tissue expansion. It is interesting to note that the first reported case of medical skin expansion was performed by Neumann in 1956. He used a rubber balloon which he inflated by air. And the patient? The patient had sustained traumatic amputation of the upper two thirds of his right ear many years before. Neumann introduced the balloon under the skin in the temporo-parietal region. He subsequently removed this and inserted a C-shaped costal cartilage graft. Neumann conceded that much work needed to be done before such a reconstruction could become accepted by the Plastic Surgical community at large, but a concept had been born [18].

Over twenty-five years ago I went to Harvard as a Research Fellow in Pathology and was determined to find out more about tissue expansion and was able to track down another pioneer in the field, Professor Jaime Planas [12]. I communicated with Professor Planas and he was gracious enough to share with me the following medical history.

"In 1975, a boy aged 17, came to my office asking for the correction of the congenital absence of one ear, which had been operated on twice. The area was scarred. I saw no possible correction other than bringing new tissues from other sources. Flaps for ear repair, at that time, gave always bad cosmetic results, and I thought again about the expansion of the skin. Dr Arion, a French plastic surgeon, whose father had the SIMAPLAST factory (French inflatable prosthesis) made two small balloons for me. The valves had not been yet discovered at the time. Moreover, the balloons were not elastic at all, so the two balloons were introduced superposed under the skin of the mastoid, and

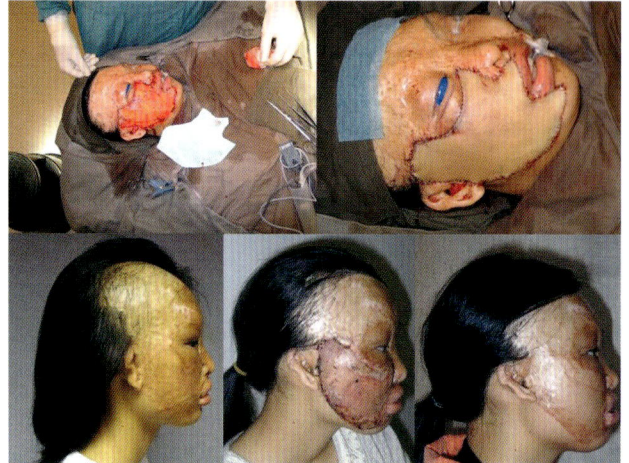

Fig. 21. The malposition of the right ear shown in Fig. 7 is corrected with a full-thickness graft to resurface the right face. A post-auricular flap has also been used to 'open' up the ear. The follow up picture is four years after the operation

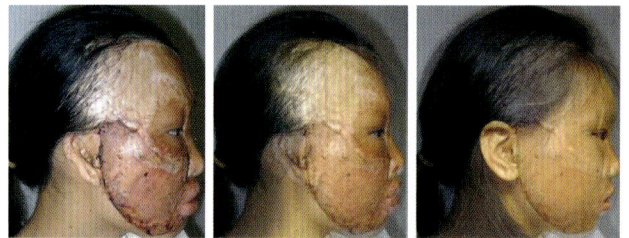

Fig. 22. Computer generated overlays to demonstrate the change in position and appearance of the right side of the face

the tubes buried under the scalp of the temporal region. The superficial balloon was inflated with 15 cc of saline and tied. Three months later the second balloon was filled with 10cc of saline. No more liquid was admitted. Four months later the balloons were removed and a cartilagenous frame, according to Tanzer's recommendations, was introduced. Some months later the new ear was separated from the mastoid and covered by a free skin graft. This was not published as I was waiting for the evolution as well as to have, at least a second case.

I think it was at the 1978 meeting in Miami that I saw the presentation of an interesting paper by Radovan, the results being far superior to mine. Therefore, I forgot about my experiment and since then I have been following the new advances on this matter."

Even in busy specialized units however, taking trauma and congenital cases there is little call for tissue expansion. The details are however very clearly explained by the Mount Vernon team. They expanded the available skin and then when removing the expander, also performing a capsulectomy. This very thin skin was drawn over the preformed framework and a close attachment was created using prolonged mini-suction drains [6].

Looking at the literature regarding ear reconstruction it would be misleading to think that they will be equally useful using skin flaps compared to scar flaps. Scarred skin can be used in other parts of the body because the subdermal capillary plexus is still present if the burn was partial thickness. It is the movement that is the problem so skin can be tubed but scar cannot, or at least cannot be tubed so easily [9].

Tubing can be useful for loss of the helical rim and the lobule but when more extensive loss involving a significant cartilage deficiency occurs then the reconstruction requires a framework.

The Mount Vernon team published their experience in 1999 [13] looking at partial ear defects. In a series of 27 cases they dealt with four ears from three patients. Three involved upper defects and one a lower pole defect. This group used autologous costal cartilage covering it with local skin with and without prior tissue expansion. In three cases where there was a significant scarring of the local tissues the framework was covered with temporoparietal fascia flaps.

A more burn specific review of a case series was presented by the group from Qatar who reported a series of 22 patients who underwent subtotal reconstruction of the auricles after burns [8]. All patients had autogenous cartilage used for the framework but different techniques to cover this were used:
(1) temporoparietal flap
(2) subcutaneous pocket technique
(3) the pre-auricular skin flap
(4) the post-auricular skin flap
These papers introduce new concepts of reconstruction with specific relation to the ear.

Figure 23 shows a case of unilateral loss of the upper pole of the ear together with tethering and distortion of the lower pole (lobule). Both can be addressed with local procedures, the upper pole requiring cartilage support.

The temporoparietal flap

This flap was first described in 1898 but remained primarily overlooked until 1983 when Brent and his colleagues reported the flap as:
(1) an axial-pattern fascial flap
(2) a random-pattern fascial flap
(3) a free fascial flap
This flap is highly versatile and is unique in being the only flap consisting of a single, vascularized, fascial layer in the head and neck region. It can readily drape over the convexities and concavities of the cartilagineous framework but also is able to take a thin skin graft providing and thin providing reliable vascularized cover. Because of the rich vascularity of the flap it is sturdy and resists infection. The flap comprises the superficial temporal fascia and the superficial temporal artery and vein. An excellent description of the flap has been written by Moran in Wei & Mardini's text book [17].

Figure 24 shows a pre-operative slide of the course of the posterior branch of the superficial temporal artery which has been mapped with the Doppler. Although the patient does not have an upper pole of the right ear he has elected for a reconstruction of the right eyebrow instead. This is an important point to consider before using the temporoparietal flap for ear reconstruction: what are the patient's priorities for repair.

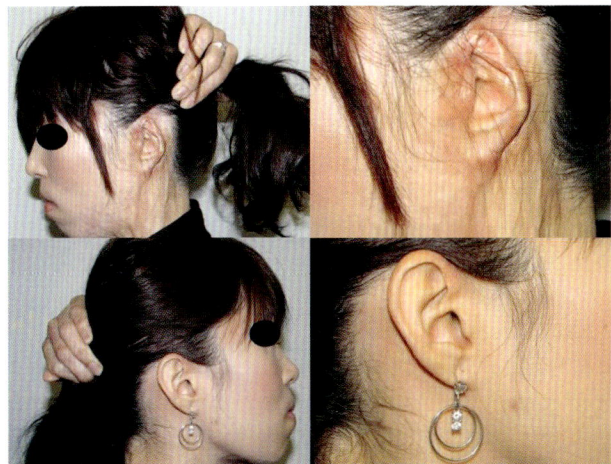

Fig. 23. Distortion of both upper and lower poles in a unilateral burn

Figure 25 shows another case where there is obviously some surviving ear cartilage but the side of the scalp has been grafted. In such cases it is not possible to harvest the flap safely and replace the overlying skin.

The subcutaneous pocket technique

The subcutaneous pocket technique has a number of applications in reconstructive and trauma surgery. Essentially it means burying something in a pocket so that viability can be achieved immediately via diffusion and subsequently by neo-vascurlarization. The group from Qatar described harvesting cartilage from the seventh and eighth costal cartilages and, after carving them, inserting them into a subcutaneous pocket. This pocket was dissected at a level that kept the subdermal plexus intact and was large enough to drape easily over the cartilaginous framework. Suction drains were used to maintain a closed space and creation of the posterior auricular groove was undertaken 3–4 months later.

Pre and post auricular skin healing flaps

The anteriorly based post-auricular flap has already been illustrated in the context of repositioning displaced ears whilst a caudally based pre-auricular skin flap can be used for lower pole/lobe, defects.

Total ear reconstruction

Total ear reconstruction following burns is a considerable challenge. Indeed there are few reported cases worldwide and even fewer where the results are aesthetically pleasing. The problem relates to the specific nature of the burn injury in that in many patients the total loss of the pinna is associated with very severe burns involving other parts of the body. The priority in these cases are to address the areas of greater functional significance first and ear reconstruction comes low in the list of priorities. Indeed in over thirty years of active postburn reconstruction I have not performed a single total ear reconstruction. It is not just the prioritization that is an issue, but also with extensive scarring the possibility of reconstructing an ear that is aesthetically acceptable is realistically limited. Although I have counselled over

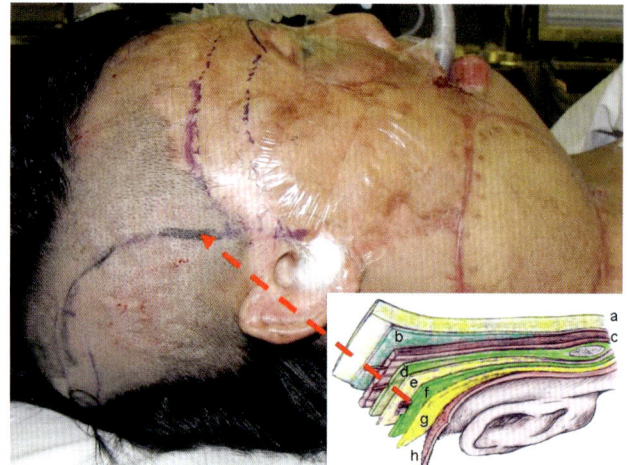

Fig. 24. The temporoparietal layer of the scalp is a multilayered complex comprising.

a) Bone
b) Pericranium
c) Temporalis muscle
d) Temporalis muscle fascia
e) Loose areola tissue
f) Temporoparietal fascia
g) Subcutaneous tissue
h) Skin

The posterior branch of the superficial temporal artery runs in the temporoparietal fascia and is marked out before raising a pedicled flap for eyebrow reconstruction

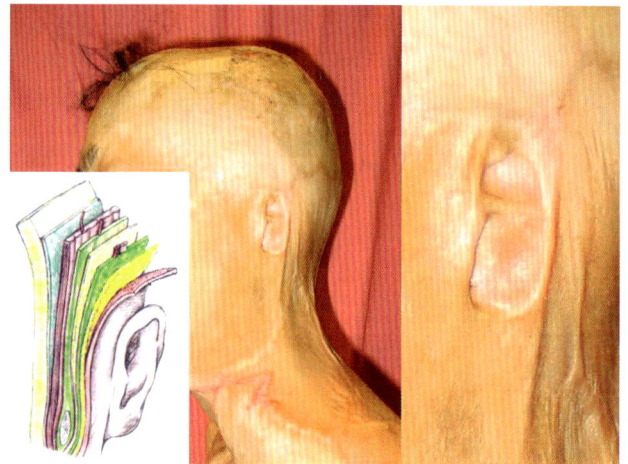

Fig. 25. In this patient the left side of the scalp has been grafted and it will not be possible to raise a temporoparietal flap

twenty patients who did have complete loss of the ear, when considering the risk-benefit analysis, all patients have opted not to have reconstruction. This decision is not affected by sex or culture.

Bhandari describes the challenge in terms of a) the framework fabrication and b) the quality and quantity of the skin available for covering the framework. On the basis of skin availability they recognize five groups of patients [1].

Group I Patients with healthy skin in the auricular region.

Group II Patients in whom the surrounding skin is either scarred or grafted but is supple.

Group III Patients with no local skin but a pedicled temporo parietal flap can be used for draping over the cartilage framework.

Group IV Patients with neither local skin nor fascial flap available but who have potential donor fascial flaps available for free microvascular transfer

Group V Patients with no donor sites for free fascial flaps or having other problems such as high anaesthetic risk. In this group ear reconstruction is not possible.

In Bhandari's paper the framework is made of cartilage, but synthetic materials have been used such as Teflon and silicone. The most popular synthetic material is a porous polyethylene available as Medpore. This is strong and flexible but also being porous it encourages both vascular and soft tissue ingrowth [16].

The design of the cartilaginous framework has been well described in the Chapter in Mathes written by Brent [2]. He describes an evolution in technique beginning first with sculpting a framework from an 'en-bloc' resection of cartilage from the ipsilateral ribs and progressing to subsequent refinements adding a tragal strut and helical run. Figure 26 is an adaptation from Brent's chapter and shows the 'en-bloc' creation of the cartilage scaffold. More recent publications have focused more on a reconstruction of the framework from several rib cartilages [15] and increasing attention is being paid to reconstituting the cartilage donor site to avoid both unpleasant scar and contour defects [11].

Nevertheless, no matter how sophisticated the technique, the results of total ear reconstruction in the post burn patient still leaves much to be desired in terms of the aesthetics [14]. Ultimately the reality of the Group V classification according to Bhandari, has to be faced. Even ectopic reconstruction using the pre-laminated ear reconstruction under an expanded radial forearm flap as illustrated by Wik-

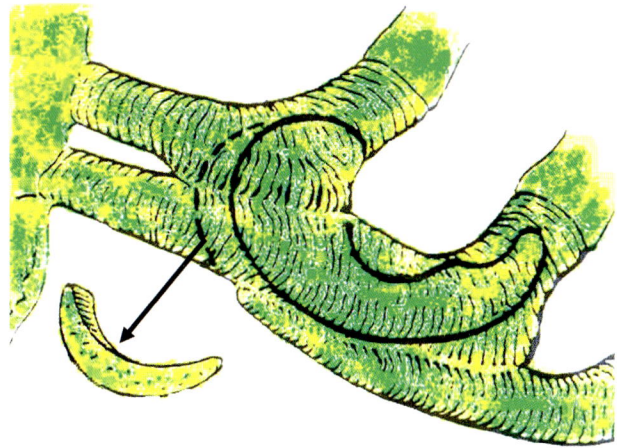

Fig. 26. The composite cartilage harvest

strom [21] is an unlikely possibility in a major burn where fascial excision of burns of the limbs may have been undertaken.

An option remains and that is to use an external prosthesis attached either with adhesive or better still using osteointegration. In a review of nearly 1,500 ear reconstruction cases, the Auricular Centre of the Plastic Surgery hospital of the Chinese Medical Sciences reported twenty four cases using titanium dowel retained prosthesis and described favourable clinical outcomes [23].

Summary

The reconstruction of the burn ear can involve a number of techniques depending upon the deformity and loss of tissue. In many cases acceptable results can be achieved with fairly simple procedures which involve repositioning and/or unfolding a deformed ear.

The total reconstruction of the ear in a patient with an extensive burn is a completely different issue and good results can hardly ever be obtained. Whilst some patients may choose to have an external prosthesis most accept the deformity and concentrate on maximizing the function and appearance of other body parts.

References

[1] Bhandari PS (1998) Total ear reconstruction in post burn deformity. Burns 24: 661–670

[2] Brent BD (2006) Reconstruction of the auricle. In: Mathes SJ, Hentz VR (eds) Plastic surgery, 2nd edn, Vol III, The Head and Neck, Part 2. Saunders, Philadelphia, pp 633–657

[3] Burd A, Ahmed K (2007) Mosquito-net burns and the prevention hexagon. Burns 33: 261–263

[4] Burd A, Chan E (2002) Keratinocyte-keloid interaction. Plast Reconstr Surg 110: 197–202

[5] Burd A, Huang L (2005) Hypertrophic response and keloid diathesis: two very different forms of scar. Plast Reconstr Surg 116: 150e-157e

[6] Chana JS, Grobbelaar AO, Gault DT (1997) Tissue expansion as an adjunct to reconstruction of congenital and acquired auricular deformities. J Plast Reconstr Aesthet Surg 50: 456–462

[7] Daya M (2009) Nostril stenosis corrected by release and serial stenting. J Plast Reconstr Aesthet Surg 62: 1012–1019

[8] El-Khatib HA, Al-Basti HB, Al-Ghoul A, Al-Gaber H, Al-Hetmi T (2005) Subtotal reconstruction of the burned auricle. Burns 31: 230–235

[9] Ellabban MG, Maamoun MI, Elsharkawi M (2003) The bi-pedicle post-auricular tube flap for reconstruction of partial ear defects. J Plast Reconstr Aesthet Surg 56: 593–598

[10] Farkas LG, Hreczko TA, Kolar JC, Munro IR (1985) Vertical and horizontal proportions of the face in young adult North American Caucasians: revision of neoclassical canons. Plast Reconstr Surg 75: 328–337

[11] Fattah A, Sebire NJ, Bulstrode NW (2009) Donor site reconstitution for ear reconstruction. J Plast Reconstr Aesthet Surg (In Press)

[12] Gorney M (2004) Prof Jaime Planas, MD, 1915 to 2004. Plast Reconstr Surg 114: 1650

[13] Harris PA, Ladhani K, Das-Gupta R, Gault DT (1999) Reconstruction of acquired sub-total ear defects with autologous costal cartilage. J Plast Reconstr Aesthet Surg 52: 268–275

[14] Ibrahim SMS, Salem IL (2008) Burned ear: the use of a staged Nagata technique for ear reconstruction. J Plast Reconstr Aesthet Surg 61: S52-S58

[15] Jiang H, Pan B, Lin L, Zhao Y, Guo D, Zhuang H (2008) Fabrication of three-dimensional cartilaginous framework in auricular reconstruction. J Plast Reconstr Aesthet Surg 61: S77-S85

[16] Jones CE, Wellisz T (1994) External ear reconstruction. Aorn Journal 59: 411–428

[17] Moran SL (2009) Temporoparietal fascia flap. In: Wei FC, Mardini S (eds) Flaps and reconstructive surgery. Saunders, UK, pp 159–173

[18] Neumann CG (1957) The expansion of an area of skin by progressive distention of a subcutaneous balloon. Plast Reconstr Surg 19: 124–130

[19] Posnick JC, Al-Qattan MM, Whitaker LA (1993) Assessment of the preferred vertical position of the ear. Plast Reconstr Surg 91: 1198–1203

[20] Sinha M, Naasan A (2007) Correction of nasal stenosis: the double cross plasty. J Plast Reconstr Aesthet Surg 60: 1368–1369

[21] Stewart K (2008) Autologous ear reconstruction – celebrating 50 years. J Plast Reconstr Aesthet Surg 61: S2–S4

[22] Tiwari VK, Sarabahi S (2006) Starplasty: an ideal method for correction of occluded external nares following burns. J Plast Reconstr Aesthet Surg 59: 1105–1109

[23] Zhao Y, Wang Y, Zhuang H, Jiang H, Jiang W, Hu X, Hu S, Wang S, Pan B (2009) Clinical evaluation of three total ear reconstruction methods. J Plast Reconstr Aesthet Surg 62: 1550–1554

Correspondence: Andrew Burd M. D., Division of Plastic, Reconstructive and Aesthetic Surgery, Department of Surgery, The Chinese University of Hong Kong, Prince of Wales Hospital, Hong Kong, E-mail: andrewburd@surgery.cuhk.edu.hk

Reconstruction of the perioral region after facial burns

Timo A. Spanholtz, Riccardo E. Giunta

Department Hand Surgery, Plastic and Aesthetic Surgery; Ludwig-Maximilians Universität München, Germany

Introduction

Etiology and pathophysiology

Deep facial burns occur for different reasons and often affect patients' outcome and life quality in a dramatic fashion. Although they are present in a minority of burned patients, they pose a greater challenge in surgical and non-surgical treatment. Chemical, electrical and thermal burns can lead to disfiguring scar formations and restrain sufficient mouth opening (impaired temporomandibular joint range of motion). The average physiological mouth opening measures 40–50 mm. An opening of 25–35 mm is still functional while an opening of less than 24 mm is severely limiting in daily life [1]. In the literature 3.7–10.8% of thermal burn admissions are complicated by reduction of the size of the oral aperture, generally called microstomia. In infants, perioral burns often occur when a child bites into or sucks on an electrical cord or the improperly connected junction of two electrical cords.

In case of electrical accidents both the enoral mucosa and the lip are damaged more extensively than the surrounding skin, as the high electrical resistance of skin tissue reduces injury to the skin while the saliva-coated lip and enoral surfaces conduct electricity very well. The soft tissue injury caused by electricity is often more extensive than initially estimated, because the current may follow the low-resistance paths of nerves, vessels and facial muscles. Coagulation necrosis with inflammation of adjacent vital tissues results in crippling scars causing hypotonicity of the circumoral muscles.

As in fact, thermal burns of 95% total body surface area (TBSA) are today associated with a 50% chance of survival in children [2] the treatment of deep facial thermal burns becomes more important to improve the quality of life in these patients. The scar contracture caused by deep facial thermal burns or electrical accidents results in several problems such as tongue cicatrization, disturbance in facial expression and microstomia. Nowhere in the body are scars more apparent than in the face.

Relevant anatomy

No cartilage or any other rigid frame supports the oral orifice nor the lips. The vermillion border flanks the oral aperture and extends to facial skin tissue to all sides. The upper lip is subdivided in 3 subunits: the philtrum and 2 lateral subunits that extend from the philtral columns to the nasolabial folds. At the oral commissure, upper and lower lip meet. Not subdivided, the lower lip stretches out to the labiomental fold inferiorly and to the nasolabial folds laterally (Figs. 1, 2).

The infraorbital nerve (V2) and the mandibular nerve (V3) assure the sensory innervation to the upper and lower lip. Oral commissures are innervated

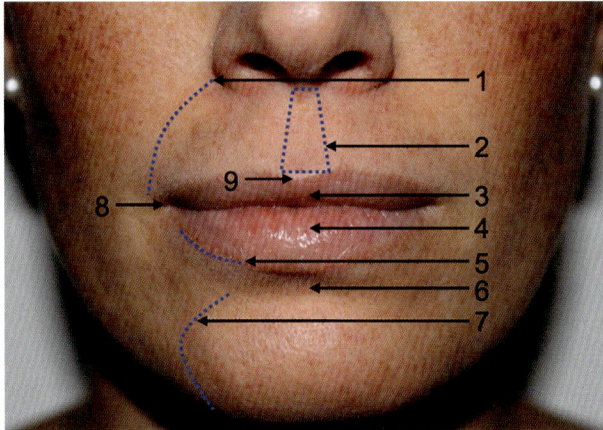

Fig. 1. Surface anatomy of the lip; 1 Nasolabial fold; 2 Philtrum; 3 Tubercle; 4 Vermilion of the lower lip; 5 Vermilion border; 6 Horizontal fold of mentum; 7 mental fold; 8 oral commissure; 9 Cupid's bow

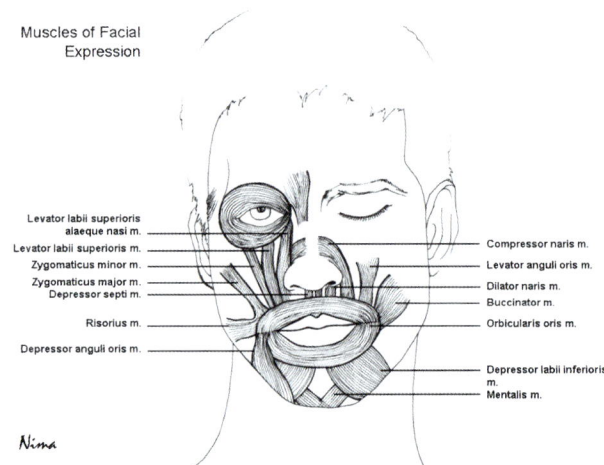

Fig. 2. Facial muscles in the perioral region

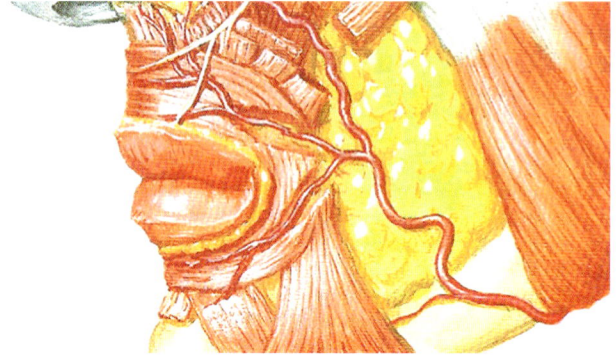

Fig. 3. Arterial and nerveous supply of the perioral region

mainly through the buccal branch of the mandibular nerve. The main arterial supply is from the labial arteries (branches from the facial artery, Fig. 3). This arterial frame forms a 360-degree loop, which allows for various flap designs. The arteries provide perforators through the orbicularis muscle to the overlying skin of the lip. Theoretically flaps in the lip area should contain one labial artery, although blood supply is so numerous in the perioral region that survival of local flaps can be secured by including one single segment of mucosa. Lymph nodes of the submandibular and submental area drain the lymph of the lower, preauricular and infraparotid nodes the lymph of the upper lip.

The orbicularis oris muscles contains of two portions: the deep portion is oriented horizontally and acts to compress the upper and lower lip and to provide sphincter function. The superficial portion is in control of finer movements for facial expression. The depressors of the lip include 4 muscles: the depressor anguli oris, mentalis, depressor labii inferioris, and the platysma muscle. Elevation of the lips is secured by the levator anguli oris, zygomaticus, and risorius muscle. Many of these muscles stretch out to the oral commissures (Fig. 2).

Presentation and classification

Dependent on the degree of tissue damage individuals with perioral burns may experience a big variety of functional symptoms such as nutritional needs with limited oral intake, articulation abnormalities with impaired communication, dental hygiene, dental treatments and abnormal development of the definition and dental arches in childhood. Restriction of mandibular motion can be hazardous when attempting to administer general anesthesia [3]. Apart from these functional restrictions, patients suffer from their facial asymmetry, disfigurement and noticeable facial expression deficits.

Ortiz-Monasterio offered a classification based on the percentage of upper and lower lip involvement [4], while Al-Qattan classified electrical commissural burns in a 3 stage grading system [5] (Table 1). A more general classification according to the involved struc-

Table 1. Classification of electrical burns to the perioral region [5]

Degree	Description	Treatment	Prognosis
Minor	2nd degree burn of the red lip only	Nil	Excellent
Moderate	Full thickness burn at the commissure involving the red lip	Early splinting plus commissuroplasty if needed	Good
Severe	Extensive tissue destruction	Flap surgery is required	Poor, with aesthetic and functional problems

tures is presented by Hashem and colleagues [6]: type I includes isolated anterior oral contractures, type II isolated posterior oral contractures and type III total contractures (anterior and posterior).

General considerations and indications

Rose outlined 5 general principles for the treatment of facial burns [7]: an undistracted "normal" look at conversational distance, facial balance and symmetry, distinct aesthetic units fused by inconspicuous scars, a doughy skin texture appropriate for corrective makeup, and a dynamic facial expression. The subunits of the face as described by Gonzalez-Ulloa [8], which are of certain interest in perioral burns, are the following:

► Cheek unit (medial subunit; zygomatic subunit; lateral subunit; buccal subunit)
► Upper lip unit (with the philtral columns and the Cupid's bow which is the concave or dipped portion of the vermillion border in the center of the upper lip.)
► Lower lip unit (central subunit; mucosal subunit)
► Mental unit

Crossing these units will always lead to disfiguring scars for the patient. Scars should always be positioned into the lines connecting these units, what will make them most unimpressive.

Focusing on perioral burn injuries, the commissures should form an acute angle at a vertical perpendicular dropped from the patient's pupil and need to be positioned symmetric with the opposite side. The ratio of the height of the upper lip to that of the lower one is ideally 1:1.4. These principles should guide the surgeon when planning both, conservative therapy and reconstructive surgery.

In accordance to any deep burn injury, facial burns are treated by excision and soft tissue reconstruction. Aesthetic subunits are excised in their entity. Mesh grafting should always be avoided to gain satisfying aesthetic results. Fraulin et al. provide the largest study on this issue, finding that patients with extensive deep facial burns fared best with tangential excision and split-thickness skin grafting [9]. Unlike the rest of the face, where excision and grafting can avoid poor skin texture, primary (or early) excision of perioral burns is generally not recommended, as it may result in overresection of indispensable tissue or underresection of necrotic skin and muscle [2,10].

A bride variety of techniques have been described to reconstruct the upper and lower lip. Most important in addressing reconstruction are two basic principles: reconstruct lost tissues with tissues of the same kind ("like-with-like") and respect aesthetic units of the face.

The external lip consists of four layers: skin and subcutaneous tissue, the underlying orbicularis oris muscles, the lip mucosa, and the vermilion (visible portion of the lip), which is distinct from the mucosa in its colour, texture and appearance. All techniques of vermilion reconstruction by using other tissues will lead to unsatisfying results. Whenever planning reconstructive surgery to the lip, the most important factor is therefore the amount of residual lip vermilion as it shows an unique light reflection and can hardly be replaced.

If either upper or lower lip is not injured, healthy tissue can be transferred from one unit to the other. The planning should always prefer to reconstruct lip tissue with lip tissue ("like-with-like"). Two techniques available to achieve like-with-like reconstruction are the Abbe-flap and the reverse-Abbe-flap. Both are lip-switch flaps with two advantages: they have no impact on the oral commissure and they tighten the donor lip and thereby redress the balance with the (also tightened) reconstructed lip. Another approach to reconstruction is to slide parts of the uninjured lip through the commissure to the recipient side: flaps that follow this concept are for example

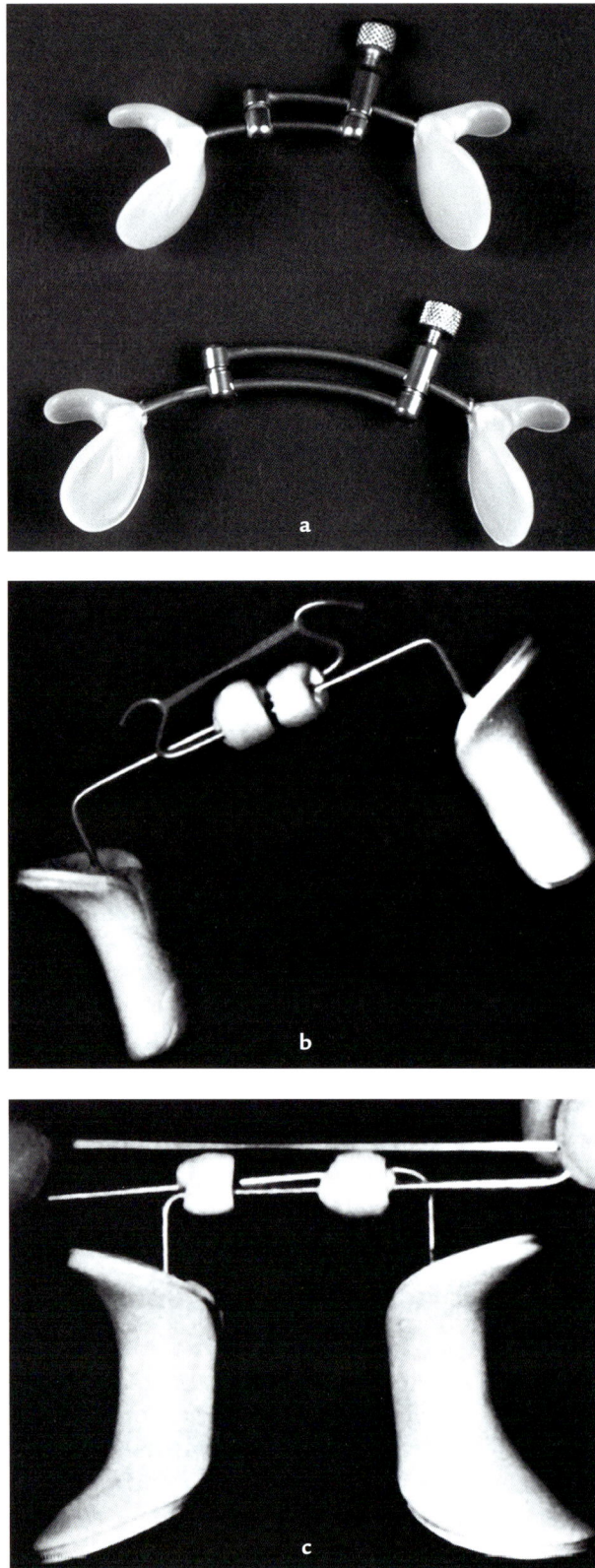

Estlander-flaps, Gilles-flaps, and Karapandzic-flaps. Not pedicled, they do not need any secondary flap division, but always affect the oral commissure and therefore often need secondary corrective procedures to restore normal lip architecture.

In presurgical decision-making it is important to know, that defects of > 40 % of the total available upper- and lower-lip surface (or > 80 % of either lip) cannot be reconstructed with local flaps but need other techniques. For these cases different authors described pedicled and free flaps for soft tissue reconstruction, such as DIEP flaps [11], bilateral pedicled forehead flaps [12] and free gracilis flaps [13].

Particuliar attention should be drawn to deep burns of the oral commissure that may result in microstomia – the most challenging complication from perioral burn injuries. Apart from early non-surgical therapies, reconstruction of the oral commissure can become necessary. Principles for commissuroplasty are based on the idea of reconstructing a symmetrical appearance and a decent function. Therapy is composed of non-surgical and surgical approaches. Anyway, as the skin is relatively mobile in the perioral region, scar maturation can take from 6 months to over a year [2]. Early and effective conservative (non-surgical) treatment is important and can prevent microstomia and the need of delayed reconstructive surgery. If microstomia developed, the surgical procedure must be fitted to the patients need and performed by a plastic surgeon experienced in burn surgery. One important principle for surgery is that the commissure needs to be in a symmetrical position with the opposite member. This requires optimal measurement to determine this location and some overcorrection to prevent relapse. Another important detail is the fact, that the oral commissure is not triangular. The short vertical component of the lateral margin needs consideration. Again, when planning surgery, local tissues are primarily used, and lost tissues are replaced by tissues of the same kind ("like-with-like").

Fig. 4. Different microstomia prevention devices

Treatment of facial burns

Microstomia: acute and non-surgical treatment

Early therapy of perioral burns includes some sort of appliances to prevent microstomia and is non-surgical at first. Moreover, conservative treatments for the prevention and management of microstomia include compression therapy [3, 14], mouth splinting [3, 5, 15, 16], scar massage [17], contact media [15], exercise [3, 16], patient education, and neck splinting [3, 15].

Devices used in burn patients having circumoral burns need vertical, horizontal and oblique stretch vectors in order to prevent contracture in more than one plane [18]. While adults find putting on these devices tolerable, it can be challenging to satisfy children and toddlers, in particular over the extended period of time necessary for obtaining satisfying results. There are many appliances available, categorized as intraoral vs. extraoral and removable vs. fix and to provide force in a vertical, horizontal or circumferential direction [3] (Fig. 4 a – c).

The efficacy of many different types was reported [2, 3, 5, 6, 15, 16]. Obviously, neither perfect tool nor generally accepted protocol has been agreed upon. In general, the device should be simple to fabricate, easy to handle and well tolerated by the patient, as the compliance is known to be the most limiting factor [3]. It is generally recommended to use the splints continuously over a period of 6 months even after scar maturation [2, 3].

Stretching devices are but one aspect of the treatment: exercise, local pressure and massage are mandatory and must be implied early as well for optimal outcome [3]. Scar contracture can be very forceful and early splinting alone may not prevent contracture of the oral commissures [1].

Microstomia: reconstruction of the oral commissure

Aim of the surgical procedure (named "commissuroplasty" or "commissurotomy") is the restoration of the oral commissure by correction of the oral commissure contracture. Indication for commissuroplasty is found in patients with manifest microstomia, impairment of function and aesthetic appearance as

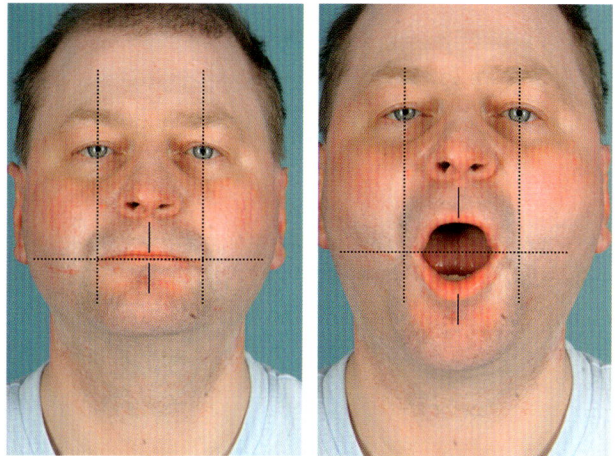

Fig. 5. Patient with microstomia and oral commissure medial to the perpendicular of the pupil; left: mouth closed; right: maximum opening of the mouth with significant microstomia

those described above. There are no contraindications for correction of microstomia. Depending on the technique all scarred contractures are either released or excised and the apex of the oral commissure is redefined. The emerging soft tissue defect is then covered with local adjacent tissues. Mucosal flaps taken from the enoral cheek proved to be more reliable and successful than advancement of the remaining vermilion toward the defect for closure. This last procedure usually resulted in shortening of the oral orifice on the affected side.

Landmarks to plan the new position of the commissure can be determined by examining the contralateral anatomy or – if both sides are affected – according to the general anatomical landmarks. In this case a slight overcorrection is sensible so that the commissural apex is positioned between the medial limbus and the midpupillary perpendicular of the eye (Fig. 5), allowing a slight overcorrection of 1–2 mm but taking care to avoid macrostomia.

Numerous technical variants of surgical procedures have been put forth in the literature, but none has proven ideally suited to address all problems associated with commissural contractures. Although Dieffenbach was the first author to present a surgical technique in 1831 [19], today's common procedures were initially described by Converse [20] and Fairbanks [21] in 1972. Converse described a commissuroplasty whereby a dermal triangle was excised at

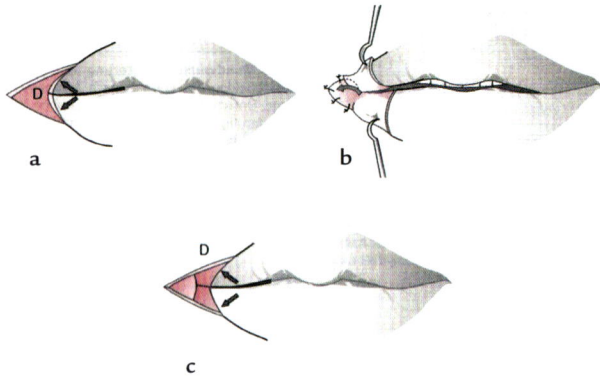

Fig. 6. Converse technique to correct microstomia: a: pink zone to be deepitheliased; b: full thickness horizontal Y-shaped dissection of the deepitheliased zone; c: advancement of the intraoral portion of mucosa to replace the vermilion

Fig. 7. a: left part of the picture: Fairbanks technique to correct microstomia with two flaps facing each other on the oral commissure; right part of the picture: expected soft tissue defect of the donor site after lateral rotation of the flaps; b: intraoral mucosa rotation flap to cover the donor site defect of the vermillion and to shift the scar contracture away from the commissural zone

the contracted commissures which was then deepened by full thickness incision to the new apex position. Buccal mucosa flaps were then wrapped out to meet the skin edges (Fig. 6a–c). The small flap in the commissure is crucial to the success of this technique. Several authors presented a modification of this technique that pays respect to the vertical component of the lateral margin. Brent Egeland introduced a modified technique without resection of any tissue. Instead he releases all intrinsic and extrinsic contractures and used a "Y to V" musculomucosal advancement flap to cover the soft tissue defect [2].

Fairbanks and Dingman used 2 small triangular mucosal flaps, one with a superior base and one with an inferior base [21]. After dissection these flaps were transposed for a lengthening effect while the buccal mucosa was advanced to the commissure to cover the soft tissue defect (Fig. 7a). Spanholtz et al. modified this technique and covered the soft tissue defect of the lateral lip with an additional rotation flap raised from the mucosa of the enoral lower lip. Resulting scars were thereby shifted to the enoral side of the lower lip, which caused less contracture in the region of the oral commissure [22] (Fig. 7).

Some others presented more experimental ideas using composite grafts harvested and reshaped from the ear lobule [23]. A major shortcoming of all techniques is the difficulty of precisely reconstructing the vermillion border.

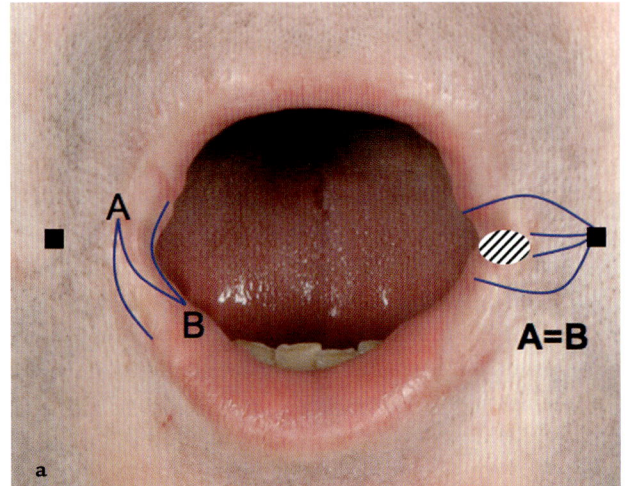

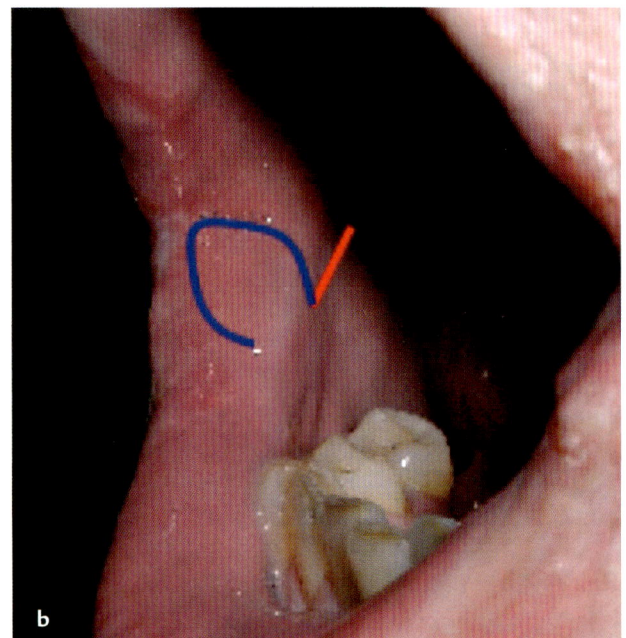

It can be useful to combine surgical correction with splinting devices as described by Koymen and colleagues, who found an increase of the interincisal opening by an average of 5 mm when Converse' technique was combined with postoperative splinting for 3 months [24].

Table 2.

	Defect size	Tissue quality/ Defect localization	Involvement of lip tissue	Technique
Lower lip	< 1/3	Primary closure		
	1/3–2/3	sufficient lip tissue	Commissure involved	Karapandzic (1st choice) Estlander
			Commissure not involved	Abbe (1st choice) Karapandzic
		insufficient lip tissue		Bernards-Burrow´s
	> 2/3	sufficient cheek tissue		Karapandzic
		insufficient cheek tissue		distal flap or free flap
Upper lip	< 1/3	Central		perialar crescentic closure
		vermillion intact		local flap from nasolabial fold
		Lateral		primary closure
	1/3–2/3	Central		Abbe (1st choice) Karapandzic
		Lateral	commissure and philtrum intact	Abbe
			commissure and/or philtrum involved	Estlander with/without perialar crecentic exzision
	> 2/3	sufficient cheek tissue	Central	Bernards-Burrow's
			Lateral	Bernards-Burrow's plus contralat. perialar crecentic exzision
		insufficient cheek tissue		distal flap or free flap

On some occasions, one procedure may not be sufficient to manage large deformities, and numerous surgical procedures are necessary over the years to eliminate functional and aesthetic impairment. In these cases it is advisable to delay reconstruction until scar contracture is complete and the scar and surrounding tissue are adequately softened. Between reconstructive procedures, months may elapse before considering a result final, requiring great patience for all parties involved.

Complications of surgical correction include flap failure with partial or complete flap necrosis. Bleeding and infection can be considered as general risks of any surgical procedure.

The most important complication is represented by the recurrent contracture with subsequent microstomia. Also unfavorable cosmetic results may occur at the mouth or donor site. Seldom one can see cases of postoperative incomplete mouth closure with leakage of fluids when swallowing increases intraoral pressure (macrostomia). This can result from overcorrection or false technique and needs surgical correction after an adequate period of time.

Reconstruction on the upper and lower lip

Flowchart for surgical planning (Table 2)

The goal when using healthy adjacent lip tissue for reconstruction is to evenly distribute the remaining lip tissue between the upper and lower lip.

The upper lip

With regards to the subunits of the upper lip, defects are classified as central defects and lateral defects. Superficial central defects of the philtrum need wedge resection if they involve less than half of the central segment. If the defect exceeds the philtral borders, the whole subunit can be replaced by (haired) skin from retro- or preauricular full-thickness skin grafts.

If the orbicularis muscles is involved and the surgeon is facing a full-thickness defect, damaged structures need to be fixed layer by layer. Defects up to 30% can be managed by primary closure via advancement of adjacent tissue. Full-thickness defects

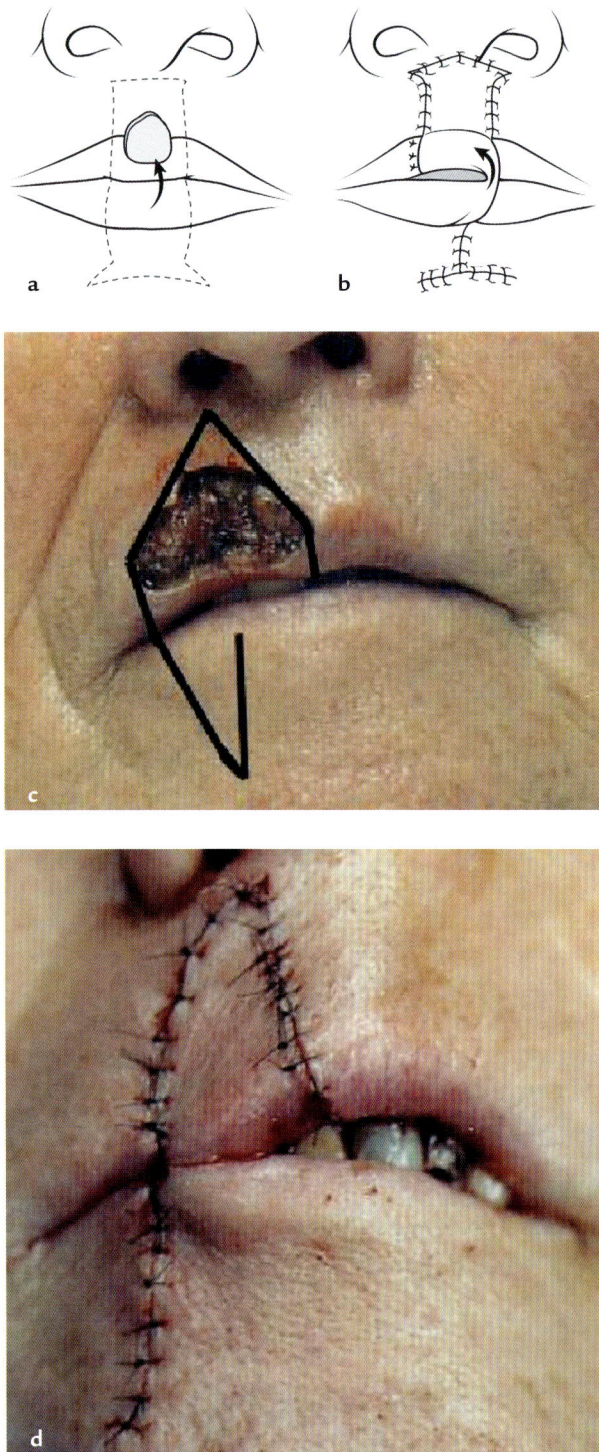

Fig. 8. The Abbe-flap (lip-switch procedure) for defects of the upper and lower lip; it can either be raised to cover central or lateral defects; a: defect and planning of the flap; b: after 180° rotation of the flap with left-sided pedicle; c: clinical example of soft tissue defect of the upper lip; d: clinical picture after soft tissue coverage with Abbe-flap

within the philtrum and affecting up to half of the philtrum width can be managed by direct closure. For wide defects Abbe-flap gives best results, although bridging of one column will result in asymmetry. Described 1898 by Robert Abbe who was plastic surgeon and radiologist in New York City, the flap was initially used as a complete reconstruction technique for the relief of the bilateral cleft lip deformity. It can be raised from upper and lower lip and its size and shape are dependent on the corresponding defect (Fig. 8). The flap can be based on the labial artery. A portion of the uninjured lip is rotated across the oral orifice and into the defect of the burned lip. An accurate closure of all three layers at the recipient site is standard. A second stage is required to ligate the pedicle and inset at around 2–3 weeks after the initial procedure. From our experience, this flap has an excellent cosmetic result when it is used to replace the entire philtrum of the upper lip.

If the defect is located on the lateral site of the upper lip and involves the oral commissure, the Estlander flap is a reasonable procedure (Fig. 9). This flap, too, is a lip switch flap but designed at the lateral part of the lip. It uses a medially based full-thickness portion of the upper lip. Upon realignment of the vermillion border, the mucosa needs to be advanced to match the thickness of the recipient site. This technique may result in a typical rounding of the oral commissure and therefore often needs corrective procedures earliest 12 weeks after the initial operation. A triangular part of the flap can be incised and the oral commissure can be reconstructed based on available techniques (see above).

The Gillies flap allows for subtotal or total lip reconstruction and is an extension of the Estlander flap. Tissues laterally to the commissures are advanced and the flap is rotated to create new commissures while tissue is advanced medially to fill the defect (Fig. 10). This technique surely has the disadvantage of sensory loss of the flap caused by surgical denervation as well as vermillion deficiency.

Large defects that need functional reconstruction can instead be addressed with the Karapandzic flap, which takes the disadvantages of the Gillies flap into account. It was described in 1974 and is based on the idea of reconstructing the lost lip tissues with tissues from the adjacent lip and cheek. Two flaps are raised from the neighbourhood skin with a width

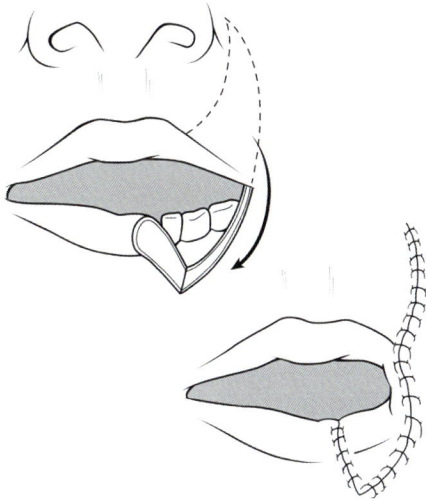

Fig. 9. The Estlander flap (rotation flap procedure) for defects of the upper and lower lip; it is rotated through the commissure and thereby shifts the commissure and thereby reduces the oral orifice

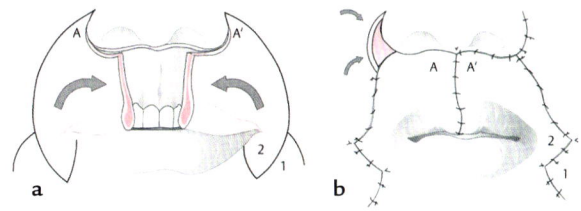

Fig. 10. Gillies flap to cover hugh central defects of the upper lip. Philtrum is sacrificed by this procedure. To spare out the paranasal skin, a sickle-shaped piece can be excised lateral to the alae nasi

equal to the height of the defect. These full-thickness musculocutaneous flaps are then slid towards each other and stitched to one another (Fig. 11). The neurovascular supply (facial artery and facial nerve branches) are dissected out and spared. For advancement it can be necessary to gradual cut the peripheral muscle fibres without the need to dissect the mucosa. Philtrum relief will commonly be lost and needs second-stage reconstruction. Perialar crescentic cheek excision is applied in large defects of the upper lip that need extensive advancement from the cheek. Because simple advancement would result in bunching at the perialar folds, a prialar elliptical skin excision is carried out with the upper part shifted laterally to avoid the nostril.

Defects affecting more than 80 % of the upper lip can only be covered with the help of nonlip tissues (local flaps from surrounding skin or free flaps [25, 26], e. g. free gracilis [27] or free radial forearm flap folded to also reconstruct the inner lining of the mouth [28]) and seldom appear naturally, especially when the lip if moving.

The distinct contour of the upper lip is difficult to create and maintain for correction. Diligent study of the surface anatomy of the upper lip is required. The sophisticated realignment of the vermillion is para-

mount. If vermillion is lost, it can be reconstructed with tattooing or buccal mucosa grafting. If relevant parts of the philtrum are affected, resurfacing of the entire aesthetic subunit should be considered [29]. Philtrum can be reconstructed with ear composite cartilage grafts. It must be located centrally in relation to the nasal columella.

The lower lip

The reconstruction of the lower lip is not as complicated as the upper lip as it tolerates wedge resection in the majority of cases. Moreover, Abbe and Estlander flaps can be used in a reverse manner to cover defects of the lower lip with tissues from the upper lip.

In most of the cases wedge resection and direct closure leads to satisfying results. If more than 50 % of the central portion are deeply burned and need reconstruction, Schuchard's technique or Karapandzic flap is to use. Schuchard's technique utilizes the tissue from the lower lip/cheek region to close central defects by advancement with bilateral inferior incisions along the labiomental folds the mandibular border (Fig. 12 a). This sliding-lip-procedure

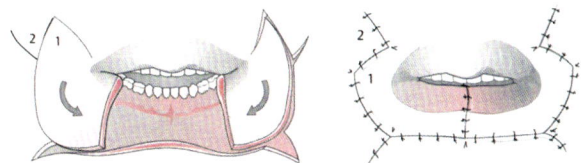

Fig. 11. Karapandzic flap to cover hugh soft tissue defects of the lower lip; musculocutaneous flaps a raised bilaterally and slid forward each other and stitched up in the midline

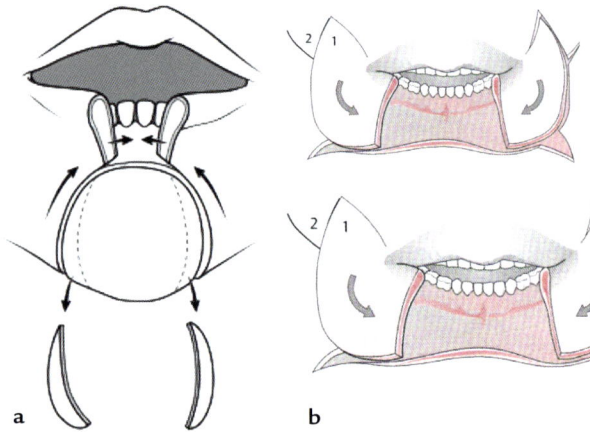

Fig. 12. Schuchard flap to cover hugh defects of the lower lip by rotating skin from the lower cheek around the chin

Fig. 13. Bilateral (reverse) Abbe flap to cover hugh defects of the lower lip by replacing vermillion with vermillion from the upper lip; sickle-shaped parts of surplus tissues; a: 2 medial pedicled Abbe flaps are raised from the upper lip; b: after 180° rotation the flaps a stitched to the defect in the lower lip

has the advantage of minimal scarring most of which lie in between the aesthetic units. The Karapandzic techniques preserve the nerves to the orbicularis muscle and the lip stays innervated. Bilateral flaps can be used to cover defects with up to 80% of tissue loss. Disadvantage is the risk of microstomia and the rounding of the commissure that might need corrective procedures afterwards (Fig. 12 b).

For larger or paramedian defects, the (bilateral) reverse-Abbe flap allows like-with-like reconstruction with primary closure of the upper lip, which serves as donor site (Fig. 13). This technique gives best results, when the flap is harvested from the lateral aspect of the upper lip and thereby does not include the philtrum. The calculated width of the flap should account for half of the defect width. It must not affect more than one-third of the upper lip, so the donor defect can be closed primarily. Literature differentiates between a central and a lateral reverse-Abbe flap. The central reverse-Abbe flap is primarily used for median tissue loss of the lower lip and differs from the lateral flap in that it does not involve the perialar crescents and is based on a medial vascular pedicle.

There are also two sliding procedures available for the reconstruction of the lower lip. The Estlander flap as described above for reconstruction of the upper lip provides good amounts of mucosa for reconstruction of the vestibulum oris and also matches with rectangular defects in the lower lip. Like the Abbe flap the Estlander technique can be combined

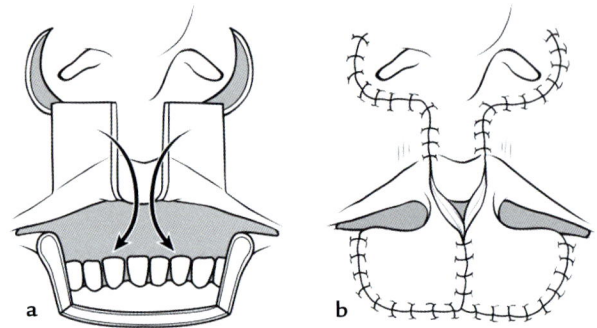

with the step technique in defects involving more than two-thirds of the lip and in cases with involvement of the commissure. Estlander full-thickness flap matches well with the remaining lower lip tissue but has a tendency to produce microstomia especially when performed bilaterally. A reasonable modification was provided by Balch [30], minimizing the resulting deformity in the donor (upper) lip. He positioned the lateral aspect of the flap into the nasolabial fold and thereby preserved the natural course of the fold and prevents philtrum disturbance. Moreover, this procedure pays respect to the oral commissure more than the classic Estlander technique (Fig. 14).

Based on the procedure described by Gillis, Karapandzic modified this technique by preserving the nerve supply to the lower lip and thereby replaced the technique of Gillis completely. The flap pivots at the commissure and upper lip and slides along the nasolabial fold. It must be classified a rotation-advancement flap and is the most useful flap for large defects.

Also described for large defects of the lower lip, the Bernard-Burrow flap allows reconstruction with advancement of adjacent cheek tissue (Fig. 15). Lateral triangular flaps based at the level of the commissures are flipped over to reconstruct defects of the central portion of the lower lip. Webster modified this technique and described incision through skin and subcutaneous tissue to preserve underlying neuromuscular structures.

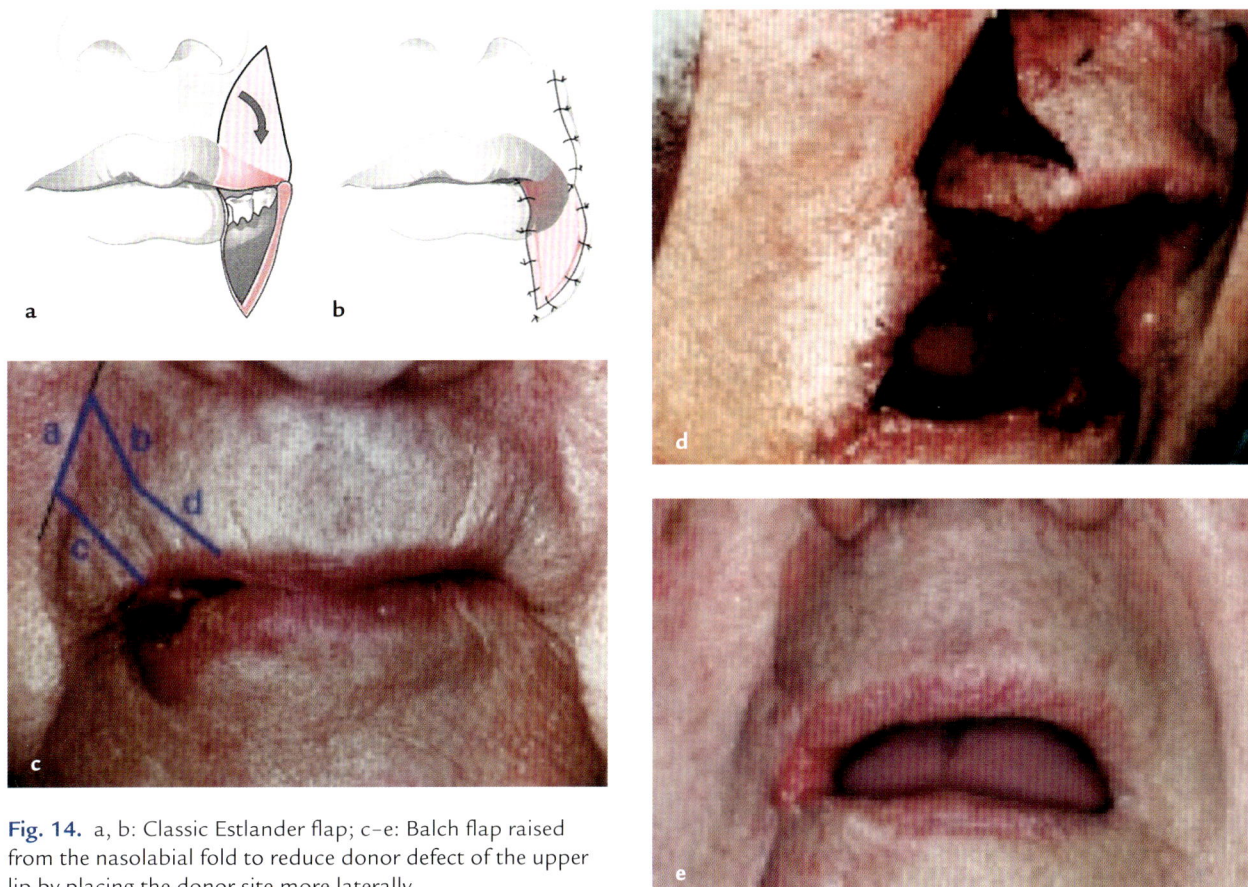

Fig. 14. a, b: Classic Estlander flap; c–e: Balch flap raised from the nasolabial fold to reduce donor defect of the upper lip by placing the donor site more laterally

Large defects of the lower lip that make the use of local solutions impossible can be challenging and demanding for the treating surgeon [31]. Distant flaps include submandibular, anterior cervical, deltopectoral, sternocleidomastoidal, as well as forehead flaps. Also free tissue transfer [26] (e. g. radial forearm flap [28, 32] or gracilis flap [27]) has been described [26].

Summary and conclusion

Patients with facial burns often suffer from perioral loss of tissue with subsequent facial scarring. Some individuals present with nutritional needs with limited oral intake, articulation abnormalities with impaired communication, dental hygiene, dental treatments and abnormal development of the definition and dental arches in childhood. Early treatment options are different stretching devices that positively influence contract scarring in the perioral region. The treating physician must not forget to apply such a device even in mechanically ventilated patients. Externally placed devices may not be able to be used too early because of open wounds or recently transplanted skin grafts. Important: early splinting decreases the need for surgical reconstruction.

In general, surgical treatment is not indicated directly after injury, because the extent of necrotic tissue cannot be defined accurately. If microstomia develops and surgery is needed, different techniques are available for the reconstruction of the oral commissure. A detailed preoperative planning according the opposite (uninjured) side or to typical established landmarks should be carried out. Most techniques are based on the idea of recruiting a mucosal flap from the cheek and transferring it to the commissure. Aesthetic and functional results are sometimes not optimal and make subsequent surgery necessary.

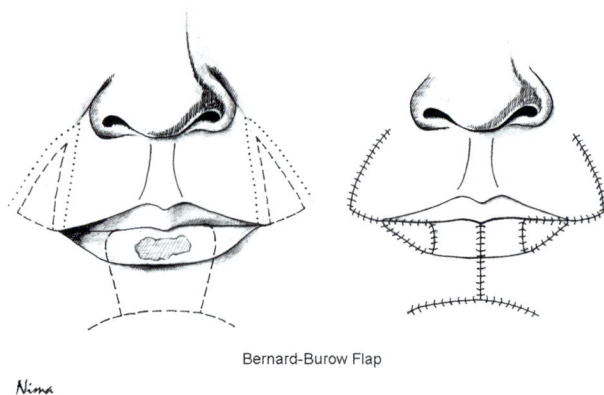

Bernard-Burow Flap

Nima

Fig. 15. Bernard-Burow flap to cover defects of the lower lip with the use of adjacent cheek tissue rotated from the nasolabial fold into the defect

When analysing lip defects and planning reconstructive procedure, the amount of remaining vermillion is the most important assessment. It is distinct in colour and texture and can hardly be replaced. Reconstruction of the function is more critical in the lower lip, whereas it can generally tolerate wedge resection in the majority of defects.

Aim of all reconstructive procedures is a well-balanced length of upper and lower lip. The two lips should generally share the remaining tissue. Lip switch procedures are accompanied by lip sliding procedures. Most of the techniques a single-step procedures but might need corrective surgery in some cases. All techniques show advantages and disadvantages. To pick the appropriate procedure for specific defects and the individual needs of patients ensures best functional and aesthetic outcomes.

References

[1] Zweifel CJ, Guggenheim M, Jandali AR, Altintas MA, Kunzi W, Giovanoli P (2010) Management of microstomia in adult burn patients revisited. J Plast Reconstr Aesthet Surg 63(4): e351–357. Epub 2009 Nov 25

[2] Egeland B, More S, Buchman SR, Cederna PS (2008) Management of difficult pediatric facial burns: reconstruction of burn-related lower eyelid ectropion and perioral contractures. J Craniofac Surg 19(4): 960–969

[3] Dougherty ME, Warden GD (2003) A thirty-year review of oral appliances used to manage microstomia, 1972 to 2002. J Burn Care Rehabil 24(6): 418–431; discussion 410

[4] Ortiz-Monasterio F, Factor R (1980) Early definitive treatment of electric burns of the mouth. Plast Reconstr Surg 65(2): 169–176

[5] al-Qattan MM, Gillett D, Thomson HG (1996) Electrical burns to the oral commissure: does splinting obviate the need for commissuroplasty? Burns 22(7): 555–556

[6] Hashem FK, Al Khayal Z (2003) Oral burn contractures in children. Ann Plast Surg 51(5): 468–471

[7] Rose EH (1995) Aesthetic restoration of the severely disfigured face in burn victims: a comprehensive strategy. Plast Reconstr Surg 96(7): 1573–1585; discussion 1586–1577

[8] Gonzalez-Ulloa M (1987) Regional aesthetic units of the face. Plast Reconstr Surg 79(3): 489–490

[9] Fraulin FO, Illmayer SJ, Tredget EE (1996) Assessment of cosmetic and functional results of conservative versus surgical management of facial burns. J Burn Care Rehabil 17(1): 19–29

[10] Pitts W, Pickrell K, Quinn G, Massengill R (1969) Electrical burns of lips and mouth in infants and children. Plast Reconstr Surg 44(5): 471–479

[11] Jin X, Teng L, Zhao M et al (2009) Reconstruction of cicatricial microstomia and lower facial deformity by windowed, bipedicled deep inferior epigastric perforator flap. Ann Plast Surg 63(6): 616–620

[12] Fan J, Liu L, Tian J, Gan C, Lei M (2009) Aesthetic full-perioral reconstruction of burn scar by using a bilateral-pedicled expanded forehead flap. Ann Plast Surg 63(6): 640–644

[13] Ninkovic M, Spanio di Spilimbergo S (2007) Lower lip reconstruction: introduction of a new procedure using a functioning gracilis muscle free flap. Plast Reconstr Surg 119(5): 1472–1480

[14] Stewart R, Bhagwanjee AM, Mbakaza Y, Binase T (2000) Pressure garment adherence in adult patients with burn injuries: an analysis of patient and clinician perceptions. Am J Occup Ther 54(6): 598–606

[15] Neale HW, Billmire DA, Carey JP (1986) Reconstruction following head and neck burns. Clin Plast Surg 13(1): 119–136

[16] Ward RS (1991) Pressure therapy for the control of hypertrophic scar formation after burn injury. A history and review. J Burn Care Rehabil 12(3): 257–262

[17] Gallagher J, Goldfarb IW, Slater H, Rogosky-Grassi M (1990) Survey of treatment modalities for the prevention of hypertrophic facial scars. J Burn Care Rehabil 11(2): 118–120

[18] Gay WD (1984) Prostheses for oral burn patients. J Prosthet Dent 52(4): 564–566

[19] Berlet AC, Ablaza VJ, Servidio P (1993) A refined technique for oral commissurotomy. J Oral Maxillofac Surg 51(12): 1400–1403

[20] Converse JM (1972) Orbicularis advancement flap for restoration of angle of the mouth. Plast Reconstr Surg 49(1): 99–100

[21] Fairbanks GR, Dingman RO (1972) Restoration of the oral commissure. Plast Reconstr Surg 49(4): 411–413

[22] Spanholtz TA, Theodorou P, Phan V, Perbix W, Spilker G (2007) [Reconstruction of the oral commissure in microstomia patients with deep dermal facial burns: a modified technique]. Handchir Mikrochir Plast Chir 39(5): 350–355

[23] Ayhan M, Aytug Z, Deren O, Karantinaci B, Gorgu M (2006) An alternative treatment for postburn microstomia treatment: composite auricular lobule graft for oral comissure reconstruction. Burns 32(3): 380–384

[24] Koymen R, Gulses A, Karacayli U, Aydintug YS (2009) Treatment of microstomia with commissuroplasties and semidynamic acrylic splints. Oral Surg Oral Med Oral Pathol Oral Radiol Endod 107(4): 503–507

[25] Bozikov K, Arnez ZM (2008) Reconstruction of large upper lip defects by free tissue transfer. Acta Chir Plast 50(2): 51–53

[26] Ueda K, Oba S, Nakai K, Okada M, Kurokawa N, Nuri T (2009) Functional reconstruction of the upper and lower lips and commissure with a forearm flap combined with a free gracilis muscle transfer. J Plast Reconstr Aesthet Surg 62(10): e337–340

[27] Cordova A, D'Arpa S, Moschella F (2008) Gracilis free muscle transfer for morpho-functional reconstruction of the lower lip. Head Neck 30(5): 684–689

[28] Daya M, Nair V (2009) Free radial forearm flap lip reconstruction: a clinical series and case reports of technical refinements. Ann Plast Surg 62(4): 361–367

[29] Neale HW, Billmire DA, Gregory RO (1985) Management of perioral burn scarring in the child and adolescent. Ann Plast Surg15(3): 212–217

[30] Balch CR (1978) Modification of cross-lip flap. Plast Reconstr Surg 61(3): 457–458

[31] Rifaat MA (2006) Lower lip reconstruction after tumor resection; a single author's experience with various methods. J Egypt Natl Canc Inst 18(4): 323–333

[32] Daya M (2010) Simultaneous total upper and lower lip reconstruction with a free radial forearm-palmaris longus tendon and brachioradialis chimeric flap. J Plast Reconstr Aesthet Surg 63(1): e75–76. Epub 2009 Apr 3

Correspondence: Timo Alexander Spanholtz, Senior Consultant, M. D. Department Hand Surgery, Plastic and Aesthetic Surgery, Universitätsklinik, Ludwig-Maximilians-Universität München, Pettenkoferstraße 8a, 80336 Munich, Germany, E-mail: timo@spanholtz.net

Nasal reconstruction

Lars-Peter Kamolz[1, 2], Maike Keck[1], Harald Selig[2], David B. Lumenta[1]

[1] Medical University of Vienna, Department of Surgery, Division of Plastic and Reconstructive Surgery, Vienna, Austria
[2] State Hospital Wiener Neustadt, Department of Surgery, Section of Plastic, Aesthetic and Reconstructive Surgery, Wiener Neustadt, Austria

The nose has a central position in the face and serves as the key anatomic area for aesthetic and facial balance. Due to its central position the nose is very often involved in facial burns. Due to its importance nose reconstruction plays a major role in regaining quality of life, but beside its aesthetic impact the nose also plays a major role as a functional organ in the upper airway.

Advances in the philosophy, approach, and techniques for nasal reconstruction have resulted in increasingly refined aesthetic and functional results. This has been achieved by adhering to the paradigm of replacing missing tissue with like tissue.
The tenets include replacing the:

▶ Lining,
▶ Framework, and
▶ Cover of the nose

with material that matches the deficient tissues as close as possible.

Achauer has described a nasal deformity according to the following schema [1]:

▶ Burn scar deformity without major tissue loss (hypertrophic scars, hypo- and hyperpigmentation, asymmetry),
▶ Ectropium (e. g. due to the loss of the alar rim),
▶ Subtotal tissue loss,
▶ Extensive tissue loss,
▶ Nostril stenosis.

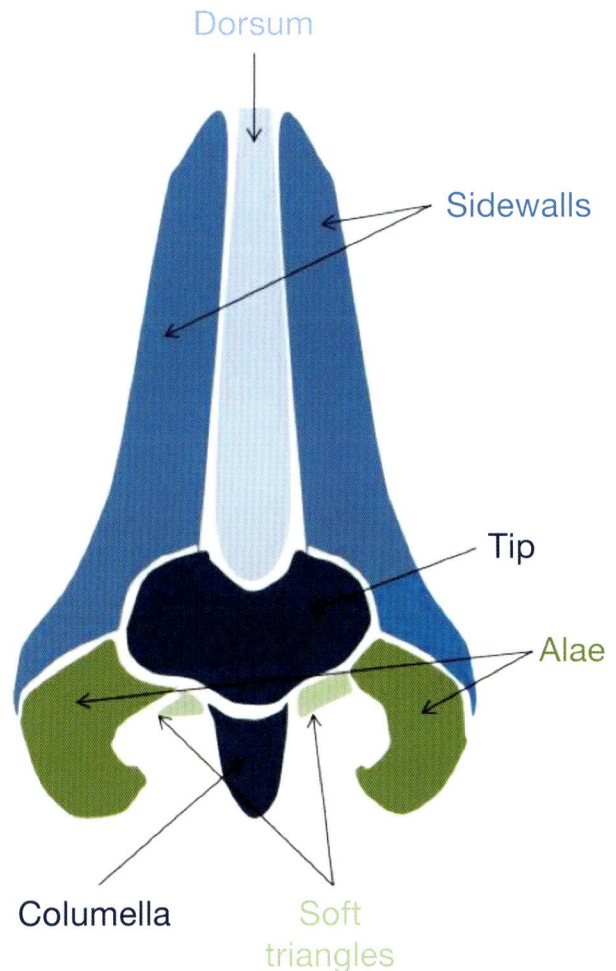

Fig. 1. Aesthetic subunits of the nose

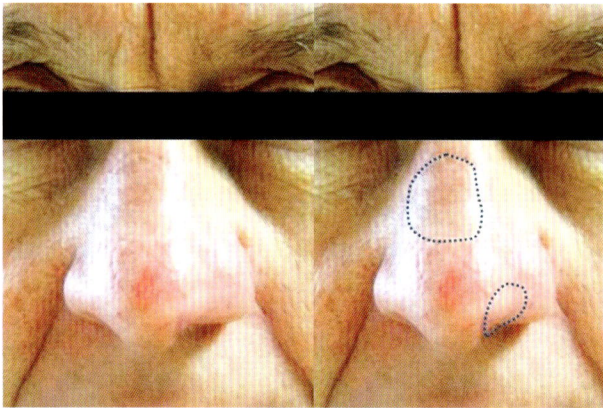

Fig. 2. Late results after defect coverage (frontal view):
Dorsum: full thickness graft
Tip – Alar Region: tunneled nasolabial island flap

Principles of nasal reconstruction

Nasal reconstruction in patients suffering from burns is similar to nasal reconstruction in patients suffering from cancer. The most important factors are soft tissue coverage, lining and skeletal support. Therefore an exact analysis of the missing tissue has to be performed prior to surgery in order to understand the tissue needs.

If there is only a need for skin coverage an unmeshed split thickness or full thickness skin graft is required. Don't forget to take the aesthetic subunits of the nose into account (Fig. 1) [2, 3]. In case of

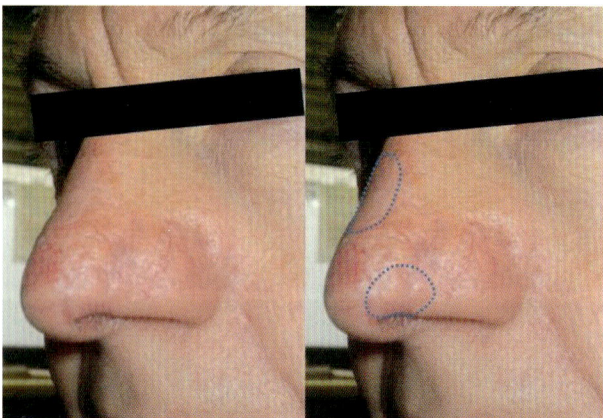

Fig. 3. Late results after defect coverage (lateral view):
Dorsum: full thickness graft
Tip – Alar Region: tunneled nasolabial island flap

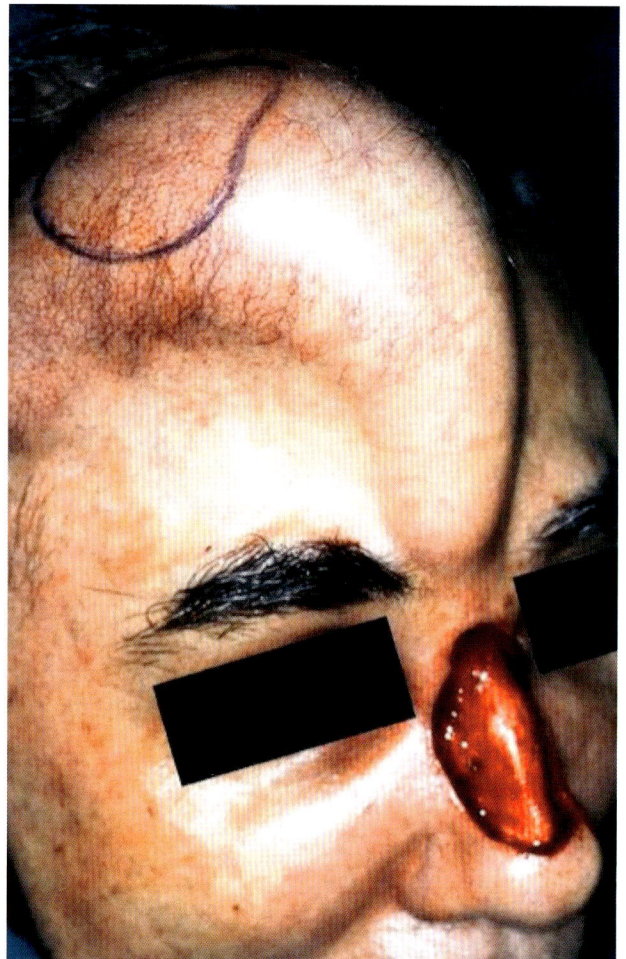

Fig. 4. Preexpanded forehead flap

small defects and good quality of the surrounding tissue a local flap can be used to solve the problem (Figs. 2, 3).

In case of extensive or subtotal tissue loss, autologous material and alloplastic material can be used for bony augmentation or bony reconstruction. Concerning to the literature, autologous material seems to be superior than alloplastic material due to their possible complications, which are associated with use of alloplastic materials [4–10], but in both cases an adequate soft tissue coverage is of utmost importance. Bone and cartilage are really optimal for replacing the framework of the nose. Generally free grafts harvested from the rib, calvarium, nasal, septum or ear can provide the foundation for the internal lining and external coverage. Occasionally, composite grafts from the ear can serve as a re-

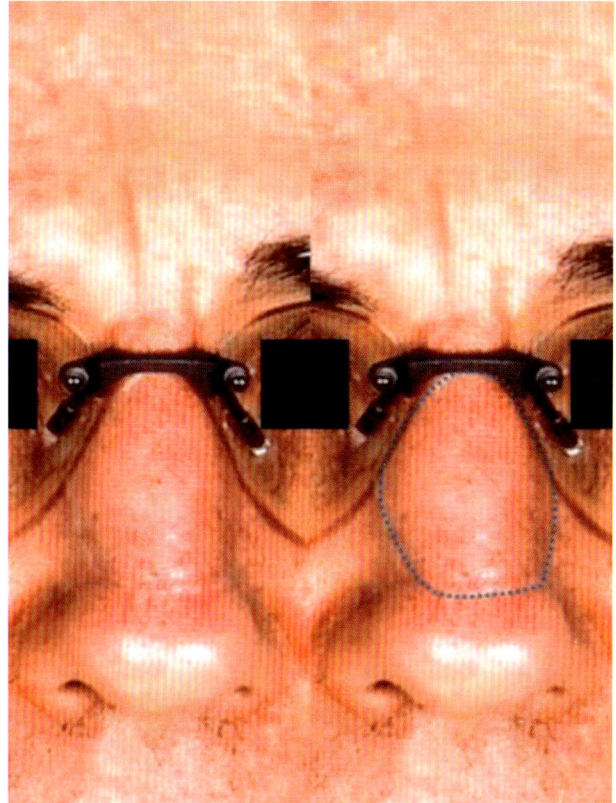

Fig. 6. Final result after forehead flap procedure

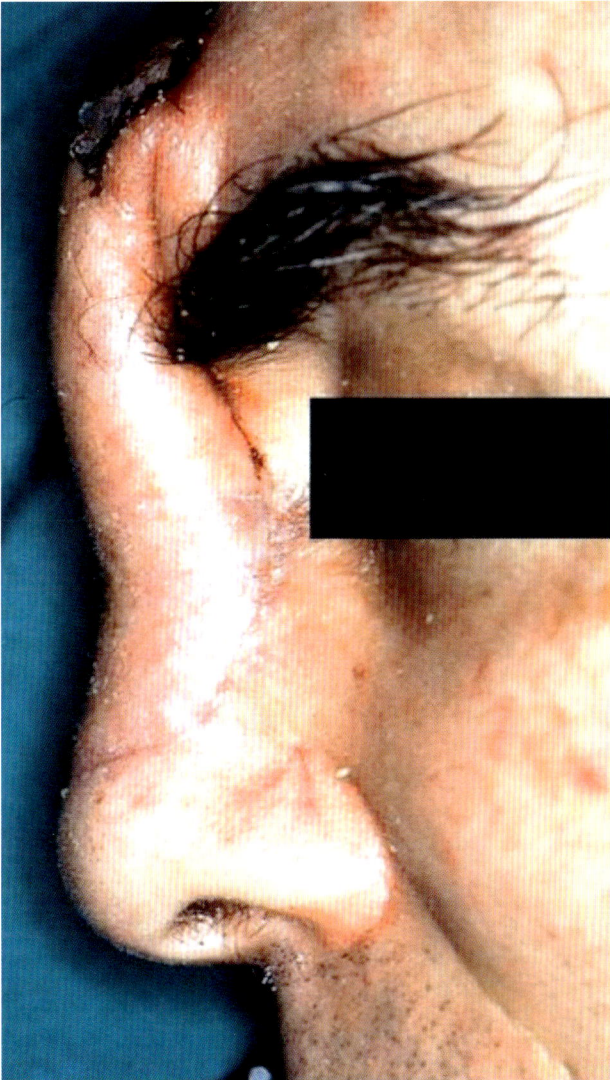

Fig. 5. Forehead flap in position

placement for full thickness defects of the lower nose [11], but also free composite auricular flaps have been used to cover larger defects in the lower part of the nose [12].

The workhorse for nasal reconstruction in case of larger defects is the forehead flap [13, 14] (Figs. 4–6) and for inner lining the septal mucoperichondrium [15].

A total nasal defect including all layers of tissue, from skin to bone might be reconstructed with a prelaminated free flap. Prelamination includes additional tissues into a flap in a multistage fashion. The forearm has been cited as a common donor site.

Skin, mucosa and cartilage grafts are inserted prior to flap raising. After lining, support and coverage have formed a stable unit, they are raised and an microvascular anastomosis performed [16].

In future allotransplantation might gain importance for large and complex defects of the face [17–19]. Moreover, the use of tissue engineering and engineered products like cartilage will improve future possibilities for nasal reconstruction [20, 21].

Summary

Reconstruction of the nose continues to progress to new level that allows plastic surgeons to restore near normal form and function to the majority of nasal defects. These advances are based on the concepts of respecting the borders of the aesthetic units (Fig. 1) and replacing missing tissue with like tissue. In future allotransplantation and tissue enginnering will gain importance for nasal reconstruction.

References

[1] Achauer BM (1991) Burn reconstruction. Thieme Medical, New York

[2] Manson PM, Hoopes JE, Chambers REG et al (1979) Algorithm for nasal reconstrction. Am J Surg 138: 528

[3] Gonzales-Uloa M (1987) Regional aesthetic units of the face. Plast Reconstr Surg 79: 489

[4] Adams JS (1987) Grafts and implants in nasal augmentation: a rational approach to material selection. Otolaryngol Clin North Am 29: 913–930

[5] Schuller D, Bardach J, Krause D (1997) Irreadiated homogenous costal cartilage for facial contour restoration. Arch Otolaryngol 103: 12–15

[6] McCollough EG, Weol C (1979) Augmentation of facial defects using Mersilene mesh implants. Otolaryngol Head Neck Surg 87: 515–521

[7] Brown BL, Neel HB, Kern E (1979) Implants of supramid, proplast, plasti-pore, and silastic. Arch Otolaryngol 104: 605–609

[8] Berman M, Pearce W, Tinnin M (1986)Theo sue of Gore-Tex E-PTFE bonded to silicone rubber as an alloplastic implant. Laryngoscope 96: 480–483

[9] Chou TD, Lee WT, Chen SL et al (2004) Split calavarial bone graft for chemical burn associated nasal augmentation. Burns 20: 380–385

[10] Neel HB (1983) Implants of Gore-Tex. Arch Otolaryngol 109: 427–433

[11] Haug MD, Rieger UM, Witt P, Gubisch W (2009) Managing the ear as a donor site for composite graft in nasal reconstruction: update on technical refinements and donor site morbidity in 110 caes. Ann Plast Surg 63: 171–175

[12] Pribas JJ, Falco N (1993) Nasal reconstruction with auricular microvasular transplant. Ann Plast Surg 31: 289–297

[13] Mennick FJ (2004) Nasal reconstruction. Forehead flap. Plast Reconstr Surg 113:100–111

[14] MCCarthy JG, Lorenc ZP, Cutting C et al (1989) The median forehead flap: the blood supply. Plast Reconstr Surg 84: 189

[15] Burget GC, Menick FJ (1989) Nasal support and lining: The marriage of beauty and blood supply. Plast Reconstr Surg 84: 189

[16] Taghina AH, Pribas JJ (2008) Complex nasal reconstrcution. Plast Reconstr Surg 121: 15e-27e

[17] Decauchell B, Badet L, Lengele B et al (2006) First human face allograft: early report. Lancet 368: 203–209

[18] Alam DS, Papay FP, Djohan R (2009) The technical and anatomical aspects of the worlds first near-total human face and maxilla transplant. Arch Facial Plast Surg 11: 369–377

[19] Semionow M, Papy F, Alam D et al (2009) Near totel human face transplantation for aseverely disfigured patient in the USA. Lancet 374: 203–209

[20] Watson D (2009) Tissue engineering for rhinoplasty. Facial Plast Surg North AM 17: 157–165

[21] Sage A, Chang AA, Schumacher Bl et al (2009) Cartilage outgrowth in fbrin scaffolds. Am J Rhinol Allergy 23: 486–491

Correspondence: Lars-Peter Kamolz, M.D., Ph.D., M.Sc., Medical University of Vienna, Department of Surgery, Division of Plastic and Reconstructive Surgery, Vienna, Austria, E-mail: kamolz@plastchirurg.info

Reconstruction/Correction of burn alopecia

Lars-Peter Kamolz[1, 2], Maike Keck[1], Harald Selig[2], David B. Lumenta[1]

[1] Medical University of Vienna, Department of Surgery, Division of Plastic and Reconstructive Surgery, Vienna, Austria
[2] State Hospital Wiener Neustadt, Department of Surgery, Section of Plastic, Aesthetic and Reconstructive Surgery, Wiener Neustadt, Austria

Burn alopecia is a significant disfigurement and its sequelae includes not only physical problems, but also psychological problems, such as low self-esteem, unhappiness, and dissatisfaction. Therefore, burn alopecia is a significant challenge for plastic surgeons concerning reconstruction and rehabilitation. The primary goal of reconstruction for burn alopecia is to recreate a natural hair-bearing appearance on the reconstructed scalp.

Generally, there are 2 basic principles available to achieve this:
▶ First, scalp tissue should be replaced by scalp tissue, if possible.
▶ Second, the reconstructive procedure must restore and preserve hair growth patterns and hairlines for a cosmetically appealing result [1].

Based on these principles, numerous reconstructive methods, including hair grafting, serial excision, local scalp flaps, as well as scalp extension and expansion procedures have been described in literature [2–12].

To facilitate an easy and good assessment of the burn alopecia and formulation of a reconstructive algorithm, burn alopecia was classified by Seong-HO J et al. based on the area, scar quality, and location [13].

They classified burn alopecia as small (50 cm²), medium (50–100 cm²), and large (>100 cm²) based on the surface area involved.

Second, they classified burn alopecia as good, moderate, and poor based on its scar quality, mainly based on its pliability and elasticity. Good quality referred to a burn scar that was pliable and had adequate elasticity. Moderate quality indicated pliability, but reduced elasticity. Poor quality signified that the scar was not pliable, but fibrotic and hard.

Finally, they classified the scars as frontal and parietal scars (including temporal, occipital, and vertex scars) based on their location (Fig. 1).

Hair grafting

Hair grafting is a simple technique that redistributes the patient's existing hair, but having a densely populated donor area is essential to the procedure. Due to the fact that in case of burn alopecia available donor area is often limited, the reconstruction of burn alopecia using hair grafting may be impossible, if the alopeceic area is too large.

Therefore, hair grafting is mainly used for reconstruction of small or medium burn alopecia, in case of the fact that scar quality is good, and the burn alopecia location is frontal or parietal. Hair grafting is a safe procedure and reasonably good results can be obtained in a single session (Fig. 2) [14].

For the reconstruction of the anterior hairline in the frontal or parietal areas, hair grafting is the best option because the hairs can be easily grafted into the desired position. Even though it is a very tedious process for the surgeon, we consider hair grafting as

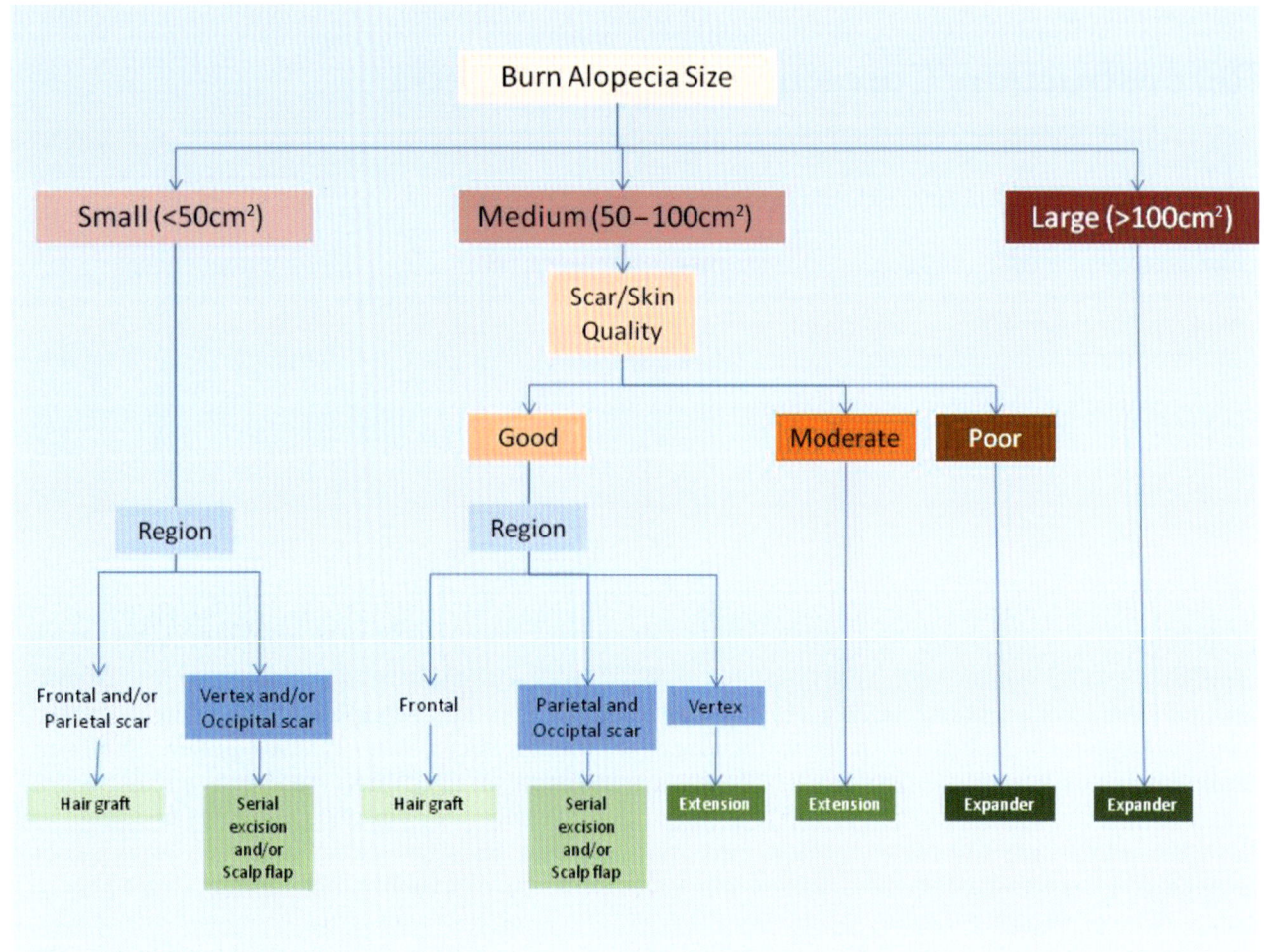

Fig. 1. Algorithm for the reconstruction of post burn alopecia in dependency of size, scar quality and location

an optimal reconstructive option in patients with small, good-quality burn alopecia (Fig. 3).

Scalp reduction
(Serial excision and local scalp flap)

Scalp reduction in this study includes serial excision and the local scalp flap. This method is mainly performed for reconstruction, if the area of burn alopecia is small or medium, and if the scar quality is good. Serial excision is an easy and effective method to remove the burn scar within the alopecic area.

Although the scalp is not very elastic, its mobility can be increased by the surrounding scalp, and if necessary, criss-cross incisions can be made in

the underlying galea to further increase the elasticity [6].

Therefore, small burn alopecia can be totally excised, and moderate burn alopecia can be diminished to an inconspicuous size by repeated excisions, if the scar quality is good. However, this method cannot be used for large, burn alopecia of poor quality [7]. reported that burn alopecic areas up to 15 % of the total scalp can be surgically removed by serial excisions. Generally, the resulting minimized scar is easily hidden with the hair. Local scalp flaps are useful for reconstruction of relatively small burn alopecia [15]. Generally, successful local flap mobilization requires a well-vascularized donor site, which is free of scars and contractures. In burn alopecia, neighboring scalp tissue is often fibrotic as a result of burn damage, thereby severely limiting the

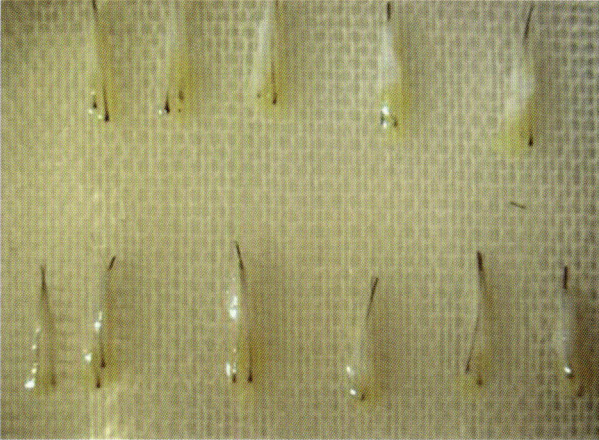

Fig. 2. Hair micrografts

use of local flaps. Moreover, local scalp flaps can be accompanied by some aesthetic problems, including incisional scars, iatrogenic alopecia, and unnatural hair growth patterns.

Scalp extension

Scalp extension surgery was first introduced by Frechet [16]. This technique uses a stretchable device that consists of an elastic silicone band with several hooks on the distal ends. With time, the memory of the silastic band pulls the hair-bearing tissues closer together via the property of biologic creep [17]. The most useful component of scalp extension is that it eliminates the stretch-back phenomenon postoperatively and can reduce the number of repetitions [18]. In addition, this method proves more socially presentable and minimizes social limitations. Moreover, this method reduces the length of hospitalization and total treatment time, as well as the number of checkups required to perform periodic pumping [8]. Nevertheless, this procedure produces is associated with more complications than scalp reduction or hair grafting.

Scalp expansion

Scalp expansion surgery is mainly used when the area of burn alopecia is large and the scar quality is poor (Figs. 4–6). Scalp expansion is the most popular

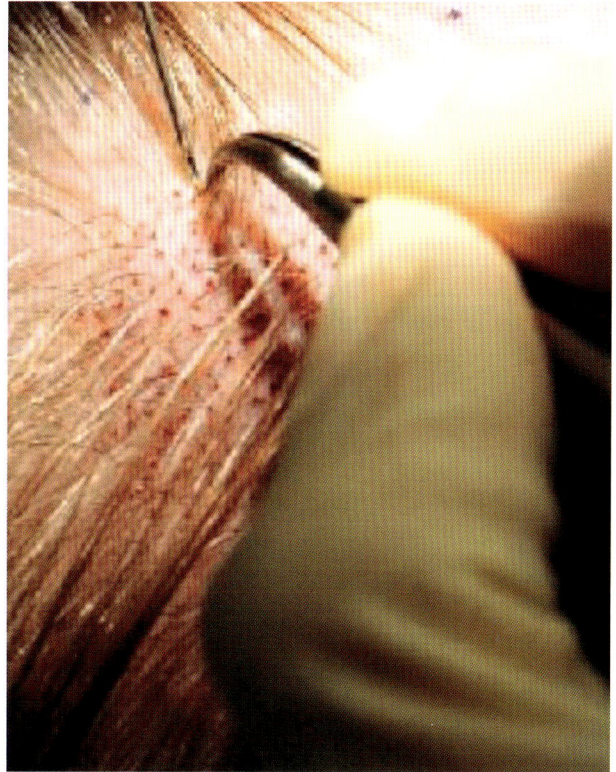

Fig. 3. Technique of hair grafting in a small frontal area

way to reconstruct the burned scalp and it has produced satisfactory results in most patients [9–12]. It provides hair-bearing scalp to the alopecic region with minimal donor site morbidity and huge alopecic regions of up to 50 % of the scalp can be recon-

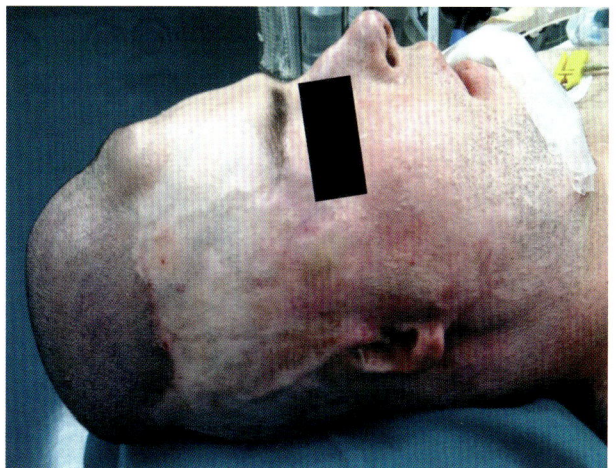

Fig. 4. Large area with moderate to poor scar/skin quality

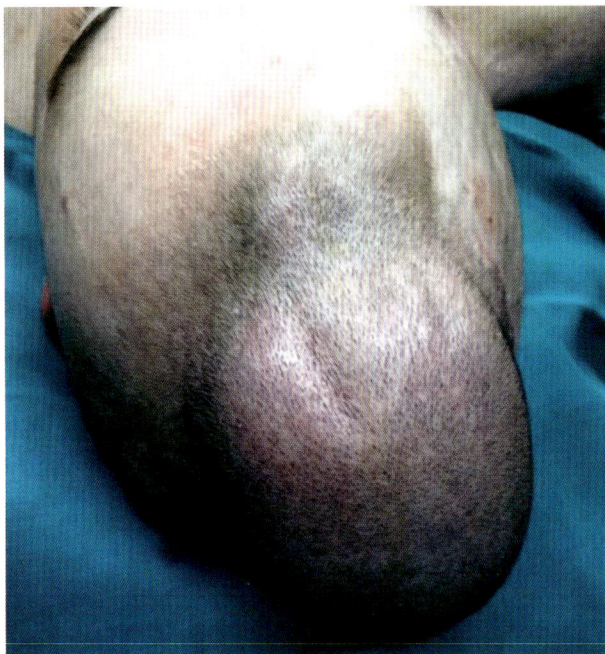

Fig. 5. "bubble head like" appearance of the expanded scalp

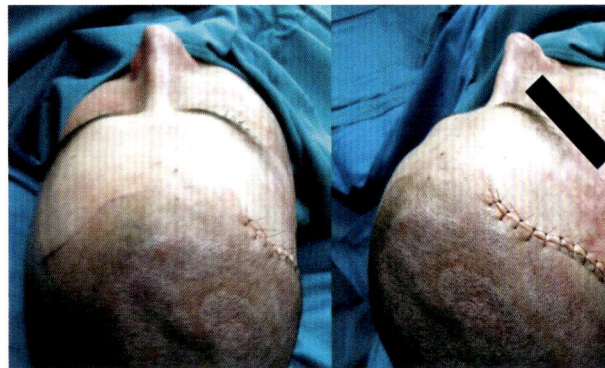

Fig. 6. Reconstruction of large alopecia area including frono-parietal hairline

lesion and the patient's preference. We suggest an algorithm based on the conditions of burn alopecia, including the size, scar quality, and location of the burn alopecia. The algorithm may not be perfect, but this approach can offer a reliable guideline to achieve satisfactory results.

structed using this method without an appreciable change in hair density [19, 20]. However, scalp expansion places a foreign body beneath the skin over a long period of time. Inevitably, this technique has a greater chance of complications than other techniques, including infections, implant exposure, and seromas. Moreover, it does have the disadvantage of requiring multiple hospital visits and the accompanying "bubble head-like" appearance (Fig. 5).

In summary, size of alopecia, scar quality, and location of the burn alopecia are important determinants for choosing a reconstructive method for burn alopecia. Generally, it takes a long time to correct burn alopecia because it usually requires repetitive procedures. Therefore, it is very important to discuss the advantages and disadvantages of each of the reconstructive methods with the patients and select an appropriate method after considering patient's needs and desires.

Conclusions

The method for reconstruction of burn alopecia should be tailored to the conditions of the alopecic

References

[1] Leedy JE, Janis JE, Rohrich RJ (2005) Reconstruction of acquired scalp defects: an algorithmic approach. Plast Reconstr Surg 116: 54e–72e

[2] Barrera A (2003) The use of micrografts and minigrafts in the aesthetic reconstruction of the face and scalp. Plast Reconstr Surg 112: 883–890

[3] Barrera A (1999) The use of micrografts and minigrafts for the treatment of burn alopecia. Plast Reconstr Surg 103: 581–584

[4] Moreno-Arias GA, Camps-Fresneda A (1999) Hair grafting in postburn alopecia. Dermatol Surg 25: 412–414

[5] Emsen IM (2008) The use of micrografts and minigrafts together with advancement of temporalis fascia and its periosteum on the treatment of burn alopecia. J Craniofac Surg 19: 907–909

[6] Vallis CP (1982) Surgical treatment of cicatricial alopecia of the scalp. Clin Plast Surg 9: 179–196

[7] Huang TT, Larson DL, Lewis SR (1977) Burn alopecia. Plast Reconstr Surg 60: 763–767

[8] Rosati P (1995) Extensive head burns corrected by scalp extension. Dermatol Surg 21: 728–730

[9] Voulliaume D, Chichery A, Chekaroua K et al (2007) Tissue expansion in surgical treatment of burn scars of the scalp. Ann Chir Plast Esthet 52: 590–599

[10] Fan J, Yang P (1997) Aesthetic reconstruction of burn alopecia by using expanded hair-bearing scalp flaps. Aesthetic Plast Surg 21: 440–444

[11] Silfen R, Hudson DA, Soldin MG et al (2000) Tissue expansion for frontal hairline restoration in severe alopecia in a child. Burns 26: 294 –297

[12] Buhrer DP, Huang TT, Yee HW et al (1988) Treatment of burn alopecia with tissue expanders in children. Plast Reconstr Surg 81: 512–515

[13] Jeong SH, Koo SH, H SK, Kim WK (2010) An algorithmic approach for reconstruction of burn alopecia. Ann Plast Surg 65: 330–337

[14] Barrera A (1998) The use of micrografts and minigrafts for the correction of the postrhytidectomy lost sideburn. Plast Reconstr Surg 102: 2237–2240

[15] Panje WR, Minor LR (1995) Reconstruction of scalp. In: Baker SR, Swanson NA (eds) Local flaps in facial reconstruction, 1st edn. Mosby, St Louis, pp 481–515

[16] Frechet P (1993) Scalp extension. J Dermatol Surg Oncol 19: 616–622

[17] Dzubow LM (1993) Hair today, gone tomorrow. J Dermatol Surg Oncol 19: 602

[18] Brandy DA (1996) Circumferential scalp reduction with a suture-in-place silasticdacron extender. Dermatol Surg 22: 137–147

[19] Mark DW (2006) Scalp reconstruction in plastic surgery. In: Mathes J, Hentz VR (eds) Plastic surgery, vol 3, 2nd edn. Saunders Elsevier, Philadelphia, pp 607– 632

[20] Sharony Z, Rissin Y, Ullmann Y (2009) Postburn scalp reconstruction using a self-filling osmotic tissue expander. J Burn Care Res 30: 744–746

Correspondence: Lars-Peter Kamolz, M.D., Ph.D., M.Sc., Medical University of Vienna, Department of Surgery, Division of Plastic and Reconstructive Surgery, Vienna, Austria, E-mail: kamolz@plastchirurg.info

Burn reconstruction: Breast

Eva Koellensperger, Guenter Germann

ETHIANUM, Clinic for Plastic, Aesthetic & Preventive Medicine at Heidelberg University Hospital, Heidelberg, Germany

Introduction

Thermal injuries to the anterior chest wall with affection of the breast can cause major functional and aesthetic problems, especially when burns are full thickness and happen early in childhood.

Thermal burns can result in damage of overlying skin, glandular breast tissue itself and postburn scar contractures that may lead to asymmetries and functional growth disturbances.

Reconstructive procedures encompass the entire spectrum of reconstructive breast surgery, including scar release, split and full thickness skin grafting – potentially combined with dermal templates, the use of local flaps, pedicled flaps and free flaps with or without a prostheses, tissue expanders, nipple areola reconstruction, balancing reduction or augmentation mammaplasty, and various techniques of mastopexy.

Reconstructive principles

The trunk is the second most frequently injured body area in burn injuries [1]. The breast is the part of the trunk, where complex reconstructive procedures are often required. Breast reconstruction begins with preserving as much breast tissue as possible during the acute phase of burn treatment. Excision of eschar should be handled carefully. In general, today early excision in acute burn care is considered to be the procedure of choice. However, when the breast is involved in the burned areas, especially during adolescence, a more delayed and conservative approach with regard to the nipple areola complex (NAC) has been shown to be beneficial for the later breast development [2]. The extent of breast tissue in young children is often underestimated while the depth of the burn injury is easily overestimated. The rudimentary breast lies directly underneath the NAC in the subcutis, is 4–8 mm of size, and should be preserved during eschar excision whenever possible. Even if the NAC is lost due to the burn injury, the immature breast is often not damaged and should be carefully preserved. The regeneration of nipple-like structures from proliferating epithelium of the milk ducts in children with third degree burns of the NAC has also been documented [2–6]. When general deep fascial excision of the anterior chest wall needs to be performed in children, a complete or partial lack of breast development has to be expected.

Compared to patients with congenital pediatric breast anomalies, patients with burn injuries to the breast usually need more procedures to reach a satisfactory reconstructive outcome [7]. Kunert et al. proposes the differentiation between scald and burn injuries regarding the surgical procedures in patients with thermal injuries in childhood. They state that scalds result in a deep second to superficial third degree burn which does not harm the underlying subcutaneously located mammary gland tissue [6].

Consequences of burns of the anterior chest wall with involvement of the breast in all ages are: asymmetry, deformity, lack of any breast, lack of projection, lack of NAC, inhibition of normal breast development, unpleasant skin texture, and psychological problems. Problems associated with thermal breast injury are related to direct damage of breast tissue and the overlying skin as well as contracture of scar tissue and development of a restrictive skin envelope. The aim of reconstructive surgery should be:

▶ to release scar contractions,
▶ to re-establish breast volume and shape,
▶ to reposition and recreate the NAC,
▶ and to restore the self image and confidence of the patient.

Reconstructive procedures depend on:

▶ the severity of the trauma,
▶ the type and amount of tissue lacking,
▶ the quality of the surrounding soft tissue,
▶ the distribution and amount of burned surface area
▶ and – in particular – the age and demands of the patient.

However, reconstructive procedures should not be performed until wounds are fully healed and scars are stable and mature.

Simultaneous combined procedures bear the advantage of a high immediate benefit with limited downtime, hospital stay, and anesthesia. However, one needs to address the fact that the definitive outcome of one procedure needs to be anticipated if the following operative step is planned to be processed simultaneously. This implicates a high level of experience with those kinds of procedures. One such example would be NAC reconstruction and contralateral reduction mammaplasty, two procedures that – at least in our opinion – should be planned with a minimum of 6 month in between to allow the opposite breast to reach a stable situation with only minor upcoming changes in shape and position of NAC. Otherwise the long-term outcome is at risk to be unsatisfactory.

Scar release

Scar release is often the first step of breast reconstruction after a burn injury. It should be performed as early as breast development is inhibited in adolescent girls, especially when surrounding healthy tissue is beginning to bulge. Release is also indicated when a significant limitation in the range of motion, unstable wound situations, and functional or subjective discomfort is present. In most pediatric patients scar release is undertaken between 14–16 years. It is recommended to excise all scarred tissue completely and cover the resulting defect with a thick split thickness skin graft or full thickness skin graft. If scaring is very severe, it is often necessary to incise scarred skin down to the deep fascia of the chest or abdomen to fully release all inhibiting contractures. When the whole breast is affected from scars it is recommended to incise 5/8 of the total circumference, and to proceed with the incision into unburned areas. An inframammary incision is the most common location for a scar release. However, if scarring involves the whole breast and contractures are located around the breast, supra-, intra- or intermammary release might be necessary [5, 6, 8, 9].

Depending on the location of the contractures local or distant flaps may be required to reconstruct the resulting soft tissue deficit in order to achieve the best possible aesthetic outcome.

Split thickness skin graft

Split thickness skin grafts (STSG) have been used not only in primary wound care after excision of burned tissue but also for secondary procedures in combination with scar release. Unfortunately STSG have a tendency to contract. If the total burn surface is small enough non-meshed STSG sheets should be used preferably for coverage of breast and décolleté regions with regard to aesthetic issues. In comparison to STSG mesh grafts, sheets have a better aesthetic outcome creating a more homogenous surface and no visible mesh pattern. Most authors use and recommend STSG with a thickness of 0.016–0.02 mm for best results in burned breasts [9].

Full thickness skin grafts

Full thickness skin grafts (FTSG) are used for reconstruction of NAC, reconstruction of the inframammary fold after scar release, and resurfacing of burned breast soft tissue [10]. Skin grafts have a tendency to shrink and contract, however, FTSG have a comparatively lower tendency than STSG. Shelley et al. have proposed the use of full FTSG from aesthetic procedures, such as abdominoplasty or reduction mammaplasty, for reconstructive purposes in burn patients. Thus donor site morbidity of skin harvesting for FTSG could be minimized with a dual benefit of improved functional and aesthetic outcome [11]. Mueller et al. have shown a case of breast resurfacing with a full thickness abdominal skin graft with good results in a patient with no loss of glandular tissue. They propose abdominal skin as a good donor site for breast resurfacing procedures because of similar skin color and texture [12].

Combination of split or full thickness grafts with dermal substitutes (Matriderm®, Integra®)

Integra® is a dermal regeneration template consisting of collagen and chondroitin-6-sulfate. It has been shown to gain a stable vascularization from the wound bed within 28 days if placed in a well vascularized environment after meticulous hemostasis. Integra® has been used successfully for the management of breast postburn contractures in combination with split thickness grafts [13, 14]. The clinical and functional outcome was convincing. When used by Palao et al. for thermal breast injuries in combination with overlying STSG, a statistically significant improvement in the Vancouver scar scale score after one year and a high level of satisfaction in treated patients with lasting improvements in breast contour and shape could be demonstrated. No contracture of the skin grafts overlaying Integra was seen. Integra® was completely replaced by host collagen and elastic fibers within one year [15]. Groos et al. have used Integra in 10 children with a medium of 45 % TBSA including breast burns, preferably with unmeshed skin grafts. After 12–45 days the initially placed Integra® was covered with a 0.15–0.2 mm thin STSG. The final outcome was described as functionally and cosmetically improved [16]. Tsoutsos et al. expanded non-meshed integra combined with a STSG for the coverage of a soft tissue breast defect after excising scars and releasing contractures with insertion of a subpectorally placed expander. After 17 month no re-contracture or distor-

tion was seen [14]. Clinically, it has been shown that Integra® needs at least 3 weeks to produce a stable neodermis suitable for skin grafting [17].

Integra® and Matriderm®, a non-cross linked collagen-elastin matrix with bovine collagen type I, III and V, have been compared in a recent animal study. It has been shown that there is no difference regarding vascularization, building of a neo-dermis, and graft take between the two matrices. The combined use of both with skin grafts leads to a significantly more and better structured neo-dermis in comparison to skin grafting alone [17].

To our knowledge the use of Matriderm® for the reconstruction of burns in the breast area has not yet been published. However, we think that it could be a worthwhile option, as its use in burns demonstrated significant advantages in other delicate regions of the body, such as burned hands and face. Combining split thickness grafts with Matriderm® leads to a significant improvement of skin elasticity, measured with Vancouver Burn Skin Score, with a consistent survival of applied skin grafts [14, 18–22]. We could show, that a one stage procedure combining Matriderm® and split thickness skin grafts simultaneously, can be performed safely in regard to skin take [20].

Local flaps

Z-plasties
When breast development is normal and only breast shape or position is disturbed by local band-like contractures, single or multiple Z-plasties are a useful option for scar release [6, 23].

Transposition flaps
Local flaps are especially used for the reconstruction of the inframammary fold in combination with scar releasing procedures. Payne et al. have used a Ryan-type thoracic advancement flap. McCauley demonstrated longitudinal abdominal transposition flaps [2, 24]. Hsiao et al. have used a lateral chest rotation flap to reconstruct breast tissue insufficiency [25].

Compared with split thickness skin grafts local flaps possess the advantage of a lower tendency for contracture and no need for postoperative splinting to maintain the correction of breast deformity [2, 26].

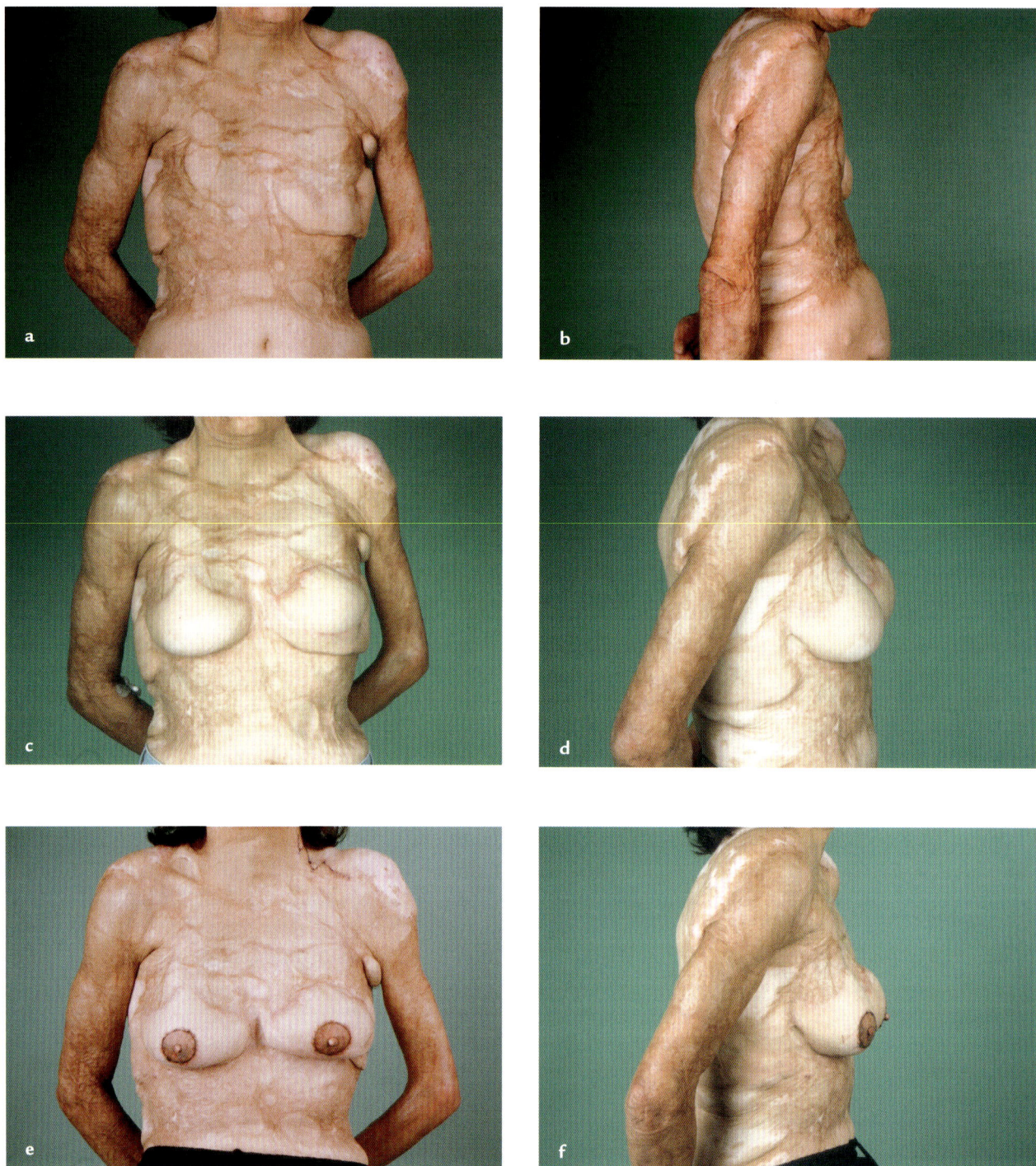

Fig.1. 35 years old woman with a deep burn injury of 80 % total body surface including total fascial excision of both breasts at the age of 17 (Fig. 1a and b). 12 years after the injury breast volume was reconstructed with a bilateral TRAM flap. 8 month later the inframammary fold on the left side was lifted with fixing sutures to the chest wall. Nipple reconstruction was performed simultaneously on both sides using a skate flap and inguinal FTSG. In the same procedure liposuction was performed on the lateral chest wall on both sides. **a/b** Patient before breast reconstruction with bilateral TRAM flap. **c/d** Patient seven months after breast reconstruction with bilateral TRAM flap. **e/f** Patient seven days after NAC reconstruction with skate flap, FTSG and bilateral liposuction on the lateral chest walls

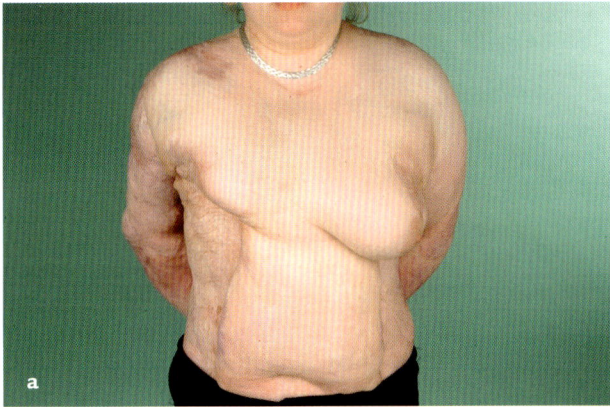

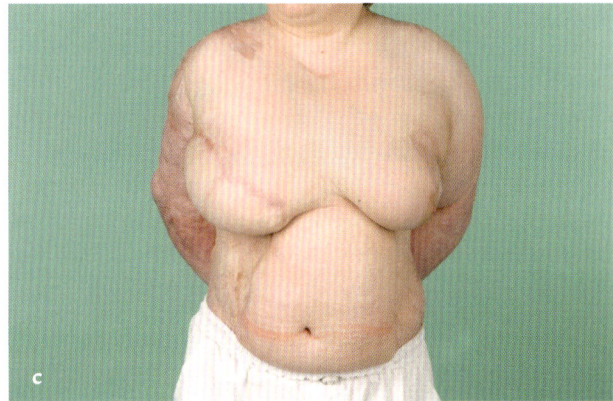

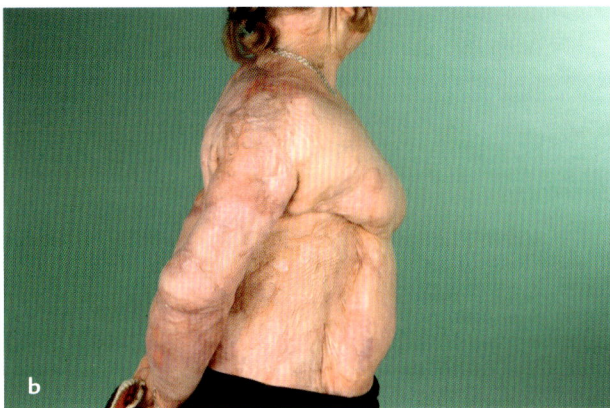

Fig. 2. 22 year old female presented with a 78 % full thickness burn. Deep fascial excision was performed on the right chest wall with ablatio mammae and coverage with STSG. A free DIEP flap was performed for reconstruction of her right breast four years after the injury. The patient was satisfied with the result and did not show up for further reconstructive procedures, such as nipple-areola complex reconstruction. **a/b** Patient before breast reconstruction with DIEP flap on the right side. **c** Patient six weeks after breast reconstruction with DIEP flap on the right side

Pedicled flaps

Transverse Rectus Abdominis Muscle (TRAM)

TRAM flaps have been used by several authors for the reconstruction of lacking breast volume not only in burned patients. With using a TRAM flap for breast reconstruction one gains enough volume and skin to rebuild a totally destroyed breast. However, the known disadvantages and risks, such as instable abdominal walls, herniation and prolonged postoperative pain, need to be addressed carefully. Furthermore, most young patients lack a sufficient abdominal laxity to easily and safely perform a TRAM flap, and often the abdominal area is also affected by the burn injury and thus not available. Patients of child-bearing age should also not be considered for a TRAM flap as pregnancy can enhance the risk of unwanted abdominal wall side effects [9, 23, 27].

M. lattissimus dorsi flap (LD)

The pedicled myocutaneous LD flap can be used for the reconstruction of the breasts soft tissue envelope or for mid-size volume deficits. Especially when most of the breast tissue has been destroyed and the opposite breast is rather large, LD flaps almost always lack enough volume to reconstruct a breast size equal to the non-injured normal breast. Therefore they often need to be combined with a permanent implant [5, 9, 10, 23, 28].

Free flaps

Free TRAM flap

Deep inferior epigastric artery perforator flap (DIEP)/ superior (SGAP)/inferior (IGAP) gluteal artery perforator flap

The use of the free TRAM flap has decreased in recent years. However in selected cases it is still a valuable option (case 1) DIEP or SGAP/IGAP flaps in general provide enough volume to restore full breast size in patients who experienced total breast loss. To our knowledge their use for the reconstruction of burned breast has not been published before. Here we show for the first time one case (see case 2) of breast reconstruction with a free DIEP flap. We think that the use of these free flaps for this indication will become more and more popular, regarding their excellent outcome in other patients with total loss of breast volume.

Anterior lateral thigh flap

Tsai et al. have published the use of a free ALT flap, split in two equal skin paddles for the reconstruction of breast volume in one patient [8]. It could also be a possible option to use super-thin cutaneous ALT flaps to restore a soft tissue envelope over adequate existing breast tissue.

Nipple-areola complex reconstruction

Nipple areola complex (NAC) reconstruction is the final step of breast reconstruction and a very important issue to restore patients self confidence and feeling of femininity. It includes restoration of the nipple and the surrounding areola with adequate projection and pigmentation. There are multiple different methods for NAC reconstruction, however, they all have in common that they should not be performed unless the newly formed breast has fully settled to its final shape and position. Such prior procedures mandating an adequate waiting time, usually 6–12 months, may include scar release, reconstruction of the inframammary fold, and augmentation or reduction mammaplasty.

Skin for NAC reconstruction can be obtained from the opposite NAC, by excising the outer half circumferentially as full thickness skin graft or full nipple and areola sharing, or from the inner upper portion of the thigh or the labia majores. Best match in texture and pigmentation is achieved by transplanting parts of the opposite NAC. Further options are local flaps or transplants from the toe pulps, ear lobes, or rib cartilage. The latter can be used especially when free flaps are used for the reconstruction of the breast mound and the anastomosis is performed at the internal mammary artery which includes partial resection of rib cartilage. After

trimming it can be banked near the wound borders underneath the flap for approximately 6 month until tissue settling has finished and NAC reconstruction is performed with the banked cartilage [5, 9, 28, 29].

AlloDerm® has been used in non burned patients to improve long term nipple projection in nipple reconstruction with local flaps with promising results. AlloDerm® was rolled together and placed in the center of the new nipple [30–32]. Nipple reconstruction in burns with AlloDerm® has not yet been published to our knowledge. However it could be a useful and supportive alternative.

For simple repositioning of a distorted but existing NAC in breast burn injuries Mohmand et al. have shown a double U-plasty technique with good results [33]. The ductal system is thought to be preserved with this technique.

Tattoo

Tatooing for aesthetic medical purposes is also named "micropigmentation" or "dermatography". The micropigments are placed between superficial and middle dermal layers and are initially fixed intracellular and gradually become extracellular [34]. After NAC reconstruction with local skin or skin transplants tattooing is often required to achieve a satisfactory pigmentation matching the opposite NAC. It should be performed with a delay of at least 8 weeks after nipple reconstruction [9, 35].

Local flaps

Local flaps for nipple restoration usually work well in breast reconstruction patients without previous burn injury. With scared burned skin, however, dermal blood supply is restricted, making local flaps more unreliable and difficult.

Bunchman et al. proposed the double bubble technique in 1974, using two concentric incisional circles within the scared skin, each one sutured with the base to the surface of the outer one, followed by epithelializing and tattooing [35]. Pensler et al. compared a local flap (quadropod flap) with earlobe grafts, the double bubble technique, split thickness skin grafts, and tattooing from the opposite areola. They found that the quadropod flap and the earlobe grafts give comparable results concerning projection, however, the quadropod flap had a lower donor-site morbidity. Tattooing gave poor long term results with fading pigments. With split thickness grafts from the contralateral areola severe hypopigmentation or hyperpigmentation associated with asymmetry was observed. The authors recommend employing local flaps for nipple reconstruction if there is adequate vascularity of the surrounding soft tissue and full thickness skin grafts for areola reconstruction [36].

Motamed and Davami have used a variation of the modified star flap for the reconstruction of the NAC in 7 females with breast burns in childhood [37]. Besides the central portion of the new nipple all flap parts are deepithelialized and buried to increase central nipple projection. This reduces the risk of skin necrosis and the amount of necessary sutures, which itself can compromise skin blood supply. With this technique a medium nipple projection of 5 +/−1 mm after a medium follow up period of 10 +/−3 month is achieved. Complications such as hematoma, necrosis or discolorations have not been reported.

Tissue expanders

In breast reconstruction after a burn injury with the loss or lack of glandular tissue, expanders are often placed under the pectoralis muscle to pre-expand the overlying soft tissue before insertion of permanent implants [7, 10]. Tissue expanders can also be inserted in a submammary position and prior to scar and contracture release with split thickness skin grafting. The expander is exchanged for a permanent implant 1–3 month after being fully inflated. Approximately 200 cc of overexpansion are recommended [23, 38, 39]. Tissue expanders have also been used underneath STSG prior to insertion of a permanent prosthesis [26] and with an overlying Integra dermal template with good results, as mentioned above [14].

Care needs to be taken when implanting expanders underneath previously burned or scarred tissue [25]. Following such procedures, general complications include skin necrosis or ulceration, exposure of the expander or injection port, wound healing problems, infections and capsule formation, or even chest wall deformations [9, 10]. However, in a breast specific study Levi et al. showed that tissue expanders

used to reconstruct burned breasts do not have a higher complication rate than those used to reconstruct congenital breast deformities. Furthermore, endoscopic placement of tissue expanders resulted in a significantly lower operative time, significantly less complications, and a significantly decreased time needed for full expansion [40].

Internal pressure due to tissue expanders or prostheses together with external pressure due to custom made compression garment can sufficiently soften existing scars and prevent further hypertrophic scarring in the breast area [25, 38].

Reduction and augmentation mammaplasty/mastopexy

Due to loss of breast volume or lack of elasticity of the skin envelope in the burned breast, asymmetry compared to the opposite breast can result. To achieve breast symmetry, reduction mammaplasty or mastopexy at the burned or contralateral breast may be indicated. Furthermore, women with burned breast can also suffer from hyperplastic breasts or macromastia requesting reduction mammaplasty.

Prior to reduction mammaplasty full scar release should be performed and full development of the breast should be allowed. The ideal reduction mammaplasty technique addresses volume and shape asymmetries, scar areas, and skin contractures as well as a possible NAC distorsion.

Payne et al. demonstrated the use of a Lejour-type reduction technique with a nearly vertical skin resection pattern in a burned breast with severe ptosis, contracting inferior scars, and inferiorly dislocated NAC. The NAC was transposed superiorly with a superior parenchymal pedicle [24]. Hunter et al. favoured a one stage procedure for the correction of a post-burn superior pole scar contracture and simultaneous reduction mammaplasty in a patient with hyperplastic breasts [41]. They used a combination of a rotational glanduloplasty with NAC transposition and a contralateral superior pedicle based reduction mammaplasty. In this case, however, a positive aesthetic outcome of the resulting scars is questionable, especially regarding possible alternative treatment options, such as a conventional reduction mammaplasty.

El-Khatib showed the reliability of an inferior pedicle in reduction mammaplasty in hyperplastic burned breasts [42]. The inferior dermal pedicle was placed in scar tissue but nevertheless showed good blood supply. The author concludes that the use of an inferior pedicle is the best technique for the reduction of hyperplastic burned breasts with a very low NAC.

Thai et al. have documented a series of 6 patients with burns to the breast in early childhood and consecutive split thickness skin grafting. 10 reduction mammaplasties were safely performed in these patients with hyperplastic or asymmetric breasts after breast burn. An inferior pedicle technique with limited undermining is recommended by the authors to avoid problems with skin blood supply [43].

Hsiao et al. and Ozgur et al. propose the simultaneous correction of functional post-burn scar release procedures and aesthetically indicated augmentation mammaplasty by using the excess skin as FTSG for scar release [23, 25]. Hsiao et al. state that implants should be placed under the pectoralis muscle to reduce the risk of capsular contraction and decrease palpability and visibility of the implant.

Ozgur et al. experienced skin necrosis after insertion of subglandular and submuscular placed permanent inplants [23]. He recommends the solitary use of inplants only if suitable skin coverage is available.

Burned breasts in which the soft tissue envelope has not been fully restored, often lack the natural developing ptosis. Therefore mastopexy of the contralateral breast might be necessary in unilateral breast burn injuries when the contralateral breast is at least moderately ptotic [1].

Conclusion

Burn injury to the anterior chest wall can cause contracting and hypertrophic scarring, breast deformity and asymmetry, lack of breast tissue, distortion or lack of nipple areola complex and thus functional, aesthetic and psychosocial problems. Long term follow up and surveillance of patients with breast burns is required to achieve the best possible outcome and address all rising problems at an adequate point in time. Correction of these problems in general requires multiple serial procedures that have to be cautiously fitted into a reliable timetable.

Take home message

1) Breast reconstruction starts with breast saving in acute burn care. Precaution should be taken with excision of eschar in the area of the breast and the NAC in children and adolescents.
2) Wounds should be closed and scars be allowed to mature before further reconstructive procedures are undertaken.
3) Wearing a custom made compression garment until scars are mature is essential for optimal outcome and can, in part, prevent invasive procedures.
4) Scar release should be performed extensively and as soon as breast development is inhibited or breast deformity is induced.
5) Reconstruction of breast volume can be achieved with local, pedicled or free flaps as well as with permanent implants, depending on the amount of lacking volume, the quality of the surrounding tissue, available donor sites, and patients' desires.
6) Contralateral and ipsilateral reduction or augmentation mammaplasty, contralateral mastopexy, and balancing procedures may be necessary to achieve aesthetically pleasing results.
7) Reconstruction of the nipple areola complex should not be performed until the breast has fully developed and prior reconstructive steps have achieved a stable long term result.
8) Long term follow up is necessary with all burn patients, especially in females with breast burns, due to life-long changes in breast shape.

References

[1]   McCauley RL (2002) Reconstruction of the trunk and genitalia. In: Herndon DN (ed) Total burn care. W. B. Saunders, Philadelphia, 2nd edition, pp 707–710
[2]   McCauley RL et al (1989) Longitudinal assessment of breast development in adolescent female patients with

burns involving the nipple-areolar complex. Plast Reconstr Surg 83(4): 676–680

[3] al-Qattan MM, Zuker RM (1994) Management of acute burns of the female pediatric breast: delayed tangential excision versus spontaneous eschar separation. Ann Plast Surg 33(1): 66–67

[4] Foley P et al (2008) Breast burns are not benign: long-term outcomes of burns to the breast in pre-pubertal girls. Burns 34(3): 412–417

[5] Neale HW et al (1982) Breast reconstruction in the burned adolescent female (an 11-year, 157 patient experience). Plast Reconstr Surg 70(6): 718–724

[6] Kunert P, Schneider W, Flory J (1988) Principles and procedures in female breast reconstruction in the young child's burn injury. Aesthetic Plast Surg 12(2): 101–106

[7] Sadove AM, van Aalst JA (2005) Congenital and acquired pediatric breast anomalies: a review of 20 years' experience. Plast Reconstr Surg 115(4): 1039–1050

[8] Tsai FC et al (2004) Free split-cutaneous perforator flaps procured using a three-dimensional harvest technique for the reconstruction of postburn contracture defects. Plast Reconstr Surg 113(1): 185–93; discussion 194–195

[9] Ogilvie MP, Panthaki ZJ (2008) Burns of the developing breast. J Craniofac Surg 19(4): 1030–1033

[10] Loss M et al (2002) The burned female breast: a report on four cases. Burns 28(6): 601–605

[11] Shelley OP et al (2006) Dual benefit procedures: combining aesthetic surgery with burn reconstruction. Burns 32(8): 1022–1027

[12] Mueller M, Boorman JG (2002) Post-burn breast resurfacing using an abdominal full-thickness skin graft. Br J Plast Surg 55(2): 148–150

[13] Shariff Z, Rawlins JM, Austin O (2007) Burned breast reconstruction by expanded artificial dermal substitute. J Burn Care Res 28(6): 929

[14] Tsoutsos D et al (2007) Burned breast reconstruction by expanded artificial dermal substitute. J Burn Care Res 28(3): 530–532

[15] Palao R, Gomez P, Huguet P (2003) Burned breast reconstructive surgery with Integra dermal regeneration template. Br J Plast Surg 56(3): 252–259

[16] Groos N et al (2005) Use of an artificial dermis (Integra) for the reconstruction of extensive burn scars in children. About 22 grafts. Eur J Pediatr Surg 15(3): 187–192

[17] Schneider J et al (2009) Matriderm versus Integra: a comparative experimental study. Burns 35(1): 51–57

[18] Haslik W et al (2010) Management of full-thickness skin defects in the hand and wrist region: first long-term experiences with the dermal matrix Matriderm. J Plast Reconstr Aesthet Surg 63(2): 360–364

[19] Kolokythas P et al (2008) [Dermal subsitute with the collagen-elastin matrix Matriderm in burn injuries: a comprehensive review]. Handchir Mikrochir Plast Chir 40(6): 367–371

[20] Ryssel H et al (2008) The use of MatriDerm in early excision and simultaneous autologous skin grafting in burns–a pilot study. Burns 34(1): 93–97

[21] Boyce A et al (2010) The use of Matriderm in the management of an exposed Achilles tendon secondary to a burns injury. J Plast Reconstr Aesthet Surg 63(2): e206–207

[22] Atherton DD et al (2010) Early excision and application of matriderm with simultaneous autologous skin grafting in facial burns. Plast Reconstr Surg 125(2): 60e–61e

[23] Ozgur F et al (1992) Reconstruction of postburn breast deformities. Burns 18(6): 504–509

[24] Payne CE, Malata CM (2003) Correction of postburn breast asymmetry using the LeJour-type mammaplasty technique. Plast Reconstr Surg 111(2): 805–809

[25] Hsiao YC et al (2009) Are augmentation mammaplasty and reconstruction of the burned breast collateral lines? Experience in performing simultaneous reconstructive and aesthetic surgery. Burns 35(1): 130–136

[26] Guan WX, Jin YT, Cao HP (1988) Reconstruction of postburn female breast deformity. Ann Plast Surg 21(1): 65–69

[27] Psillakis JM, Woisky R (1985) Burned breast: treatment with a transverse rectus abdominis island musculocutaneous flap. Ann Plast Surg 14(5): 437–442

[28] Bishop JB, Fisher J, Bostwick J 3rd (1980) The burned female breast. Ann Plast Surg 4(1): 25–30

[29] Heitland A, Markowicz M, Koellensperger E (2006) Long-term nipple shrinkage following augmentation by an autologous rib cartilage transplant in free DIEP-flaps. J Plast Reconstr Aesthet Surg 59(10): 1063–1067

[30] Chen WF, Barounis D, Kalimuthu R (2010) A novel cost-saving approach to the use of acellular dermal matrix (AlloDerm) in postmastectomy breast and nipple reconstructions. Plast Reconstr Surg 125(2): 479–481

[31] Holton LH et al (2005) Improving long-term projection in nipple reconstruction using human acellular dermal matrix – an animal model. Ann Plast Surg 55(3): 304–309

[32] Garramone CE, Lam B (2007) Use of AlloDerm in primary nipple reconstruction to improve long-term nipple projection. Plast Reconstr Surg 119(6): 1663–1668

[33] Mohmand H, Naasan A (2002) Double U-plasty for correction of geometric malposition of the nipple-areola complex. Plast Reconstr Surg 109(6): 2019–2022

[34] Garg G, Thami GP (2005) Micropigmentation: tattooing for medical purposes. Dermatol Surg 31(8 Pt 1): 928–31; discussion 931

[35] Bunchman HH 2nd et al (1974) Nipple and areola reconstruction in the burned breast. The "double bubble" technique. Plast Reconstr Surg 54(5): 531–536

[36] Pensler JM, Haab RL, Parry SW (1986) Reconstruction of the burned nipple-areola complex. Plast Reconstr Surg 78(4): 480–485

[37] Motamed S, Davami B (2005) Postburn reconstruction of nipple-areola complex. Burns 31(8): 1020–1024

[38] Versaci AD, Balkovich ME, Goldstein SA (1986) Breast reconstruction by tissue expansion for congenital and burn deformities. Ann Plast Surg 16(1): 20–31

[39] Slator RC, Wilson GR, Sharpe DT (1992) Postburn breast reconstruction: tissue expansion prior to contracture release. Plast Reconstr Surg 90(4): 668–671; discussion 672–674

[40] Levi B, Brown DL, Cederna PS (2010) A comparative analysis of tissue expander reconstruction of burned and unburned chest and breast using endoscopic and open techniques. Plast Reconstr Surg 125(2): 547–556

[41] Hunter JE, Gilbert PM, Dheansa BS (2009) Correction of postburn superior pole breast deformity and macromastia–a novel approach. Burns 35(5): 746–749

[42] El-Khatib HA (1999) Reliability of inferior pedicle reduction mammaplasty in burned oversized breasts. Plast Reconstr Surg 103(3): 869–873

[43] Thai KN et al (1999) Reduction mammaplasty in postburn breasts. Plast Reconstr Surg 103(7): 1882–1886

Correspondence: Guenter Germann, M.D., Ph.D. – Professor of Plastic Surgery, ETHIANUM, Clinic for Plastic, Aesthetic & Preventive Medicine at Heidelberg University Hospital, Bergheimer Straße 89/1, 69115 Heidelberg, Germany, E-mail: guenter. germann@urz-uni-heidelberg. de

Reconstruction of burn deformities of the lower extremity

Christian Ottomann[1], Bernd Hartmann[2]

[1] Plastische Chirurgie, Handchirurgie, Intensiveinheit für Schwerbrandverletzte, Universitätsklinikum Schleswig-Holstein Campus Lübeck, Lübeck, Germany
[2] Zentrum für Schwerbrandverletzte mit Plastischer Chirurgie, Unfallkrankenhaus Berlin, Germany

Introduction

In addition to reconstructive surgery to restore form, the main goal of reconstructive burn surgery is to re-integrate the patient into professional and social life [1]. Although the stigmatizing scars which result from burns to the lower extremities can be covered by clothing, functional restrictions are particularly noticeable due to changes in the patient's gait [2]. As a result, the goal of reconstructive surgery on patients who have suffered burn trauma is to both restore the skin's surrounding soft tissue in order to improve form as well as to restore function. Acute treatment applied to the lower extremity is similar to that applied to the body's remaining surface, with the exception that the exposed tendons and bones in the area of the tibia and foot are only protected by extremely thin soft skin tissue. Problems in reconstructing the skin's soft tissue often already arise during acute treatment, and they often result in secondary healing and subsequent scarring [3]. As a result, post-burn contractures and unstable scars occur with some frequency on the lower extremities [4]. Unfortunately, a post-burn contracture still does not only result from the trauma which causes the tissue damage, but also – particularly in elderly patients – as a result of immobilizing the area within the scope of providing initial treatment. As is the case in the entire field of plastic reconstructive surgery, reconstruction of the burned extremity should be oriented along the reconstructive ladder.

Reconstructive ladder stage 1: Z-plasty

The Z-plasty technique represents a form of plastic surgery in which two triangular skin flaps across from each other are mobilized. By rotating these flaps, tension is reduced along the central limb. This technique makes use of the area's width, which means that sufficient tissue must be available on each side of the scar. If more length is needed, or if the available tissue elasticity in the lateral skin areas is not sufficient for a single z-plasty, several small z-shaped incisions can be strung together (Figs. 1, 2). Necrosis in the tips of the flaps, which occurs in small flaps whose angles are too acute, and old scars running perpendicular to the

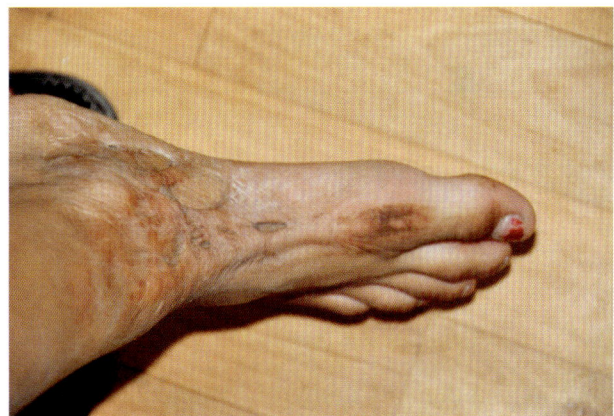

Fig. 1. Post burn-contracture on the dorsum of the right foot with consecutive restrictions to mobility

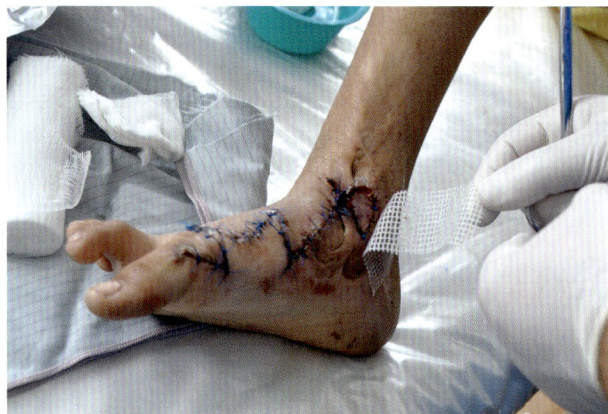

Fig. 2. Result after scar adhesiolysis and z-plasty

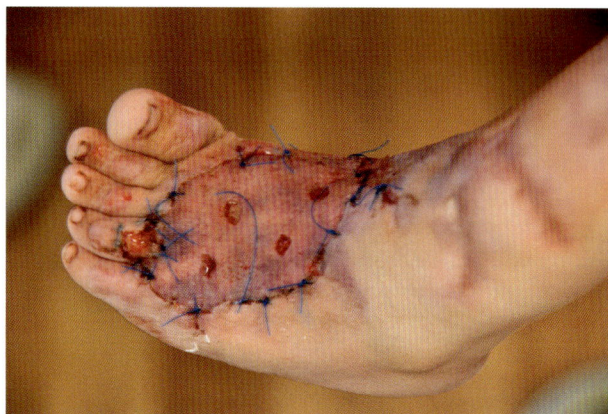

Fig. 4. Result after scar excision and full-thickness skin graft

base of the flap, which have a negative effect on blood circulation, represent the primary complications in this case. In addition to the actual z-plasty technique, there are also other modified versions of the flap triangles which can be selected in special cases, for example incisions with the opposite alignment (such as the butterfly or jumping man) [5].

Reconstructive ladder stage 2: Skin graft transplantation

Reconstruction of an excision scar is carried out using a skin graft transplantation. Healthy subcutaneous fatty tissue, uninjured peritendineum, healthy muscle fascia, or healthy muscle tissue are suitable

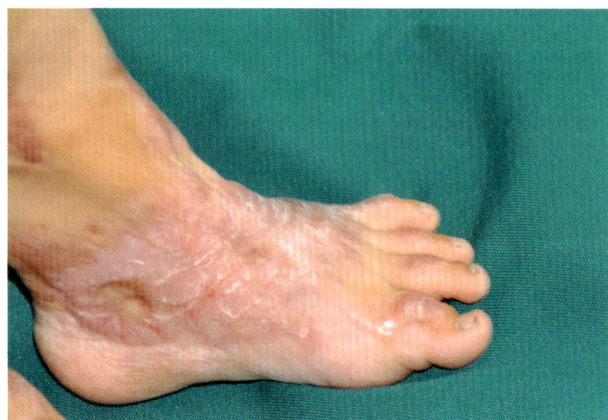

Fig. 3. Scarring on the dorsum of the left foot after a scald

for receiving a skin graft (Fig. 3). Debrided granulation tissue or tissue conditioned with an artificial dermal substitute can also serve as the recipient site. Free skin grafts differ in their thickness, and thick split-skin or full-thickness skin is suitable for scar reconstruction (Fig. 4). The individual grafts all have advantages and disadvantages, both as they pertain to the donor site and their characteristics at the recipient site. With thick split-skin grafts, one must take factors into consideration ranging from poor reepithelialization of the donor site with the possibility of subsequent scarring to the possibility of keloid scarring. In addition, the area of full-thickness skin which can be used as donor tissue is limited. At the recipient site, free skin grafts heal better the thinner they are, however the thickness of the layer of skin used corresponds with the desired result. A sufficient dermal layer must be used, particularly when grafting on the soles of the feet, since a three-dimensional network of fine fibroelastic tendons, which form a multitude of small cushioning elements, pervade the plantar fat pad. This unique anatomical configuration makes the sole of the foot the perfect shock absorber while walking. Preserving this tissue – particularly since this area of the foot often exhibits repeated bruising after suffering a burn – represents an important reconstructive goal. In this case, one must always consider the use of skin grafts. Another factor which must be noted is the tendency of free skin grafts to shrink. For example, thick split-skin grafts can shrink by up to 30 %. In addition, artificial dermal substitutes are available for use in modern reconstructive treatment. The advantages lie in the reduction in donor morbidity from full-thickness skin grafts and the benefits from their wide availability in comparison with full-thickness skin grafts. As a result of the graft, improved dermal regeneration is achieved, which reduces the formation of new scar tissue [7]. Dermal substitutes promote the formation of a vascularized neodermis, which can be covered with an extremely thin autologous epidermal split-skin graft or with cultivated keratinocytes after 14–21 days [8].

Reconstructive ladder Stage 3: Pedicle flaps

Selecting the skin flap to use in reconstructive surgery on the lower extremities is done according to different principles than for the upper extremities. In the upper extremities, a large portion of all muscles are needed to ensure that the arms and hands can function sufficiently, and removing a single muscle can cause a significant loss of function in this area. In contrast, the lower extremities have a number of different muscles which all have the same function. For example, the four individual muscles which form the quadriceps femoris are responsible for extending the knee joint. Using one of these individual muscles as a graft will not affect the active extension of the knee joint. Based on the same principle, the individual muscles which form the hamstring or those used for dorsiflexion or plantarflexion can also be used. The following is a list of flaps which used most often:

Tensor Fascia Lata flap (TFL)

The tensor fascia lata flap is located in the area of the lateral circumflex femoral artery. It is comprised of a muscular and fascial portion. It can measure up to 15 cm wide and up to 40 cm long. Vascularization of the distal portion can sometimes be problematic, but can be improved through bilateral elevation. This flap is particularly suited to reconstructive procedures in the upper third of the thigh. The TFL flap can also be used as a free microsurgical flap or as a perforator flap [9].

Anterolateral Thigh flap (ALT)

The ALT is a flap with a relatively constant vascular supply. It can be harvested as a myocutaneous or perforator flap. It is mainly indicated for use with defects in the upper and middle third of the thigh. In addition, the ALT can also see application as a free microsurgical flap, and in this case can also be used as a myocutaneous or perforator flap [10].

Gracilis flap

The myocutaneous gracilis flap is a thin flap for defects in the upper third of the thigh. It can be up 24 cm long, and this length can be extended to 32 cm by including the tendon. Its width is limited to 6–8 cm. This graft exhibits very constant and secure vascularization. A further benefit is that with this graft, primary closure is usually feasible [11].

Vastus lateralis flap

The vastus lateralis flap, as part of the quadricips femoris, is supplied by numerous vascular pedicles which primarily stem from the profunda femoris artery. It is vascularized proximally by one or two branches of the lateral circumflex femoral artery, the middle third is supplied by the perforating arteries of the profunda femoris, and the distal third receives branches from the popliteal artery. The two branches of the lateral circumflex femoral artery are sufficient to supply the entire muscle. Defects in the proximal section of the thigh, particularly with unstable scars in the area of the trochanter, are an indication for the use of the vastus lateralis flap in reconstructive surgery for burns to the lower extremity [12].

Soleus muscle flap

Soleus muscle flaps are particularly suited for use in the reconstruction of lower leg defects. This muscle is located in the superficial posterior compartment of the leg. The muscle is triangular, and its length differs from person to person, which is an important factor as it pertains to the potential radius of rotation. Secure proximal vascularization is supplied by a main branch of the tibialis posterior artery, which allows it to be mobilized at its isolated proximal vascular pedicles. An indication for its use in the scope of reconstruction of a burned lower extremity is soft-tissue reconstruction in the middle third of the lower leg, especially if the tibial ridge is exposed [13].

Gastrocnemius muscle flap

The gastrocnemius muscle has a medial and a lateral head, and is supplied by the sural arteries, which arise from the popliteal artery. Each head can be harvested individually at its proximal vascular pedicle (Figs. 5, 6). This flap is particularly suited to reconstruction of the knee joint and the proximal third of the lower leg [14].

Saphenous flap

The saphenous flap is a fasciocutaneous flap that is harvested from the medial area of the calf. The skin of the calf is supplied by branches of the great saphenous vein, which runs along the saphenous nerve [15].

Sural flap

The distal sural pedicle flap is supplied by the sural arteries. It is a relatively thin flap, and is primarily used in the area around the ankle, Achilles tendon, and heel. The donor site defect usually needs to be covered with a split-skin graft. In certain cases, a bi-

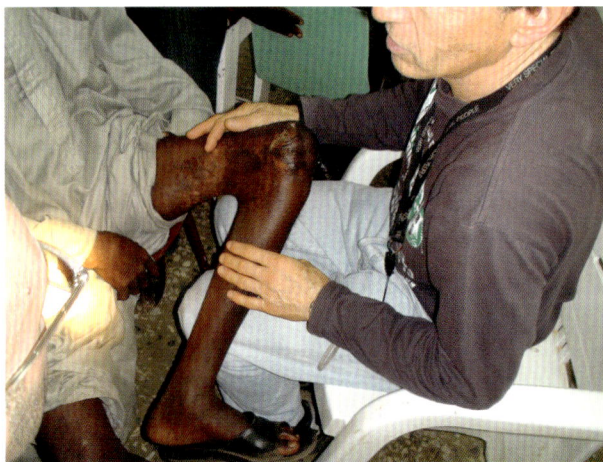

Fig. 6. Intraoperative contracture release and reconstruction with a rotation flap

lateral approach is required which calls for modifying the primary flap by cutting it in advance [16].

Dorsalis pedis flap

The dorsalis pedis flap is a neurovascular flap which can also be used as a free flap. It is mainly supplied by the dorsalis pedis artery, which is a continuation of the anterior tibial artery. The tendons of the extensor hallucis longus muscle serve as a point of reference and run medial to the artery, while the tendons of the extensor digitorum muscle run lateral to the artery. In the proximal area, the artery perforates plantar, anastomosing with the plantar arch. Harvesting the flap is extremely difficult. An indication for the use of this flap is if reconstruction is necessary in the area of the distal third of the lower leg as well as the foot [17].

Reconstructive ladder stage 4: Free flaps

Free microsurgical flaps are indicated especially for use in reconstruction of burned extremities, since due to the subsequent scarring after a burn trauma, adequate local or pedicle flaps are not available in this area [18].

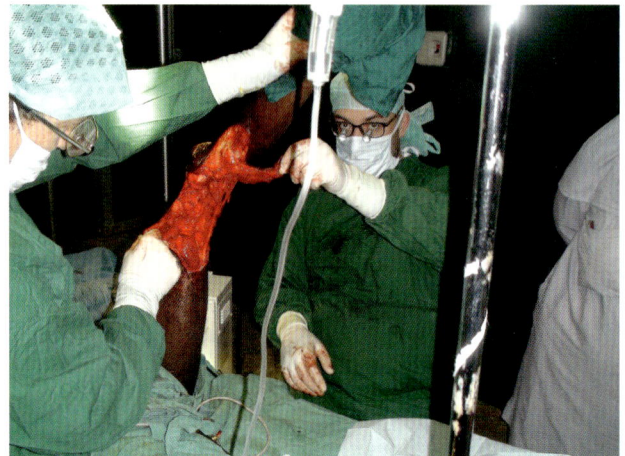

Fig. 5. Severe contracture on the inside of left knee after III° burn trauma

Latissimus dorsi flap

Due to its flap volume and the fact that it can be used anywhere, the latissimus dorsi flap is one of the most important. It can be elevated both as a myocutaneous or osteocutaneous flap. In addition, a functional reconstruction can also be carried out at the same time, for example using a muscle transposition flap from the posterior tibialis muscle. At the same time, the muscle flap can also serve as free neurovascular flap for restoring motor function. This allows it to be used to cover defects and to restore the function of the quadriceps femoris [19].

Scapular and parascapular flap

The scapular flap is adipocutaneous flap which is fed by the circumflex scapular artery. Primary closure can usually be used on the donor site defect. The flap is indicated for large defects in the entire lower leg and ankle region. In case of extremely large defects, it can be combined with a latissimus dorsi flap [20].

Lateral arm flap

The lateral upper arm flap is a septocutaneous flap. It is supplied by the posterior radial collateral artery and the deep brachial artery. Its benefit lies in the consistent neurovascular pedicle, which allows it to transplanted as a sensitive flap [21].

Radial artery flap

The fasciocutaneous radial artery flap is particularly well-suited to reconstruction in the area of the ankle and/or Achilles tendon, as well as the heel and dorsum of the foot (Fig. 7). In addition, the flap can also be used for limited defects in the area of the patella. The preoperative Allen Test is obligatory. A significant drawback to this flap is the obvious donor site [22].

Reconstructive ladder stage 5: Perforator flap

As a modern variation of free microsurgical reconstruction, all musculocutaneous and adipocutaneous flaps can be elevated as perforator flaps. In pri-

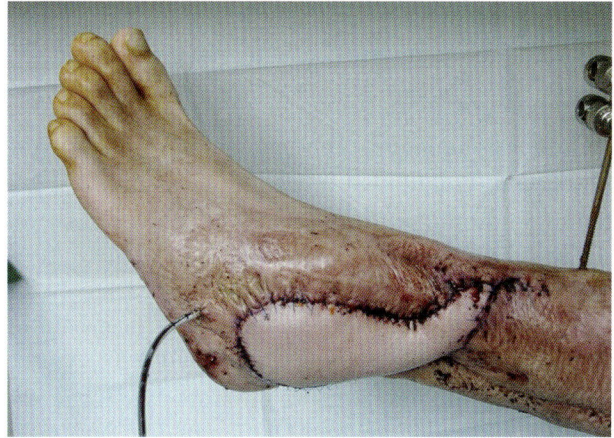

Fig. 7. Result after free flap reconstruction with an unstable scar on the left upper ankle joint

mary patients with severe burn wounds, a healthy island of skin is often not available, which means the ability to harvest a flap is limited. Using this technique, however, defects in all areas of the body can be reconstructed with particularly flexible and thin flaps. Perforator flaps are an important advancement in reconstructive surgery for patients with severe burn injuries, especially from an aesthetic standpoint [23].

Discussion

Platt et al. report that 3.6 % of all their burn victims which receive acute treatment in an inpatient setting require a free flap reconstruction. Figures on the percentage of patients requiring free flaps solely in the scope of reconstructive surgery on the lower extremity are not available. Reconstruction of burned extremities represents a particular challenge to reconstructive surgeons, since they must cover defects of various sizes and depths. Correction of burn scar contractures for the purpose of restoring function is the primary indication for secondary reconstructive surgery, as well as treating unstable scars and scar carcinoma resulting in lesions of different sizes. In addition, amputation stumps often need to be stabilized. Soft tissue reconstruction is carried out based on principles set forth in the reconstructive ladder which are adapted to the individual situation, from simple to complex free flap surgery [24]. The skin tissue which borders the defect is often scarred, however, which means that a local or rotation flap often cannot be used within the reconstructive ladder. In order to achieve the goal of restoring form, function, and aesthetics in the best way possible, a number of indications require mastery of the entire microsurgical spectrum. The selection of a free microsurgical flap can also be limited by a scarred donor site, however, which requires the surgeon to use their second or third choice. As a result, when performing reconstructive surgery on a burned lower extremity, the entire spectrum of plastic surgical methods must be considered when selecting the operative procedure, which means that procedures must also be considered which appear obsolete in reconstructive surgery on patients which have not suffered burn injuries. Cross leg flaps and the use of Kirschner wire in the case of an exposed tibial ridge are often successful when other reconstructive procedures have been ruled out [26,27]. In primary reconstruction of a burned extremity, the distal extremity is the most often affected anatomical area, since the tibial ridge and the foot are only protected by a thin subcutaneous layer, which means tendons and bones are affected and/or are exposed after debridement at above-average rates. In contrast, the proximal extremity of the thigh offers better protection thanks to the soft tissue pad found in this area, which means that reconstructive flap surgery is carried out on the thigh less often. Due to its thin layer of soft-tissue, the foot presents significant challenges to reconstruction as it pertains to restoring a sufficient level of function, especially when plantar structures are involved. Flaps used on the foot must be thin, yet still offer a secure sheath for the tendons. A number of authors prefer to use thin fascia flaps which are then covered with split-skin grafts. These can be wrapped around the extensor tendons using the sandwich technique to create a layer of connective tissue [28]. As an alternative to a thin flap, De Lorenzi et al. describes arterialized venous flaps which are harvested from along the great saphenous vein [29]. Their reliability as a standard procedure is still open to debate, however, but they represent a viable alternative with a small harvesting defect. Furthermore, adipocutaneous flaps are suitable for use in reconstructive surgery, especially for thin patients, since they offer excellent

skin elasticity. As a classical microsurgical flap, the radial or lateral upper arm flaps can be used for small areas, and the scapular and parascapular flaps can be used for larger defects. In reconstructive procedures on the foot, one must generally differentiate between stress-bearing and non-stress-bearing areas. When operating on a stress-bearing area, muscular flaps should be preferred, since these flaps offer stable coverage that can withstand shear stress [30].

Within the scope of primary reconstruction carried out after suffering a burn, flap surgery is conducted earlier on patients with electrical injuries than those with thermal trauma. In addition to superficial burns, injuries from high-voltage current also cause electricity to flow through deep tissue. The current flows through the path of least resistance, primarily through the body's vasculature, nerves, and muscles (Fig. 8). Concealed deep tissue lesions occur as a result, particularly periosteal lesions in the muscles [31–33]. Radical debridement after an electrical injury also leads to exposure of deeper structures. When dealing with lesions from electrical injuries that require the use of free flaps, the assumption of progressive necrosis exists, meaning that the extent of the tissue damage is first demarcated after several debridements (principle of progressive awareness) [34,35]. In this context, there is always the danger that even when performing radical debridement, if the reconstructive procedure is carried out too early, necrosis could persist. In these

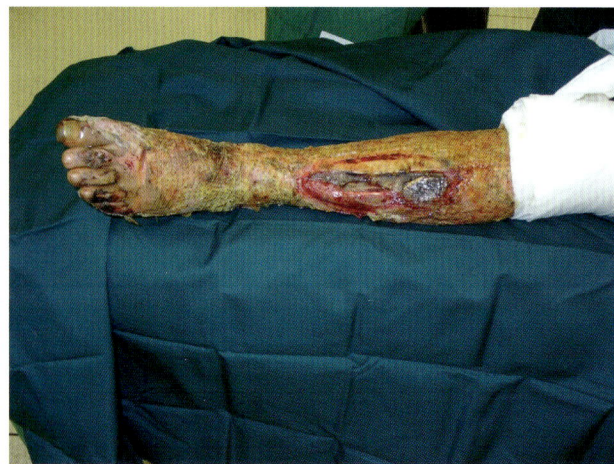

Fig. 8. Primary reconstruction necessary after III° high-voltage burn

case, large-size muscular flaps are indicated, as they are better at terminating infections thanks to their vascularization [36]. The latissimus dorsi flap is particularly suited for this purpose, since it can be harvested with a size of up to 26 cm in women and 33 cm in men [37]. For smaller defects which require sufficient vascularization from a muscle, we recommend the microsurgical gracilis flap, which can be harvested with close to zero donor morbidity [38]. If needed, the serratus anterior flap can also be harvested for even smaller defects [39]. When covering defects which involve bone, in some cases a vascularized bone transplant may be required [40]. In particularly severe contractures as a result of a burn to the lower extremity, Bar-Meir et al. describe the combination of using an Ilizarov apparatus and a free flap [41].

Concrete data comparing the complication rate of local, pedicle, or microsurgical flaps used in the scope of secondary reconstruction to those used in reconstruction in the primary stage is not available. Baumeister et al. were able to detect a relationship between the time reconstructive surgery was carried out and the complication rate, however [42]. In their study on reconstruction of burned extremities through transplantation of free flaps in primary reconstructive surgery, they report that 80 % of flap losses occurred when the flap surgery was conducted between the 5th and 21st day post-trauma. In contrast, flap losses did not occur in elective secondary reconstruction.

Summary

As a result of the specific anatomical conditions found in the knee, lower leg, and foot (which exhibit a thin soft-tissue covering), a thermal trauma to the lower extremity often results in scarred contractures which affect the patient's gait and necessitate secondary reconstruction. When treating a patient with a severely burned lower extremity, functional structures often become exposed in the initial stages after radical debridement, which then require early stage primary reconstruction. Regardless of when reconstructive surgery on the lower extremity is carried out, the reconstructive ladder should be followed. Due to changes to the local area caused by scarring, it is often impossible to use treatment methods which are used on unburned tissue as a standard procedure, which means that modified operative procedures can be successful, as well as operative techniques which would otherwise be viewed as obsolete. Due to these reasons, a reconstructive surgeon should possess knowledge of the entire range of plastic surgical methods, since treating high-grade burn contractures of the lower extremity poses a significant challenge to even the most experienced surgeons.

References

[1] Wrigley M et al (1995) Factors relating to return to work after burn injury. J Burn Care Rehabil 16(4): 444–450

[2] Silverberg R, Lomardo G, Gorga D et al (2006) Gait variables of patients after lower extremity burn injuries. J Burn Care Rehabil 21(3): 259–267

[3] Barbour JR, Schweppe M (2008) Lower extremity burn reconstruction in the child. J Craniofac Surg 19(4): 976–988

[4] Ezoe K, Yotsuyanagi T, Saito T et al (2009) A circumferential incision technique to release wide scar contracture. JPRAS 61(9): 1059–1064

[5] Ulkur E, Acikel C et al (2006) Use of rhomboid flap and double z plasty technique in the treatment of chronic postburn contractures. Burns 32(6): 765–769

[6] Jauss MH, Michelson JD, Desai P (1992) Investigations into the fat pads of the sole of the foot: anatomy and histology. Foot Ankle Int 13: 233

[7] Wainwright D et al (1996) Clinical evaluation of an acellular allograft dermal matrix in full-thickness burns. J Burn Care Rehabil 17(2): 124–136

[8] Stern R, Mc Pherson, Longaker MT (1990) Histologic study of artifical skin used in the treatment of full-thickness thermal injury. J Burn Care Rehabil 11: 7–13

[9] Kimura N, Satoh K, Hosaka Y (2004) Tensor fasciae latae flap. Clin Plast Surg 30(3): 439–446

[10] Wong CH, Wie FC (1967) Anterolateral thigh flap. Head and Neck 32(4): 529–540

[11] Redett RJ, Robertson BC, Chang B et al (2006) Limb salvage of lower extremity wounds using gracilis muscle reconstruction. Plast Reconstr Surg 106(7): 1507–1513

[12] Mathes SJ, Nahai F (eds) (1982) Clinical application for muscle and musculocutaneous flaps. Mosby, St. Louis, pp 482–483

[13] Rios-Luna A, Fahandezh-Saddi H et al (2009) Pearls and tips in coverage of the tibia after a high energy trauma. Int J Orth 42(4): 387–394

[14] Withney T, Heckler F, White M (1995) Gastrocnemius muscle transposition to the femur: how high can you go? Ann Plast Surg 34: 415

[15] Thatte MR, Thatte RL (1993) Venous flaps. Plast Reconstr Surg 91: 747

[16] Loonen MP, Kon M, Schuurman AH (2009) Distally based sural flap modifications. Ann Plast Surg 64(1): 128

[17] Ritz M, Mahendru S, Somia N et al (2009) The dorsalis pedis fascial flap. J Reconstr Microsurg 25(5): 313–317

[18] Yücel A, Senyuva C, Aydin Y et al (2004) Soft tissue reconstruction of sole and heel defects with free tissue transfers. Ann Plast Surg 44(3): 268

[19] Segev E, Wientroub S, Kollender Y et al (2007) A combined use of a free vascularised flap and an external fixator for reconstruction of lower extremity defects. J Orth Surg 15(2): 207–210

[20] German G, Bickert B, Steinau HU, Sauerbier M (2000) Versatility and reliability of combined flaps of the subscapular system. Plast Reconstruct Surg 103: 1386–1399

[21] Song R, Song Y, Yu Y, Song Y (1982) The upper arm free flap. Clin Plast Surg 9: 27

[22] Steinau HU, Clasbrummel B, Josten C et al (2004) The interdisciplinary approach in reconstructive surgery of the extremities. Chirurg 5(4): 390–398

[23] Feng CH, Yang JY, Chuang SS et al (2010) Free medial thigh perforator flap for reconstruction of the dynamic and static complex burn scar contracture. Burns 36(4): 565–571

[24] Platt AJ, McKiernan MV, McLean NR (1996) Free tissue transfer in the management of burns. Burns 22: 474–476

[25] Turner AJ, Parkhouse N (2006) Revisiting the reconstructive ladder. Plast Reconstr Surg 118(1): 267–268

[26] Ruano-Ravina A, Jato Díaz M (2003) Autologous chondrocyte implantation: a systematic review. Osteoarth Cartilage 14(1): 47–51

[27] Zao L, Wan L, Wang S (2006) Clinical studies on maintenance of cross-leg position through internal fixation with Kirschner wire after cross leg flap procedure. Chin J Rep Reconstr Surg 20(12): 1211–1213

[28] Upton J, Rogers C, Durham-Smith G, Swartz WM (1986) Clinical applications of free flaps in reconstruction. J Hand Surg (AM) 11: 475–483

[29] De Lorenzi F, Boeck W et al (2001) Free flaps in burn reconstruction. Burns 27: 603–612

[30] Baumeister S, Germann G (2001) Soft tissue coverage of the extremely traumatized foot and ankle. Foot Ankle Clin 6: 867–903

[31] Luce EA, Dowden WL, Hoopes JE (1978) High tension electrical injury of the extremity. Surg Gynecol Obstet 147: 38–42

[32] Lewis GK (1958) Electrical burns of the upper extremities. J Bone Joint Surg 40: 27–32

[33] Mann RJ, Wallquist JM (1975) Early decompression fasciotomy in the treatment of high-voltage electrical burns of the extremities. South Med J 68: 1103–1108

[34] Robson MC, Murphy RC, Heggers JP (1984) A new explanation for the progressive tissue loss in electrical injuries. Plast Reconstr Surg 73: 431–437

[35] Zelt RG, Daniel RK, Brisette Y et al (1988) High-Voltage electrical injury: chronic wound evolution. Plast Reconstr Surg 82: 1027–1041

[36] Chang N, Mathes SJ (1982) Comparison of the effect of bacterial inoculation in musculocutaneous and random-pattern flaps. Plast Reconstr Surg 70: 1–10

[37] Serafin D (1996) Atlas of microsurgical composite tissue transplantation, 1st edn. WB Saunders, Philadelphia

[38] Menktelow RT (1986) Microvascular reconstruction. New York, Springer, pp 37–44

[39] Gordon L, Levinsohn DG, Finkemeier C et al (1993) The serratus anterior free-muscle transplant for reconstruction. An analysis of the donor and recipient sites. Plast Reconstr Surg 92: 97–101

[40] Tu YK, Yen CY (2007) Role of vascularized bone grafts in lower extremity reconstruction. Orth Clin North Am 38(1): 37–49

[41] Bar-Meir E, Yaffe B, Winkler E et al (2006) Combined Ilizarov and free flap for severe recurrent flexion – contracture release. J Burn Care Research 8: 529–534

[42] Baumeister S, German G, Gielser G et al (2004) Wiederherstellung der verbrannten Extremität durch Transplantation freier Lappenplastiken. Chirurg 75: 568–578

Correspondence: Dr. med. Christian Ottomann, Facharzt für Plastische und Ästhetische Chirurgie, Plastische Chirurgie, Handchirurgie, Intensiveinheit für Schwerbrandverletzte, Universitätsklinikum Schleswig-Holstein Campus Lübeck, Ratzeburger Allee 160, 23560 Lübeck, Germany, Tel: +49 451 500 2061, Fax: +49 451 500 3555, E-mail: Christian.Ottomann@uk-sh.de

Thermal injuries to the foot

Thilo Schenck[1], Riccardo E. Giunta[2]

[1] Klinik und Poliklinik für Plastische Chirurgie und Handchirurgie, Klinikum rechts der Isar, Technische Universität München, München, Germany
[2] Handchirurgie, Plastische Chirurgie und Ästhetische Chirurgie, Klinikum der Ludwig-Maximilians Universität München, München, Germany

Introduction

Thermal injuries to the foot, in particular isolated burns, are less common than burn injuries to other body parts such as the face or the hand. One reason for this low number of injuries is due to the fact that most of the time our feet are protected by shoes. Despite the foot's relatively small percentage of the total body surface area (TBSA) of approximately 3.5 %, special attention should be paid on foot burns because the sequelae of these injuries can dramatically reduce the patients' quality of life [1]. The significance of foot injuries becomes obvious when we consider how much of our daily-life depends on the main function of our feet, i. e. to statically and dynamically carry body-weight. The long-term impairments of thermal foot injuries can include anything from problems with shoe fit to recurrent ulcerations, and from gait disturbances to inability of standing and walking.

Many different causes can lead to thermal injuries of the feet. Especially children, the elderly and disabled persons are at risk [2] (Fig. 1). Burns of the feet in children are often caused by scalds [1]. Neuropathy due to diabetes puts the elderly at risk for burn injuries [3]. Burns of the feet are also common in electrical injuries because the electric current exits the body through the feet. The risk factors for thermal foot injuries also depend on geographical and cultural factors. In tropical or subtropical geo-

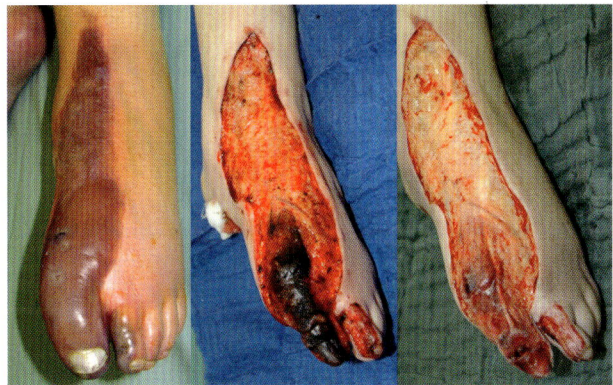

Fig. 1. Third degree burn of the forefoot including the toes in a paraplegic patient who burned herself with a powersupply pack of her computer. This case demonstrates how lack of protective sensibility leads to increased risk for thermal injuries of disabled patients. Exact debridement with careful preservation of the paratendon of the extensor hallucis longus tendon could achieve a wound bed which was suitable for skin graft transplantation

graphic areas walking on hot road surfaces or sand without adequate footwear can lead to severe injuries, especially in children [4]. Fire walking rituals, as being performed particularly in India are a frequent cause of isolated foot burns as well [5]. The aim of acute therapy and reconstruction is to allow patients to return to normal gait and ambulation. Additionally, follow-up care of patients with burn wounds of the feet is necessary. Long term consequences like foot deformities, scarring and contractures can lead

269

to impaired walking, ulceration, chronic problems in wearing shoes and secondary injuries after falls. Compared to burn injuries of other body areas, injuries of the feet can lead to rather long hospital stays as pressure on the injured areas has to be avoided.

Anatomy

Knowing the anatomy and understanding the function of the foot is essential for the surgeon to perform reconstruction of the foot. Similar to the hand, the plantar and dorsal soft tissue of the foot have different functions and therefore have different anatomic structures. The dorsum of the foot has tendons and veins lying superficially under the skin. Since the skin of the dorsum is not prone to mechanical stress it is relatively thin. In contrast, the plantar side of the foot has to carry the weight of the body and serves as a shock-absorbing cushion. Carrying the body weight without developing pressure sores highly depends on intact sensibility.

Vulnerable structures such as blood vessels, nerves and the plantar fascia are protected by strong layers of subcutaneous fat with fibrous septa which provide adherence to the deep structures. Special emphasis should be put on the weight-bearing surfaces of the foot which include the heel, the metatarsal heads, the lateral arch and parts of the medial arch. Vascularisation and skin coverage above the Achilles tendon make the ankle region a challenge for reconstruction.

Three major arteries provide blood supply to the foot. Similar to the vascular anatomy of the hand, the major arteries of the foot communicate with each other through numerous anastomoses [6]. The three main arteries of the foot divide the foot and ankle region into six angiosomes [7]. The peroneal artery has two major branches that supply the anterolateral portion of the ankle and the rear foot. The anterior tibial artery continues into the dorsalis pedis artery and then builds up the dorsal system which supplies blood to the dorsum of the foot and later on breaks up into the dorsal metatarsal arteries. The posterior tibial artery is responsible for the plantar system which consists of the medial and the lateral plantar artery.

Venous drainage of the lower extremities including the feet is provided by a deep and a superficial venous system, which are connected to each other by perforator veins [8]. Due to our upright body position the hydrostatic pressure is highest in the veins of the lower extremities, which are therefore vulnerable for venous insufficiency. The veins of the deep system accompany the arteries and are named accordingly. The course of the superficial venous system is independent of the arteries and consists of the great and the small saphenous vein and their branches.

Lymphatic vessels of the lower extremity and foot run with the veins and share the principle of a deep and superficial system. The superficial lymphatic vessels of the foot are divided into a small dorsolateral bundle which accompanies the small saphenous vein and a ventromedial bundle that accompanies the great saphenous vein [9]. While the dorsolateral bundle is responsible for the lateral border of the foot, the ventromedial bundle is responsible for the rest of the foot.

Innervation of the foot is provided exclusively by branches of the sciatic nerve except for the medial malleolus which is innervated by the saphenous nerve, the continuation of the femoral nerve [10]. The tibial nerve follows the course of the posterior tibial artery and correspondingly breaks up into a medial and lateral plantar nerve to innervate the sole of the foot. Dorsal innervation, of the foot is mainly provided by branches of the superficial peroneal nerve. Sensation to the first interdigital web space is provided by the deep peroneal nerve. The lateral side of the foot, from the lateral malleolus to the little toe, is innervated by the sural nerve. Compared to the nerves of the sole, the branches of the superficial peroneal nerve, the sural nerve and the saphenous nerve are located relatively superficially what puts them at higher risk for injury.

Burn therapy

General assessment

The long-time result of burn therapy is mostly influenced by the extent and severity of the burn wound, the involvement of certain specialized areas and the quality of the initial therapy. Except for minor injuries, treatment should be managed by specialized burn care facilities [11]. In combination with further burn injuries, burns of the feet are sometimes not given enough attention from the beginning, as they are thought to have less severe consequences compared to burns of the face and the hands for instance.

Similar to burns of other locations, wound conditions including size and depth of the wound and type of damaged or exposed structures must be evaluated before selecting therapy. Special focus should be put on possible involvement of weight-bearing surfaces, damaged bones, tendons, vessels and nerves. In the later phase of treatment, weight-bearing patterns by Harris mat prints and mapping of plantar sensation can be required [12].

Prior to treatment, the general situation of the patient and the relevance of the burn injury to the foot have to be evaluated thoroughly. This information is required to choose the right reconstructive strategy. In addition to accurate evaluation of all injuries, including the burned proportion of total body surface area, the patient's medical history plays an important role, as well. To assess the possible goals of therapy, general risk factors like diabetes, obesity, smoking, age and specific risk factors for the lower extremities like e. g. peripheral artery disease, chronic venous insufficiency and peripheral polyneuropathy should be taken into account. Additional diagnostic efforts such as arteriography and Doppler sonography might be required when preparing complex reconstructive approaches. In spite of the benefits of these convenient and quantifiable methods, the fast, simple and cheap method of examining the pedal pulses should not be disregarded. When considering flaps with defined blood supply such as free, pedicled or axial flaps, existence and patency of the chosen vessels should be evaluated in advance. It should be always kept in mind that vessels could be unavailable due to trauma or anatomic variations. One example is the congenital absence of the dorsalis pedis artery which occurs in 2 % of the population, leading to unavailability of the numerous standardized dorsalis pedis artery flaps [13]. For proximally based flaps, arteries of the plantar and dorsal systems have to be uninterrupted and communicating anastomoses open. Clinical examination of the vessels, angiography and Doppler sonography are crucial. Especially in the preparation of perforator flaps the Doppler sonography plays an important role [14]. Although the possibilities of reconstruction and micro-

surgery have tremendously increased in the last decades, considerations in primary burn care should not exclude amputation as an option in some injuries [15]. The basic principle of "life before limb" remains a pillar of any reconstructive procedure.

Goal of therapy

The main goal in the treatment of thermal feet injuries is to restore the function of the foot, which is to carry body weight and the ability to stand and walk. The functional outcome of reconstruction can be estimated by the parameters ulceration, pain and footwear [16, 17]. The patient's daily activities, capability to return to work and quality of life is highly affected by pain, which therefore serves as an appropriate parameter for the outcome of the reconstruction [18]. Incidence of ulcers is a suitable parameter as well, because it indicates durability of soft tissue coverage. Ulcers are also a measure of quality of life because repetitive changes of dressings interfere with daily activities. Although aesthetic goals are of minor importance in extensive injuries to the feet, an adequate contour should be aimed at to allow the patient to use normal footwear. Hence the ability to use normal footwear acts as an indicator of a good flap shape [18]. Another goal is to maintain sensation at the sole of the foot. Without sensibility, especially to pressure, in the reconstructed foot the patient has similar risks for secondary injuries as known from patients suffering from neuropathic feet [18]. In the early phase of therapy, fast skin coverage should be achieved to protect the subjacent structures and to prevent infections. The long-term outcome of skin coverage can be rated by occurrence of contractions and hypertrophic scars.

Primary treatment

The first steps of acute treatment of thermal feet injuries should not differ from other burn injuries. At first, the vital threat of the injury and the overall situation of the patient have to be evaluated. The goal of acute treatment of the wound is cleaning, debridement, necrosectomy and if possible early closure of the wound (Figs. 1 and 2). Besides, management of foot burns in the acute phase should consist of pain control, foot elevation to prevent swelling, wound

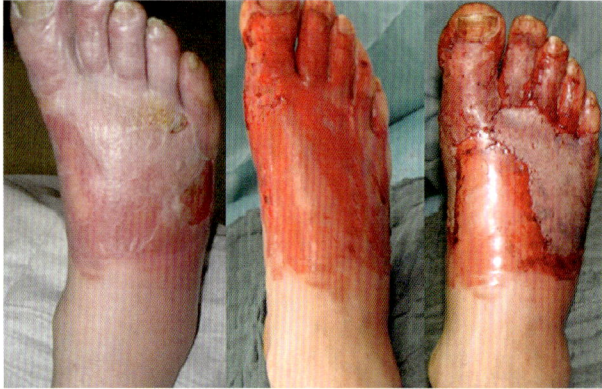

Fig. 2. This second degree burn injury of the foot resulted from spilling hot water in the kitchen. The patient came to the emergency department with a delay of five days. Debridement revealed a combination of deep and superficial dermal injury. For injuries without exposure of vulnerable structures, bones or tendons, such as this deep dermal injury, skin grafting is the best treatment option. Before skin transplantation, the wound needs careful cleaning and debridement. Skin grafting is a fast and easy method with very limited harvesting defects. If applied on larger defects contractions can occur

dressings with antiseptic agents, frequent observations and depending on the extend of the wound prophylactic systemic antibiotics [1, 19, 20]. Superficial partial thickness burns are often underestimated. Treating them aggressively is often a worthwhile procedure to prevent the progression from a superficial to a deep partial thickness burn injury [2]. However, necrosectomy has to be performed very carefully so that vulnerable structures like peritendineums, superficial veins and lymphatic vessels which are crucial to defect coverage remain intact. Hospital treatment should be rigorously indicated to avoid infections. In some cases early skin grafting as temporary or final defect coverage can be considered (Fig. 2). In the acute treatment of foot burns the use of splints should be considered to prevent deformities due to contractions. Although the aim of the treatment is to rescue as much structures of the foot as possible, indications for amputation should be checked already in the beginning. Delay of amputation in cases where it is unavoidable often leads to unnecessary operations and more psychological stress. It has to be evaluated if the patient might have a higher benefit from a good prosthesis than from an insufficiently reconstructed foot [21]. In addition, amputation often allows faster return to ambulation than complex reconstruction. In the decision process for or against amputation, the extent of the injury, the presence and severity of wound infections and the situation of the patient as a whole have to be considered. If one or more toes are severely damaged, amputation is often indicated because the loss of function is relatively negligible. An exception to this is the great toe, which is of higher importance to gait stability. If the forefoot or midfoot is severely damaged or severe proximal injury of the lower extremity is present, Chopart, Lisfranc or even more proximal amputation can be indicated. Even though amputation is a destructive procedure, it has to be performed accurately and can only be considered successful if the resulting stump has a stable, well cushioned soft tissue coverage, is free from pain and allows good ambulation.

Bridging the time to final reconstruction

Fast and definitive closure of wounds should be the goal of treatment. But if defects are more complex, reconstruction of the injured foot often becomes a more than one stage approach. In cases of foot injuries occurring as a concomitant injury, its treatment is often postponed until the patient is out of vital danger and co-existing injuries of higher importance such as injuries of the face or hand have been treated. Reconstructing at a later point gives time for thorough evaluation– and accurate repetitive debridement, but also bears the risk of developing complications. Attention should be paid to the development of soft-tissue infections. Sample collection for microbiological analysis should be performed to allow specific antibiotic treatment. Microbiological analysis should be generously indicated as the foot is a very susceptible region for infections. In cases where bone structures are not covered, osteomyelitis is a feared complication, which can be ruled out by plain radiographs. In cases of osteomyelitis or wound infection the use of muscle flaps can be advantageous [22, 23]. During the time span until final defect coverage is achieved, wound treatment aims at preserving stable wound conditions, preventing infections and limiting fluid and protein loss. Infections of the wounds have to be ruled out or treated successfully before the final defect coverage.

For skin defects, skin grafts can be helpful in this phase but synthetic or biologic wound coverage has gained popularity, as well. Especially in cases when donor skin is unavailable due to extensive burn injury or when the wounds are not ready for autografting, temporary skin substitutes are valuable [24]. Many temporary artificial skin replacement products such as collagen-glycosaminoglycan matrix, acellular allogenic dermis or collagen/elastin matrix are available on the market and their number is constantly growing [25]. If deeper structures are exposed vacuum assisted closure devices can help to temporarily close the wound. Similar to burns to the hand, the complex anatomic structure of the foot makes the application of temporary wound dressings a challenge. For the hand a temporary wound dressing in the shape of a glove has been developed [26]. So far, no analog for feet is available on the market but in some cases the existing glove can be used for the foot as well.

Skin grafting

Skin grafts are a good and frequently applied option for burn injuries if the extent of the injury is limited (Fig. 2). Split skin grafts are fast and easily applicable and leave only very limited harvesting defects [27]. Full skin grafts are thought to have better mechanical properties, but are limited in availability. If skin grafts serve the demands of the defect, it has to be evaluated if the defect serves the demands of the skin graft, as well. For successful graft take, the area to be covered must be able to supply the skin graft with nutrition and oxygen. This can be successfully provided in most soft tissue defects. Exposed bones and tendons without peritendineum cannot sufficiently meet the needs of skin grafts, hence a different approach should be chosen. If vulnerable structures like vessels or nerves are exposed, skin grafts will usually not provide enough mechanical protection. Even though bare bones are generally considered a contraindication for skin grafts, they can be tolerated if their contribution to the whole defect is just minor. In these cases debridement of the wound bed should include decortication of the exposed bones to stimulate the formation of granulation tissue before skin graft transplantation can be carried out as a next step [21]. Prior to grafting, infections of the recipient site should be ruled out or sufficiently treated surgically and with antimicrobial agents. Preparation of the recipient site should include sufficient debridement to achieve good perfusion. In the early phase after transplantation nutrition and oxygen are provided by diffusion. To allow diffusion the graft must be well attached to the wound ground. Because the hydrostatic pressure is highest in the feet, leaking of arterioles, venous capillaries and lymphatic vessels bring the risk of fluid accumulation under the graft. For this reason, constant pressure should be applied to the graft for the first days after transplantation and the wounded foot should be elevated at all times. The use of vacuum assisted closure (V. A. C.® therapy) devices to fix split-thickness-skin-grafts and to withdraw fluid from the transplanted area has risen steadily in the last decade [28]. Thin split skin grafts and mesh grafts should be avoided on the foot because they show higher risks for contraction and the aesthetic outcome is lower than in unmeshed grafts [29]. However, it is advantageous to make some incisions in the graft to avoid accumulation of wound fluid under the transplant.

Even though skin grafts often need corrections including re-grafting, skin grafting is an effective method to cover defects fast and easily or at least to reduce them significantly in size. Skin grafting can also help to bridge the time from acute treatment to further complex reconstructive approaches. Frequent problems seen with skin grafts on the foot are hyperkeratosis at the borders of the grafts, ulcerations and contractions. Although skin grafting remains the gold standard for skin lesions, the development of bioartificial skin is proceeding constantly and dermal replacement products based on collagen already show satisfying results in burn patients [30].

Postoperative care

Successful treatment of thermal foot injuries highly depends on postoperative care. Most of the surgical efforts take place in the first couple of weeks after the accident but the postoperative care may be necessary for a much longer time. Postoperative care should therefore be accurately planned and multidisciplinary approached. Its extent depends on the extent of the injury and the complexity of the reconstructive efforts.

In the early phase after reconstruction, the focus lays on monitoring, appropriate wound dressings, medication and bed rest with elevation of the operated foot. For sufficient monitoring frequent changes of wound dressings combined with accurate cleaning are necessary. Maximum attention has to be paid to signs of infections and delayed wound healing. If free flaps are applied perfusion has to be monitored frequently. Monitoring devices such as external and laser Doppler are increasing but most frequent visual controls including recapillarisation time remain the gold standard.

Medication should address antibiotic coverage, pain medication, fluid management and anticoagulation until full ambulation. Systemic comorbidities like diabetes, peripheral artery disease, chronic venous insufficiency and malnutrition should be treated as well. Time of bed rest, leg elevation and time until weight bearing depend on the chosen defect coverage. When patients return to ambulation, pressure treatment and orthopedic footwear, such as thermoplastic boot splints become necessary. In case of split skin transplantation accumulation of fluid under the graft and shear forces have to be avoided. This works best by applying pressure on split skin grafts with elastic bandages for at least 5 days. Pressure should not be applied on skin grafts which are used on top of free flaps. In this case dressings with pressure would impair perfusion and make monitoring difficult.

Hydrostatic pressure as in a standing position sets free flaps of the lower extremity at risk for venous and lymphatic congestion. Three to five days after free flap transfer, the strict elevation can be started to be periodically interrupted. In order to protect the foot from fluid congestion elastic bandages have to be applied. This procedure is started for a duration of 15 minutes per day and is increased within approximately one week to three times three hours per day. As soon as wounds are stable and post-operative swelling has decreased, an orthopedic pressure stocking is customized which replaces the elastic bandages in the following months. Intensive physical therapy is of great importance to return to ambulation and to regain or maintain joint flexibility. Beside selection of an adequate reconstructive approach, detailed education about foot care and frequent follow-up visits play an im-

portant role in maintaining reconstructed feet healthy and the flap intact [31]. The patient has to learn that a loss of sensation has to be replaced by frequent self examinations [32]. Treatment of scars with silicon-sheets, compression garment and scar reduction creams can be started when defect coverage is accomplished and wounds have reached a stable level.

Secondary reconstruction

Defects of the foot and the lower one third of the leg are challenging subjects for reconstruction. Since thermal injuries to the feet occur in a countless number of variations, each defect has to be evaluated individually. Depending on the extent of the injury, treatment can reach from conservative treatment with wound dressings to multi-step operational approaches [33]. A multidisciplinary team and accurate planning of all reconstructive efforts are crucial for success and can only be managed if the medical team is capable of the full surgical armamentarium [34].

For the thermally injured foot a broad spectrum of methods has been described that includes almost all options of defect coverage. It spans from skin graft, skin and muscle flaps to free flaps. The challenge for the plastic surgeon is to choose the most adequate strategy according to general principles for reconstruction. Form and function of injured structures should be restored by replacing them with structures of similar properties. When doing so, the gain of function at the recipient-site must outweigh the loss of function at the donor-site. If different options remain, the least complicated and traumatizing should be applied. Accurate planning of flap contour in the beginning can reduce amount and extent of later flap debulking procedures which become necessary in many cases [32].

To achieve a reconstruction providing the proper weight-bearing surfaces, reconstruction efforts should aim at re-establishing the bone architecture including its longitudinal and transverse arches. In the long-term, bony prominences are a high risk factor for the development of ulcers and should be removed if possible [32]. According to the different needs of the anatomic regions, different reconstructive approaches should be chosen.

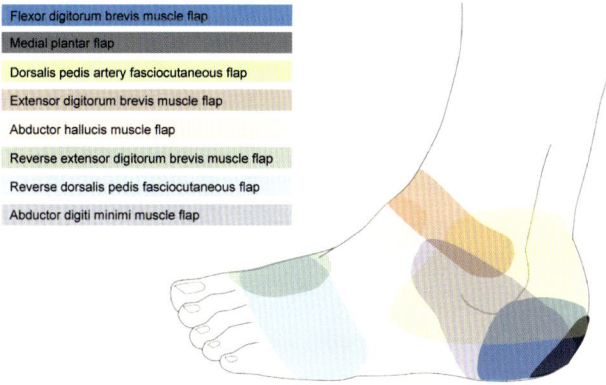

Fig. 3. Local fasciocutanoeus and muscle flaps for the dorsum and the lateral ankle region. If defects are too extensive for local solutions, regional or free flaps have to be considered

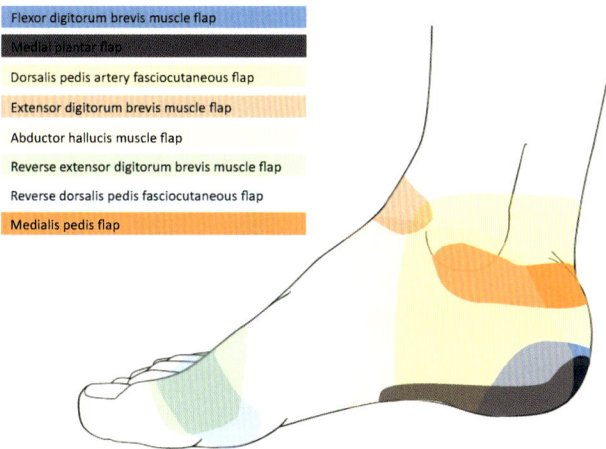

Fig. 4. Local fasciocutanoeus and muscle flaps for the dorsum and the medial ankle region. If defects are too extensive for local solutions, regional or free flaps have to be considered

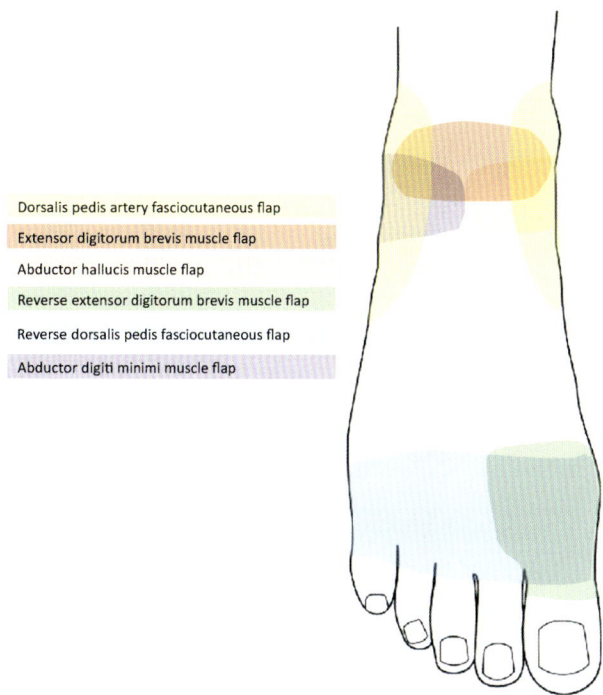

Fig. 5. Local fasciocutanoeus and muscle flaps for the dorsum of the foot. If defects in this area are superficial and the peritendineum of the extensor tendons is uninjured split skin coverage brings good results

Defects of the dorsum of the foot and ankle

The dorsum of the foot and ankle is more frequently involved in burn injuries than the sole. In the majority of cases, burns are superficial and the extensor tendons and the bones remain covered with subcutaneous tissue. In these cases, split skin grafts are suitable. If the peritendineum of the extensor tendons is destroyed or even deeper structures are involved, flap coverage becomes necessary. In the region of the Achilles tendon and the dorsum of the foot, the skin is thin and mobile. Any form of coverage of these areas must maintain or restore the unrestricted motion of the underlying structures. Flap coverage can be managed by local, regional and free flaps (Figs. 3–6). Local fasciocutaneous and muscle flaps from the dorsalis pedis artery are useful for medium size defects of the complete dorsum, the ankle and malleoli (Table 1). Small defects of the proximal dorsum and the proximal sides of the foot can also be covered with local muscle flaps from the posterior tibial artery (Table 1). Fasciocutaneous flaps from the posterior tibial artery have been described for the posterior aspect of the heel and the insertion of the Achilles tendon. For large defects or if defects are too proximal for local flaps of the foot, regional flaps from the lower leg and individual flaps ("freestyle flaps", "propeller flaps") can serve as coverage. Large and complex defects usually require the application of free flaps (Table 2).

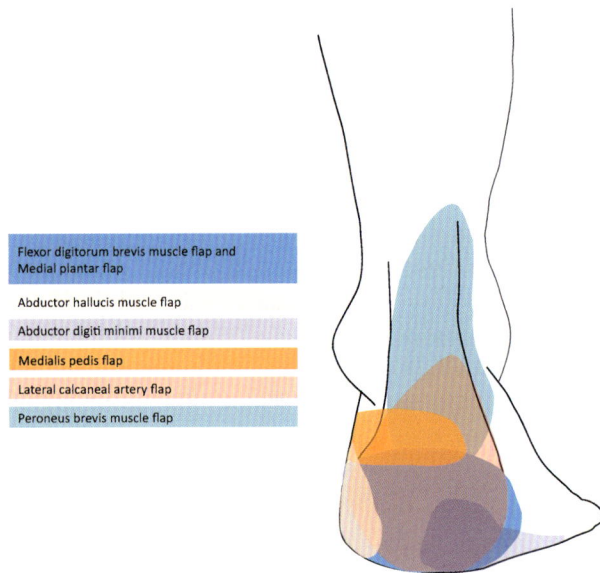

Fig. 6. The posterior aspect of the foot can often be covered by local muscle and fasciocutanous flaps. These flaps do not reach the height of the malleoli. In cases of more proximal or larger defects regional flaps from the lower leg or free flaps are used

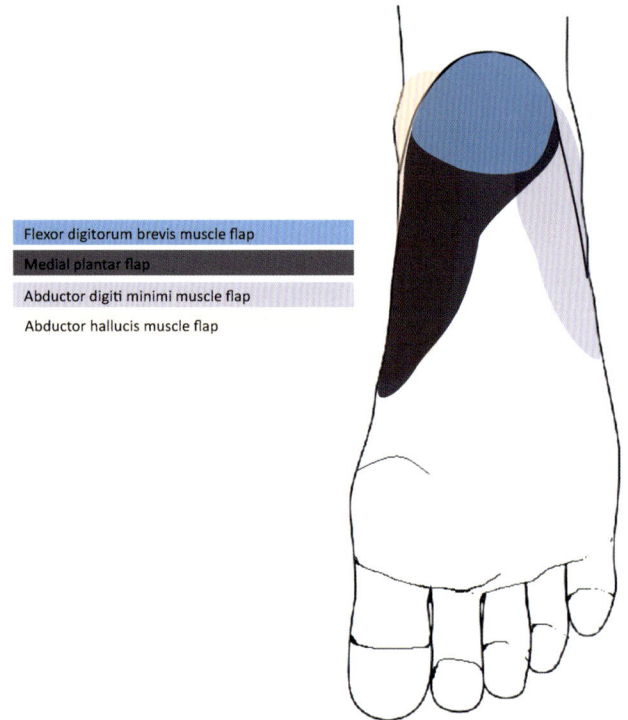

Fig. 7. The sole of the foot, especially the weight-bearing parts are a delicate area for coverage. Only few local muscle flaps are available. In many cases split-skin covered free flaps have to be used

Defects of the sole

Injuries of the sole are not as frequent as injuries of the dorsum of the foot. One reason is that shoe soles offer some protection to our feet. Another reason is that in burns due to spilling of hot liquids, the liquids usually damage the dorsum and rinse off the feet without getting in contact with the sole. Thermal injuries to the sole are seen more frequently in patients with neuropathies e. g. due to diabetes and as exit wounds in patients that suffer from high voltage injuries. The reconstruction of the sole is challenging because the reconstructed site must be very durable and able of bearing weight load. If wounds do not involve deeper structures skin grafts can achieve stable wound conditions. For defects of the proximal sole and the heel, a group of local muscle flaps from the posterior tibial artery has been described (Fig. 7). The distal half of the foot, including the weight-bearing areas is a difficult place to reach with local flaps. For these defects, just like for any other sole defects that expose deeper structures, free flaps covered with split-skin grafts are used (Table 2).

Local flaps

For small and moderate defects coverage with local tissue transfer is a recommendable option if involvement of bones, joints or tendons is absent or of limited extend. Availability of local tissue on the foot which is suitable for transfer is limited due to relatively tight skin and poor vascularity. If local flap coverage is possible it has the advantage of being a simple, safe and economical solution with shorter operation and hospitalization time than free flaps [35]. Since many patients with foot burns have additional injuries, local coverage of defects has the advantage of avoiding additional trauma by flap harvesting [35]. Small defects of the foot can be covered with transposition flaps, advancement flaps, rotation flaps or Z-plasties. Z-plasties and W-plasties play also an important role in the correction of postburn contractions (Fig. 8). If small skin flaps are not sufficient for defect coverage, local fasciocutaneus and muscle flaps are applied. These flaps can be classified according to their vascular origin into the

276

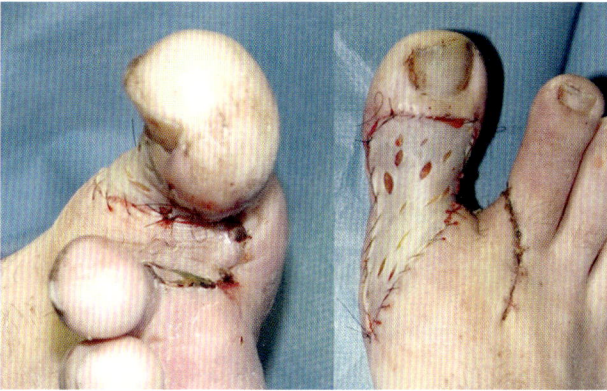

Fig. 8. Reconstruction of first web space by rotation flap and skin grafting

groups of dorsalis pedis artery flaps and posterior tibial artery flaps (Table 1).

Local flaps from the dorsalis pedis artery

The dorsalis pedis artery is used for the dorsalis pedis artery fasciocutaneous flap, which can be applied in defects of the malleoli and the ankle region [36]. By including the superficial or deep peroneal nerve a sensory flap can be created. Even burn injuries of the distal foot and toes including the web spaces can be covered with flaps of the dorsalis pedis artery. For this purpose, the dorsalis pedis artery fasciocutaneous flap can be harvested as a reverse dorsalis pedis flap [37, 38] or its continuation, the first dorsal metatarsal artery, can be included in a flap [39].

A variant of the dorsalis pedis flap for defects, which require muscle for coverage, is the extensor digitorum brevis muscle flap [40]. It can be used distally or proximally based for defects of the forefoot and the ankle region including the distal tibia [41, 42].

Local flaps from the posterior tibial artery

The posterior tibial artery divides into two major branches below the medial malleolus, the medial and the lateral plantar artery. Both arteries, or one of their branches can be used in a number of fasciocutaneous, musculocutaneous or muscle flaps.

The medial plantar artery can be used for flaps that have their origin at the medial border of the foot including the non-weight-bearing portion of the plantar arch. They can be used to cover defects of the weight-bearing plantar skin of the heel with tissue from the non-weight-bearing parts of the foot. The medial plantar flap and the medialis pedis flap are both fasciocutaneous flaps from the medial plantar artery. The medial plantar flap can also be used as a musculocutaneous or as a muscle flap with skin graft coverage [43, 44]. For treatment of burn defects it has been described as both, an antegrade or retrograde flap [45]. The medial plantar artery is accompanied by the medial plantar nerve which makes harvesting of a sensory flap possible [46]. Plantar flaps can be raised in a level below or above the plantar fascia. Including the plantar fascia makes flaps very suitable for heel defects because the fascia adheres well to the calcaneus [47]. Planning of medial plantar artery flaps should include angiography because the artery can have alterations in their course or even be completely missing. The medialis pedis flap has a cutaneous branch of the medial plantar artery as a pedicle. It is a small and thin fasciocutaneous flap which has not been described for the use in burns but can be used for the cranial part of the medial malleolus and for the area superficial to the insertion of the Achilles tendon [48].

For heel and malleolar defects a group of local muscle flaps originating from the posterior tibial artery has been described [49].

The posterior tibial artery provides blood support for three local muscle flaps, the abductor hallucis muscle flap, the flexor digitorum brevis muscle flap and the abductor digiti minimi muscle flap. They are used for defects of the heel pad and the malleoli but also for the proximal dorsum. They are frequently covered with skin grafts and in some cases it is indicated to use them in combination. The abductor hallucis muscle flap and the abductor digiti minimi muscle flap have their pedicles arising from the lateral and medial side of the hindfoot, so that their arc of rotation allows using these flaps for dorsal and plantar defects. The blood supply of the abductor hallucis muscle is derived from several branches from the medial plantar artery [50]. The abductor hallucis flap can be harvested with the medial plantar artery or with one of its branches [51]. In this way a proximal pedicle is created that arises below the medial malleolus. The flap can be

Table 1. Summary of the local and regional flaps classified by vascular supply and type of flap

Local fasciocutaneous flaps		Region	General Literature	Burn specific Literature
Dorsalis pedis artery fasciocutaneous flaps:				
	Dorsalis pedis artery fasciocutaneous flap	Malleoli and ankle region	McCraw and Furlow 1975 [36]	Shah 2002 [2]
	Reverse dorsalis pedis fasciocutaneous flap	Distal foot and Web spaces	Ishikawa et al. 1987 [37]	Schwabegger and Wechsel-berger 1996 [38]
	First dorsal metatarsal artery fasciocutaneous flap	Distal foot and Web spaces	Hayashi et al. 1993 [39]	Goldberg 2000
Posterior Tibial Artery fasciocutaneous flaps:				
Medial plantar artery:	Medial plantar flap	Weight bearing and posterior aspect of the heel	Shanahan and Gingrass 1979 [46]	Uygur et al. 2008 [45]
	Medialis pedis flap	Medial malleolus, Achilles tendon insertion	Masquelet and Romana 1990 [48]	
Local muscle flaps		**Region**	**General Literature**	**Burn specific Literature**
Dorsalis pedis artery muscle flaps:				
	Extensor digitorum brevis muscle flap	Proximal dorsum, Malleoli and ankle region	Landi 1985 [40]	Goldberg 2000
	Reverse Extensor digitorum brevis muscle flap	Distal forefoot	Kurata 1992 [41]	Shah 2002
Posterior tibial artery muscle flaps:				
Medial plantar artery	Abductor hallucis muscle flap	Heel, medial malleolus proximal dorsum and medial side of the midfoot	Ger 1986 [50]	Goldberg 2000
Medial and lateral plantar artery	Flexor digitorum brevis muscle flap	Heel defects, both malleoli, Achilles tendon insertion	Bostwick 1976 [88]	Goldberg 2000
Lateral plantar artery	Abductor digit! minimi muscle flap	Heel, lateral malleolus and proximal dorsum	Ger 1976 [52]	Goldberg 2000
Regional flaps from the lower leg		**Region**	**General Literature**	**Burn specific Literature**
Peroneal artery:	Lateral supramalleolar flap	Complete dorsum and lateral aspect of the foot, distal Achilles tendon	Masquelet et al. 1988 [58]	Goldberg 2000
	Distally based sural island flap	Ankle, Heel, distal Achilles tendon	Jeng and Wei 1977 [59]	Sood 2006 [67]
	Lateral calcaneal artery flap	Dorsal aspect of the heel	Grabb and Argenta 1981 [60]	Goldberg 2000
	Peroneus brevis muscle flap	Achilles tendon insertion	Jackson and Scheker 1982 [61]	

Anterior tibial artery	Tibialis anterior muscle flap	Distal third of tibial crest	Ger 1970 [62]	Sood 2006 [68]
	Distally based anterior tibial fasciocutaneous flap	Complete dorsum and sides of the foot	Morrison and Shen 1987 [63]	Sood 2006
Posterior tibial artery				
	Distally based posterior tibial fasciocutaneous flap	Complete dorsum, sides and sole of the foot	Hong et al. 1989 [64]	Goldberg 2000
	Distally based posterior tibial fasciocutaneous flap	Complete dorsum, sides and sole of the foot	Hong et al. 1989 [64]	Goldberg 2000

rotated in an upward direction to cover proximal dorsal defects or even the medial malleolus. It can be also rotated downward to the sole in order to cover defects of the medial aspects of the midfoot and the heel.

The abductor digiti minimi muscle flap is quite similar to the abductor hallucis muscle flap but located at the lateral border of the foot [52]. It is based on the lateral plantar artery and can be used for defects of the proximal dorsum and the lateral malleolus. If rotated downward to the sole, the lateral aspects of the midfoot and the heel can be reached. For distal foot coverage a distally based abductor digiti minimi muscle flap has been described [53]. The largest local muscle flap in this group is the flexor digitorum brevis muscle flap. Its blood support is

provided by branches of the lateral and medial plantar artery and it can be used as a muscle or musculocutaneous flap [54]. It is not used for dorsal defects but serves for covering the posterior aspect of the heel, the medial and lateral malleoli and the lower part of the achilles tendon [55].

Regional flaps from the lower leg

If the extent of injury makes local flaps not suitable for defect coverage, flaps from the lower leg, especially reverse-flow flaps have to be considered. The three arteries of the lower leg, the anterior tibial, the posterior tibial and the peroneal artery can serve as base for flaps if left intact by the trauma and can also serve for classification of the flaps. Most of the prox-

Table 2. Summary of free flaps which have been described for the use in reconstruction of severe burn injuries to the foot and ankle [21]

Free flaps		Region
Frequently used free flaps:	Latissimus dorsi muscle flap	Sole, complete dorsum and sides of the foot.
	Rectus abdominis muscle flap	Complete dorsum, sides of the foot and ankle region
	Anterolateral thigh flap	Heel, dorsum, sides of the foot and ankle region
	Radial forearm flap	Heel, dorsum, sides of the foot and ankle region
	Gracilis muscle flap	Sides of the foot and ankle region
Less frequently used free flaps:	Lateral arm flap	Heel, dorsum, sides of the foot and ankle region
	Medial arm flap	Heel, dorsum, sides of the foot and ankle region
	Temporalis fascia flap	Dorsum, sides of the foot and ankle region
	Scapular flap	Dorsum, sides of the foot and ankle region
	Deltoid flap	Heel, complete dorsum, sides of the foot and ankle region
	Serratus anterior muscle flap	Sole, complete dorsum, sides of the foot and ankle region

imally based flaps from the lower leg do not reach the foot and ankle region. Hence, only the most relevant flaps from the lower leg are presented. The proximally based flaps serve as a good addition to the local flaps from the foot. In the challenging region of the malleoli and the Achilles tendon, most of the local flaps do not reach much higher than to the level of the malleoli. Above that level the proximally based flaps can be valuable. The distally based flaps can cover relatively large defects of almost any part of the foot but it has to be evaluated very thoroughly whether scarifying one of the three arteries of the lower leg is justified. Preoperatively, the blood flow through the anastomosis has to be assured.

Regional flaps from the peroneal artery

For the dorsum of the foot a group of flaps originating from the peroneal artery can provide defect coverage. The lateral supramalleolar flap has become the most commonly used flap of this group [56, 57]. This large cutaneous perforator flap is based on a branch of a perforator of the peroneal artery [58]. The perforator is found proximal to the superior extensor retinaculum, where it perforates the interosseus membrane and from thereon has a cranial and a caudal branch. The cranial branch supplies a large area of skin on the lateral aspect of the lower leg and therefore is ideal for flap harvesting. Because of the anastomosis of the caudal branch with the anterior lateral malleolar artery, which originates from the anterior tibial artery, the flap can be used as a distally based flap. Its axis of rotation is centered at the midtarsal joint. With its rather long pedicle it can be used as a pedicled flap and as an island flap. In this way its range of coverage reaches to the distal dorsum of the foot, the achilles tendon and the whole lateral side of the foot. Even though the flap can reach the weight-bearing areas it is not indicated for those areas because, since it originates from the lower leg, it is composed of relatively thin skin.

The distally based sural island flap is an adaptation of the lateral supramalleolar flap. It has the same pedicle but includes the lateral sural cutaneous nerve, making it a sensory flap [59]. The lateral calcaneal artery flap is a reliable flap for coverage of the dorsal aspect of the heel. It is designed with a neurovascular pedicle consisting of the continuation of the peroneal artery, the lesser saphenous vein and the sural nerve for sensation. Its axis for rotation lies dorsal to the lateral malleolus [60]. Defects over the insertion of the Achilles tendon into the calcaneus can be covered by a peroneus brevis flap which has not been described in the context of burn injuries to the foot. It gets its blood supply from small branches of the peroneal artery [61].

Regional flaps from the tibialis anterior artery

The tibialis anterior muscle supplied by branches of the anterior tibialis artery can be used for the middle third of the tibial crest [62]. A distally based anterior tibial fasciocutaneous flap was described to reach the complete dorsum and the sides of the foot [63].

Regional flaps from the tibialis posterior artery

Based on the posterior tibial artery, the reverse posterior tibial fasciocutaneous and myofasciocutaneous flap have been described [64, 65].

The reverse posterior tibial flaps have their axis of rotation at the height of the medial malleolus and can reach the complete dorsum, the lateral and medial aspects and the sole of the foot [66].

Cross-leg flaps

Since the introduction of microsurgical free flap transplantation, the use of cross-leg flaps has become more or less outdated. In rare occasions, such as complete unavailability of recipient vessels, cross-leg flaps could be indicated [69]. For coverage of the weight-bearing areas, a cross-foot skin flap of the sole has also been described [70].

Free flaps

Large or complicated defects with exposure of bones or other deep structures require free tissue transfer for defect coverage [102]. Since burn injuries of the foot are very variable, using a free flap gives the surgeon maximum flexibility in defect coverage. The advantage of free flaps is that they are independent of uninjured vascular anatomy because they can be connected to further proximal vessels. When free

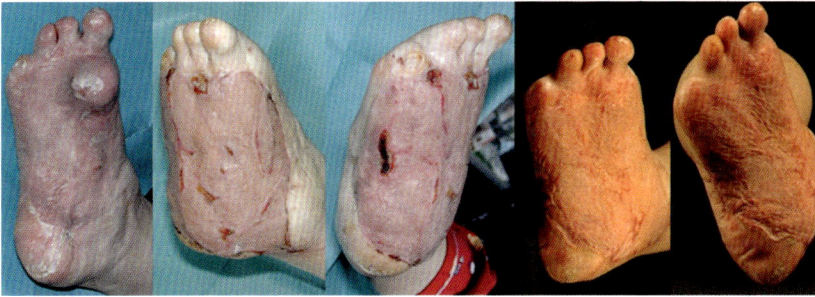

Fig. 9. Free rectus abdominis flap with split-skin graft for reconstruction of the sole. Instable wound as a sequelae of a burn injury (left) made this reconstruction necessary. High effort was put into good cushioning of the prominent first metatarsal bone

flaps are indicated, the broad majority of defects can be covered by standard free flaps, such as the latissimus dorsi or rectus abdominis flap [21] (Table 2). Many more free flaps have been described and may be indicated in special situations but for the choice of flap it is also legitimate to take into account which flap the individual surgeon is familiar with and has the most experience with. With the trend to perforator flaps and better understanding of the anatomy of the septocutaneous vessels of the lower leg, the popularity of fasciocutanoeus flaps has risen [72]. Free flaps can be used in the weight-bearing areas but the ulceration rate is three times higher and the time to full ambulation is significantly longer when the flap is used in the weight-bearing areas compared to non-weight-bearing areas [73]. For the weight-bearing areas flaps with a broad and flat shape like e.g. the latissimus dorsi muscle flap, the serratus anterior muscle flap, the rectus abdominus muscle flap or the gracilis muscle flap plus split skin graft are most commonly used in sole reconstruction. Choice of free flap should also include considerations of the required length of the pedicle to reach uninjured and suitable recipient vessels.

Two strategies for reconstruction with free flaps have been discussed thoroughly in literature and can be used successfully for foot reconstruction in weight-bearing areas: split-skin grafted muscle flaps and innervated fasciocutaneous flaps [31, 74]. Many authors state that flap insensitivity is a risk factor for ulcer development [77, 79]. To avoid insensitivity, many neurosensory flaps have been described which are thought to prevent ulceration and injuries to the flap similar to the injuries known to occur in patients with neuropathic feet [80, 82]. Long term sensory evaluation shows that almost all of the sensory and non-sensory flaps develop sensitivity for

deep pressure [73]. Sensation to light touch occurs much less frequent in both groups [73]. Ulceration rate as a measure of flap quality could not show superiority of sensory flaps [32]. Successful reconstruction correlates only with restored deep pressure sensibility, while light touch sensation does not correlate with successful reconstruction [32, 80]. Skin graft covered muscle flaps show the advantage of being more adjustable to the demand of contours and lessen the necessity of debulking procedures [83, 84]. This is mainly due to the lack of excessive subcutaneous fat, which also leads to unstable gait [32]. Despite the discussed benefits of neurosensory flaps, the split-thickness skin graft covered muscle flaps remain the most successful method for defects of the sole [21, 73] (Fig. 9).

For many large defects of the foot the latissimus dorsi flap with its broad and flat shape provides excellent coverage [85] (Fig. 9). Due to its size it can be adjusted to fit almost any shape of defect. If defects are smaller, rectus abdominis muscle flaps, radial forearm flaps, anterolateral thigh flaps and gracilis muscle flaps are frequently used [21]. The final shape of the flap becomes visible months after reconstruction, when muscle atrophy due to denervation is complete.

Long-time sequelae

The success of foot burn treatment has to be evaluated in the long run. Inadequate sensitive protections, poorly shaped contours or bony prominences can lead to recurrent ulcerations and pain. Due to lymphatic destruction edema can occur as long-term consequences affecting especially the dorsum of the foot. Return to pain-free, unimpaired ambulation is the goal. Especially contracture deformities of

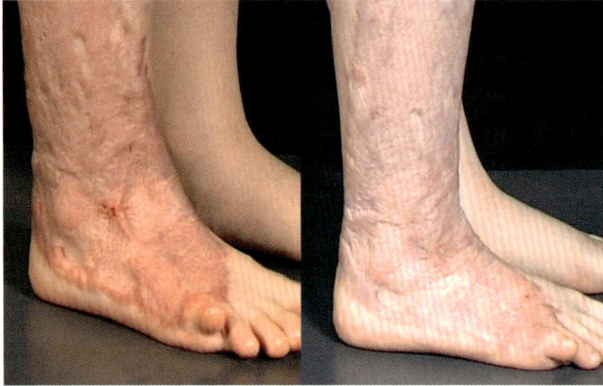

Fig. 10. A burn injury of the dorsum of the foot and the lateral lower leg was initially treated by transplantation of meshed split skin grafts. Several months after defect coverage, the patient suffered from problems with plantar flexion of the foot and hyperextension deformity of the fifth toe. Since hyperextension was mild and metatarsophalangeal luxation was absent, treatment of the toe consisted of scar release and transplantation of a full skin graft. The plantar flexion of the foot could be improved by scar release by a Z-plasty on the proximal dorsum

the soles of the feet can make this goal harder to achieve [87]. Wound contraction, a physiologic process to lessen the size of the wound, leads to contractures in the wounded area, which is accompanied by severe static and dynamic problems in the long run. Without prevention and treatment of contractures, the success of a good reconstruction can easily be diminished, leading to a prolonged convalescence [88]. Splints and physical therapy are very useful in preventing contractures. If foot burn contractures are mild, basic plastic techniques like single or multiple Z-plasties or W-plasties can be used to release tension of the scar [89]. Dorsal scar contractures can be successfully treated by a transverse and/or longitudinal burn scar release in combination with a skin graft [29, 90] (Fig. 10). Dorsal foot burn contractures are often accompanied by syndactyly of the toes which can be treated with Z- or W-plasties, V-Y Advancement flaps or skin grafts [91]. The most common sequelae of dorsal foot burn scar contractures is hyperextension and metatarsophalangeal subluxation of the toes leading to the rocker bottom deformity [89, 92]. It can be corrected by closed capsulotomies and K-wire fixation [90]. In the treatment of hyperextension or hyperflexion a moderate hypercorrection is recommended to achieve an enduring

result [87]. In the treatment of chronic burn deformities, especially dorsiflexion deformities, the Ilizarov fixateur is frequently used [93]. If postburn contractures are very severe, free flaps must be considered [94].

Thermal injuries of feet in children

Infants and children are a special risk group for foot burns [1]. Due to their thinner skin especially infants are at increased risk to suffer from full-thickness thermal injuries [2]. Again, the success of treatment has to be evaluated by the return to normal gait and ambulation but also by the incidence of contractures and other late sequelae [87]. Treatment of burns in children is different due to higher regeneration potential, lack of cooperation and different risk profile for long-time consequences including psychological factors [95, 96].

Especially plantar burns in children show unique characteristics and their treatment, particularly the decision between conservative and surgical treatment, is subject to controversial debate. Skin grafts are often used and it has been shown that in children even deep burns of the weight bearing parts of the sole can be sufficiently covered by split thickness skin grafts [97]. It has been stated that early excision and grafting results in a reduction of reconstructive needs [98]. Then again it has been reported that there is no difference in outcome between early excision followed by autografting and conservative treatment [99]. A widely accepted treatment protocol for plantar burns proposes conservative treatment together with progressive weight-bearing rehabilitation, active physiotherapy and stretching of the burned skin [96]. It also includes that wounds which do not heal within three weeks should be excised and covered by skin grafts. This protocol shows a negligible complication rate and significantly reduced incidence of contractures and late sequelae. Children are exceptionally at risk for contractures because growth brings additional tension to the scarred areas. If contractures in children are not corrected in time, they can lead to deformities of bones and joints, such as equinus or equinovarus deformity [87, 100]. In these cases scar release and skin grafting is insufficient. Osteotomy, tendon lengthening and soft tissue flaps must be considered. The contracture recurrence rate in childrens' feet, unlike other parts of their body, does not differ between full-thickness skin grafts, unmeshed split-thickness skin grafts or meshed split-thickness skin grafts [101, 102].

Summary and conclusion

Thermal injuries to the feet may not be underestimated because a lack of their function can dramatically reduce the patients' quality of life. The importance of adequate treatment becomes obvious when we think of how many of our daily activities depend on ambulation. Thermal wounds can occur in a wide range of variations. This makes individual evaluation of each case necessary. Accurate assessment of the wounds and of the overall situation of the patient is important to choose the right treatment. For the choice of reconstruction the location of the defect on the foot plays an important role. Especially weight-bearing areas are challenging fields. Profound knowledge of the foot's complex anatomy and availability of the full armamentarium of therapeutic options are prerequisites for a successful treatment. Hence, treatment should be managed by specialized burn care facilities. Long-term pain-free ambulation is the goal of therapy. Depending on the extent of the injury, treatment can reach from conservative approaches with wound dressings to multi-step operational approaches. In the acute phase of treatment cleaning of the wounds and fast coverage with skin or dermal replacements is intended. Similar to other burn wounds, skin grafts play an important role in covering defects which do not expose deeper structures. If defects are deeper or more complicated the surgeon can choose between different options of local, regional and free flaps. Treating burn wounds of children's feet is different not only because the regenerative potential is higher but also because special attention must be paid to the prevention of long-time sequelae such as contraction deformities.

References

[1] Hemington-Gorse S, Pellard S, Wilson-Jones N, Potokar T (2006) Foot burns: Epidemiology and management. Burns 33: 1041–1045

[2] Shah BR (2002) Burns of the feet. Clin Podiatr Med Surg 19(1): 109–123

[3] Djikstra S, vd Bent MJ, vd Brand HJ, Bakker JJ, Boxma H, Tjong Joe Wai R, Berghout A (1997) Diabetic patients with foot burns. Diabetic Medicine 14: 1080–1083

[4] Winfield RD, Chen MK, Langham MR Jr, Kays DW, Beierle EA (2008) Ashes, embers, and coals: significant sources of burn-related morbidity in children. J Burn Care Res 29(1): 109–113

[5] Sayampanathan SR, Ngim RC, Foo CL (1997) Fire walking in Singapore: a profile of the burn patient. J R Coll Surg Edinb 42(2): 131–134

[6] Harold E (2006) Clinical anatomy, 11th edn. Blackwell Publishing Ltd., Maiden Oxford Carlton, p 247

[7] Attinger, CE, Evans KK, Bulan E, Blume P, Cooper P (2006) Angiosomes of the foot and ankle and clinical implications for limb salvage: reconstruction, incisions and revascularization. Plast Reconstr Surg 117(7): 261–293

[8] Harold E (2006) Clinical anatomy, 11 th edn. Blackwell Publishing Ltd., Maiden Oxford Carlton, p 248

[9] Schünke M, Schulte E, Schumacher U (2005) Prometheus Lernatlas der Anatomie. Allgemeine Anatomie und Bewegungssystem. Georg Thieme, Stuttgart New York, p 468

[10] Schünke M, Schulte E, Schumacher U (2005) Prometheus Lernatlas der Anatomie. Allgemeine Anatomie und Bewegungssystem. Georg Thieme, Stuttgart New York, p 421

[11] Giunta RE, Kamholz LP, Mailander P (2007) Management of burn injuries. Handchir Mikrochir Plast Chir 39(5): 301

[12] Hidalgo DA, Shaw WW (1986) Reconstruction of foot injuries. Clin Plast Surg 13(4): 663–680

[13] Harold E (2006) Clinical anatomy, 11 th edn. Blackwell Publishing Ltd., Maiden Oxford Carlton, p 213

[14] Giunta RE, Geisweid A, Feller AM (2000) The value of preoperative Doppler sonography for planning free perforator flaps. Plast Reconstr Surg 105(7): 2381–2386

[15] Hallock GG (1986) Severe lower extremity injury. The rationale for micro-surgical reconstruction. Orthop Rev 15: 465

[16] Gidumal R, Carl A, Evanski P, Shaw W, Waugh TR (1986) Functional evaluation of nonsensate free flaps to the sole of the foot. Foot Ankle 7: 118

[17] Durham JW, Saltzman CL, Steyers CM, Miller BA (1994) Outcome after free flap reconstruction of the heel. Foot Ankle 15: 250

[18] Sonmez A, Bayramicli M, Sonmez B, Numanoglu A (2003) Reconstruction of the weight-bearing surface of the foot with nonneurosensory free flaps. Plast Reconstr Surg Ill: 2230–2236

[19] Daeschlein G, Assadian O, Bruck JC, Meinl C, Kramer A, Koch S (2007) Feasibility and clinical applicability of polihexanide for treatment of second-degree burn wounds. Skin Pharmacol Physiol 20: 292–296

[20] Zachary LS, Heggers JP, Robson MC, Smith DJ Jr, Ma-niker AA, Sachs RJ (1987) Burns of the feet. J Burn Care Rehabil 8(3): 192–194

[21] Goldberg DP, Kucan JO, Bash D (2000) Reconstruction of the burned foot. Clin Plast Surg 27(1): 145–161

[22] Mathes SJ, Alpert BS, Chang N (1982) Use of the muscle flap in chronic osteomyelitis: experimental and clinical correlation. Plast Reconstr Surg 69(5): 815–829

[23] Mathes SJ, Feng LJ, Hunt TK (1983) Coverage of the infected wound. Ann Surg 198(4): 420–429

[24] Saffle JR (2009) Closure of the excised burn wound: temporary skin substitutes. Clin Plast Surg 36(4): 627–641

[25] Rennekampff HO (2009) Skin graft procedures in burn surgery. Unfallchirurg 112(6): 543–549

[26] Busche MN, Herold C, Schedler A, Knobloch K, Vogt PM, Rennekampff HO (2009) The Biobrane glove in burn wounds of the hand. Evaluation of the functional and aesthetic outcome and comparison of costs with those of conventional wound management. Handchir Mikrochir Plast Chir 41(6): 348–354

[27] Grube BJ, Engrav LH, Heimbach DM (1992) Early ambulation and discharge in 100 patients with burns ofthe foot treated by grafts. J Trauma 33(5): 662–664

[28] Roka J, Karle B, Andel H, Kamolz L, Frey M (2007) Use of V. A. C. therapy in the surgical treatment of severe burns: the Viennese concept. Handchir Mikrochir Plast Chir 39(5): 322–327

[29] Alison WE Jr, Moore ML, Reilly DA, Phillips LG, Mc-Cauley RL, Robson MC (1993) Reconstruction of foot burn contractures in children. J Burn Care Rehabil 14(l): 34–38

[30] Machens HG, Berger AC, Mailander P (2000) Bioartificial skin. Cells Tissues Organs 167(2–3): 88–94

[31] Potparic Z, Rajac0ic N (1997) Long-term results of weight-bearing foot reconstruction with non-innervated and reinnervated flaps. Br J Plast Surg 50(3): 176–181

[32] May JW Jr, Halls MJ, Simon SR (1985) Free microvascular muscle flaps with skin graft reconstruction of extensive defects of the foot: A clinical and gait analysis study. Plast Reconstr Surg 75(5): 627–641

[33] Haug MD, Valderrabano V, Rieger UM, Pierer G, Schaefer DJ (2008) Anatomically and biomechanically based treatment algorithm for foot and ankle soft tissue reconstruction. Handchir Mikrochir Plast Chir 40(6): 377–385

[34] Machens HG, Kaun M, Lange T, Egbers HJ, Wenzl M, Paech A, Reichert B, Mailander P (2006) Clinical impact of operative multidisciplinarity for severe defect injuries of the lower extremity. Handchir Mikrochir Plast Chir 38(6): 403–416

[35] Mozafari N, Moosavizadeh SM, Rasti M (2008) The distally based neurocutaneous sural flap: A good choice for reconstruction of soft tissue defects of lower leg, foot and ankle due to fourth degree burn injury. Burns 34: 406–411

[36] McCraw JB, Furlow LT Jr (1975) The dorsalis pedis arterialized flap. A clinical study. Plast Reconstr Surg 55(2): 177–185

[37] Ishikawa K, Isshiki N, Suzuki S, Shimamura S (1987) Distally based dorsalis pedis island flap for coverage of the distal portion of the foot. Br J Plast Surg 40(5): 521–525

[38] Schwabegger A, Wechselberger G (1997) Distally based dorsalis pedis island flap for distal lateral electrical burn of the big toe. Burns 23(5): 459

[39] Hayashi A, Maruyama Y (1993) Reverse first dorsal metatarsal artery flap for reconstruction of the distal foot. Ann Plast Surg 31(2): 117–122

[40] Landi A, Soragni O, Monteleone M (1985) The extensor digitorum brevis muscle island flap for soft-tissue loss around the ankle. Plast Reconstr Surg 75(6): 892–897

[41] Kurata S, Hashimoto H, Terashi H, Honda T, Takayasu S (1992) Reconstruction of the distal foot dorsum with a distally based extensor digitorum brevis muscle flap. Ann Plast Surg 29(l): 76–79

[42] Koul AR, Patil RK, Philip V (2009) Extensor digitorum brevis muscle flap: modified approach preserving extensor retinaculum. J Trauma 66(3): 835–839

[43] Hidalgo DA, Shaw WW (1986) Anatomic basis of plantar flap design. Plast Reconstr Surg 78(5): 627–636

[44] Harrison DH, Morgan BD (1981) The instep island flap to resurface plantar defects. Br J Plast Surg 34(3): 315–318

[45] Uygur F, Duman H, Ulkiir E, Noyan N, Celikoz B (2008) Reconstruction of distal forefoot burn defect with retrograde medial plantar flap. Burns 34(2): 262–267

[46] Shanahan RE, Gingrass RP (1979) Medial plantar sensory flap for coverage of heel defects. Plast Reconstr Surg 64(3): 295–298

[47] Morrison WA, Crabb DM, O'Brien BM, Jenkins A (1983) The instep of the foot as a fasciocutaneous island and as a free flap for heel defects. Plast Reconstr Surg 72(l): 56–65

[48] Masquelet AC, Romana MC (1990) The medialis pedis flap: a new fasciocutaneous flap. Plast Reconstr Surg 85(5): 765–772

[49] Bostwick J 3rd (1976) Reconstruction of the heel pad by muscle transposition and split skin graft. Surg Gynecol Obstet 143(6): 973–974

[50] Ger R (1986) The clinical anatomy of the intrinsic muscles of the sole of the foot. Am Surg 52(5): 284–285

[51] Scheflan M, Nahai F, Hartrampf CR (1981) Surgical management of heel ulcers – a comprehensive approach. Ann Plast Surg 7(5): 385–406

[52] Ger R (1976) The management of chronic ulcers of the dorsum of the foot by muscle transposition and free skin grafting. Br J Plast Surg 29(2): 199–204

[53] Yoshimura Y, Nakajima T, Kami T (1985) Distally based abductor digiti minimi muscle flap. Ann Plast Surg 14(4): 375–377

[54] Hartrampf CR Jr, Scheflan M, Bostwick J 3rd (1980) The flexor digitorum brevis muscle island pedicle flap: a new dimension in heel reconstruction. Plast Reconstr Surg 66(2): 264–270

[55] Ikuta Y, Murakami T, Yoshioka K, Tsuge K (1984) Reconstruction of the heel pad by flexor digitorum brevis musculocutaneous flap transfer. Plast Reconstr Surg 74(1): 86–96

[56] Beveridge J, Masquelet AC, Romana MC, Vinh TS (1988) Anatomic basis of a fascio-cutaneous flap supplied by the perforating branch of the peroneal artery. Surg Radiol Anat 10(3): 195–199

[57] Okazaki M, Ueda K, Kuriki K (1998) Lateral supramalleolar flap for heel coverage in a patient with Werner's syndrome. Ann Plast Surg 41(3): 307–310

[58] Masquelet AC, Beveridge J, Romana C, Gerber C (1988) The lateral supramalleolar flap. Plast Reconstr Surg 81(1): 74–81

[59] Jeng SF, Wei FC (1997) Distally based sural island flap for foot and ankle reconstruction. Plast Reconst Surg 99(3): 744–750

[60] Grabb WC, Argenta LC (1981) The lateral calcaneal artery skin flap. Plast Reconstr Surg 68: 723

[61] Jackson IT, Scheker L (1982) Muscle and myocutaneous flaps on the lower limb. Injury 13(4): 324–330

[62] Ger R (1970) The management of open fracture of the tibia with skin loss. J Trauma 10(2): 112–121

[63] Morrison WA, Shen TY (1987) Anterior tibial artery flap: anatomy and case report. Br J Plast Surg 40(3): 230-235

[64] Hong G, Steffens K, Wang FB (1989) Reconstruction of the lower leg and foot with the reverse pedicle posterior tibial fasciocutaneous flap. Br J Plast Surg 42: 512

[65] Costa H, Malheiro E, Silva A (1996) the distally based tibial myofasciocutaneous island flap for foot reconstruction. Br J Plast Surg 49: 111

[66] Emsen IM (2008) An alternative and new approach to free flap in treatment of calcaneal region and lower third of the lower extremity reconstruction: reverse flow posterior tibial fasciocutaneous skin island flaps. J Trauma 64(3): 780–785

[67] Sood R, Achauer BM (2006) Achauer and Sood's burn surgery, reconstruction and rehabilitation. Elsevier Health Sciences, New York, pp 349–350

[68] Sood R, Achauer BM (2006) Achauer and Sood's burn surgery, reconstruction and rehabilitation. Elsevier Health Sciences, New York pp 330

[69] Agarwal P, Raza H (2008) Cross-leg flap: Its role in limb salvage. Indian J Orthop 42(4): 439–443

[70] Mir y Mir L (1954) Functional graft of the heel. Plast Reconstr Surg 14(6): 444–450

[71] Tolhurst DE, Haeseker B, Zeeman RJ (1983) The development of the fasciocutaneous flap and its clinical applications. Plast Reconst Surg 71: 597–605

[72] Carriquiry C, Costa MA, Vasconez LO (1985) An anatomic study for the septocutaneous vessels of the leg. Plast Reconstr Surg 76: 354–363

[73] Goldberg JA, Adkins P, Tsai TM (1993) Microvascular reconstruction of the foot: weight-bearing patterns, gait analysis, and long-term follow-up. Plast Reconstr Surg 92(5): 904–911

[74] Sinha AK, Wood MB, Irons GB (1989) Free tissue transfer for reconstruction of the weight-bearing portion of the foot. Clin Orthop 242: 269–271

[75] Kuran I, Turgut G, Bas L, Ozkan T, Bayry O, Gulgonen A (2000) Comparison between sensitive and nonsensitive free flaps in reconstruction of the heel and plantar area. Plast Reconstr Surg 105(2): 574–580

[76] Noever G, Briiser P, Kohler L (1986) Reconstruction of heel and sole defects by free flaps. Plast Reconstr Surg 78(3): 345–352

[77] Lister GD (1978) Use of an innervated skin graft to provide sensation to the reconstructed heel. Plast Reconstr Surg 62(2): 157–161

[78] Serafin D, Voci VE (1983) Reconstruction of the lower extremity: Microsurgical composite tissue transplantation. Clin Plast Surg 10(1): 55–72

[79] Wood MB, Irons GB, Cooney WP (1983) Foot reconstruction by free flap transfer. Foot Ankle 4(1): 2–7

[80] Sommerlad BC, McGrouther DA (1978) Resurfacing the sole: Long-term follow-up and comparison of techniques. Br J Plast Surg 31(2): 107–116

[81] Chang KN, Buncke HJ (1986) Sensory reinnervation in reconstruction of the foot. Foot Ankle 7(2): 124–132

[82] Rautio J (1990) Patterns of recovery of sensibility in free flaps transferred to the foot: A prospective study. J Reconstr Microsurg 6(1): 37–41

[83] May JW Jr, Lukash FN, Gallico GG 3rd (1981) Latissimus dorsi free muscle flap in lower-extremity reconstruction. Plast Reconstr Surg 68(4): 603–607

[84] Gordon L, Buncke HJ, Alpert BS (1982) Free latissimus dorsi muscle flap with split-thickness skin graft cover: a report of 16 cases. Plast Reconstr Surg 70(2): 173–178

[85] Clark N, Sherman R (1993) Soft-tissue reconstruction of the foot and ankle. Orthop Clin North Am 24(3): 489–503

[86] Fernandez-Palacios J, De Armas Diaz F, Deniz Hernandez V, Rodriguez Aguirre M (1996) Radial free flaps in plantar burns. 22(3): 242–245

[87] Shakirov BM, Tursunov BS (2005) Treatment of severe foot burns in children. Burns 31(7): 901–905

[88] Pap GS (1966) Hot metal burns of the feet in foundry workers. J Occup Med 8(10): 537–539

[89] Leung PC, Cheng JC (1986) Burn contractures of the foot. Foot Ankle 6(6): 289–294

[90] Dhanraj P, Owiesy F, Phillips LG, McCauley RL (2002) Burn scar contractures of the feet: efficacy of bilateral simultaneous surgical correction. Burns 28(8): 814–819

[91] Krizek TJ, Robson MC, Flagg SV (1974) Management of burn syndactyly. J Trauma 14(7): 587–593

[92] Kucan JO, Bash D (1992) Reconstruction of the burned foot. Clin Plast Surg 19(3): 705–719

[93] Shen YM, Huang L, Hu XH, Li M, Zhang GA (2008) Treatment of burn cicatricial foot drop with Ilizarov fixator. Chinese Journal of Burns 24(4): 287–289

[94] Uygur F, Duman H, Ulkur E, Celikoz B (2008) Are reverse flow fasciocutaneous flaps an appropriate option for the reconstruction of severe postburn lower extremity contractures? Ann Plast Surg 61 (3): 319–324

[95] Lohmeyer JA, Eich U, Siemers F, Lange T, Mailander P (2007) Psychological and behavioural impairment following thermal injury in childhood. Handchir Mikrochir Plast Chir 39(5): 333–337

[96] Barret JP, Herndon DN (2004) Plantar burns in children: epidemiology and sequelae. Ann Plast Surg 53(5): 462–464

[97] Heimburger RA, Marten E, Larson DL, Abston S, Lewis SR (1973) Burned feet in children. Acute and reconstructive care. Am J Surg 125(5): 575–579

[98] Singh K, Prasanna M (1995) Tangential excision and skin grafting for ash burns of the foot in children: a preliminary report. J Trauma 39(3): 560–562

[99] Gore D, Desai M, Herndon DN (1988) Comparison of complications during rehabilitation between conservative and early surgical management in thermal burns involving the feet of children and adolescents. J Burn Care Rehabil 9: 92–95

[100] Steinwender G, Saraph V, Zwick EB, Uitz C, Linhart W (2001) Complex foot deformities associated with soft-tissue scarring in children. J Foot Ankle Surg 40(l): 42–49

[101] Waymack JP (1986) Release of burn scar contractures of the neck in paediatric patients. Burns Incl Therm Inj 12(6): 422–426

[102] Waymack JP, Fidler J, Warden GD (1988) Surgical correction of burn scar contractures of the foot in children. Burns Incl Therm Inj 14(2): 156–160

Correspondence: Prof Dr. med. Riccardo E. Giunta, Handchirurgie, Plastische Chirurgie und Ästhetische Chirurgie, Klinikum der Ludwig-Maximilians Universität München, Pettenkoferstraße 8a, München, Germany, Tel: +4989 5160 2697, Fax: +4989 5160 4401, E-mail: r.giunta@med.uni-muenchen.de

Burn reconstruction: Hand and upper extremity

Hugo Benito Kitzinger, Birgit Karle, Manfred Frey

Vienna Burn Centre, Division of Plastic and Reconstructive Surgery, Department of Surgery, Medical University of Vienna, Vienna, Austria

Introduction

Although hand burns affect less than 3 % of the total body surface area (per hand), they are classified to be severe injuries, which will require the treatment in a specialized burn centre. In more than 80 % of severely burned patients the hand is involved [49]. Even if hand burns do not play a major role concerning mortality, they are important factors for a successful reintegration into society and professional life after discharge from hospital [26]. An adequate treatment of the hands is often neglected in the acute phase in favour of the treatment of other body parts or intensive care, but already in this acute phase the course for a successful restoration of hand function is set. At the end of the 1940s, surgeons pointed out that failing to mobilize fingers will lead to early stiffening of the fingers and therefore to a loss of hand function [7]. Apart from functional rehabilitation, the aesthetic outcome is also essential since hands cannot, similar to the face, be hidden by clothes so easily.

An optimal hand burn management demands a number of major decisions concerning: necessity of a escharo- or fasciotomy in the early posttraumatic phase, time and type of surgical debridement, type of wound coverage, as well as immobilization and rehabilitation. These efforts primarily aim to restore hand function or as Peacock et al. (1953) [57] stated it, the preservation and not the restoration of finger and hand function. Sheridan et al. (1995) [69] succeeded in regaining normal hand function in 97 % of the patients with superficial dermal burns, whereas in patients with deep dermal and full-thickness burns the success rate was only 81 %.

Mechanisms of the injury and anatomic characteristics

Most of the deep dermal and full-thickness hand burns affect the dorsum of the hand. Full-thickness palmar burns occur relatively rarely, mostly infants, who have just started grabbing things. The low incidence of palmar involvement in adults is due to the fact that hands are used to protect the face against a severe burn trauma and thereby only the dorsal parts of the hands are exposed. Moreover the skin of the palm has a higher tolerance for thermal energy due to its thickness and its well-developed stratum corneum.

There are some special characteristics in the hand's anatomy. Its physical sturdiness, the sensory qualities and the high capillary density in the stratum papillare are making this skin unique. The proportion between skin surface and tissue volume is extraordinary: there is a disproportional shift in favour of the hand. A volume of 1 cm³ correlates with a skin surface of 2,5 cm², whereas this value decreases already in the forearm to 0,5 cm² [53].

There are distinctive differences between the dorsum of the hand and the palm. The skin at the extensor side of the hand is thin and mobile, thus facilitating the flexion of the finger joints. The palmar skin is sturdy and resistant against pressure, contains essential sensory endorgans and adheres strongly to the palmar aponeurosis. A density of Merkel's tactile disks, Meissner's tactile corpuscles, Vater-Pacini's lamellated corpuscles and free nerve ends are found in the skin. That is the reason why hand burns may cause severe sensory deficits [67]. In contrast to other body parts, blood vessels, tendons and joints are located very close to the skin surface. This circumstance makes theses structures extremely vulnerable when exposed to high thermal energy.

Aims and principles of treatment

An optimal treatment of a hand burn can only be provided by a close interdisciplinary co-operation among surgeons, physiotherapists, occupational therapists, psychologists and motivated health care personnel [11]. A fast healing wound must be the primary aim [32] in order to achieve a well-functioning hand, which will facilitate a rapid re-integration of the burn patient into society and normal life. According to Robson et al. (1992) [63], treatment of hand burn trauma can be divided into aims and principles.

The key aims are:
▶ Prevention of additional or deeper injuries
▶ Rapid wound closure
▶ Preservation of active and passive motion
▶ Prevention of infection or loss of functional structures
▶ Early functional rehabilitation

The following aims should be gained by applying basic treatment principles:
▶ Determination of dimension and depth of the burn
▶ Escharotomy (if indicated)
▶ Application of adequate wound dressings
▶ Decision upon conservative or surgical treatment
▶ Surgical management (necrosectomy, skin grafts, skin substitutes, free flaps etc.)

▶ Early hand therapy with splinting
▶ Functional rehabilitation by early active and passive motion due to physiotherapy
▶ Secondary and tertiary corrections (if indicated)

Determination of burn depth

After stabilizing the burn patient's vital functions, a clinical examination should provide exact information about the severity of trauma (e. g. burn depth, secondary injuries).

Clinical assessment remains the most frequent technique to measure the depth of a burn wound although this has been shown to be accurate in only 60–75 % of the cases, even when carried out by an experienced burn surgeon. But there are more and more modalities available, which are useful to provide an objective assessment of burn wound depth. These modalities range from simple clinical evaluation to biopsy and histology and to various perfusion measurement techniques such as thermography, vital dyes, video angiography, video microscopy, and laser Doppler techniques [14, 22, 30, 39, 40, 46, 52, 56, 79]. Concerning recent literature Laser Doppler imaging seems to be the only technique that has shown to be accurate in predicting wound outcome with a large weight of evidence. Moreover this technique has been approved for burn depth assessment by regulatory bodies including the FDA.

Indication for escharotomy

The maintenance of perfusion is the first and foremost aim in the acute treatment of hand burns. During the acute phase, deep dermal, circular or nearly circular burns should be cared for most attentively because they can cause circulatory impairment. Tissue underneath a deep dermal or full-thickness burn will expand due to the increasing edema and the pressure within the compartment will rise. The escharotomy will lead to a decompression, the compartment pressure will decrease and the tissue perfusion will increase. The presence of a nearly circular or circular deeper burn and an increasing edema should be an indicator for immediate escharotomy. Missing pulse of the radial or ulnar artery under adequate resuscitation is a sign of a progressed ischemia and requires immediate escharotomy. Delayed decompression may cause circulatory disorders, nerve damage, extensive muscle necrosis and a consecutive function loss. Even for experienced surgeons it is sometimes extremely difficult to determine whether an escharotomy of the hand will be necessary or not. In case fingers are circularly firmly strained regardless of burn depth, the dorsum of the hand appears pale white, the recapillarisation of the nail bed is deregulated and a loss of sensibility can be observed, an escharotomy will be inevitable [84] (Fig. 1).

When determining the need for escharotomy, it should be noted that the edema can increase for up to 36 hours after injury due to the increased vascular permeability. Thus the risk for the development of a compartment syndrome in massive burns is much higher. In such cases a prophylactic escharotomy might be indicated. The evaluation of a burned hand must always be carried out in the context to the other burned areas [69].

Escharotomy

In urgent cases, an escharotomy can be carried out bedside under sterile conditions, but it is recommended to do it in the operating room. An incision on arm and hand is best carried out by electrocau-

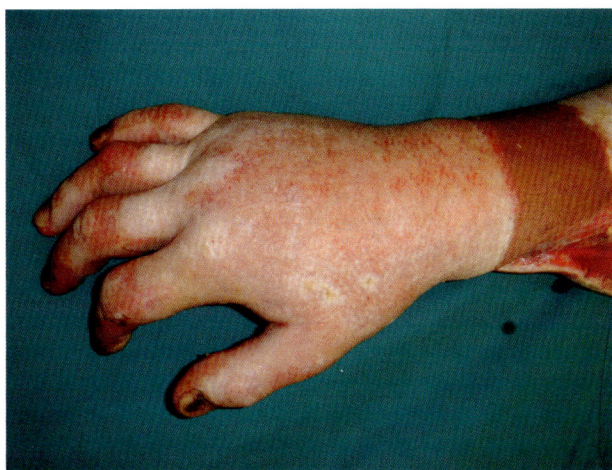

Fig. 1. Full-thickness hand burn: fingers are firmly strained and appear pale white

tery in order to reduce bleeding. During incision attention should be paid to the ulnar nerve at the medial epicondyle, to the superficial branch of the radial nerve and to the tendon of the flexor carpi radialis muscle at the distal forearm due to their superficial location. At the wrist it is obligatory to decompress the carpal tunnel. In the finger area the monopolar needle or a No. 15 blade can be used to split the necrosis completely without injuring the extensor tendons or the lateropalmar neurovascular bundle [81]. In order to achieve as few motion-limiting scars as possible, the line of incision is radial on thumb and little finger and ulnar on the other fingers [70]. This line can be defined well by putting the fingers in maximum flexion, marking the lateral extensions of the finger joint flexor wrinkles and completing them to a continuous line. Salisbury and Levine (1976) [64] have shown that the number of finger amputations could be significantly reduced by carrying out an adequate digital escharotomy.

An ischemic necrosis of the intrinsic muscles is accompanied by a significant functional impairment because the fingers will develop an intrinsic-minus position [65]. In deep hand burns and in case of an intrinsic tightness, the intrinsic compartment should always be decompressed. An intrinsic tightness is diagnosed by securing the metacarpophalangeal joint in a 0° position and flexing the finger passively in the proximal or distal interphalangeal joints. Resistance is an indication for intrinsic tightness, which requires an additional fasciotomy of the intrinsic muscles. For that purpose the area between the metacarpals II/III and IV/V is incised longitudinally whereby the extensor tendons remain covered. From there a fasciotomy of the intrinsic compartments can be carried out easily. To prevent desiccation of the free structures, wounds are covered temporarily by skin substitutes, e. g. Epigard®.

Formally, fasciotomy has to be distinguished from escharotomy. In an escharotomy, necrosis is cut up to the subcutaneous fat tissue, whereas in case of a fasciotomy the muscle fascia is also opened. This intervention is indicated in case an escharotomy did not provide the desired increase in perfusion or if the patient suffers from electrical [70].

Treatment of edema

Immediately after a burn trauma it is reasonable to cool the hand by applying cold water in order to eliminate the high thermal energy and to reduce pain. In most favorable cases cooling also reduces the edema formation and thereby burn wound progression [62]. Massive burns should not be cooled in order to avoid a massive decrease of body temperature, which will lead consecutively to burn wound progression. An effective and simple way to prevent or to decrease the development of edema is a continuous elevation of the hand above heart level.

Splinting

Joint contractures inhibit free movement of the finger joints. This is extremely evident in claw hand deformity. The deformation is caused by the trauma, wound infection, inadequate wound coverage, long time immobilization and inappropriate bedding and positioning of the hand.

In patients with severe burns the incidence of edema is significantly increased. The reason for the intrinsic-minus position of the hand is an increased fluid accumulation in the joints with distension of the joint capsule and imbibition of the collateral ligaments and subsequent ligament contraction. The intrinsic-minus position is a wrist flexion with a simultaneous hyperextension of the metacarpophalangeal joints (MCP), a flexion of the proximal and distal interphanlangeal joints [59] and a thumb adduction. This defective position emanates in the MCP joints. If the MCP joints are extended, joint capsule and collateral ligaments flag [44]. The joint is relatively unstable with a high degree of freedom for rotation, abduction and adduction. The contact areas of the corresponding joint surfaces are minimized. The combination of these factors will provide the biggest volume capacity for interstitial fluid accumulation. In flexion, the collateral ligaments are tightened with maximum contact of joint surfaces, which reduces the possibility of fluid accumulation in the joint. In the presence of the burn edema, the intra-articular fluid increase causes an extension of the MCP joint, similar to a hydraulic pump. In this position, the tension of the flexors increases whereas the tension of the extensors decreases. This causes a flexion in the

proximal as well as in the distal IP joints. In contrast to the MCP joints, the volumetric capacity of the IP joints in flexion and extension is nearly identical, so that there is no hydraulic effect. Thus the flexion of the IP joints is the immediate consequence of the extension of the MCP joints (Fig. 2).

So, the therapeutic principle must be an optimal positioning of the hand in order to avoid permanent contractures and deformities [60]. Ideally, a thermoplastic fixation device should be fitted in intrinsic-plus position already on the day of injury. The hand should be slightly extended in the wrist with 20°–30°, flexed in the MCP joint with approximately 80° and completely extended in the IP joints. The thumb is placed in maximum abduction to prevent adduction contractures.

In awake and cooperative patients a night splint is often sufficient. Active and passive exercises with the hand should be carried out twice a day. Only in deep dermal or full-thickness burns, in which there

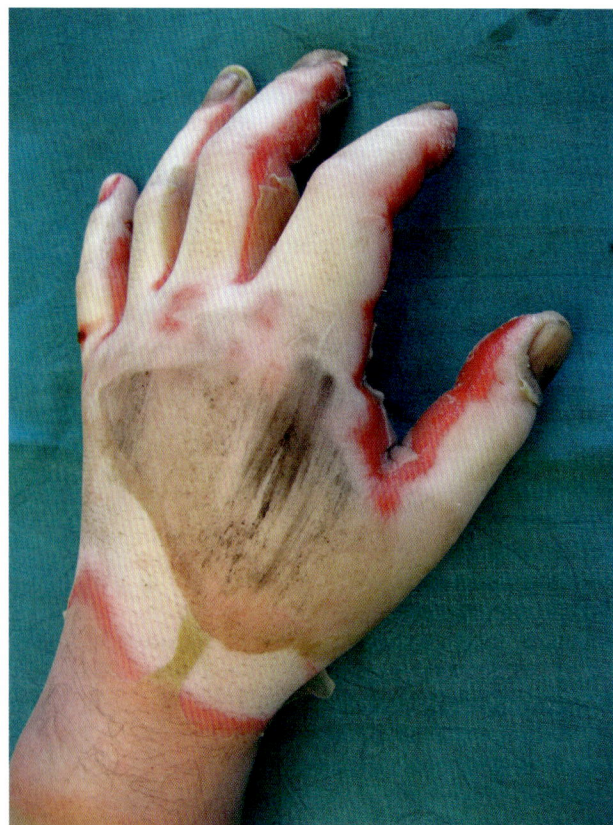

Fig. 2. Edema with hyperextension of the MCP joints and flexion in the IP joints

is suspicion of an injured extensor tendon apparatus, a flexion of the proximal IP joint should be avoided to prevent a rupture of the central slip and thus a Boutonnière or buttonhole deformity.

Wound management

The acute burn wound has to be cleaned and debrided. Until some years ago, blisters were not removed because it was believed that they serve as a biological wound dressing. Recent studies showed though that the blister's secretion contains prostaglandines and other pro-inflammatory cytokines as for example interleukine-6 and interleukine-8 [29, 55]. Therefore it is recommended to remove the blisters or at least the fluids [70].

Superficial hand burns are treated with special lipid regulating ointments (e. g. Bepanthen®) for a few days. It is important to familiarize the patient with the immediate active mobilization of the hand.

Superficial partial thickness burns require dressings, which protect the wound against infection and reduce pain at the same time. Paraffin gauze dressings (e. g. Bactigras®, Grassolind®) provide maximum mobilization of the hand and avoid painful adherence to the wound. Alternatively, epidermal substitutes, as for example Biobrane® or Suprathel® can be applied. Advantages are an accelerated epithelialisation and pain reduction.

In deep dermal and full-thickness burns, antiseptic agents, which can penetrate into deeper layers, as for example silversulfadiazine (Flammazine®) should be applied [12]. The released silver ions bind to the microbial genes (DNA) and inhibit the reproduction of bacteria and fungi. The sulfadiazine inhibits the production of folic acid which is necessary for the reproduction of bacteria [45]. In case of later surgical debridement an unfavorable effect of silversulfadiazine is that it softens the necrosis thus complicating a tangential excision. If applied broadly, the systemic resorption of silver ions may cause an impaired acid-base-balance, leukopenia as well as liver and kidney damage [77]. In smaller burns, povidone iodine (Betaisodona®-ointment) can be used alternatively [85]. Povidone iodine stains the burn wound thus complicating the determination of burn depth. In large burns, the application of povidone iodine is contraindicated due to a potential induction of hyperthyreosis or the risk of an acute iodine-intoxication. According to a study by Homann et al., a new formula for ointments with hydrogel and povidone iodine (Repithel®) has lead to a faster healing in superficial burns [35].

In general, burn wound dressings should be changed at least once a day – in the presence of heavy wound secretion even more often. It is particularly important to keep hand dressings as thin as possible in order to allow mobilization. This also includes the supply of thumbs and fingers with tube dressings. Alternatively, a thread glove can be used, which has been previously filled with the desired ointment.

Surgical treatment

As soon as the burn depth can be determined exactly – usually on the second or third day post trauma – the wounds should be excised and covered [70]. During the first five days, the burn wound is defined as "sterile" and thus optimal for surgery. After these five days there is a higher risk for infection and graft failure [20]. In case of the fact that a surgical intervention is not possible in the initial phase, it is recommended to postpone the coverage until the infection has been treated sufficiently. Adequate splinting and physical therapy should be provided in order to achieve results nearly as good as after early surgical debridement and coverage [47].

Superficial burns that heal spontaneously within two weeks do not require surgical treatment but daily wound care, as described above. Goodwin et al. (1983) [23] showed that a hypertrophic scar formation is very rare in these cases and that the functional outcome is very good. In full-thickness burns, especially in contact burns e. g. caused by hot metals or tar, there is no need to wait days to start excision and grafting. But in most of the burn wounds it is difficult to determine the burn depth and its potential progression exactly immediately after trauma. In these cases the question remains if there is still enough dermal tissue left to ensure conservative healing within two weeks or if the waiting period justifies the risk for the development of hypertrophic scars and scar contractures [15].

The strategies that have been applied over the last decades have considerably changed. Until the

1960s, a conservative treatment with antimicrobial ointments used to be the standard treatment. Functional outcomes were poor. That changed with the early 1970s when early debridement and early grafting led to much better results [28, 38].

The treatment and grafting strategies for deep dermal burns are still developing: e. g. covering the wound with biosynthetic epidermal substitutes like Suprathel® leads to results as good as after traditional skin grafting [73]. In predominantly deep dermal and full-thickness hand burns, an early debridement and skin grafting is still the method of choice.

The surgical therapy that is most often applied on hand burns is tangential excision: the necrotic skin is abraded in layers until capillary hemorrhage occurs. In isolated hand burns the blood loss can be reduced significantly by use of a tourniquet [9]. In these cases, the surgeon can not rely on the capillary bleeding but has to pay attention to other characteristics as the whitish color of vital dermis and the yellow color of vital fat tissue.

Palm burns

Contact burns in toddlers are often palmar burns. Surgical intervention is very rarely indicated because the skin of the palm is thick and well-protected. A surgical debridement is difficult to carry out due to the palm's distinct anatomy and the tight coherence to the palmar aponeurosis. A substitution is only applicable to a limited degree. These factors justify a conservative treatment for three to four weeks. In case of the fact that a necrosectomy is required, a sparing debridement is important. Since the palm is used excessively in daily life, thick split thickness or full thickness grafts should be used [37]. After surgical treatment, scar contractures of the palm are often occurring long-term complications . . . [4].

Methods of coverage

The method of choice for the coverage of the hand are autologous split skin grafts applied as unmeshed sheet graft [48]. The sometimes observed fluid retention underneath the graft with the risk of graft loss can be avoided by scarifying with a No. 11 blade

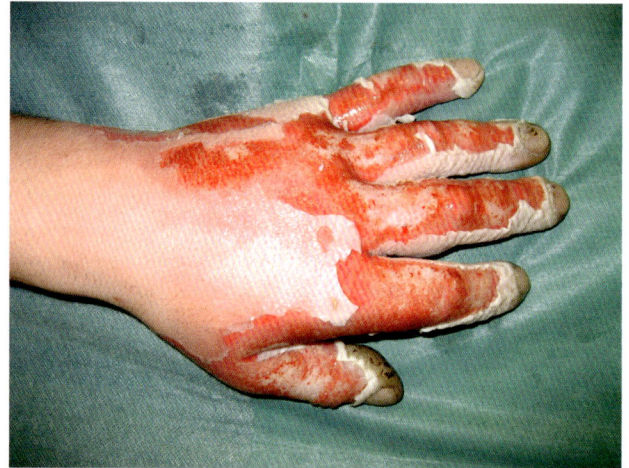

Fig. 3a. Deep dermal hand burn prior to surgery

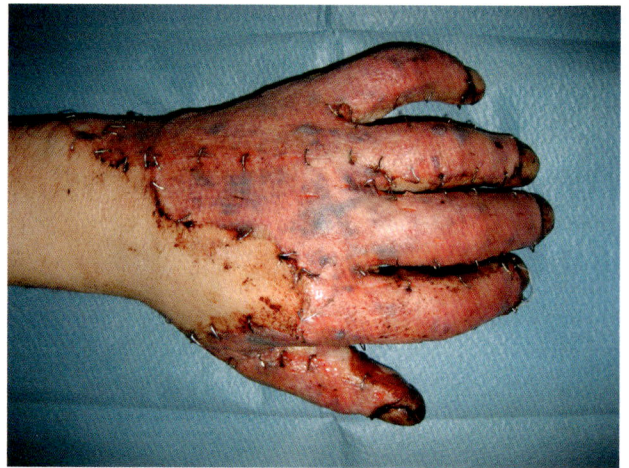

Fig. 3b. After debridement and split thickness skin graft

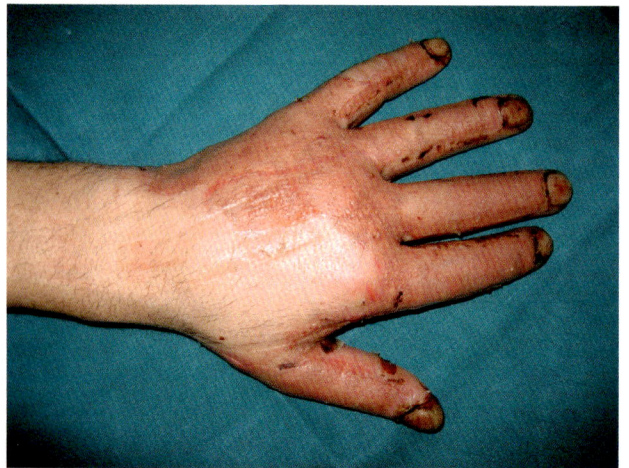

Fig. 3c. Early result three weeks after surgery

(Fig. 3 a – c). Alternatively, split skin grafts can be processed into mesh grafts with various expansion levels or used in Meek technique [61]. These techniques should only be applied in case that there are not enough autologous donor sites available. In comparison with mesh grafts, sheet grafts show a lower tendency to shrink and provide better aesthetic outcome. In the post-operative stage the hands are put in intrinsic-plus position by a palmar forearm splint; hand therapy will be determined as early as possible dependent on the wound condition.

Skin substitutes

In general there are two types of skin substitutes: temporary and permanent substitutes. It must further be decided whether an epidermal, a dermal or a combined dermal-epidermal substitute material is indicated [76]. The following section will only deal with those skin substitutes that are well-established in the treatment of hand burns.

The authors apply biological active epidermal skin substitutes, as for example allogeneic human keratinocytes, in infant deep dermal hand burns [41] in order to achieve faster healing and better cosmetic outcome. In teenagers and adults, synthetic epidermal skin substitute materials e. g. Biobrane® and Suprathel® are used.

Biobrane® is constructed of a semipermeable silicone film with a nylon fabric partially embedded into the film. Porcine collagen type I is also incorporated. Biobrane® is suggested for use in superficial partial-thickness burns [82]. Ready-made Biobrane® gloves facilitate the application. Benefits of Biobrane® are pain reduction, avoiding dressing changes, possibility of immediate active and passive mobilization of the hand and continuous observation of the wound due to the transparent material. After complete epithelialisation, the film can be easily removed. In comparison to Flammazine® dressings, the healing time is reduced up to seven days in wounds treated with Biobrane® [5]. Downsides of this material are the relatively high costs and the fact that also small fluid accumulations underneath the membrane have to be punctured in order to avoid infection [80].

Suprathel® is a copolymer consisting of polyactide, trimethylene carbonate and caprolactone. It is supplied as a membrane, whose properties are similar to those of Biobrane®. Benefits of Suprathel® are painless dressing changes, faster epithelialisation and the possibility of an early hand therapy [68]. First studies have demonstarted that Suprathel® provides good healing of deep dermal burns within three weeks after trauma [74]. After healing Suprathel® will degrade.

Integra® has been the most popular dermal equivalent in the field of permanent dermal replacements. Integra® is a matrix consisting of bovine collagen and glycosaminoglycans. Integra® must be applied in a two-step procedure. The reasons why Integra® is used primarily in the field of reconstruction these days are that the hand remains immobile for a longer period of time. Moreover the risk of infection is elevated [10, 31].

Another new dermal substitute is Matriderm®, which consists of bovine collagen and elastin. A distinctive advantage of Matriderm® is that it can be applied in a one-step procedure. First studies in hand burns could confirm this one-stage skin reconstruction [27]. Scar quality and viscoelasticity are as good as the functional outcome (Fig. 4 a–d), but there is a need for more studies to confirm these results.

Combined skin substitutes as for example allogeneic skin or Epigard® are applied in those cases where the period between trauma and definite coverage has to be bridged. The advantage of allogeneic skin is the fact that it is a biological scaffold which supports wound bed preparation. Moreover it reduces the risk of infection and protects the wound from water loss [59].

Exposed joints

The areas above the extensor-sided PIP joints must be particularly well observed. If primary skin transplantation is not successful, an infection of the joint accompanied by cartilage erosion and finally ancylosis will follow. In this phase the formation of granulation tissue is gained. In these cases the best achievable acute result will be an instable scar, which can be replaced later by adequate tissue e. g. a dorsal metacarpal artery flap (DMCA-flap) [19].

In case tendons, joints and bones are also affected by the burn trauma, these structures must be de-

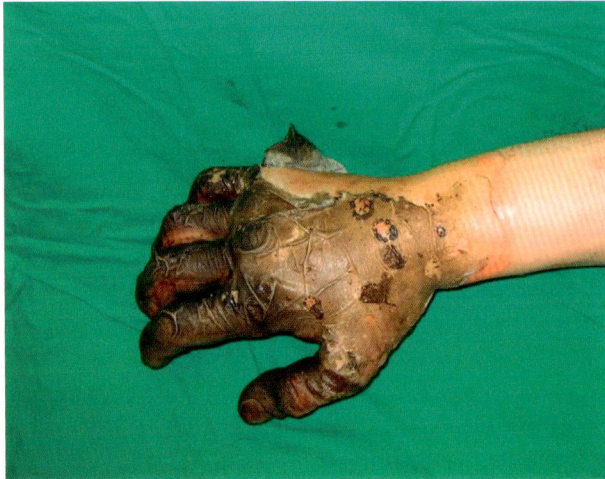

Fig. 4a. Full-thickness burn of the hand

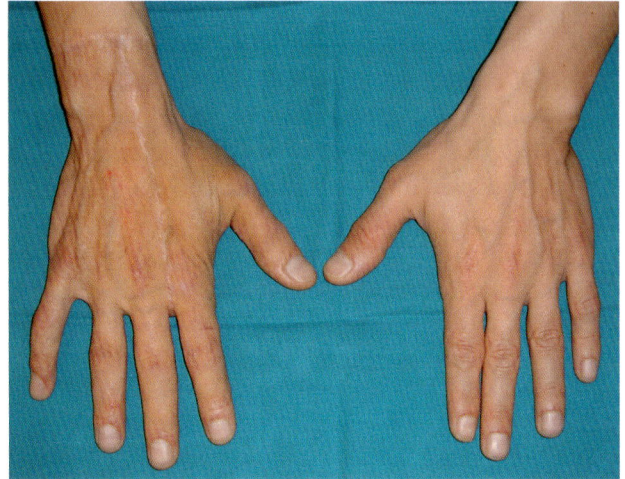

Fig. 4c. Long-term result (1 year after surgery) after single step reconstruction and compression therapy

brided, regardless of their function. A reconstruction which adheres to the principle of the reconstructive ladder is justified in these situations. When choosing flaps, it should be kept in mind that more reconstructive interventions will become necessary later on. Larger defects on the dorsum of the hand with exposed tendons and bones are treated in the acute phase with groin flaps, even today [51]. The temporary immobilization of the shoulder joint is well tolerated and the donor site of the flap is cosmetically inconspicuous. In case that the trauma is an isolated severe hand burn or the patient's general condition is stable, free microvascular tissue transfer are an ex-

cellent means of coverage [6, 9, 66]. Excellent cosmetic outcome is achieved by using lateral upper arm flaps or gracilis muscle flaps. If there is also a peritendineum necessary due to an injured paratenon, solutions can be found by use of serratus or other fascial flaps [16, 17].

Reconstruction

An adequate treatment of the hand burn in the acute phase determines the functional outcome. Due to the complex trauma accompanied by the destruction of highly specific soft tissue, deformities sometimes cannot be avoided even under an optimal therapy. The deformities after hand burn trauma were outlined by Achauer (1987) [1]:

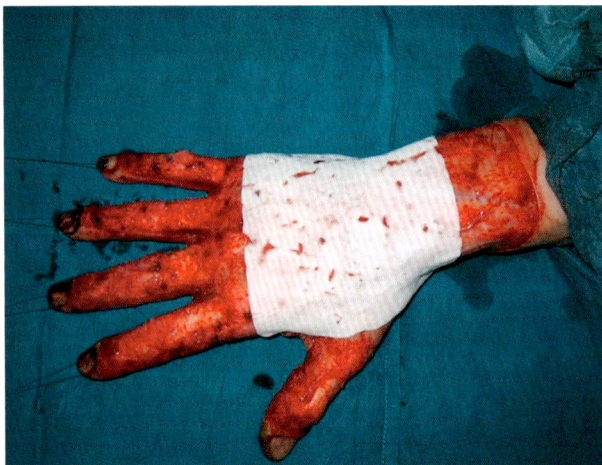

Fig. 4b. After debridement and application of Matriderm®

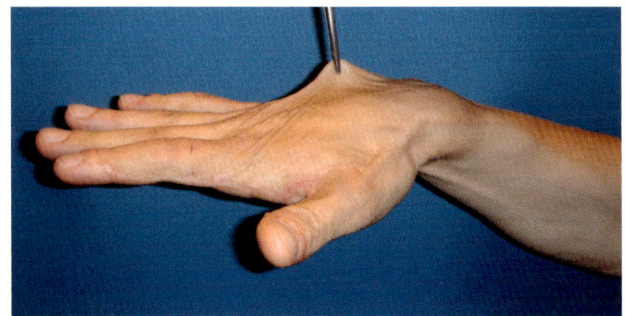

Fig. 4d. Skin elasticity

- ▶ claw deformity
- ▶ palmar contracture
- ▶ web space deformity
- ▶ hypertrophic scars
- ▶ amputation deformity
- ▶ nail bed deformity

Numerous surgical techniques have been described for the treatment of these deformities. Generally, the patient suffers from a combination of various deformities. The most frequent problems following hand burns are scar and soft tissue contractures, as they might appear following spontaneously healed deep burns, split skin grafting of inadequate size and thickness, with missing and/or not correctly positioned splints or inadequate physical therapy.

Claw deformity

Hypertrophic linear scars or scarred areas on the dorsum of the hand can lead to a hyperextension in the MCP joints, in rare cases even to a dislocation of the joint and to limited flexion. Buttonhole deformities are often seen at the PIP joints in deeper burns. The central extensor denaturizes due to the direct heat damage or desiccates following a longer period of exposition. That makes the side slips move into the palmar direction, which are situated now at the flexor side of the central joint. So, an attempted extension causes a flexion of the central joint. Whereas there are numerous treatments for buttonhole deformity in a non-burned hand, attempts to reconstruct this deformity in a burned hand are often not promising. A good alternative is the arthodesis of the joint in functional position. Functionally inhibiting defective positions of the distal joints are rare but can be corrected by arthodesis if necessary.

In large and thick scars which cause a hyperextension of the MCP joints, an excision of the scar with subsequent skin grafting is required. In case of the fact that a resection of the scarred and contracted subcutaneous tissue is required, Matriderm® as a dermal skin substitute has shown good results in combination with split thickness skin grafts [27]. In deep dermal burn wounds, contractures are not only due to scars but also due to defective extensor aponeurosis, defective tendons, defective joint capsules and muscles. Depending on the extent of the scar excision, an adequate coverage of the defect according to the reconstructive ladder should facilitate high quality soft tissue coverage. For this purpose there are numerous options available: the groin flap, the radial forearm flap and the interossea posterior artery flap and/or free muscular and fasciocutaneous flaps. In case joint contractures have already developed (due to a longer persisting defective position of the MCP joints) an artholysis should only be carried out after creating sufficient soft tissue coverage.

Palmar contractures

Posttraumatic contractures of the palm can develop due to secondary healing or due to inadequate positioning of the hand. They might also occur after a successful primary surgical treatment. Tendency to developing a tendon contracture in the wrist and the fingers as well as developing an adduction contracture in the thumb require splinting with slight wrist extension and 80° flexion of the MCP joints with extended PIP and DIP joints (intrinsic plus position) and maximum abduction of the thumb. In case contractures develop, a surgical incision or excision of the scar followed by full-thickness grafting is the method of choice [36]. Isolated, linear scars with sufficient tissue in the vicinity can be dissolved by one or multiple z-flap plasties. In the presence of a longer existing tendon contracture of the MCP or PIP joint, a release of the periarticular structures, as for example the articular capsule, the collateral tendons and the palmar plate is often required to achieve a complete extension of the joint [33]. In these cases a digital ischemia distal of the mobilized joint might occur due to traction of the lateropalmar vessels. For a definitive arthrodesis of the joint, the phalanges have to be shortened in this situation in favor of a functionally beneficial arthrodesis angle with still good perfusion.

An early physiotherapy and particularly a consequent nightly splinting over a period of at least six months are the decisive factors in avoiding a contracture relapse.

Web space deformities

Syndactylia or web space deformities are commonly observed following conservative treatment of deep burns, but also after surgery. In an intact hand, the web space goes in a 45° angle from the extensor-sided MCP joints in the palmar direction until the center of the basic phalanx. This anatomy can change considerably in burned web spaces. A palmar scar contracture can be distinguished from a dorsal scar contracture, which stretches – like a roof – over the commissure (syndactylia). A correction by using local flaps is generally successful [34]. In very severe cases the combination of local flaps and full-thickness grafts are the method of choice [25].

The span of the first web space is of particular importance for the grip function of the hand. In addition to scar contracture, a possible cause for a limited grip function might be adduction contracture of the thumb. Such a contracture is caused by a secondary fibrosis of the adductor pollicis and the dorsal first interosseus muscle. In case of a slight scar contracture, a z-plasty or butterfly plasty is sufficient. In more distinct contractures, full-thickness grafts are used. Depending on the intraoperative findings an additional release of the adductor pollicis muscle may be required. Hereby, the muscle is detached at its root at the third metacarpal or from its inset at the base of the thumb [82]. In rare and intense cases, a reconstruction of the first web space supported by a flap is necessary.

Hypertrophic scars

In burn injuries it takes the scars at least one year until they are healed and mature. Thus, corrections of scars should be carried out ideally after that period. In case of scar-related, functional constraints, e. g. in the finger joints, an early correction is necessary. Isolated scars with extensive surrounding soft tissue can be dissolved by small, local flaps, e. g. a z-plasty. Alternatively, numerous other flaps, as for example a cross-finger or reversed cross-finger-flap [24] or full-thickness grafts, can be used [75]. The application of a tailor-made compression glove, possibly with silicone inlets, can reduce hypertrophic scarring and scar contractures significantly [43, 58].

Amputation deformity

In severe burns, e. g. caused by high voltage, a loss of thumbs or fingers might be possible. The numerous techniques for a reconstruction of the trauma-related isolated amputation injury can be adopted only to a limited extend for a burned hand. The desired functional outcome is limited due to a combined defect of essential structures. Generally, hand function can be improved by a phalangization with deepening of the web space [72], by a distraction osteogenesis of the metacarpalia [50], by a pollicization [78] or by a toe transfer [2]. The precondition for these interventions is a high quality soft tissue coverage. For this purpose free tissue transfer is often necessary to create a good soft tissue surrounding.

Nail bed deformity

A defective nail growth following burn trauma of the hand is frequently observed. In very few cases the reason for that is a direct impairment of the nail bed or the germinative matrix. More often the reason is a secondary contracture of the soft tissue proximal to the nail bed. This leads to an eversion of the nail bed with proximal dislocation and to a loss of contact between dorsal nail matrix and nail and/or eponychium and nail. This causes coarse nails with longitudinal furrows. Injuries of the nail bed occur very often even after slight trauma. The extent of the nail bed eversion and the defective growth are proportional. A defect in the germinative matrix causes a cleft nail and/or a completely missing nail.

Various techniques have been published for the treatment of nail bed eversion, including dissolution of the underlying contractures by wrapping local flaps or skin grafts with subsequent reposition of the nail bed. Bilateral and proximal pedicle skin flaps are often used to create sufficient tissue at the extensor side [3]. That causes an unnatural diminution at the donor site. A newer technique is described by Donelan and Garcia (2006) [14].

Rehabilitation

The best treatment of burn scars is their prevention, an appropriate timing and burn depth specific surgery, and well-fitting pressure garments worn as soon as the skin grafts are stable. Silicone sheets [42, 58] have been useful on the dorsum of fingers and webspaces, placed under the pressure garment glove. Pressure garments are worn 24 h a day at least for an initial period of approximately 6 months in burns with prolonged healing time or burns that have required skin grafting [43]. Subsequent pressure garment use is individualized depending on scar quality and response. The exact mechanism by which pressure garments alter scar formation is not clear [70]. They do, however, seem to improve the quality of scars in both texture and colour in the long term [21]. Other scar manipulation techniques, such as steroid injection [54, 71], can be used as indicated. Heat and ultrasound is used to assist with joint mobilization and scar contracture treatment, but also Laser is used to improve scar quality [18]. Physical and occupational therapy progress from the acute phase to rehabilitation. Hand therapy continues until function returns to normal or treatment is no longer providing improvement. A maintenance hand therapy program is then continued.

Summary

Burn injuries very often affect the hands. Small burns can already cause severe deformities accompanied by loss of function. A fast wound closure is of utmost importance because the risk of infection, of hypertrophic scar formations and contractures increases with a prolonged healing time. Important parts of the treatment include early excision and early coverage within the first days post trauma. The success of the treatment also depends heavily on infection control and the preservation of the active and passive motion of the hand as well as on an early splinting and functional rehabilitation. The interdisciplinary teamwork of surgeons, physio- and occupational therapists, psychologists, motivated health care personnel and consequent treatment strategies can contribute to regaining normal hand function.

References

[1] Achauer BM (1987) Management of the burned patient. Appleton & Lange, East Norwalk

[2] Achauer BM (1999) The burned hand. In: Green DP, Hotchkiss RN, Pederson WC (eds) Operative hand surgery. Churchill Livingstone, Philadelphia

[3] Achauer BM, Welk RA (1990) One-stage reconstruction of the postburn nailfold contracture. Plast Reconstr Surg 85: 937–940; discussion 941

[4] Barret JP, Desai MH, Herndon DN (2000) The isolated burned palm in children: epidemiology and long-term sequelae. Plast Reconstr Surg 105: 949–952

[5] Barret JP, Dziewulski P, Ramzy PI, Wolf SE, Desai MH, Herndon DN (2000) Biobrane versus 1 % silver sulfadiazine in second-degree pediatric burns. Plast Reconstr Surg 105: 62–65

[6] Baumeister S, Germann G, Giessler G, Dragu A, Sauerbier M (2004) Wiederherstellung der verbrannten Extremität durch Transplantation freier Lappenplastiken. Chirurg 75: 568–578

[7] Braithwaite F, Watson J (1949) Some observations on the treatment of the dorsal burn of the hand. Br J Plast Surg 2: 21–31

[8] Cartotto R, Musgrave MA, Beveridge M, Fish J, Gomez M (2000) Minimizing blood loss in burn surgery. J Trauma 49: 1034–1039

[9] Chick LR, Lister GD, Sowder L (1992) Early free-flap coverage of electrical and thermal burns. Plast Reconstr Surg 89: 1013–1019; discussion 1020–1011

[10] Dantzer E, Queruel P, Salinier L, Palmier B, Quinot JF (2001) [Integra, a new surgical alternative for the treatment of massive burns. Clinical evaluation of acute and reconstructive surgery: 39 cases]. Ann Chir Plast Esthet 46: 173–189

[11] Deb R, Giessler GA, Przybilski M, Erdmann D, Germann G (2004) Die plastisch-chirurgische Sekundärrekonstruktion von Schwerstbrandverletzten. Chirurg 75: 588–598

[12] Dimick AR (1971) Management of patients with thermal injuries. Am Surg 37: 637–641

[13] Donelan MB, Garcia JA (2006) Nailfold reconstruction for correction of burn fingernail deformity. Plast Reconstr Surg 117: 2303–2308; discussion 2309

[14] Droog E, Steenbergen W, Sjöberg F (2001) Measurement of depth of burns by laser Doppler perfusion imaging. Burns 27: 561–568

[15] Edstrom LE, Robson MC, Macchiaverna JR, Scala AD (1979) Prospective randomized treatments for burned hands: nonoperative vs. operative. Preliminary report. Scand J Plast Reconstr Surg 13: 131–135

[16] Flügel A, Kehrer A, Heitmann C, Germann G, Sauerbier M (2005) Coverage of soft-tissue defects of the hand with free fascial flaps. Microsurgery 25: 47–53

[17] Fotopoulos P, Holmer P, Leicht P, Elberg JJ (2003) Dorsal hand coverage with free serratus fascia flap. J Reconstr Microsurg 19: 555–559

[18] Gaida K, Koller R, Isler C, Aytekin O, Al-Awami M, Meissl G, Frey M (2004) Low Level Laser Therapy – a conservative approach to the burn scar? Burns 30(4): 362–367

[19] Germann G, Funk H, Bickert B (2000) The fate of the dorsal metacarpal arterial system following thermal injury to the dorsal hand: A Doppler sonographic study. J Hand Surg [Am] 25: 962–968

[20] Germann G, Steinau HU (1993) Aktuelle Aspekte der Verbrennungsbehandlung. Zentralbl Chir 118: 290–302

[21] Giele HP, Liddiard K, Currie K (1984) Direct measurement of cutaneous pressure generated by pressure graments. Burns 10: 154–163

[22] Godina M, Derganc M, Brcic A (1978) The reliability of clinical assessment of the depth of burns. Burns 4: 92–96

[23] Goodwin CW, Maguire MS, McManus WF, Pruitt BA, Jr (1983) Prospective study of burn wound excision of the hands. J Trauma 23: 510–517

[24] Groenevelt F, Schoorl R (1985) Cross-finger flaps from scarred skin in burned hands. Br J Plast Surg 38: 187–189

[25] Gülgönen A, Ozer K (2007) The correction of postburn contractures of the second through fourth web spaces. J Hand Surg [Am] 32: 556–564

[26] Harvey KD, Barillo DJ, Hobbs CL, Mozingo DW, Fitzpatrick JC, Cioffi WG, McManus WF, Pruitt BA, Jr (1996) Computer-assisted evaluation of hand and arm function after thermal injury. J Burn Care Rehabil 17: 176–180; discussion 175

[27] Haslik W, Kamolz LP, Nathschlager G, Andel H, Meissl G, Frey M (2007) First experiences with the collagen-elastin matrix Matriderm as a dermal substitute in severe burn injuries of the hand. Burns 33: 364–368

[28] Haynes BW, Jr (1969) Early excision and grafting in third degree burns. Ann Surg 169: 736–747

[29] Heggers JP, Ko F, Robson MC, Heggers R, Craft KE (1980) Evaluation of burn blister fluid. Plast Reconstr Surg 65: 798–804

[30] Heimbach D, Afromowitz M, Engrav L, Marvin J, Perry B (1984) Burn depth estimation – man or machine. J Trauma 24: 373–378

[31] Heitland A, Piatkowski A, Noah EM, Pallua N (2004) Update on the use of collagen/glycosaminoglycate skin substitute-six years of experiences with artificial skin in 15 German burn centers. Burns 30: 471–475

[32] Hentz VR (1985) Burns of the hand. Thermal, chemical, and electrical. Emerg Med Clin North Am 3: 391–403

[33] Hintringer W (2002) Arthrotenolyse der Mittelgelenke (PIP). Technik und Ergebnisse. Handchir Mikrochir Plast Chir 34: 345–354

[34] Hirshowitz B, Karev A, Rousso M (1975) Combined double Z-plasty and Y-V advancement for thumb web contracture. Hand 7: 291–293

[35] Homann HH, Rosbach O, Moll W, Vogt PM, Germann G, Hopp M, Langer-Brauburger B, Reimer K, Steinau HU (2007) A liposome hydrogel with polyvinyl-pyrrolidone iodine in the local treatment of partial-thickness burn wounds. Ann Plast Surg 59: 423–427

[36] Iwuagwu FC, Wilson D, Bailie F (1999) The use of skin grafts in postburn contracture release: a 10-year review. Plast Reconstr Surg 103: 1198–1204

[37] Jang YC, Kwon OK, Lee JW, Oh SJ (2001) The optimal management of pediatric steam burn from electric rice-cooker: STSG or FTSG? J Burn Care Rehabil 22: 15–20

[38] Janzekovic Z (1970) A new concept in the early excision and immediate grafting of burns. J Trauma 10: 1103–1108

[39] Jeng JC, Bridgeman A, Shivnan L, Thornton PM, Alam H, Clarke TJ et al (2003) Laser Doppler imaging determines need for excision and grafting in advance of clinical judgement: a prospective blinded trial. Burns 29(7): 665–670

[40] Kamolz L, Andel H, Haslik W, Donner A, Winter W, Meissl G et al (2003) Indocyanine green video angiographies help to identify burns requiring operation. Burns 29: 785–791

[41] Kamolz LP, Luegmair M, Wick N, Eisenbock B, Burjak S, Koller R, Meissl G, Frey M (2005) The Viennese culture method: cultured human epithelium obtained on a dermal matrix based on fibroblast containing fibrin glue gels. Burns 31: 25–29

[42] Katz BE (1995) Silicone gel sheeting in scar therapy. Cutis 56: 65–67

[43] Kealey GP, Jensen KL, Laubenthal KN, Lewis RW (1990) Prospective randomized comparison of two types of pressure therapy garments. J Burn Care Rehabil 11: 334–336

[44] Kitzinger HB, Lanz U (2004) Die Anatomie der Fingergelenke. DAHTH 6: 3–11

[45] Klasen HJ (2000) A historical review of the use of silver in the treatment of burns. II. Renewed interest for silver. Burns 26: 131–138

[46] La Hei E, Holland A, Martin H (2006) Laser Doppler imaging of paediatric burns: burn wound outcome can be predicted independent of clinical examination. Burns 33: 550–553

[47] Levine BA, Sirinek KR, Peterson HD, Pruitt BA, Jr (1979) Efficacy of tangential excision and immediate autografting of deep second-degree burns of the hand. J Trauma 19: 670–673

[48] Logsetty S, Heimbach DM (2000) Modern techniques for wound coverage of the thermally injured upper extremity. Hand Clin 16: 205–214

[49] Luce EA (2000) The acute and subacute management of the burned hand. Clin Plast Surg 27: 49–63

[50] Matev IB (1980) Thumb reconstruction through metacarpal bone lengthening. J Hand Surg [Am] 5: 482–487

[51] McGregor IA, Jackson IT (1972) The groin flap. Br J Plast Surg 25: 3–16

[52] Monstrey S, Hoeksema H, Verbelen J, Pirayesh A, Blondeel P (2008) Assessment of burn depth and burn wound healing potential. Burns 34: 761–769

[53] Morel Fatio D (1961) Surgery of the skin. In: Tubiana R (ed) The hand. WB Saunders, Philadelphia, pp 224–225

[54] Oikarinen A, Autio P (1991) New aspects of the mechansim of costicosteroid-induced dermal atrophy. Clin Exp Derm 16: 416–419

[55] Ono I, Gunji H, Zhang JZ, Maruyama K, Kaneko F (1995) A study of cytokines in burn blister fluid related to wound healing. Burns 21: 352–355

[56] Pape S, Skouras C, Byrne P (2001) An audit of the use of laser Doppler imaging (LDI) in the assessment of burns of intermediate depth. Burns 27: 233–239

[57] Peacock EE (1953) Management of conditions of the hand requiring immobilization. Surg Clin North Am: 1297–1309

[58] Perkins K, Davey RB, Wallis KA (1983) Silicone gel: a new treatment for burn scars and contractures. Burns Incl Therm Inj 9: 201–204

[59] Philipp K, Giessler GA, Germann G, Sauerbier M (2005) Die akzidentelle thermische Verletzung der Hand. Unfallchirurg 108: 179–188

[60] Prasad JK, Bowden ML, Thomson PD (1991) A review of the reconstructive surgery needs of 3167 survivors of burn injury. Burns 17: 302–305

[61] Raff T, Hartmann B, Wagner H, Germann G (1996) Experience with the modified Meek technique. Acta Chir Plast 38: 142–146

[62] Raine TJ, Heggers JP, Robson MC, London MD, Johns L (1981) Cooling the burn wound to maintain microcirculation. J Trauma 21: 394–397

[63] Robson MC, Smith DJ, Jr, VanderZee AJ, Roberts L (1992) Making the burned hand functional. Clin Plast Surg 19: 663–671

[64] Salisbury RE, Levine NS (1976) The early management of upper extremity thermal injury. In: Salisbury RE, Priutt BA (eds) Burns of the upper extremity. WB Saunders, Philadelphia, pp 36–46

[65] Salisbury RE, McKeel DW, Mason AD, Jr (1974) Ischemic necrosis of the intrinsic muscles of the hand after thermal injuries. J Bone Joint Surg Am 56: 1701–1707

[66] Sauerbier M, Ofer N, Germann G, Baumeister S (2007) Microvascular reconstruction in burn and electrical burn injuries of the severely traumatized upper extremity. Plast Reconstr Surg 119: 605–615

[67] Schmidt H-M, Lanz U (2003) Chirurgische Anatomie der Hand. G. Thieme, Stuttgart

[68] Schwarze H, Kuntscher M, Uhlig C, Hierlemann H, Prantl L, Noack N, Hartmann B (2007) Suprathel, a new skin substitute, in the management of donor sites of split-thickness skin grafts: results of a clinical study. Burns 33: 850–854

[69] Sheridan RL, Hurley J, Smith MA, Ryan CM, Bondoc CC, Quinby WC, Jr, Tompkins RG, Burke JF (1995) The acutely burned hand: management and outcome based on a ten-year experience with 1047 acute hand burns. J Trauma 38: 406–411

[70] Smith MA, Munster AM, Spence RJ (1998) Burns of the hand and upper limb – a review. Burns 24: 493–505

[71] Tang YW (1992) Intraoperative and postoperative steroid injection for keloids and hypertrophic scars. Br J Plast Surg 45: 371–373

[72] Tubiana R, Roux JP (1974) Phalangization of the first and fifth metacarpals. Indications, operative technique, and results. J Bone Joint Surg Am 56: 447–457

[73] Uhlig C, Rapp M, Dittel KK (2007) Neue Strategien zur Behandlung thermisch geschädigter Haut unter Berücksichtigung des Epithelersatzes Suprathel®. Handchir Mikrochir Plast Chir 39: 314–319

[74] Uhlig C, Rapp M, Hartmann B, Hierlemann H, Planck H, Dittel KK (2007) Suprathel-an innovative, resorbable skin substitute for the treatment of burn victims. Burns 33: 221–229

[75] Ulkur E, Uygur F, Karagoz H, Celikoz B (2007) Flap choices to treat complex severe postburn hand contracture. Ann Plast Surg 58: 479–483

[76] Vogt PM, Kolokythas P, Niederbichler A, Knobloch K, Reimers K, Choi CY (2007) Innovative Wundtherapie und Hautersatz bei Verbrennungen. Chirurg 78: 335–342

[77] Wang XW, Wang NZ, Zhang OZ, Zapata-Sirvent RL, Davies JW (1985) Tissue deposition of silver following topical use of silver sulphadiazine in extensive burns. Burns Incl Therm Inj 11: 197–201

[78] Ward JW, Pensler JM, Parry SW (1985) Pollicization for thumb reconstruction in severe pediatric hand burns. Plast Reconstr Surg 76: 927–932

[79] Watts A, Tyler M, Perry M, Robberts A, McGrouther D (2001) Burn depth and its histological measurement. Burns 27: 154–160

[80] Weinzweig J, Gottlieb LJ, Krizek TJ (1994) Toxic shock syndrome associated with use of Biobrane in a scald burn victim. Burns 20: 180–181

[81] Weinzweig J, Weinzweig N (2004) Burns of the hand and upper extremity. In: Berger RA, Weiss A-PC (eds) Hand surgery. LWW, Philadelphia, pp 1073–1084

[82] Whitaker IS, Prowse S, Potokar TS (2008) A critical evaluation of the use of Biobrane as a biologic skin substitute: a versatile tool for the plastic and reconstructive surgeon. Ann Plast Surg 60: 333–337

[83] Witthaut J, Leclercq C (1998) Anatomy of the adductor pollicis muscle. A basis for release procedures for adduction contractures of the thumb. J Hand Surg [Br] 23: 380–383

[84] Wong L, Spence RJ (2000) Escharotomy and fasciotomy of the burned upper extremity. Hand Clin 16: 165–174, vii

[85] Zellner PR, Bugyi S (1985) Povidone-iodine in the treatment of burn patients. J Hosp Infect 6 Suppl A: 139–146

Correspondence: Hugo Benito Kitzinger, MD, Vienna Burn Centre, Division of Plastic and Reconstructive Surgery, Department of Surgery, Medical University of Vienna, Waehringer Guertel 18–20, 1090 Vienna, Austria, Tel: +43 1 40 400 6986, Fax: +43 1 40 400 6988, E-mail: hugo@kitzinger.de

Burn reconstruction
(Future perspectives)

Burn reconstruction – Future perspectives: Facial transplantation

Maria Siemionow[1], Fatih Zor[2]

[1] Department of Plastic Surgery, Cleveland Clinic, Cleveland, OH, USA
[2] Gulhane Military Medical Academy, Department of Plastic Surgery, Etlik, Ankara, Turkey

Introduction

Only a few fields in burn care are a greater challenge than the management of the burned face. The aesthetic and functional outcomes are critical to the patients' daily lives and are intimately related to their self-esteem. Many variables contribute to the ultimate aesthetic outcome, including the extent and depth of the injury, and preservation of critical areas, such as the oral commissure, mental crease, and canthal region. We will discuss face allotransplantation as an option for patients with severe facial burn injuries.

Burn injury in the 21st century

It has been estimated that there are around 500 000 burn victims requiring medical treatment each year in the United States, accounting for 40 000 hospitalizations per year [17]. Acute burn care, rehabilitation and reconstruction remain a major problem worldwide. Today, due to an advancement of acute burn wound coverage, intensive care management, new drug protocols and a better understanding of the pathophysiology of the burn wound, there was a significant decrease of burn related mortality. Patients with severe burn injuries, which were fatal in the past, now survive with deformities, opening a new reconstructive challenge. The anatomical regions most commonly involved in burn injuries are: upper extremities (70 %),

and head and neck region (50 %), which frequently results in long-term morbidity [26]. There are many patients who, despite the best efforts in burn resuscitation, treatment and rehabilitation, are not able to return to their normal social life and activities. Patients with severe facial burn injury exclude themselves from their professional and social lives.

The face is an extremely important medium through which one interacts with the rest of the world. The unique character of the facial skin and close anatomical and functional association with the underlying muscles allow for facial expression of emotions which is critical to social interactions. Since a person's identity is bound to the appearance of the face, sustaining major facial deformity is thus one of the most devastating injuries one can suffer from in terms of social interaction and quality of life.

Reconstruction of head and neck following burn injury is a great challenge but also opens great opportunities. Successful treatment of burn patients requires surgical judgment and technical expertise, as well as understanding of burn wound pathophysiology and development of wound contractures. Burn injuries constrict and deform the face, distorting its features, proportions and expression. Burns also alter the surface of the facial mask due to scarring as well as due to alteration of facial skin texture and pigmentation. These changes of the skin surface need reconstruction, however the real challenge is created by the changes in facial proportion, and functional expression [14].

Table 1. Stigmata of facial burn injury

- Ectropion of lower eyelid
- Short nose
- Alar flaring of the nose
- Short and retruded upper lip
- Eversion and inferior displacement of lower lip
- Flat and stiff facial features
- Loss of jawline

Evaluation of facial burn deformities

Facial burn reconstruction should be based on an overall strategy and clear understanding of the underlying functional deformity. Following a deep second- and third-degree burn injury of the face, the wound healing process involves epithelialization and wound contraction. The degree of contraction depends on the severity of the injury and treatment modalities. Due to the effect of contracting forces, facial structures are gradually deformed resulting in the characteristic appearance of a burned face. These severe deformities are to a variable degree similar for all facial burns and constitute the stigmata of facial burn injury (Table 1). The eyelids are distorted by ectropion, the nose is shortened with flaring of the ala, the upper lip is shortened and retruded with loss of the philtral contour, the lower lip is everted and inferiorly displaced, and the lower lip is wider than the upper lip on the anterior view. The tissues of the face and neck appear in the same plane with loss of jaw line definition. The severity of these changes is proportional to the severity of the burn trauma. Fortunately, the majority of facial burn injuries are not severe and do not involve the entire face. Patients with facial burn injuries can be divided into two different categories according to the severity of the injury as described in Table 2. Type I deformities consist of essentially normal facial features with localized scarring with or without contractures. Type II deformities are found in a much smaller number of patients and represent "pan-facial" burn deformities presenting some or all characteristics of facial burn stigmata [12]. There are many techniques which have been described for the reconstruction of facial subunits such as nose [5, 6], ears [7, 28], eyelids [30], scalp [21], mouth [27] and neck [23, 25]. However, only a few articles report a total reconstruction of the

Table 2. Facial burn categories

Type I:	Essentially normal faces with local burn scarring with or without contractures
Type II:	Pan-facial burn deformities with some or all stigmata of facial burns

burned face [3, 8]. The functional and aesthetic outcomes of conventional techniques are less than optimal and the management of most severe injuries is challenging and outcomes are often questionable.

Conventional reconstructive methods

The human face is a demanding structure to reconstruct because it represents unique subunits, texture, and functions. The face also plays a central role in our daily interactions through its expression of feelings, beauty, and identity. Therefore, it is essential in social interaction. As a result, face trauma and disfigurement caused by burns, tumor resection, and congenital malformations have deleterious effects on a person's life. Reconstruction of severe facial deformities following deep burns is a challenge for surgeons, who wish to reliably restore facial function and appearance. Current reconstructive procedures for facial deformity include combinations of standard skin grafting, application of local flaps, tissue expansion, prefabrication, and free tissue transfers (Table 3) [2, 4, 9, 15, 20, 27, 29, 34]. Although these severely injured patients are subjected to multiple surgical interventions, the functional and aesthetic outcomes of currently available conventional reconstructive procedures are less than optimal. Particularly difficult are long term follow-ups since quite often the result is a tight, mask-like face with a lack of facial expression and an unsatisfactory cosmetic outcome [8]. In cases involving large and wide areas of the burned face including scarring of the adjacent tissue there are only limited options to provide reconstruction with soft, thin and pliable tissue. The best result of facial reconstruction was reported following replantation of the avulsed scalp and face where normal animation and facial expression were achieved as well as adequate hair growth on the scalp [37]. Current methods of face reconstruction fail when tissue loss is considerable, because the body does not

Table 3. Techniques available for burn reconstruction

1. Without deficiency of tissue

    Excision and primary closure

    Z-plasty

2. With deficiency of tissue

    Simple reconstruction
    – Skin graft
    – Transposition flaps (Z-plasty and modifications)

    Reconstruction of skin and underlying tissues
    – Axial and random flaps
    – Myocutaneous flaps
    – Tissue expansion
    – Free flaps

provide tissue possessing the texture, pliability, and complexity of the human face. For this reason, in severe cases the only option for restoring facial features and functions in severely disfigured patients remains the transplantation of a face from a human donor.

Composite tissue allotransplantation and face transplantation

Composite tissue allotransplantation (CTA) involves transplantation of tissue, derived from ectoderm and mesoderm. It typically contains skin, fat, muscle, nerves, lymph nodes, bone, cartilage, ligaments, and bone marrow as opposed to a single tissue organ which is the case in conventional solid organ transplantation (SOT). An example of CTA is limb transplantation, in which the transplanted graft includes skin, muscle, nerve, blood vessels, and bone. The function and the immunologic properties of the composite tissue transplant are more difficult to define, because each individual component has its own unique characteristics that ultimately affect the successful outcome of the transplantation. Most applications of CTA predominantly improve the quality of life for non-life-threatening conditions and aim to restore anatomic, cosmetic, and functional integrity. The benefits gathered by such procedures have to be balanced against the morbidity of the surgical procedure itself and a long-term immunosuppression therapy.

Advances in composite tissue allograft transplantation have opened a new era in the field of re-

constructive surgery. In 1998, after report on the first successful hand transplantation in France, the field of CTA has further developed opening new alternatives for facial reconstruction [13].

On 27 November 2005, in Amiens, France, a surgical team led by Dr. Bernard Devauchelle and Jean-Michel Dubernard announced that they had performed a partial face transplant on a 38-year-old female, whose face had been disfigured by a dog bite [11]. Up to now, a total of 9 face transplantations have been performed worldwide in France, China, USA and Spain [16, 18, 35, 36].

The world's first near total face transplantation was performed in Cleveland in December, 2008 by a team led by Dr. Maria Siemionow [31]. The patient was a 45-year-old woman who suffered from severe facial trauma to her midface from a close-range shotgun blast in September 2004. Her facial deformities included absence of nose, nasal lining and underlying bone; contracted remnants of the upper lip; loss of orbicularis oris and orbicularis oculi muscle functions; distorted and scarred lower eyelids with ectropion; right-eye enucleation supported by eye prosthesis and facial nerve deficit manifested by the lack of midface function. Before face transplantation, the patient had undergone 23 major autologous reconstructive operations that included correction of bone defect by free fibula and split-calvaria/rib grafts, soft-tissue defect by anterolateral free flap, temporalis muscle flap, paramedian forehead flap, and radial forearm free flap and skin defect by multiple split-thickness skin grafts. The donor was a brain-dead woman who matched the patient in age, race, and skin complexion. The allograft was designed to cover the recipient's anterior craniofacial skeleton, and it included about 80 % of the surface area of the anterior face. It was based on a Le Fort III composite tissue allograft containing total nose, lower eyelids, upper lip, total infraorbital floor, bilateral zygomas, and anterior maxilla with incisors, and included total alveolus, anterior hard palate, and bilateral parotid glands [31, 32] (Fig. 1). The allotransplant inset to the recipient started with the adjustments of a Le Fort III composite allograft to the recipient's skeletal defect. Once bone components of the facial allograft were secured and stable, bilateral microvascular anastomoses of both arteries and veins were performed. Once craniofacial skeleton was intact, the

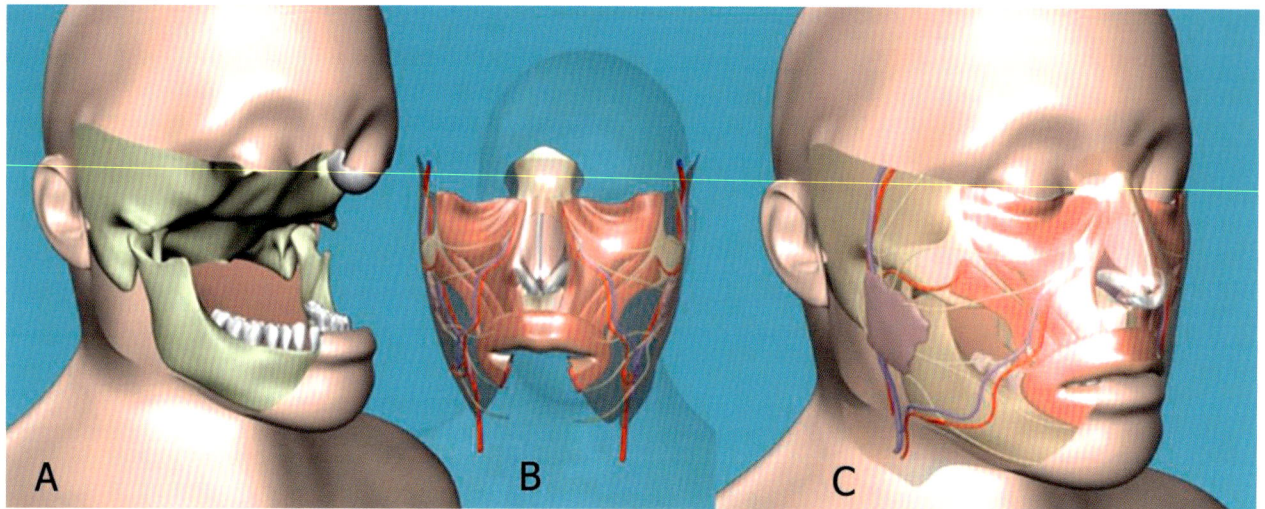

Fig. 1. Illustration of the first U. S. near -total human face transplantation.
A. Facial defect following resection of the scars.
B. Composite tissue allograft including nose, lower eyelids and upper lip.
C. Reconstruction of the facial defect.

bilateral facial nerves were connected using standard epineural repair. First, the donor's vagus nerve, taken as an interpositional graft, was attached to the upper division of the trunk of the right side of the recipient's facial nerve. On the left side, the donor's hypoglossal nerve, used as an interpositional graft, was attached to the upper division of the trunk on the recipient's facial nerve. Both grafts were connected to the main trunk of the donor nerve. Then, porous polyethylene implants were used to reconstruct orbital floors. Finally, the lower eyelids, including the recipient's conjunctiva and lash lines, were reconstructed bilaterally using donor eyelid skin. The composite facial allograft inset was completed after skin closure. Induction of immunosuppression was carried out with rabbit anti-thymocyte globulin (1×2 mg/kg intravenously once a day for 9 days) in combination with methylprednisolone 1000 mg bolus intravenously on the day of transplant, and rapidly tapered thereafter. The immunosuppressive regimen was maintained with tacrolimus, mycophenolate mofetil, and low-dose oral prednisone.

After 9 months, sensory discrimination returned to the entire facial skin, as measured by pressure-specified sensory device presence of two-point sensory discrimination at the area under the lower eye-

lids, upper lip, and the tip of the nose on both sides of the graft. Motor recovery included improved facial mimetics with asymmetric smile and upper lip occlusion.

Functional recovery of this three-dimensional facial defect is excellent, with restoration of major missing functions such as eating solid food without the need of a gastric-tube, drinking from a cup, and restoration of intelligible speech after hard palate reconstruction with composite allograft and palatal obturator support. At 1 year post-transplant aesthetic outcome is improved by excision of the redundant skin and subcutaneous tissues. Psychologically, the patient is doing well without symptoms of depression or post-traumatic stress disorder. Finally, her pain level was significantly reduced since scarred and contracted tissue within the face were removed during face transplantation [31].

The first application of face transplantation in burn patient was reported by Dr. Lantieri in April 2009 in Paris. The entire upper face including nose, eyelids, forehead, scalp and ears as well as bilateral hands were transplanted to a burn victim from a male donor [19]. Unfortunately, nearly 2 months after transplantation, the patient died due to complications including severe infection and heart failure [10].

Face transplantation in facial burn reconstruction

Based on current reports on successful face transplantation, it is obvious that face transplantation meets all criteria needed for an excellent reconstruction of a burned face. However, both the face transplantation as well as facial burn reconstruction bring about very unique challenges and issues: facial transplantation involves immunological, psychological and ethical issues which may interfere with burn reconstruction. On the other hand, the conventional reconstruction of a burned face is limited by timing of the reconstruction, by development of scar tissue and skin contracture and by the need for reconstruction of specific functional units which may interfere with facial transplantation.

Indications for burned face reconstruction

It is helpful to categorize facial plastic surgery procedures in burned patients as urgent, essential and desirable. Urgent procedures are commonly performed during the acute phase. These include flap reconstruction to cover exposed bones and vital organs or to allow for mouth opening to facilitate feeding. Essential procedures are carried out to restore function. Examples include e. g. neck release and ectropion repair. It is most desirable for the patients to restore the normal facial appearance. Examples are nasal reconstruction, ear reconstruction and scalp reconstruction. Today, face transplantation is still considered an experimental procedure and may be indicated as the last therapeutic option for severely disfigured patients to restore major functional deficits of the burned face.

For this reason face transplantation should not be considered as an emergency procedure neither in trauma nor in the burn patient.

Timing of burned face reconstruction

The timing of reconstructive plastic surgery following facial burn injuries falls into three separate phases: acute, intermediate and late phase. Acute reconstructive surgery takes place during the first months after burn injury and includes urgent procedures which are required to facilitate patient care or

to prevent the development of contractures, which could lead to permanent functional damage. Acute reconstructive intervention is most frequently indicated in the eyelid, perioral and cervical regions. Intermediate reconstructive surgery is performed months or years after burn injury when wounds are closed and scar maturation process is completed. Finally, late phase reconstruction is performed many years after burn injury. Considering reconstructive ladder in burn patient, face transplantation seems to be appropriate for late phase reconstruction in cases where conventional options have failed. With current advances in composite tissue allotransplantation, indications for face transplantation in burn patients may be considered during intermediate or even acute phase of treatment in the near future.

Reconstruction of specific facial regions

Facial deformity can be divided into three categories: peripheral only, central only or combined peripheral and central [33]. Although many techniques are described for reconstruction of peripheral and central deformities, no satisfying method for facial reconstruction after burn injury is available today. This is even more challenging when considering burn injury in the central face which includes the most important aesthetic units as the lower lip and chin, upper lip, nose, and bilateral upper and lower eyelids. These facial units have both aesthetic and functional features and the surgical outcome is directly related to the number and function of the units which are involved.

Large facial burn deformities are almost always a combined type of deformities affecting both the peripheral and central areas of the face. Usually, following burn injury, there is a limited access to the normal facial skin which is left for potential reconstruction. Currently, tissue expansion and microsurgical tissue transfer are the only reconstructive options in these complex cases. However, these techniques are useful for the coverage of skin defect and are far from meeting the actual need for functional reconstruction of the facial burn. Functional units such as nose, periorbital and perioral areas are hard to reconstruct by means of tissue expansion and microsurgical tissue transfer because of the limited availability of donor tissue and texture mismatch.

Facial transplantation provides a unique opportunity to reconstruct the structures of a burned face with the same structures coming from a human donor. Today, only one patient with facial burn was reconstructed using face allograft transplantation [19]. The allograft included the entire upper face, nose, eyelids, forehead, scalp and ears. In addition due to amputation of both hands during burn accident, this patient received simultaneously bilateral hand transplantation from the same donor. Unfortunately, the patient died at 2 months post-transplant due to severe infection and cardiac arrest [10]. It is clear that more clinical cases are needed to address the long term outcomes of facial transplantation in burn patients. Mathes et al performed a survey on North American burn and plastic surgeons on their attitudes toward facial transplantation. The survey report concluded that CTA should be supported in reconstruction of complex facial deformities [22].

Immunological issues

The major concern in composite tissue allotransplantation is to prevent rejection of the transplanted allograft. Although there are different immunosuppressive protocols used to overcome rejection, the ultimate goal is to develop a donor specific tolerance to avoid the need for life-long immunosuppression. The immunologic status of the patient is quite important for the success of the CTA. In this context burn patients are different from other trauma patients since extensive burn injury affects all organs including the immune system. During the acute period following burn injury a systemic immunosuppression develops. During this early period skin allograft take without additional immunosuppression was reported [1]. There is however, a lack of studies describing immunological challenges following burn injury. Patients with major burns are often subjected to transfusion of blood and blood products such as fresh frozen plasma. The long term effect of these therapies on immunological responses in case of face transplantation is still unknown. The same is true for early wound coverage with cadaver skin allograft which may result in patient presensitization and have potential impact on the outcome of CTA. So far, there is only one study reporting delayed immunosuppression up to 3.5 months following major burn injury.

So, more research and clinical studies are needed to further evaluate immunological sequel of severe burn injury [24].

Conclusion

Severe burn injuries at the head and neck region often result in deep tissue damage with development of scarring, contracture, and functional loss. Thus, the primary goal of facial burn reconstruction should be functional restoration and optimal aesthetic outcome. Currently available techniques are limited in providing complex tridimensional craniofacial reconstruction due to the lack of facial-like tissues and lack of facial subunits in our own body.

Facial transplantation would provide such a unique reconstructive option, however life-long immunosuppression is required afterwards.

With the advancements in the transplant immunology and development of the donor specific tolerance, face transplantation may replace most of conventional reconstructive methods and may be considered as an alternative reconstructive option for severely burned patients.

References

[1] Achauer BM, Hewitt CW, Black KS, Martinez SE, Waxman KS, Ott RA, Furnas DW (1986) Long-term skin allograft survival after short-term cyclosporin treatment in a patient with massive burns. Lancet 1(8471): 14–15

[2] Achauer BM (1992) Reconstructing the burned face. Clin Plast Surg 19: 623–636

[3] Angrigiani C, Grilli D (1997) Total face reconstruction with one free flap. Plast Reconstr Surg 99: 1566–1575

[4] Baumeister S, Koller M, Dragu A, Germann G, Sauerbier M (2005) Principles of microvascular reconstruction in burn and electrical burn injuries. Burns 31: 92–98

[5] Benmeir P, Neuman A, Weinberg A, Rotem M, Eldad A, Lusthaus S, Kaplan H, Wexler MR (1991) Reconstruction of a completely burned nose by a free dorsalis pedis flap. Br J Plast Surg 44: 570–571

[6] Bernard SL (2000) Reconstruction of the burned nose and ear. Clin Plast Surg 27: 97–112

[7] Bhandari PS (1998) Total ear reconstruction in post-burn deformity. Burns 24: 661–670

[8] Birgfeld CB, Low DW (2006) Total face reconstruction using a preexpanded, bilateral, extended, parascapular free flap. Ann Plast Surg 56: 565–568

[9] Celikoz B, Deveci M, Duman H, Nisanci M (2001) Reconstruction of facial defects and burn scars using large size freehand full-thickness skin graft from lateral thoracic region. Burns 27: 174–178

[10] Daily Telegraph webpage. Website home page. http://www.dailytelegraph.com. au/news/world/worlds-first-face-and-and-double-hand-transplant-patient-dies-in-france/story-e6frev00-1225736077918. Accessed 2009, November 26

[11] Devauchelle N, Badet L, Lengele B, Morelon E, Testelin S, Michallet M, D'Hauthuille C, Dubernard JM (2006) First human face allograft: early report. Lancet 368: 203–209

[12] Donelan MB (2007) Reconstruction of head and neck. In: Herndon D (ed) Total burn care, 3rd edn. Elsevier, pp 701–718, ISBN: 978-1-4160-3274-8

[13] Dubernard JM, Owen E, Herzberg G, Lanzetta M, Martin X, Kapila H, Dawahra M, Hakim NS (1999) Human hand allograft: report on first 6 months. Lancet 353: 1315–1320

[14] Engrav L, Donelan MB (1997) Face burns: Acute care and reconstruction. Operative Techniques in Plastic and Reconstructive Surgery 4: 53–85

[15] Feldman JJ (1990) Facial burns. In: McCarthy JG (ed) Plastic surgery, vol 3. Philadelphia, PA, Saunders, pp 2153–2236

[16] Guo S, Han Y, Zhnag X Lu B, Yi C, Zhang H, Ma X, Wang D, Yang L, Fan X, Liu Y, Lu K, Li H (2008) Human facial allotransplantation: A-2 year follow-up study. Lancet 372: 631–638

[17] http://www.ameriburn. org/resources_factsheet. php, American Burn Association, Burn Incidence Fact Sheet, Accessed: August 23, 2009

[18] International Registry of Hand and Composite Tissue Transplantation. Hand Registry home website page. http://www.handregistry.com. Accessed 2009, November 28

[19] Lantieri L, Meningaud JP, Grimbert P, Bellivier F, Lefaucheur JP, Ortonne N, Benjoar MD, Lang P, Wolkenstein P (2008) Repair of the lower and middle parts of the face by composite tissue allotransplantation in a patient with massive plexiform neurofibroma: a 1-year follow-up study. Lancet 372: 639–645

[20] Latifoglu O, Ayhan S, Atabay K (1999) Total face reconstruction: Skin graft versus free flap. Plast Reconstr Surg 103: 1076–1078

[21] Mangubat EA (2008) Scalp reconstruction and repair. Facial Plast Surg 24: 428–445

[22] Mathes DW, Kumar N, Ploplys E (2009) A survey of North American burn and plastic surgeons on their current attitudes toward facial transplantation. J Am Coll Surg 208: 1051–1058

[23] Ninkovic M, Moser-Rumer A, Ninkovic M, Spanio S, Rainer C, Gurunluoglu R (2004) Anterior neck reconstruction with pre-expanded free groin and scapular flaps. Plast Reconstr Surg 113: 61–68

[24] Parment K, Zetterberg A, Ernerudh J, Bakteman K, Steinwall I, Sjoberg F (2007) Long-term immunosuppression in burned patients assessed by in vitro neutrophil oxidative burst (Phagoburst). Burns 33: 865–871

[25] Parrett BM, Pomahac B, Orgill DP, Pribaz (2007) The role of free-tissue transfer for head and neck burn reconstruction. Plast Reconstr Surg 120: 1871–1878

[26] Prasad JK, Bowden ML, Thomson PD (1991) A review of the reconstructive surgery needs of 3167 survivors of burn injury. Burns 17: 302–305

[27] Pribaz JJ, Weiss DD, Mulliken JB, Eriksson E (1999) Prelaminated free flap reconstruction of complex central facial defects. Plast Reconstr Surg 104: 357–365

[28] Rosenthal JS (1992) The thermally injured ear: A systematic approach to reconstruction. Vogt PM. Clin Plast Surg 19: 645–661

[29] Santanelli F, Grippaudo FR, Ziccardi P, Onesti MG (1997) The role of pre-expanded free flaps in revision of burn scarring. Burns 23: 620–625

[30] Sassoon EM, Codner MA (1999) Eyelid reconstruction. Operative Techniques in Plastic and Reconstructive Surgery 6: 250–264

[31] Siemionow M, Papay F, Alam D, Bernard S, Djohan R, Gordon C, Hendrickson M, Lohman R, Eghtesad B, Coffman K, Kodish E, Paradis C, Avery R, Fung J (2009) Near-total human face transplantation for a severely disfigured patient in the USA. Lancet 374: 203–209

[32] Siemionow M, Papay F, Djohan R, Bernard S, Gordon CR, Alam D, Hendrickson M, Lohman R, Eghtesad B, Fung J (2009) First U. S. near-total human face transplantation – a paradigm shift for massive complex injuries. Plast Reconstr Surg Nov 13 [Epub ahead of print]

[33] Spence RJ C (2008) The challenge of reconstruction for severe facial burn deformity. Plast Surg Nurs 28: 71–76

[34] Teot L, Cherenfant E, Otman S, Giovannini UM (2000) Prefabricated vascularised supraclavicular flaps for face resurfacing after postburns scarring. Lancet 355: 1695–1696

[35] Usatoday webpage. Website home page. http://www.usatoday.com/news/health/2009-08-22-spain-face-transplant_N.htm Accessed 2009, November 28

[36] Usatoday webpage. Website home page. http://www.usatoday.com/news/nation/2009-04-10-face-transplant_N.htm Accessed 2009, November 28

[37] Wilhelmi BJ, Kang RH, Movassaghi K, Ganchi PA, Lee WP (2003) First successful replantation of face and scalp with single-artery repair: model for face and scalp transplantation. Ann Plast Surg 50: 535–540

Correspondence: Maria Siemionow, M. D., Ph. D., D. Sc, Department of Plastic Surgery, Cleveland Clinic, 9500 Euclid Avenue, A-60, Cleveland, OH 44 195, USA, Tel: 216 445 2405, Fax: 216 444 9419, E-mail: siemiom@ccf.org

Modern myoprostheses in electric burn injuries of the upper extremity

Oskar C. Aszmann[1], Hans Dietl[2], Tatjana Paternostro[3], Manfred Frey[1]

[1] Division of Plastic and Reconstructive Surgery, Department of Surgery, Medical University of Vienna, Austria
[2] Division of Research & Development, Otto Bock HealthCare Products, Vienna, Austria
[3] Department of Physiotherapy and Rehabilitation, Medical University of Vienna, Austria

Electrical burn injuries typically comprise only a small percentage of the total admissions to major burn centers. In the Vienna Burn Unit this is about 5 % per annum. Unlike the rest of burn victims electrical burns almost always affect primarily young adult men. Most of these injuries are work related. In the US these injuries account for nearly 6 % of all occupational fatalities per year, which also reflects the severity of this injury [7]. In Europe another common way of injury is "train surfing" during which the individuals get too close to the power lines and get struck by the electric current. This is not necessarily done in a suicide attempt, but rather as a special kind of high-risk test of courage. In a recent publication 41 such accidents were reported within a 15 year period in Berlin with 14 fatalities [11].

Electrical injuries have several unique characteristics that differ from other thermal injuries and require expertise in surgical and anesthesiological management, which is described elsewhere in this book. The most momentous fact however is that they are the most frequent cause of extremity amputations in a burn service. This affects the upper and the lower extremity alike, depending what route the electric current travelled through the body [6]. In regards to the specific surgical treatment of such an injury it is of utmost importance that a fasciotomy is performed as early as possible and as ample as necessary. Since the electrical current travels through the deep tissues more readily, the surface markings are only the tip of the iceberg and do not reveal the immense damage hidden in the deep. If a fasciotomy is deemed necessary, all compartments need to be opened. In the hand all intrinsic compartments, the carpal tunnel, superficial and the deep forearm as well as the dorsal compartment need to be opened through separate incisions. These injuries all call for a second and third look until one can be sure that the climax of tissue damage is overcome. Even at this stage of treatment one must have the biological and technical reconstructive possibilities in mind. If an amputation of the upper extremity at any level is necessary one must be aware that every joint preserved adds several degrees of freedom and every inch of length adds stability to a given prosthetic device. These are not diabetic patients with recurrent ulcerations where an amputation is almost an inevitable consequence, but a sudden massive assault to an extremity of an otherwise healthy and most often young individual (Fig. 1 A, B). One should therefore tap the entire spectrum of reconstructive surgery to maintain length and definitely think twice before resecting a joint (Fig. 2 A, B). Since often both upper extremities are affected, a preserved limb, even if without any function, can at a later stage be used as a biological spare part donor site for the contralateral extremity (Fig. 3 A–D).

If all reconstructive measures fail, myoelectric prostheses are a promising resort to go to. In recent years these have been improved tremendously by in-

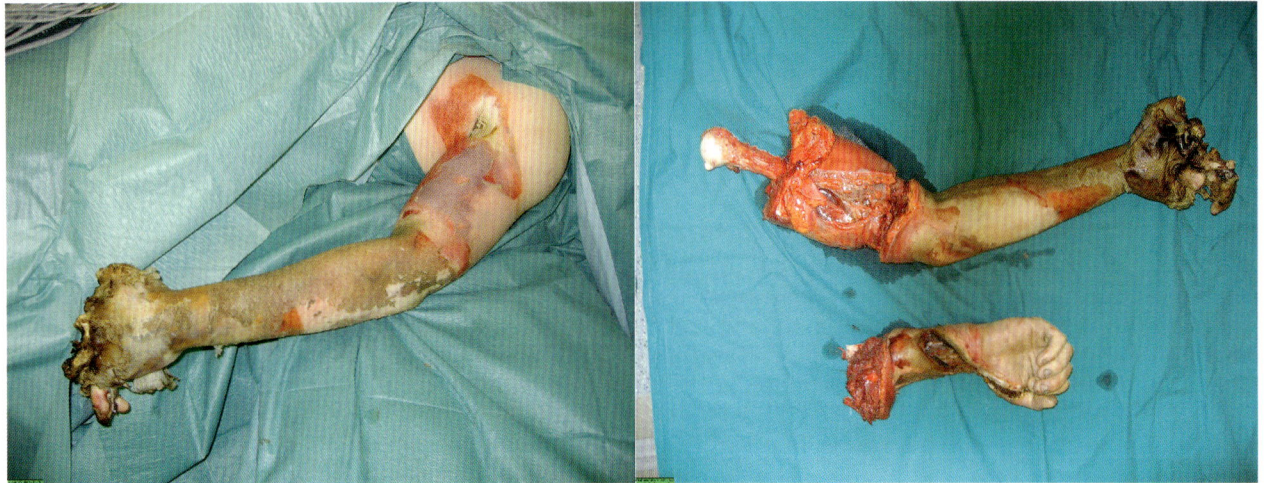

Fig. 1 A, B. Electrical burn injury of an 18 yrs old young man. All four extremities were affected, leading to multiple amputations with loss of both upper extremities

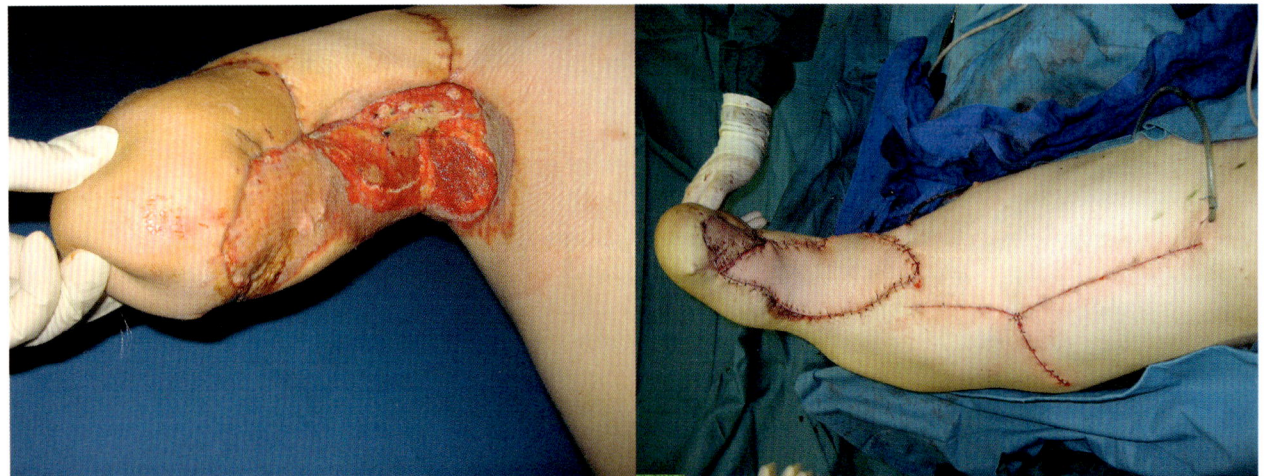

Fig. 2 A, B. Preservation of stump length by investment of fleur de lile latissimus dorsi flap

troducing targeted muscle transfers (TMR) to the armamentarium of reconstructive surgery [1, 4, 5, 8]. Depending at what level the extremity has been amputated, several options are possible to enlarge the "neurological landscape" of the amputated extremity. The more functional neuromuscular units can be established the better the myoelectric prosthesis can be governed. Modern myoelectric prostheses have multiple degrees of freedom that mandate a complex controll system to provide dependable use for the patient. To date, the movement of myoelectrical arm prostheses proceeds via two transcutaneous electrodes that are controlled by two separately innervat-

ed muscle groups. The various control levels are chosen by co-contractions of these muscles and the

Fig. 3 A–F. Work related electrical burn injury of both hands of a 20 yrs old young man. All four extremities were affected with loss of the thumb and III finger of the right hand and loss of all internal structures of the left forearm. To preserve the left hand a groin flap was invested after final debridement. At a later stage the IV finger of the left hand was used as a free graft to reconstruct the thumb of the right hand. Six months later an ALT flap was invested at the left hand to augment soft tissue coverage and reconstruct tendons to the I–III finger with vascularized fascia lata strips. Furthermore, the ulnar nerve was used to reconstruct the median nerve in the same session

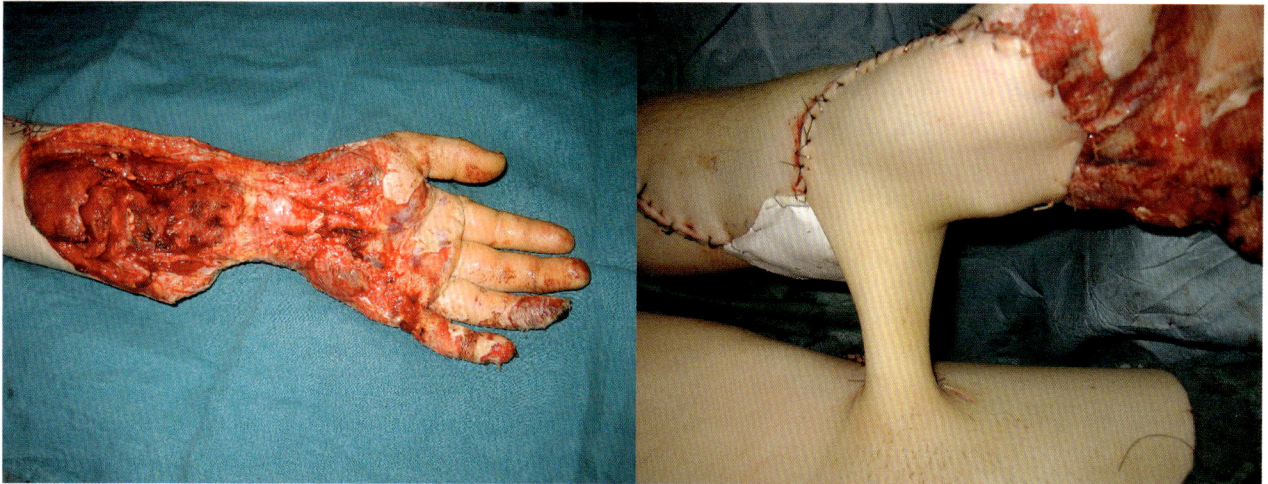

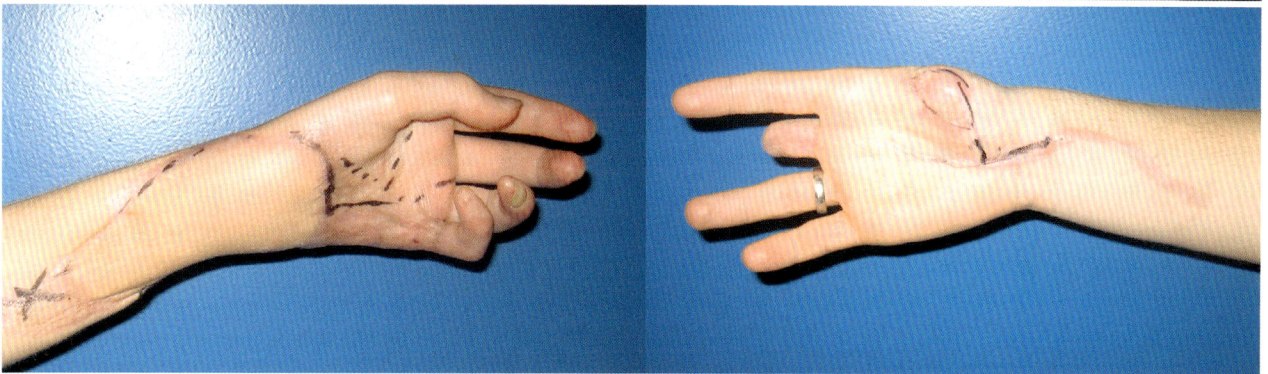

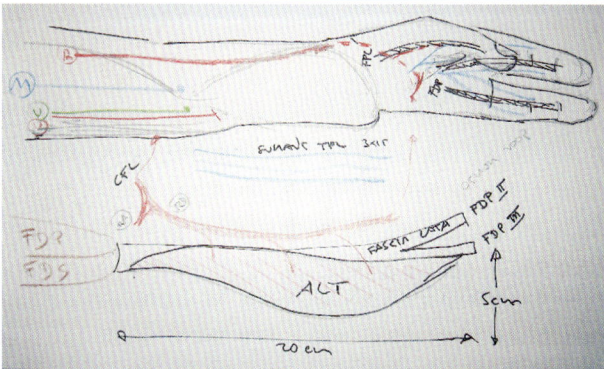

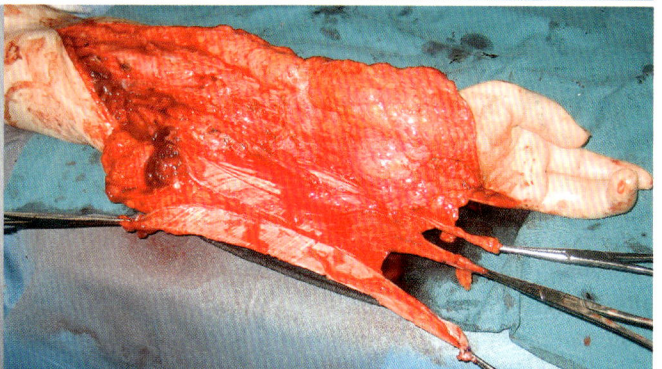

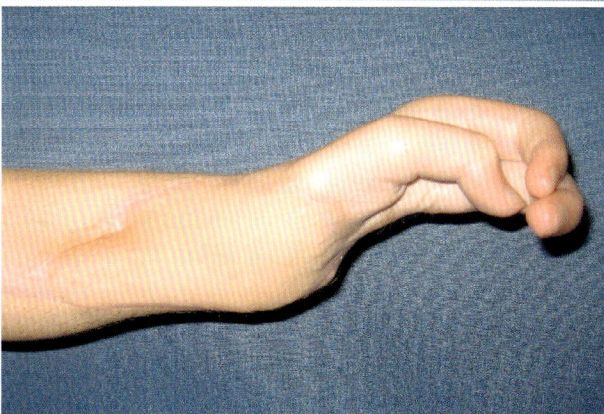

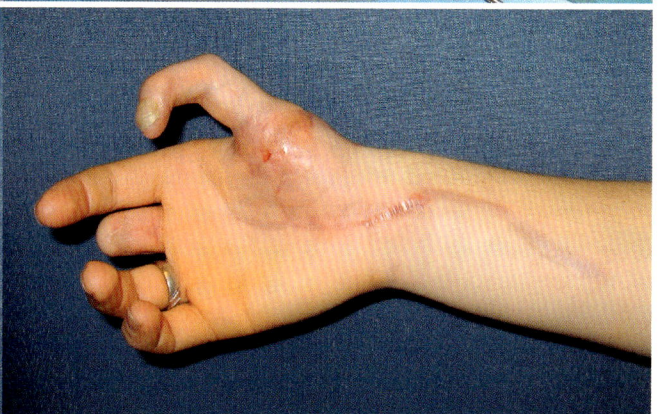

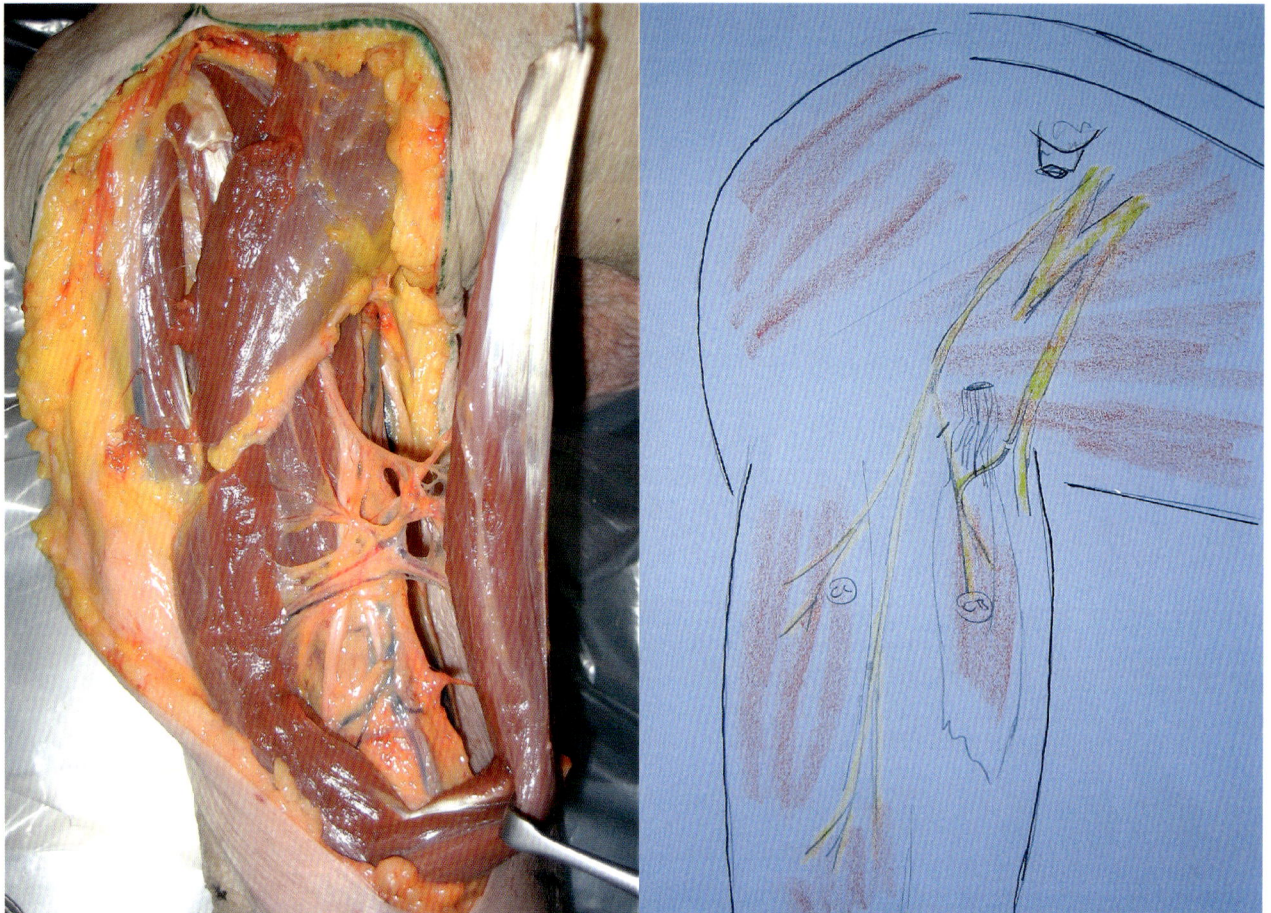

Fig. 4 A, B. Anatomical situs showing the short head of the biceps with its own neurovascular supply. The schematic drawing depicts the selective nerve transfer from the ulnar nerve to the nerve branch of the short head of the biceps

respective level is linearly controlled by the same muscles. A harmonious course of movement as in the corresponding natural pattern of motion is not possible. An appreciable improvement would be given if the individual movement levels could be governed by signals that correspond with the natural pattern of motion. Just recently, prostheses with seven degrees of freedom have been technically realised. The objective is to separate the major arm nerves, such as the musculocutaneous nerve, radial nerve, median nerve and ulnar nerve, from the proximal arm plexus and to transfer them to the residual nerve branches of remaining muscles in the environment of the stump in order to create meaningful neuromuscular units, that can serve as impulse generators for the myoelectrical prosthesis. In the transradial amputee an array of muscles is still available that suffice to

drive a prosthesis with two to four degrees of freedom. In the transhumeral amputee a maximum of six degrees of freedom is necessary to provide good intuitive function. However, only two muscle groups are available. Elbow flexors and elbow extensors. Expendable muscles are the short head of the bizeps on the ventral surface and the lateral head of the triceps on the dorsal aspect of the arm. Depending on the level of amputation possibly the brachialis muscle is still present and can also be used as a target muscle. In a recent anatomical study we have analyzed the feasibility of nerve transfers to these muscles in order to create two additional myoelectrical signals in the transhumeral amputee (Fig. 4 A, B). Similar to an Oberlin transfer, a fascicle of the ulnar nerve can be transferred to the motor branch of the short head of the bizeps. This will allow intrinsic function (grasp-

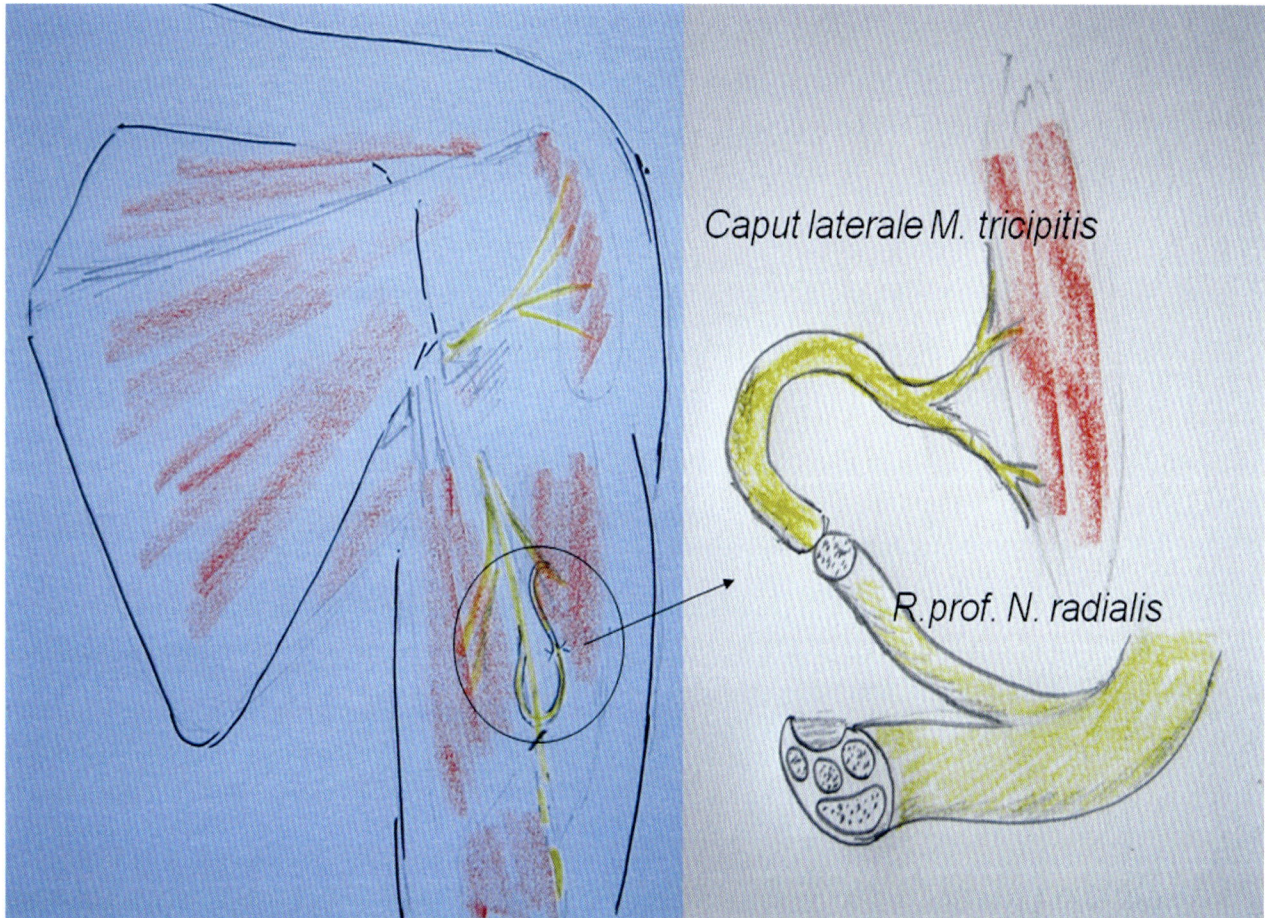

Fig. 5 A, B. The schematic drawing depicts the selective nerve transfer from the deep branch of the radial nerve to the nerve branch of the lateral head of the triceps

ing) to be represented as a signal in the arm. Respectively a part of the radial nerve can be rerouted to the motor branch of the lateral head of the triceps to establish hand/finger extension (Fig. 5 A, B). Finally, if the brachialis is still available parts of the median nerve can be coapted to this motor branch to either establish pronation or extrinsic fingerflexion. The elegance of this protocol is that all signals can be picked up with electrodes embedded in the shaft of the prostheses and allow direct, independent and intuitive control of all relevant functions of the prosthesis. Since these nerve transfers are all done very proximal, these are feasible for all transhumeral amputees without the need of nerve grafts. The limiting factor for these patients is more the length of the stump in regards to sufficient shaft stability. Anything proximal to the deltoid tuberosity will present a consider-

able challenge to the prosthetist and may benefit from a stump lengthening protocol. The goal must be unrestricted shoulder movement with sufficient active stability of the prosthesis. If this goal is not achievable, or the amputation is higher or even at the glenohumeral joint level, then the shaft of the prosthesis must also encompass the entire shoulder for reasons of stability (Fig. 6 A–D). This fitting restricts independent movement of the shoulder (if this joint should still be present) however, it opens up a greater surface with a lot more options for selective nerve transfers. The different parts of the major and minor pectoral muscles at the ventral body surface and the latissimus dorsi at the posterior body surface are accessible. In an anatomical study done a few years ago we have analyzed the detailed anatomy of the pectoral nerves and have found that the clavicular, the ster-

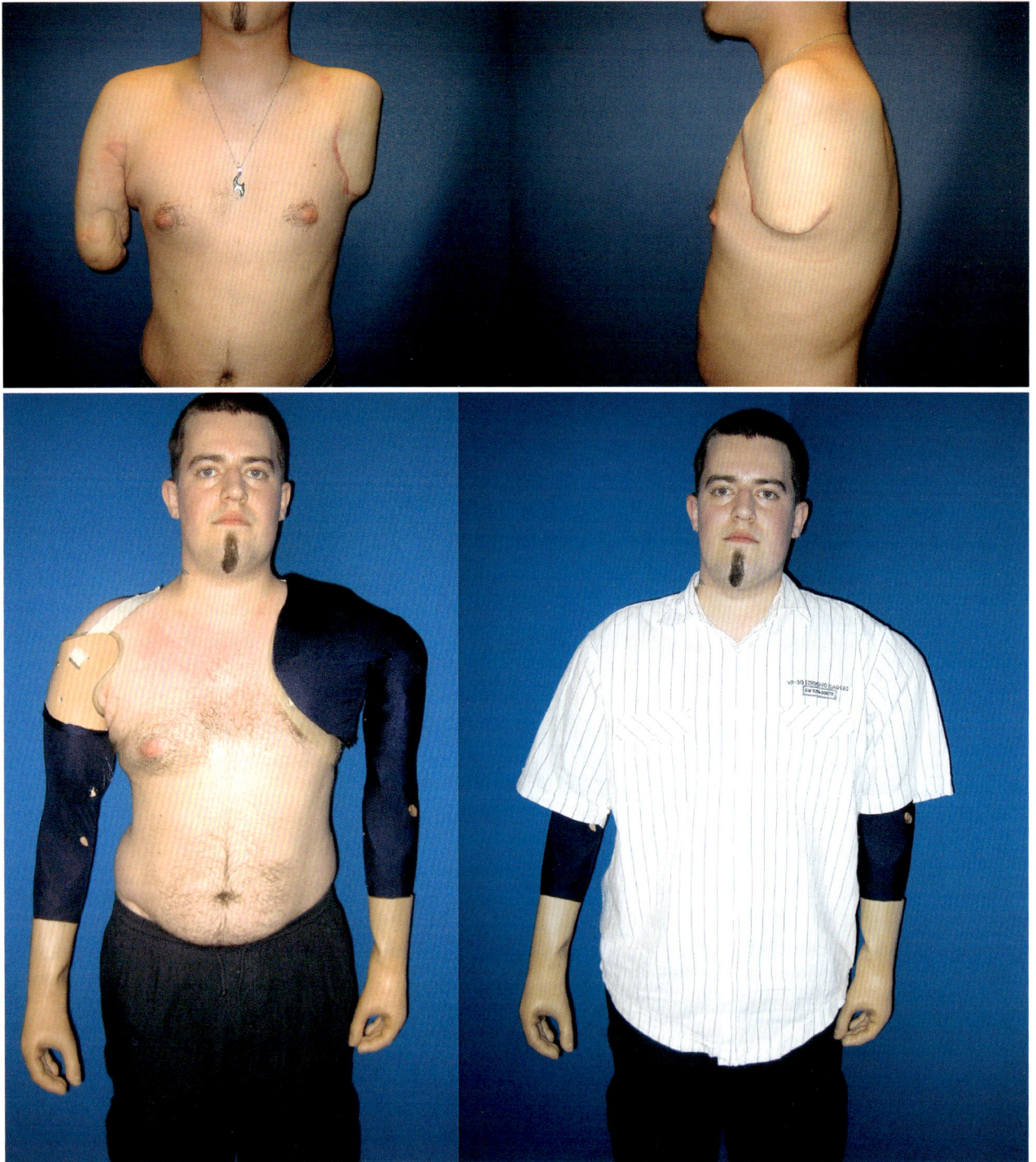

Fig. 6 A–D. Transhumeral amputation of the right arm and glenohumeral disarticulation of the left arm. The fitting of the left arm must encompass the shoulder and part of the thorax for both reasons of stability and placement of pick-up electrodes. Both fittings are connected with a shoulder strap to help balancing both prostheses. Note also that the left arm is shorter for reasons of weight and leverance

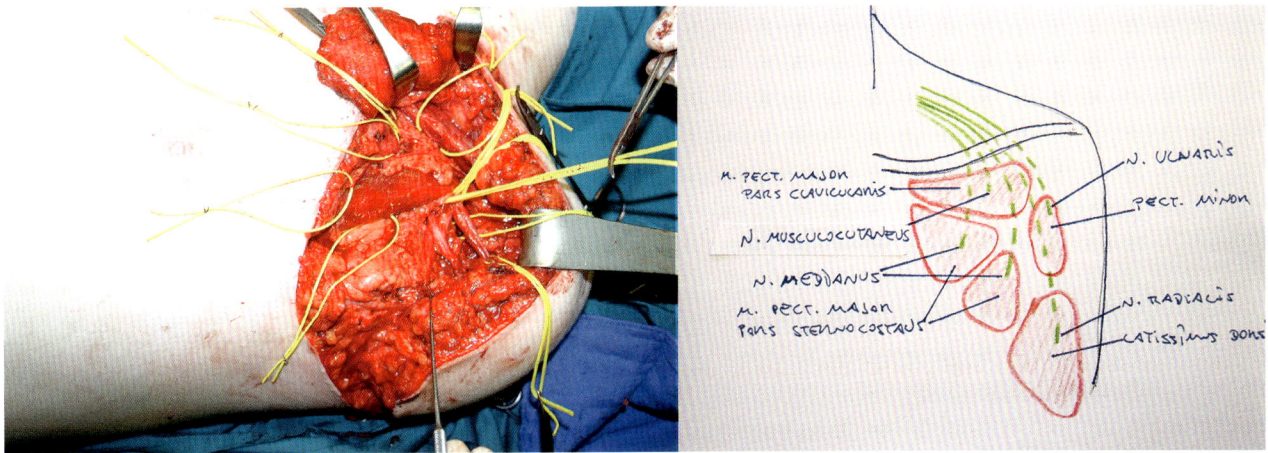

Fig. 7 A, B. Intra- operative picture and schematic drawing depicting the different nerve transfers that have been realized in this patient

nocostal, the abdominal head of the pectoralis major and the pectoralis minor have their distinct motor branches that can be used for selective distal nerve transfers in brachial plexus reconstruction [3, 10]. In reverse these neuromuscular units of the remaining chest now can be used as targets for selective nerve transfers to provide a new neurological landscape for the lost targets of the axons of the brachial plexus. Similar to the partial nerve transfers of the transhumeral amputee, here all major nerves must and can be transferred to new targets as is illustrated in Fig. 7 A, B. Before performing these nerve transfers one must carefully evaluate the remaining function of these muscles, the presence and whereabouts of the proximal nerve stumps (MRI) and rule out more proximal nerve lesions (i. e. root avulsions or supraclavicular nerve damage) Furthermore a technician well familiarized with modern myoelectric prostheses and an experienced prosthetist must be consulted to discuss the technical needs and the biological possibilities. At the end of this discussion a "nerve transfer matrix" should be established that may well also use already existing neuromuscular units as for example the axillary/deltoid system (Table 1).

After any of the above described nerve transfer procedures a closely monitored, staged TechnNeuroRehabilitation Programme must be entered (Table 2). It will take about three months for the first axons to reach their targets. The patient will slowly learn how to address his new functions. (ChannelingStrengthening) This process can be enhanced by various biofeedback systems. Some functions will be established easier and earlier than others. Elbow flexion for example is a rather simple movement that for the most part is restricted to musculocutaneous nerve function. However, fisting may prove a real challenge, since this "movement" is encoded by motoneurons of both the extrinsic and intrinsic flexors,

Table 1. Nerve transfer matrix of a glenohumeral amputee and the results after 18 months postoperatively

Source Nerve	Target Muscle	Result	Target Function
Musculocutaneous Nerve	Pars clavicularis M. pectoralis major	excellent	Elbowflexion
Median Nerve	Pars sternocostalis M. pectoralis major	excellent	Pronation Wristflexion
Median Nerve	Pars sternocostalis M. pectoralis major	excellent	Fingerflexion
Ulnaris Nerve	M. pectoralis minor	excellent	Intrinsic Function
Radialis Nerve	M. latissimus dorsi	excellent	Fingerextension
Medial Trunc C7	N. supraclavicularis	excellent	Thumb, Index, Palm of Hand

Table 2. TechNeuroRehabilitation Programme

Healing:
(1–3 Weeks postop- Patient/Surgeon)
Decrease Edema, Pain Control, Wound Healing

Channeling:
(1–3 month postop- Patient/Surgeon/OTR)
Beginn "movement" at each joint. No visible muscle activity is expected.

Strengthening:
(3–6 month postop- Patient/OTR)
When muscle activity is observed during intended movement, begin strengthening excercises

Patterning:
(6–9 months postop- Patient/OTR/Prosthetist)
Focus on "meaningful" muscle activity using specific intended movements. Virtual fitting

Early Fitting:
(9–12 months- Patient/Prosthetist/Technician)
Transfer signals of meaningful contractions to control elements of actual prosthesis

Final Fitting:
(after 15 months- Surgeon/Prosthetist/Technician)
A final fitting is provided, appropriate testing and outcome measures documented

which can be addressed with the ulnar as well as with the median nerve. However, with time and patience the patient will learn how to address certain functions with certain movements. The challenge in this time period (Patterning), which may well last for about 18 months, is that the process of nerve regeneration will change the neurological landscape not only in regards to topography but also in regards to established function. That means for example that a patient with a nerve transfer of the radial to the thoracodorsal nerve will establish the function of supination in one area of the latissimus dorsi at 9 months postoperatively. Three months later however this function may have shifted to a more distal location, whereas closeby a new function of the radial nerve, for example that of wrist extension may be present. These changes are a real challenge to the prosthetist and the technician, which may necessitate changes in shaft design, electrode positioning and software management [12]. We therefore do not advise early fitting, since this may lead to a frustrating experience for both the patient and the team taking care of the patient. However, it is of utmost importance to pro-

vide a training programme that allows the patient to perform strengthening exercises and repetitively practice relearned discrete functions using various feedback systems, best of which is a virtual arm that the patient can move with his own signals. Once these signals are stable and can be clearly addressed by the patient, a diagnostic fitting can be provided to start the early prosthetic rehabilitation programme. Clearly, the earlier the patient will learn how to incorporate this technical device in his new body image, the more natural and intuitive he will use it. On the other hand reliability of prosthetic function is the acid test of this procedure. At this stage less is more. Once the patient demonstrates consistent, independent control of four myoelectric sites more degrees of freedom can be added. Finally, about 15 months after the nerve transfers have been performed, all targets should have stable reinnervation, the patient should be able to address these functions distinctly and no major changes in the neurological landscape should be expected. At this time a final fitting should be provided that allows the patient to address the different functions of the prosthesis consistently and independently.

Another longterm goal of prosthetic development is to offer some type of proprioception. The increasing complexity of upper limb prostheses, require the provision of sensory feedback to the amputee. This has not been realized in available products so far. By way of selective sensory nerve transfers or random sensory reinnervation as a result of targeted nerve transfers, a new sensory surface will be established that can be used to provide real sensation to the artificial extremity via different specific sensory inputs (Fig. 8 A, B) [2, 9].

Different sensory parameters have been quantified and tested for feasibility to be used in a closed loop biofeedback system. Tactile gnosis, vibration and thermal thresholds were tested and appropriate technical actuators developed. A special software has been developed to integrate these stimuli in prosthesis governance.

The results show that an array of sensory information can be useful for closed loop control and sensory feedback. Stimuli are easy to register and distinguished from each other and in some cases highly intuitive. However, only light touch and pressure were the only sensory component that could

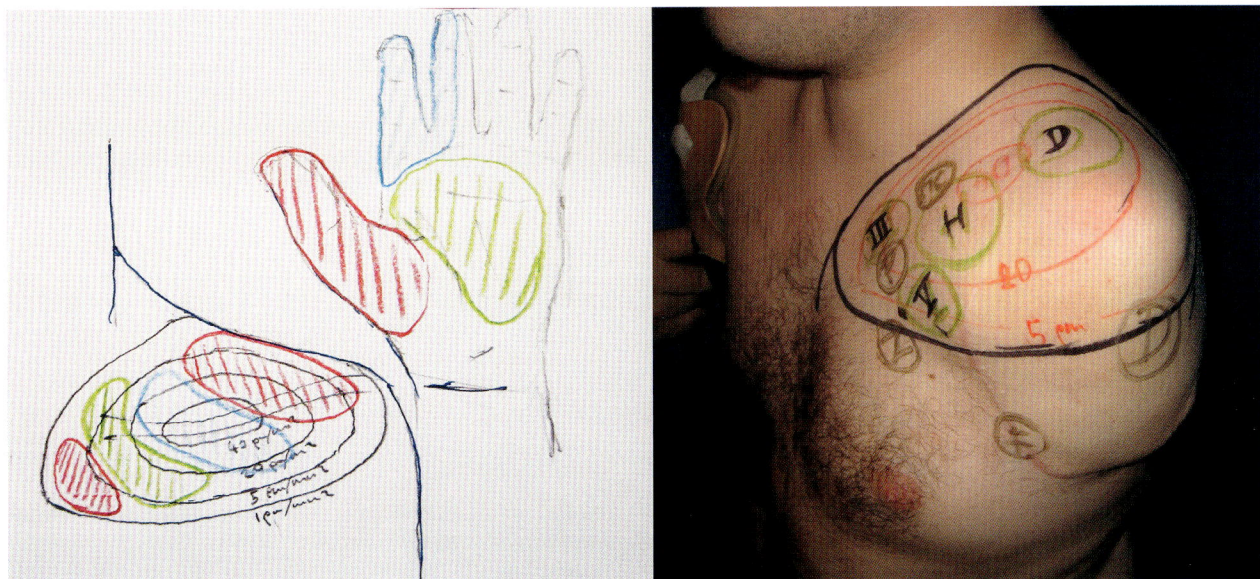

Fig. 8 A, B. Schematic drawing of the sensory map after selective sensory nerve transfer of the supraclavicular nerves to the C6 root. After 18 months a new neurological landscape was established that represented part of the patients left hand on his shoulder. The qualities of light touch, temperature and vibration (100 Hz) could all be correctly be identified and localized at thresholds similar to a normal hand. Only two-point discrimination was above 20 mm. The golden circles identify the regions of the different movements

serve as a reliable, cognitive and reproducible feedback system. Technically this has been realized with actuators that were integrated in the prosthetic fitting at a location where the patient feels his left thumb and index finger (Fig. 9 A, B).

We found that closed loop biofeedback systems are not only eminently important for the cognitive

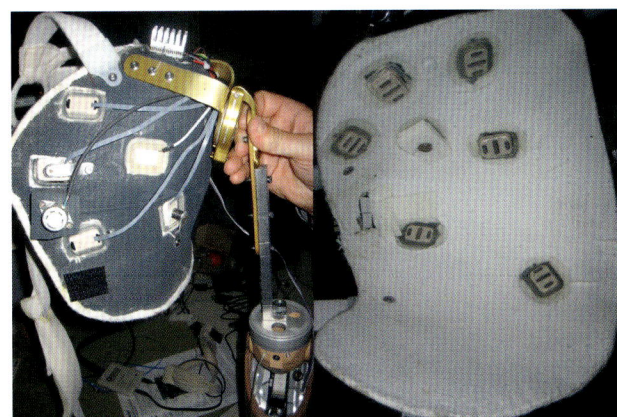

Fig. 9 A, B. Outer and inner appearance of a shaft design for the same patient with integrated pick-up electrodes for controlling of a prosthesis with 6 degrees of freedom and three different sensory feedback units

rehabilitation of high-end myoelectric prostheses but also lead to a much higher acceptance of an otherwise rather foreign technical extension.

Extremity reconstruction in the 21 century will see many new avenues to replace the loss of a limb and reconstruct the loss of function. Both biological and technical advances will provide possibilities that may well open up therapies that have been unthinkable only a few years ago. Targeted muscle reinnervation together with the provision of a myoelectric prosthesis with several degrees of freedom is such an approach and will definitely be a solid stepping stone leading to new strategies in extremity rehabilitation.

References

[1] Aszmann OC, Dietl H, Frey M (2008) Selective nerve transfers to improve the control of myoelectric arm prosthesis. Handchir Mikrochir Plast Chir 40: 60–65

[2] Aszmann OC, Muse V, Dellon AL (1996) Evidence of collateral sprouting after sensory nerve resection. Ann Plast Surg 37: 520–525

[3] Aszmann OC, Rab M, Kamolz LP, Frey M (2000) The anatomy of the pectoral nerves and their significance in brachial plexus reconstruction. J Hand Surg (Am) 25: 942–947

[4] Dumanian GA, Ho JH, O'Shaughnessy KD, Kim PS, Wilson CJ, Kuiken TA (2009) Targeted reinnervation for transhumeral amputees: current surgical technique and update on results. Plast Reconstr Surg 124: 863–867

[5] Hijjawi JB, Kuiken TA, Lipschutz RD, Miller LA, Stubblefield KA and Dumanian GA (2006) Improved myoelectric prosthesis control accomplished using multiple nerve transfers. Plast Reconstr Surg 118: 1573–1577

[6] Hunt JL, Mason AD, Masterson TS et al (1975) The pathophysiology of acute electric injuries. J Trauma 16: 335–340

[7] Janicak CA (1997) Occupational fatalaties caused by contact with overhead powerlines in the construction industry. J Occup Environ Med 39: 328–332

[8] Kuiken TA, Dumanian GA, Miller LA, Stubblefield KA (2004) The use of nerve-muscle grafts for improved myoelectric prosthesis control in a bilateral shoulder disarticulation amputee. Prosthet Orthot Int 28: 245–249

[9] Kuiken TA, Marasco PD, Lock BA, Harden RN, Dewald JPA (2007) Redirection of cutaneous sensation from the hand to the chest skin of human amputees with targeted reinnervation. Proc Nat Acad Science 104: 20061–20066

[10] Stockinger T, Aszmann OC, Manfred Frey (2008) Clinical application of pectoral nerve transfers in the treatment of traumatic Brachial Plexus Injuries. J Hand Surg (Sept) 33: 1100–1107

[11] Strauch H, Wirth I, Geserick G (1998) Fatal accients due train surfing in Berlin. Forensic Sci Int 94: 119–127

[12] Stubblefield KA, Miller LA, Lipschutz RD, Kuiken TA (2009) Occupational therapy protokol for amputees with targeted muscle. Reinnervation J Rehab Res Dev 46: 481–488

Correspondence: Oskar C. Aszmann, MD, Associate Professor of Plastic & Reconstructive Surgery, Division of Plastic and Reconstructive Surgery, Department of Surgery, Medical University of Vienna, Währinger Gürtel 18–20, 1090 Vienna Austria, Tel: +43 1 40 400 6986, Fax: +43 1 40 400 6988, E-mail: oskar.aszmann@meduniwien.ac.at

Subject index